Radiographic
Image
Analysis

FOURTH EDITION

Radiographic Image Analysis

KATHY McQUILLEN MARTENSEN, MA, RT(R)

Instructional Services Specialist, Radiologic Technology Education
University of Iowa Hospitals and Clinics
Iowa City, Iowa

ELSEVIER

ELSEVIER
SAUNDERS

3251 Riverport Lane
St. Louis, Missouri 63043

International Standard Book Number: 978-0-323-28052-5

Executive Content Strategist: Sonya Seigafuse
Content Development Manager: Laurie Gower
Content Development Specialist: Charlene Ketchum
Publishing Services Manager: Julie Eddy
Senior Project Manager: Marquita Parker
Senior Book Designer: Margaret Reid

Printed in the United States of America

Last digit is the print number: 9 8 7 6 5 4 3 2

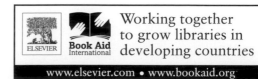

Working together to grow libraries in developing countries

www.elsevier.com • www.bookaid.org

To my parents, Pat and Dolores McQuillen,
and to my husband, Van,
and to our family, Nicole, Zachary, Adam, Phil, Haley,
Katelynn, and Alexander.

REVIEWER LIST

Laura Aaron, PhD, RT(R)(M)(QM), FASRT
Director & Professor School of Allied Health
Northwestern State University of Louisiana
Shreveport, Louisiana

Susan Anderson, MAED, RT(R)
Senior Radiographer
Dublin Dental University Hospital
Dublin, Ireland

Patricia Davis, BS, RT(R)(MR)
Assistant Clinical Professor, Clinical Liaison,
    Radiography and Medical Imaging Technology
    Programs, Allied Health Sciences
Indiana University Kokomo
Kokomo, Indiana

Catherine DeBaillie, EdD, RT(R)
Associate Professor, Radiography Program,
    Clinical Coordinator
Trinity College of Nursing & Health Sciences
Rock Island, Illinois

Becky Farmer, MSRS, RT(R)(M)
Associate Professor of Allied Health and
    Radiologic Science
Northwestern State University
Shreveport, Louisiana

Merryl N. Fulmer, BS, RT(R)(M)(MR)(QM)(CT)
Program Director
Shore Medical Center
School of Radiologic Technology
Somers Point, New Jersey

This textbook serves as a practical image analysis and procedure reference for radiography educators, students, and technologists, by providing information to correlate the technical and positioning procedures with the image analysis guidelines for common projections; adjust the procedural setup for patient condition variations, nonroutine situations, or when a less-than-optimal projection is obtained; develop a high degree of radiography problem-solving ability; and prepare for the radiography ARRT examination.

THIS EDITION

The organization of the procedures for this edition has been changed to reduce repeatable information and provide efficient access to specific data. The new format includes additional boxes and tables that summarize important details and can be used for quick reference. This edition also includes many new and updated images, with improved detail resolution.

Chapters 1 and 2 lay the foundations for evaluating all projections, outlining the technical and digital imaging concepts that are to be considered when studying the procedures that are presented in the subsequent chapters.

Chapters 3 through 12 detail the image analysis guidelines for commonly performed radiographic procedures. For each procedure presented, this edition provides the following:

- Accurately positioned projections with labeled anatomy.
- Photographs of accurately positioned models.
- Tables that provide detailed one-to-one correlation between the positioning procedures and image analysis guidelines.
- Discussions, with correlating images, on identifying how the patient, central ray, or image receptor were poorly positioned if the projection does not demonstrate an image analysis guideline.
- Discussions of topics relating to positioning for patient condition variations and nonroutine situations.
- Photographs of bones and models positioned as indicated to clarify information and demonstrate anatomy alignment when distortion makes it difficult.
- Practice images of the projection that demonstrate common procedural errors.

ACKNOWLEDGMENTS

I would like to thank the following individuals who have helped with this edition.

The University of Iowa Hospitals and Clinics' Radiologic Technology Classes of 1988 to 2014, who have been my best teachers because they have challenged me with their questions and insights.

Sonya Seigafuse, Charlene Ketchum, and the entire Elsevier Saunders team for their support, assistance, and expertise in advising, planning, and developing this project.

The professional colleagues, book reviewers, educators, and technologists who have evaluated the book, sent me compliments and suggestions, and questioned concepts in the first three editions. Please continue to do so.

—Kathy

CONTENTS

1   Image Analysis Guidelines   1

2   Digital Imaging Guidelines   37

3   Chest and Abdomen   76

4   Upper Extremity   149

5   Shoulder   234

6   Lower Extremity   278

7   Pelvis, Hip, and Sacroiliac Joints   366

8   Cervical and Thoracic Vertebrae   390

9   Lumbar, Sacral, and Coccygeal Vertebrae   423

10   Sternum and Ribs   447

11   Cranium, Facial Bones, and Paranasal Sinuses   461

12   Digestive System   486

Bibliography   517

Glossary   518

Index   523

Image Analysis Guidelines

OUTLINE

Why Image Analysis, 2
Terminology, 3
Characteristics of the Optimal
  Image, 3
  Displaying Images, 4
  Contrast Mask, 6

Display Stations, 8
Image Analysis Form, 8
  Demographic Requirements, 8
  Marking Projections, 10
  Anatomic Structure Requirements
    and Placement, 14

Collimation, 14
Anatomic Relationships, 17
Sharpness of the Recorded
  Details, 28
Radiation Protection, 32

OBJECTIVES

After completion of this chapter, you should be able to:

- State the characteristics of an optimal projection.
- Properly display projections of all body structures.
- State the demographic requirements for projections and explain why this information is needed.
- Discuss how to mark projections accurately and explain the procedure to be followed if a projection has been mismarked or the marker is only faintly seen.
- Discuss why good collimation practices are necessary, and list the guidelines to follow to ensure good collimation.
- Describe how positioning of anatomic structures in reference to the central ray (CR) and image receptor

(IR) affects how they are visualized on the resulting projection.
- State how similarly appearing structures can be identified on projections.
- Determine the amount of patient or CR adjustment required when poorly positioned projections are obtained.
- Discuss the factors that affect the sharpness of recorded details in a projection.
- Describe the radiation protection practices that are followed to limit patient and personnel dose and discuss how to identify whether adequate shielding was used.

KEY TERMS

ALARA
annotation
anterior
atomic density
backup timer
contrast mask
decubitus
detector element (DEL)
distortion
dose creep
dose equivalent limit
elongation
exposure maintenance formula
field of view (FOV)
flexion
focal spot
foreshortening

grid
grid cutoff
image receptor (IR)
inverse square law
involuntary motion
lateral
law of isometry
manual exposure
matrix
medial
midcoronal plane
midsagittal plane
nonstochastic effects
object–image receptor distance
  (OID)
picture archival & communication
  system (PACS)

pixel
posterior
profile
project
radiolucent
radiopaque
recorded detail
scatter radiation
shuttering
source–image receptor distance
  (SID)
source-skin distance (SSD)
spatial frequency
spatial resolution
stochastic effects
volume of interest (VOI)
voluntary motion

WHY IMAGE ANALYSIS?

Radiographic images are such that slight differences in quality do not necessarily rule out the diagnostic value of a projection. Radiologists can ordinarily make satisfactory adjustments by reason of their experience and knowledge, although passing less than optimal projections may compromise the diagnosis and treatment and result in additional projections at a higher expense and radiation dose to the patient. The purpose of image analysis is to teach technologists how to evaluate projections for acceptability, determine how to improve positioning and technical skills before repeating a projection, and continually improve skills.

Why should a technologist care about creating optimal projections and studying all the small details relating to image analysis? The most important answer to this question lies in why most technologists join the profession— to help people. From the patient's point of view, it provides the reviewer with projections that contain optimal diagnostic value, prevents the anxiety that occurs when additional projections or studies need to be performed, and prevents the radiation dosage that might be caused by additional imaging. From a societal point of view, it helps prevent additional increases in health care costs that could result because of the need for additional, more expensive imaging procedures and because of the malpractice cases that might result from a poor or missed diagnosis. From a technologist's point of view, it would be the preventable financial burden and stress that arise from legal actions, a means of protecting professional interest as more diagnostic procedures are being replaced with other modalities, and the personal satisfaction gained when our patients, employer, and ourselves benefit from and are recognized for our expertise.

Consider how accuracy in positioning and technical factors affect the diagnostic value of the image. It is estimated that in the United States 68 million chest imaging procedures are performed each year to evaluate the lungs, heart, and thoracic viscera as well as disease processes such as pneumonia, heart failure, pleurisy, and lung cancer. The reviewer must consider all the normal variations that exist in areas such as the mediastinum, hila, diaphragm, and lungs. Should they also have to consider how the appearance of these structures is different with preventable positioning and technical errors? It takes only 2 or 3 degrees of rotation to affect the appearance of the lungs, causing differences in brightness values along the lateral borders of the chest projection (Figure 1-1). Similarly, certain conditions such as mediastinal widening or cardiac size cannot be evaluated properly on a rotated posteroanterior (PA) chest projection. The normal heart shadow on such a projection will occupy slightly less than 50% of the transverse dimension of the thorax (Figure 1-2). This is evaluated by measuring the largest transverse diameter of the heart on the PA or anteroposterior (AP) projection and relating

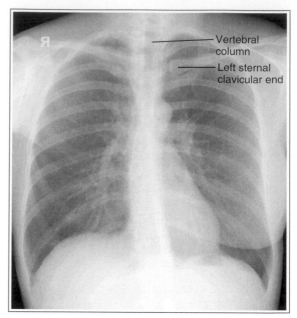

FIGURE 1-1 Rotated PA chest projection.

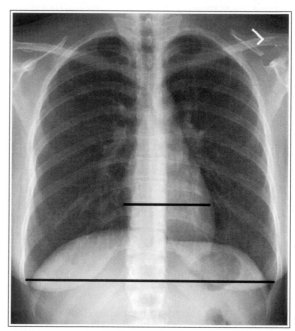

FIGURE 1-2 Evaluating a PA chest projection for mediastinal widening.

that to the largest transverse measurement of the internal dimension of the chest. When the PA chest projection is rotated, bringing a different heart plane into profile, this diagnosis becomes compromised.

If instead of being evaluated for acceptability, projections are evaluated for optimalism, could more consistent and improved diagnoses be made from diagnostic projections? For example, Figures 1-3 and 1-4 demonstrate three lateral and PA wrist projections, all of which were determined to be acceptable and sent to the radiologist for review. Note how the trapezium is visualized only on the first lateral wrist projection but is not

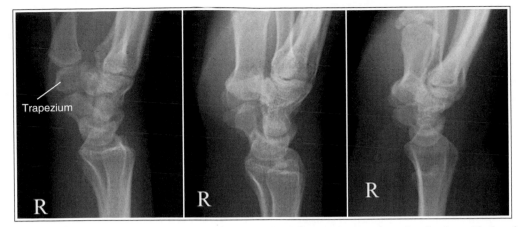

FIGURE 1-3 Lateral wrist projections demonstrating the difference in trapezium visualization with thumb depression and elevation.

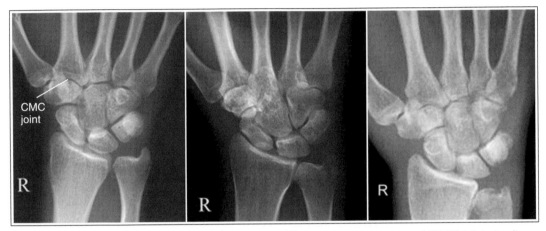

FIGURE 1-4 PA wrist projections demonstrating the difference in carpometacarpal (CMC) joint visualization with variations in metacarpal alignment with the IR.

demonstrated on the other two, and observe how the carpometacarpal joints and distal carpal bones are well visualized on the first PA wrist projection but are not seen on the other two projections. The first lateral wrist projection was obtained with the patient's thumb depressed until the first metacarpal (MC) was aligned with the second MC, whereas the other lateral wrist projections were obtained with the first MC elevated. The first PA wrist projection was obtained with the MCs aligned at a 10- to 15-degree angle with the image receptor (IR), the second PA wrist projection was taken with the MCs aligned at an angle greater than 15 degrees, and the third projection was taken with the MCs aligned at an angle less than 10 degrees. If the radiologist cannot arrive at a conclusive diagnosis from the projections that the technologist provides, he or she must recommend other imaging procedures or follow-up projections.

TERMINOLOGY

Different terms are used in radiography to describe the path of the x-ray beam, the patient's position, the precise location of an anatomic structure, the position of one anatomic structure in relation to another, and the way a certain structure will change its position as the patient moves in a predetermined direction. Familiarity with radiography terminology will help you understand statements made throughout this text and converse competently with other medical professionals. At the beginning of most chapters there is a list of key terms that should be reviewed before reading the chapter. The glossary at the end of the textbook provides definitions of these terms.

CHARACTERISTICS OF THE OPTIMAL IMAGE

The guidelines needed to obtain optimal images of all body structures are taught in radiographic procedures, image analysis, radiation protection, and radiographic exposure (imaging) courses.

An optimal image of each projection demonstrates all the most desired features, which includes the following:

- Demographic information (e.g., patient and facility name, time, date)

- Correct markers in the appropriate position without superimposing volume of interest (VOI)
- Desired anatomic structures in accurate alignment with each other
- Maximum geometric integrity
- Appropriate radiation protection
- Best possible contrast resolution, with minimal noise
- No preventable artifacts

Unfortunately, because of a patient's condition, equipment malfunction, or technologist error, such perfection is not obtained for every projection that is produced. A less than optimal projection should be thoroughly evaluated to determine the reason for error so that the problem can be corrected before the examination is repeated. A projection that is not optimal but is still acceptable according to a facility's standards should be carefully studied to determine whether skills can be improved before the next similar examination; continuous improvement is sought. A projection should not have to be taken a third time because the error was not accurately identified and the proper adjustment made from the first attempt.

This book cannot begin to identify the standards of acceptability in all the different imaging facilities. What might be an acceptable standard in one facility may not be acceptable in another. As you study the projections in this book, you may find that many of them are acceptable in your facility even though they do not meet optimal standards. You may also find that some of the guidelines listed are not desired in your facility. The goal of this text is not to dictate to your facility what should be acceptable and unacceptable projections. It is to help you focus on improving your image analysis, positioning, radiation protection, and exposure skills and to provide guidelines on how the projection may be improved when a less than optimal image results and a repeat is required.

Displaying Images

Digital images are initially displayed on the computer monitor in the manner in which they have been obtained or after a preprocessing algorithm has been applied that changes how the projection is displayed to meet the facilities' desires. For example, a left lateral chest projection may be transversely flipped to be displayed as a right lateral. Box 1-1 lists the guidelines to follow when evaluating the displaying accuracy.

Computed Radiography Image Receptor and Patient Orientation. Computed radiography IR cassettes have orientation labels that indicate to the user which end of the cassette is the "top" and which side is the "right" or "left" side. These orientation indicators align the image orientation with the computer algorithm of a patient in the anatomic position (AP projection). The top indicator is placed under the portion of the anatomy that is up when the projection is displayed and for projections of

---

| BOX 1-1 | **Image Displaying Guidelines** |

- Display torso, vertebral, cranial, shoulder, and hip projections as if the patient were standing in an upright position.
- AP, PA, and AP-PA oblique projections of the torso, vertebrae, and cranium are displayed as if the viewer and the patient are facing one another. The right side of the patient's image is on the viewer's left, and the left side of the patient's image is on the viewer's right. Whenever AP or AP oblique projections are taken, the R (right) or L (left) marker appears correct when the projection is accurately displayed, as long as the marker was placed on the IR face-up before the projection was taken (Figure 1-5). When PA or PA oblique projections are taken, the R or L marker appears reversed if placed face-up when the projection was taken (Figure 1-6).
- Accurately displayed lateral projections are displayed in the same manner as the technologist viewed the patient when obtaining the projection. For a right lateral the patient faces the viewer's left side and for a left lateral the patient faces the viewer's right side. The marker on these projections is correct as long as it was placed on the IR face-up before the projection was taken (Figure 1-7). One exception to this guideline may be when left lateral chest projections are displayed; often, reviewers prefer the left lateral projection to be displayed as if taken in the right lateral projection.
- AP/PA (lateral decubitus) chest and abdomen projections are oriented as described above in the AP-PA projection and then turned to be displayed so that the side of the patient that was positioned upward when the projection was taken is upward on the displayed projection (Figure 1-8).
- Inferosuperior (axial) shoulder and axiolateral hip projections are displayed so the patient's anterior surface is up and posterior surface is down (Figure 1-9).
- Extremity projections are displayed as if the viewer's eyes were going through the projection in the same manner the CR went through the extremity when the projection was taken. For example, a right PA hand projection is displayed with the thumb positioned toward the viewer's left side and a right lateral hand projection is displayed so the palmar side of the hand is positioned toward the viewer's left side (Figure 1-10).
- Display finger, wrist, and forearm projections as if the patient were hanging from the fingertips.
- Display elbow and humeral projections as if they were hanging from the patient's shoulder.
- Display toe and AP and AP oblique foot projections as if the patient were hanging from the toes.
- Display lateral foot, ankle, lower leg, knee, and femur projections as if they were hanging from the patient's hip.

---

the torso, vertebrae, or cranium the right side of the patient is placed over the right side indicator. When the IR is processed it is read from left to right, starting at the top, and the projection is displayed in the same manner as the IR is read. Thus, if the examination is taken in a position other than just described, the examination chosen (PA) on the workstation must indicate this variation before the projection is read for it to be displayed accurately.

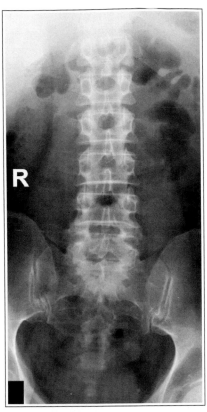

FIGURE 1-5 Accurately displayed and marked AP lumbar vertebrae projection.

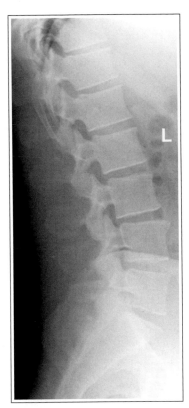

FIGURE 1-7 Accurately displayed left lateral lumbar vertebrae projection.

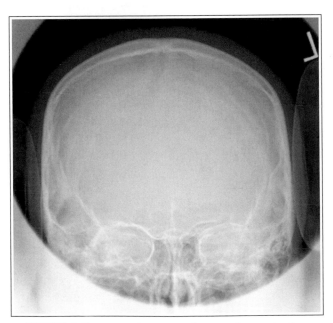

FIGURE 1-6 Accurately displayed PA cranium projection.

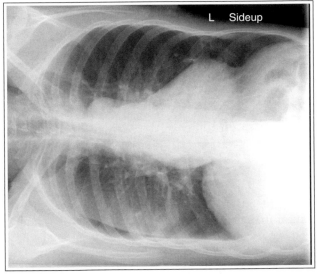

FIGURE 1-8 Accurately displayed and marked AP (right lateral decubitus) chest projection.

Direct-Indirect Capture Digital Radiography. For the digital radiography (DR) system, patient and IR orientation must also be considered when positioning the patient, and the technologist must also choose the correct examination from the workstation before exposing the projection for it to be displayed accurately. When using the table, position the patient's head at the head end of the table, on the technologist's left side, or adjust the patient orientation on the digital system to prevent the projection from being displayed upside down.

When possible avoid positioning extremities diagonally on the IR. Instead, align the long axis of extremities with the longitudinal or transverse axis of the IR (Figure 1-11). Because most digital systems only allow projection to be rotated in increments of 90 degrees, a diagonally obtained projection cannot be aligned vertically on the display computer and will be displayed diagonally.

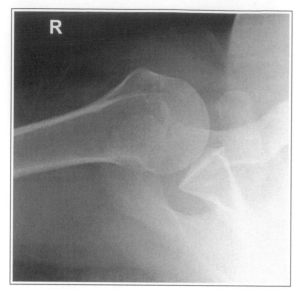

FIGURE 1-9 Accurately displayed and marked inferosuperior (axial) shoulder projection.

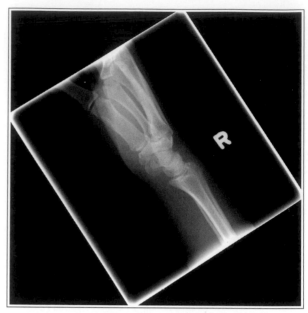

FIGURE 1-11 Diagonally displayed right lateral wrist projection.

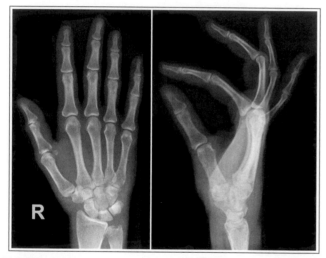

FIGURE 1-10 Accurately displayed right PA and lateral hand projections.

Adjusting for Poor Display. Digital images that have been displayed inaccurately can be flipped horizontally and vertically, and rotated 90 degrees. When poorly displayed projections are obtained, they need adjusting before being saved to the picture archival and communication system (PACS), but this must be done with great care and only if a marker was placed accurately on the projection when it was obtained because inaccurate manipulation can result in the right and left sides getting confused. The marker will provide clues to the patient's orientation with the IR for the projection (see marking images later). The first AP foot projection in Figure 1-12 was obtained using a DR system and with the toes facing the foot end of the table, which causes the foot to be displayed upside down. If the projection was vertically flipped to accurately display it, the marker will be

reversed and the foot displayed as if it were a left foot instead of a right as demonstrated in the second foot projection in Figure 1-12. If the first foot projection was rotated instead of being flipped, the marker will remain face-up and the foot will be displayed accurately as demonstrated on the third foot projection in Figure 1-12.

Contrast Mask

A contrast mask is a postprocessing manipulation that can be added to digital projections as a means of helping the viewer to better evaluate contrast resolution in the selected area. The contrast mask does so by adding a black background over the areas outside the VOI to eliminate them and provide a perceived enhancement of image contrast. *As a rule, the technologist should only mask to the exposed areas, matching the collimation borders, even though it is possible to mask into the exposed areas.* Because it is possible to mask into the exposed areas, some facilities do not allow masking or request that masking be annotated on the projection because of the possibility that the radiologist will not see information that has been included on the original projection. Masking does not replace good collimation practices and should not be used to present a perceived radiation dose savings to the patient. Figure 1-13 demonstrates two abdomen projections taken on the same patient; one that has not been masked and one that has been laterally masked to remove the arms and cover up poor radiation protection practices. Such masking may be construed as altering the patient's medical record because the images are part of the patient's record, lead to misdiagnosis, and carry legal implications. A projection that has been masked and sent to the PACS cannot be unmasked.

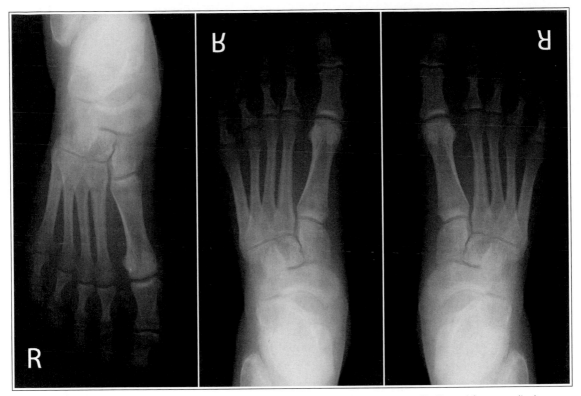

FIGURE 1-12 AP foot projection that has been displayed upside down, vertically flipped for poor display, and rotated for accurate display.

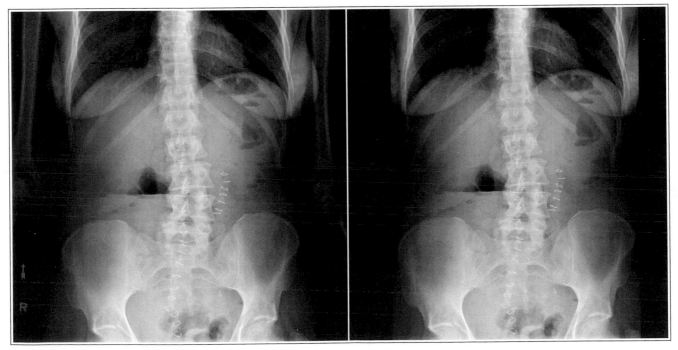

FIGURE 1-13 AP abdomen projections with and without contrast masking and demonstrating poor radiation protection practices.

Display Stations

The resolution ability of the image may be different, depending on where the image is displayed in the department. Display station resolution refers to the maximum number of pixels that the screen can demonstrate. To display images at full resolution, the display monitor must be able to display the same number of pixels as those at which the digital system acquired the image. If the digital system matrix size is smaller than the display station's matrix size, the values of surrounding pixels will be averaged to display the whole image. The technologist's workstation display monitors typically do not demonstrate resolution as high as that of the radiologist's display monitor.

IMAGE ANALYSIS FORM

Once a projection is correctly displayed, it is evaluated for positioning and technical accuracy. This should follow a systematic approach so that all aspects of the analytic process are considered, reducing the chance of missing important details and providing a structured pattern for the evaluator to use in a stressful situation. The image analysis form shown in Box 1-2 is designed to be used when evaluating projections to ensure that all aspects of the projection are evaluated. Under each item in the image analysis form, there is a list of questions to explore while evaluating a projection. The discussion in Chapters 1 and 2 will explore each of these question areas in depth. The answers to all the questions, taken together, will determine whether the projection is optimal, acceptable, or needs repeating.

Demographic Requirements

The correct patient's name and age or birthdate, patient identification number, facility's name, and examination time and date should be displayed on projections.

Computed Radiography. Each computed radiography cassette has a barcode label that is used to match the image data with the patient's identification barcode and examination request. For each examination, the cassette and patient barcodes must be scanned, connecting them with each other and the examination menu.

Direct-Indirect Capture Digital Radiography. With the DR system, the examination and patient are matched when the patient's information is pulled up on the workstation before the examination is obtained. It is important to select the correct patient and order number before

---

BOX 1-2 | Image Analysis Form

_____ Projection is accurately displayed.
- Is the correct aspect of the structure positioned at the top of the displayed projection?
- Is the marker face-up or reversed, as expected?
- If projection was flipped or rotated to improve display, does marker still indicate correct side as displayed?
- Is the long axis of the VOI aligned with the longitudinal axis of the display monitor?

_____ Demographic requirements are visualized on the projection.
- Are the patient's name and age or birthdate, and patient identification number visible and are they accurate?
- Is the facility's name visible?
- Are the examination time and date visible?

_____ Correct marker (e.g., R/L, arrow) is visualized on projection and demonstrates accurate placement.
- Is the marker visualized within the exposure field and is it positioned as far away from the center of field as possible?
- Have specialty markers been added and correctly placed if applicable?
- Is the marker clearly seen without distortion and is it positioned so it does not superimpose the VOI?
- Does the R or L marker correspond to the correct side of the patient?
- If more than one projection is on IR, have they both been marked if they are different sides of the patient?
- Are annotated markings correct?

_____ Required anatomy is present and correctly placed in projection.
- Are all of the required anatomical structures visible?
- Was the field size adequate to demonstrate all the required anatomy?

- Computed radiography: Was the IR cassette positioned crosswise or lengthwise correctly to accommodate the required anatomy and/or patient's body habitus?
- Computed radiography: Was the smallest possible IR cassette used?

_____ Appropriate collimation practices are evident.
- Is the collimated border present on all four sides of the projection when applicable?
- Is collimation within ½ inch (1.25 cm) of the patient's skin line?
- Is collimation to the specific anatomy desired on projections requiring collimation within the skin line?

_____ Relationships between the anatomical structures are accurate for the projection demonstrated.
- Are the relationships between the anatomical structures demonstrated as indicated in the procedural analysis sections of this textbook or defined by your imaging facility?
- Is the anatomical VOI in the center of the projection?
- Does the projection demonstrate the least possible amount of size distortion?
- Does the projection demonstrate undesirable shape distortion?
- Are the joints of interest and/or fracture lines open?
- Was the CR centered to the correct structure?

_____ Projection demonstrates maximum recorded detail sharpness.
- Was a small focal spot used when indicated?
- Was the appropriate SID used?
- Was the part positioned as close to the IR as possible?
- Does the projection demonstrate signs of undesirable patient motion or unhalted respiration?
- Computed radiography: Are there signs of a double exposure?
- Computed radiography: Was the smallest possible IR cassette used?

BOX 1-2 | Image Analysis Form—cont'd

_____ Radiation protection is present on projection when indicated, and good radiation protection practices were used during the procedure.

- Was the exam explained to the patient and were clear, concise instructions given during the procedure?
- Were immobilization devices used to prevent patient motion when needed?
- Was the minimal SSD of at least 12 inches (30 cm) maintained for mobile radiography?
- Was the possibility of pregnancy determined of all females of childbearing age?
- Is gonadal shielding evident and accurately positioned when the gonads are within the primary beam and shielding will not cover VOI?
- Were radiation protection measures used for patients whose radiosensitive cells were positioned within 2 inches (5 cm) of the primary beam?
- Was the field size tightly collimated?
- Were exposure factors (kV, mA, and time) set to minimize patient exposure?
- If the AEC was used, was the backup time set to prevent overexposure to the patient?
- Are there anatomical artifacts demonstrated on the projection?
- Were personnel or family who remained in the room during the exposure given protective attire, positioned as far from the radiation source as possible, and present only when absolutely necessary and for the shortest possible time?

_____ Image histogram was accurately produced.

- Is the exposure indicator within the acceptable parameters for the system?
- Was the correct body part and projection chosen from the workstation menu?
- Was the CR centered to the VOI?
- Was collimation as close to the VOI as possible, leaving minimal background in the exposure field?
- Was scatter controlled with lead sheets, grids, tight collimation, etc.?
- If collimated smaller than the IR, is the VOI in the center of the projection and are all four collimation borders seen?
- Computed radiography: Was at least 30% of the IR covered?
- Computed radiography: If multiple projections are on one IR, is collimation parallel and equidistant from the edges of the IR and are they separated by at least 1 inch (2.5 cm)?
- Computed radiography: Was the IR left in the imaging room while other exposures were made and was the IR read shortly after the exposure?
- Computed radiography: Was the IR erased if not used within a few days?

_____ Adequate exposure reached the IR.

- Were the technical factors of mAs and kV set appropriately for the projection?
- Is the required subject contrast in the VOI fully demonstrated?
- Is the EI number obtained at the ideal level or within the acceptable parameters for the digital system?
- Is the brightness level adequate to demonstrate the VOI?
- Does the projection demonstrate quantum noise?
- Does any VOI structure demonstrate saturation?

- Is there a decrease in contrast and detail visibility caused by scatter radiation fogging?
- Was a grid used if recommended, and if so, was the appropriate grid ratio and technique used for the grid?
- Are there grid line artifacts demonstrated?
- Was the correct SID used for the exposure set?
- Was the OID kept to a minimum, and if not, were the exposure factors adjusted for the reduction in scatter radiation when applicable?
- If collimation was significantly reduced, were the technical factors adjusted for the reduction in scatter radiation when applicable?
- If a 17-inch field size was used, was the thinnest end of a long bone or vertebral column positioned at the anode end of the tube?
- Was exposure adjusted for additive and destructive patient conditions?
- If the AEC was used, was the mA station set to prevent exposure times less than the minimum response time?
- If the AEC was used, was the backup time set at 150% to 200% of the expected manual exposure time for the exam?
- If the AIC was used, was the activated ionization chamber(s) completely covered by the VOI?
- If the AEC was used, is there any radiopaque hardware or prosthetic devices positioned in the activated chamber(s)?
- If the AEC was used, was the exposure (density) control on zero?

_____ Contrast resolution is optimal for demonstrating the VOI.

- If projection is less than optimal but acceptable, does windowing allow the VOI to be fully demonstrated?
- If projection is less than optimal but acceptable, does an alternate procedural algorithm improve contrast resolution enough to make the projection acceptable?

_____ No preventable artifacts are present on the projection.

- Are any artifacts visible on the projection?
- Can the artifact be removed?
- What is the location of any present artifact with respect to a palpable anatomic structure?
- Have you asked the patient about the nonremovable artifact's origin (surgical implant, foreign body)?
- Does the projection have to be repeated because of the artifact?
- Can the artifact be removed?
- Have you asked the patient about any nonremovable artifact's origin?

_____ Ordered procedure and the indication for the exam have been fulfilled.

- Has the routine series for the body structure ordered been completed as determined by your facility?
- Do the projections in the routine series fulfilled the indication for the examination, or must additional projections be obtained?

Projection is:

_____ optimal

_____ acceptable, but not optimal

_____ unacceptable

If projection is acceptable but not optimal, or is unacceptable, describe what measures should be taken to produce an optimal projection.

beginning the examination in DR so the correct algorithm is applied to the projection before displaying it. Before selecting the patient and examination, compare the patient name and order number to be certain that they match. It may also be necessary to change the examination type (PA and lateral wrist may be shown, when a PA, lateral, and oblique wrist was ordered). If necessary, change the examination type before beginning the examination so that the correct view options are available. After the examination, double-check the order number before sending to the PACS.

Once a projection is sent to the PACS, it is immediately available to whoever has access. Improperly connecting the patient and projections will make it difficult to retrieve. If the projection is associated with the wrong patient, the projection may be seen or evaluated by a physician before the misassociation is noticed, resulting in an inaccurate diagnosis and unnecessary or inaccurate treatment of the wrong patient.

If incorrect patient information is assigned to a projection, the technologist can reattribute the examination to the correct patient as long as the projection has not been sent to the PACS. If the projections are sent to the PACS with the incorrect patient assigned to the examination, the PACS coordinator must be immediately notified to correct the error before the projections are viewed.

Marking Projections

Lead markers are used to identify the patient's right and left sides, indicate variations in the standard procedure, or show the amount of time that has elapsed in timed procedures, such as small bowel studies. The markers are constructed of lead so as to be radiopaque. Whenever a marker is placed on the IR within the collimated light field, radiation will be unable to penetrate it, resulting in an unexposed white area on the projection where the marker was located. Each projection must include the correct marker. Mismarking a projection can have many serious implications, including treatment of the incorrect anatomic structure. After a projection has been produced, evaluate it to determine whether the correct marker has been placed properly on the projection. Box 1-3 lists guidelines to follow when marking and evaluating marker accuracy on projections.

BOX 1-3 | **Marker Placement Guidelines**

- Position marker in the exposure field (area within collimated light field) as far away from the center as possible.
- Avoid placing marker in an area that will cover up the VOI (Figure 1-14) or be hidden by a shield.
- Place marker directly on the IR or tabletop whenever possible in a face-up position. This placement avoids marker distortion and magnification, prevents scatter radiation from undercutting the marker, and ensures that the marker will not be projected off the IR (Figure 1-15).
- Do not place the marker directly on the patient's skin.
- For **AP and PA projections** of the torso, vertebrae, and cranium, place the R or L marker laterally on the side being marked. The patient's vertebral column is the dividing plane for the right and left sides. If marking the right side, position the R marker to the right of the vertebral column; if marking the left side, position the L marker to the left of the vertebral column (Figure 1-5).
- For **lateral projections** of the torso, vertebrae, and cranium, the marker indicates the side of the patient positioned closer to the IR. If the patient's left side is positioned closer to the IR for a lateral lumbar vertebrae projection, place an L marker on the IR (Figure 1-16). Whether the marker is placed anteriorly or posteriorly to the lumbar vertebrae does not affect the accuracy of the image's marking, although the images of markers placed posteriorly are often overexposed (Figure 1-17).
- For **AP and PA oblique projections** of the torso, vertebrae, and cranium, the marker identifies the side of the patient positioned closer to the IR and is placed on the correct side of the patient (Figure 1-18). As with the AP-PA projections, the vertebral column is the plane used to divide the right and left sides of the body.
- For **AP/PA (lateral decubitus) projections** of the torso, place the R or L marker laterally on the correct side. If marking the

right side, position the R marker to the right of the vertebral column; if marking the left side, position the L marker to the left of the vertebral column. The marker will be better visualized and less likely to obscure the VOI if the side of the patient that is positioned up, away from the cart or table on which the patient is lying is the side marked. Along with the right or left marker, use an arrow marker pointing up toward the ceiling or lead lettering to indicate which side of the patient is positioned away from the cart or table (Figure 1-8).

- For **extremity projections**, mark the side of the patient being imaged. When multiple projections are placed on the same IR, it is necessary to mark only one of the projections placed on the IR as long as they are all projections of the same anatomic structure (Figure 1-19). If projections of a right anatomic structure and its corresponding left are placed on the same IR, mark both projections with the correct R or L marker (Figure 1-20).
- For **AP and AP oblique shoulder and hip projections**, the marker indicates the side of the patient being imaged (Figure 1-21). It is best to place the marker laterally to prevent it from obscuring medial anatomic structures and to eliminate possible confusion about which side of the patient is being imaged. Figure 1-22 demonstrates an AP hip projection with the marker placed medially. Because the marker is placed at the patient's midsagittal plane, the reviewer might conclude that the technologist was marking the right hip.
- For **cross-table lateral projections**, position the marker anteriorly to prevent it from obscuring structures situated along the posterior edge of the IR. The marker used indicates the right or left side of the patient when the extremities, shoulder, or hip is imaged (Figure 1-9) and the side of the patient positioned closer to the IR when the torso, vertebrae, or cranium is imaged (Figure 1-16).

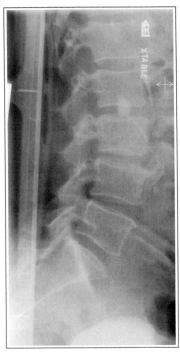

FIGURE 1-14 Left lateral lumbar vertebrae projection with marker superimposing VOI.

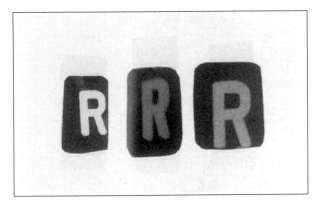

FIGURE 1-15 Marker magnification and distortion.

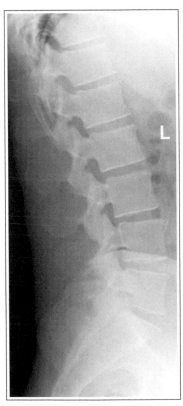

FIGURE 1-16 Marker placement for lateral lumbar vertebrae projection.

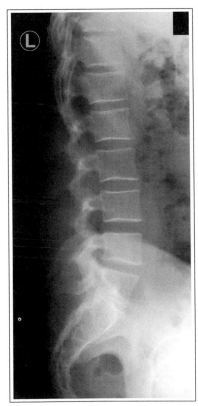

FIGURE 1-17 Poor marker placement in lateral lumbar vertebrae projection.

Using the Collimator Guide for Marker Placement with Computed Radiography. When collimating less than the size of the IR used, it can be difficult to determine exactly where to place the marker on the IR so that it will remain within the collimated field and not obscure the VOI. The best way of accomplishing this is first to collimate the desired amount and then use the collimator guide (Figure 1-23) to determine how far from the IR's midline to place the marker. Although different models of x-ray equipment have different collimator guides, the information displayed by all is similar. Each guide explains the IR coverage for the source–image receptor distance (SID) and amount of longitudinal and transverse collimation being used. If a 14- × 17-inch (35- × 43-cm) IR cassette is placed in the Bucky tray at a set SID, and the collimator guide indicates that the operator has collimated to an 8- × 17-inch (20- × 43-cm) field size, the marker should be placed 3.5 to 4 inches (10 cm) from the IR's longitudinal midline to be included in the exposure field (Figure 1-24). If the field was also longitudinally collimated, the marker would also have to be positioned within this dimension. In the preceding example, if the collimator guide indicates that the longitudinal field is collimated to a 15-inch (38-cm) field size, the marker would have to be placed 7.5 inches (19 cm) from the IR's transverse midline (Figure 1-24).

Marker Placement with Digital Radiography. The space between the tabletop and the IR is often too narrow to place the marker directly on the IR for DR images as described previously for the computed radiography system. If this is the case, place the marker either

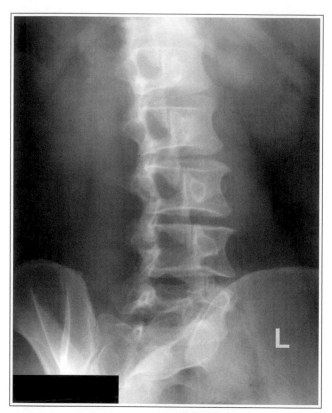

FIGURE 1-18 Marker placement for AP oblique lumbar vertebrae projection.

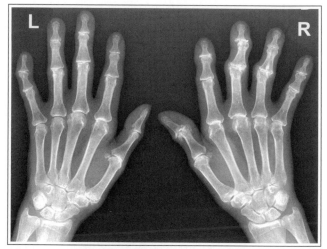

FIGURE 1-20 Marker placement for bilateral PA hand projections.

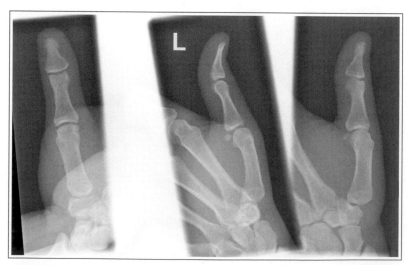

FIGURE 1-19 Marker placement for unilateral finger projections on one IR.

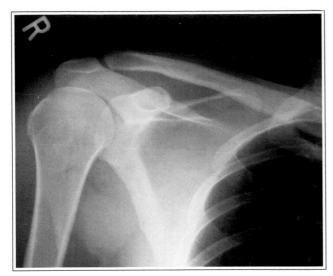

FIGURE 1-21 Marker placement for an AP projection of shoulder.

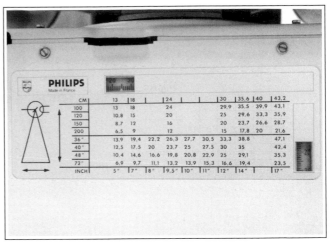

FIGURE 1-23 Collimator guide.

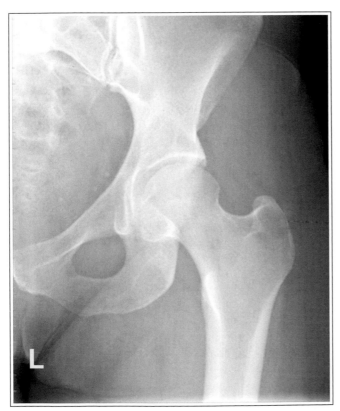

FIGURE 1-22 Poor marker placement on an AP projection of hip.

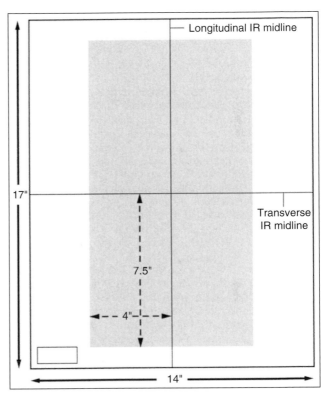

FIGURE 1-24 Marker placement for tightly collimated image.

directly on the table or upright IR or on the patient's gown. Do not place the marker on the patient's skin. The marker must be placed in the collimated light field for it to be included on the projection. It should be noted that the tape used around the marker and used to maintain the marker's placement needs to be replaced often because it may transmit bacteria from patient to patient causing additional medical issues for already compromised patients. Also, make certain that the marker does not superimpose the VOI. When low kilovolt (kV) techniques are used, the tape will be displayed on the image as an artifact.

Post-Exam Annotation. Digital imaging systems allow the technologist to add annotations (e.g., R or L side, text words) after the exposure. For example, if the original R or L side marker was partially positioned outside the collimation field during the exposure and is only partially demonstrated on the resulting projection, an annotated marker may be added (Figure 1-25). When adding annotations, the original marker should not be covered up.

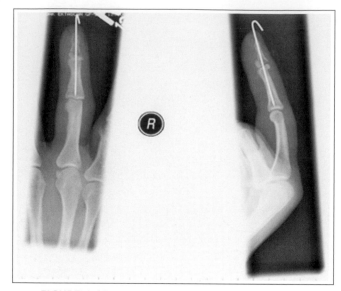

FIGURE 1-25 Partially visible marker and annotation.

Even though marker annotations can be added after processing the projection, using markers during the positioning process remains an important practice. Because projections may be flipped and rotated after processing, as described in adjusting for poor display, markers added after processing may be less reliable and may lead to misdiagnosis and legal issues.

Anatomic Structure Requirements and Placement

Each projection requires that a particular VOI is centered within the exposure field and a certain amount of the surrounding anatomic structures is included. For example, all wrist projections require that one fourth of the distal forearm be included because radiating wrist pain may be a result of a distal forearm fracture, and a lateral ankle projection includes 1 inch (2.5 cm) of the fifth metatarsal base to rule out a Jones fracture. For each projection presented in Chapters 3 through 12 there are guidelines on what should be included on the projection and a description of how to collimate so the required VOI is included. *As a general guideline, when positioning the VOI on the IR the long axis of the part is aligned with the long axis of the IR and oriented for best display and tightest collimation. The actual area of the IR that is needed to include the required anatomy is defined by accurate CR centering and good collimation practices.*
Computed Radiography. The computed radiography system uses 8 × 10 inch (18 × 24 cm), 10 × 12 inch (24 × 30 cm), and 14 × 17 inch (35 × 43 cm) size IR cassettes. The IR chosen for the procedure should be just large enough to include the required VOI and to provide a projection with the best spatial resolution. Whether the long axis of the IR is placed crosswise or lengthwise is a matter of positioning it so that all the required anatomy can fit on the chosen IR. This is mostly dictated by the body habitus and part length. To prevent a histogram analysis error, center the VOI in the center of the IR, and when placing multiple projections on one IR, place them parallel and equidistant from each other and the edges of the IR with an evenly defined unexposed space between them.
Digital Radiography. Digital radiography systems have an IR size of 16 × 16 inches (41 × 41 cm) or 17 × 17 inches (43 × 43 cm). The VOI may be placed anywhere within the IR without reducing spatial resolution or causing histogram analysis error. Part placement is dictated by accurate display requirement in DR.
Long Bones. When imaging long bones, such as the forearm, humerus, lower leg, or femur, which require one or both joints to be included on the projection, choose a large enough IR and/or extend the collimation field so it extends 1 to 2 inches (2.5 to 5 cm) beyond each joint space. This is needed to prevent the off-centered joints from being projected off the IR when they are projected in the direction in which the diverged x-ray beams that are used to record them on the projection are moving (Figure 1-26).

Projections of the humerus and lower leg may be placed diagonally on the IR to have enough length that both joints can be included on a single projection when the system's algorithm for these projections adjusts for this (Figure 1-27). This is not advisable when using computed radiography unless the system allows, because an exposure field that is not parallel with the edges of the IR may result in poor exposure field recognition and a histogram analysis error.

Collimation

Proper collimation defines the exposure field size and is accomplished when the beam of radiation is narrow enough to include only the VOI and approximately 0.5 to 1 inches (1.25-2.5 cm) of the required surrounding anatomy. Good collimation practices result in the following: (1) clearly delineates the VOI; (2) decreases the radiation dosage by limiting the amount of patient tissue exposed; (3) improves the visibility of recorded details by reducing the amount of scatter radiation that reaches the IR; and (4) reduces histogram analysis errors. *As a general guideline, each projection should demonstrate a small collimated border around the entire VOI. The only time that this rule does not apply is when the entire IR must be used to prevent clipping of needed anatomy, as with chest and abdominal projections.* This collimated border not only demonstrates good collimation practices but also can be used to determine the exact location of CR placement. Make an imaginary X on the projection by diagonally connecting the corners of the collimated border (Figure 1-28). The center of the X indicates the CR placement for the projection.

Accurate placement of the CR and alignment of the long axis of the part with the collimator's longitudinal

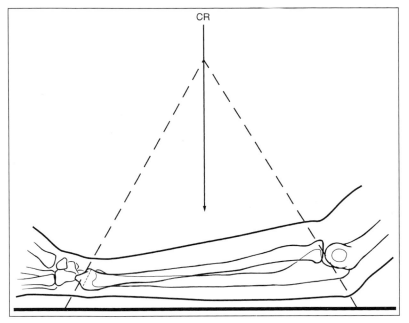

FIGURE 1-26 Proper positioning of long bones with diverged x-ray beam.

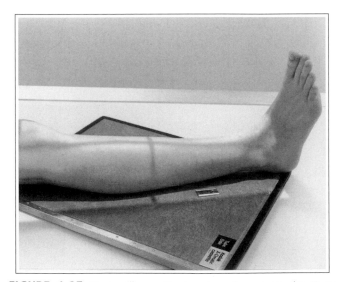

FIGURE 1-27 Diagonally positioning long bones on the IR to include both joints.

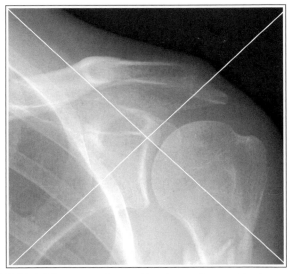

FIGURE 1-28 Using collimated borders to locate CR placement.

light line are two positioning practices that will aid in obtaining tight collimation. When collimating, do not allow the collimator's light field to mislead you into believing that you have collimated more tightly than what has actually been done. When the collimator's CR indicator is positioned on the patient's torso and the collimator is set to a predetermined width and length, the light field demonstrated on the patient's torso does not represent the true width and length of the field set on the collimator. This is because x-rays (and the collimator light, if the patient was not in the way) continue to diverge as they move through the torso to the IR, increasing the field size as they do so (Figure 1-29). The thicker the part being imaged, the smaller the collimator's light field that appears on the patient's skin surface.

On a very thick patient, it is often difficult to collimate the needed amount when the light field appears so small, but on these patients, tight collimation demonstrates the largest improvement in the visibility of the recorded details because it will cause the greatest reduction in the production of scatter radiation.

Learn to use the collimator guide (Figure 1-23) to determine the actual IR coverage. For example, when an AP lumbar vertebral projection is taken, the transversely collimated field can be reduced to an 8-inch (20-cm) field size. Because greater soft tissue thickness has nothing to do with an increase in the size of the skeletal structure, the transverse field can still be reduced the same amount when a thick patient is being imaged. Accurately center the patient by using the centering light field and then set

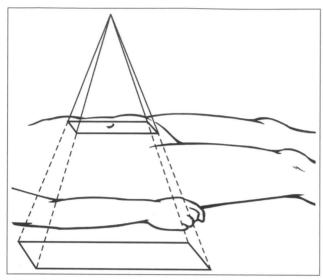

FIGURE 1-29 Collimator light field versus IR coverage.

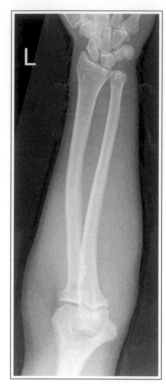

FIGURE 1-30 Proper "to skin line" collimation on an AP forearm projection.

> **BOX 1-4** | **Collimation Guidelines**
>
> - For extremity projections, collimate to within 0.5 inch (1.25 cm) of the skin line of the thickest VOI (Figure 1-30).
> - For chest and abdomen projections, collimate to within 0.5 inch (1.25 cm) of the patient's skin line (Figure 1-31).
> - When collimating structures within the torso, bring the collimated borders to within 1 inch (2.5 cm) of the VOI. Use palpable anatomic structures around the VOI to determine how close the borders are. (In Figure 1-32, the collimation field was closed to the palpable symphysis pubis and ASISs to frame the sacrum.)

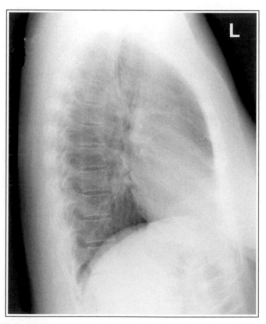

FIGURE 1-31 Proper "to skin line" collimation on a lateral chest projection.

the transverse collimation length to 8 inches by using the collimator guide. Be confident that the IR coverage will be sufficient, even though the light field appears small. Box 1-4 lists guidelines to follow when collimating and evaluating collimation accuracy on projections.

Rotating Collimator Head. The collimator head can be rotated without rotating the entire tube column on DR systems. This capability allows the technologist to increase collimation on projections when the longitudinal axis of the anatomical structure is not aligned with the longitudinal or transverse axis of the IR. Figure 1-33 demonstrates how rotating the collimator head for a leaning lateral chest can reduce radiation to a kyphotic patient's face and arms. Rotating just the collimator head does not affect the alignment of the beam with the grid; this alignment is affected only when the tube column is rotated and is demonstrated on the projection by visualization of grid lines artifacts and grid cutoff. Rotation of the collimator head should be avoided when using computed radiography because it may affect the exposure field recognition process.

Overcollimation. Evaluate all projections to determine whether the required anatomic structures have been

included. Overcollimation can result in the clipping of required anatomy (Figure 1-34). This is especially easy to have occur on a structure that is not placed in direct contact with the IR, such as for a lateral third or fourth finger or lateral hand projection. Clipping occurs because the divergence of the x-ray beam has not been taken into consideration during collimation. To prevent clipping, view the shadow of the object projected onto the IR by the collimator light (Figure 1-35). It will be magnified. This magnification is similar to the divergence that the x-ray beam undergoes when the projection is created. Allow the collimated field to remain open enough to include the shadow of the object, ensuring that the object will be shown in its entirety on the projection.

Anatomic Relationships

Evaluate each projection for proper anatomic alignment, as defined in the procedural analysis sections of this text. Each projection should demonstrate specific bony relationships that will best facilitate diagnosis. For example,

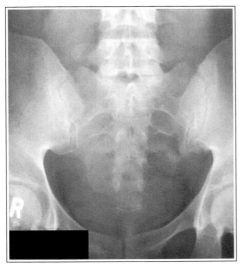

FIGURE 1-32 Proper collimation on an AP sacral projection.

an AP ankle projection demonstrates an open talotibial joint space (medial mortise), whereas the AP oblique projection demonstrates an open talofibular joint space (lateral mortise), and the lateral projection demonstrates the talar domes and soft tissue fat pads.

Positioning Routines and Understanding the Reason for the Procedure. Most positioning routines require AP-PA and lateral projections to be taken to demonstrate superimposed anatomic structures, localize lesions or foreign bodies (Figure 1-36), and determine alignment of fractures (Figure 1-37). When joints are of interest, oblique projections are also added to this routine to visualize obscured areas better. In addition to these, special projections may be requested for more precise demonstration of specific anatomic structures and pathologic conditions.

To appreciate the importance of the anatomic relationships on a projection, one must understand the clinical reason for what the procedure is to demonstrate for the reviewer. This is particularly important when obtaining special projections that are not commonly performed and require specific and accurate anatomic alignment to be useful. For example, an optimally positioned tangential (supraspinatus outlet) shoulder projection (Figure 1-38) demonstrates the supraspinatus outlet (opening formed between acromion and humeral head) and the posterior aspects of the acromion and acromioclavicular (AC) joint in profile. The technologist produces these anatomic relationships when the patient's midcoronal plane is positioned vertically and it can be ensured that the proper positioning was obtained when the superior scapular angle is positioned at the level of the coracoid tip on the projection. From this optimal projection the

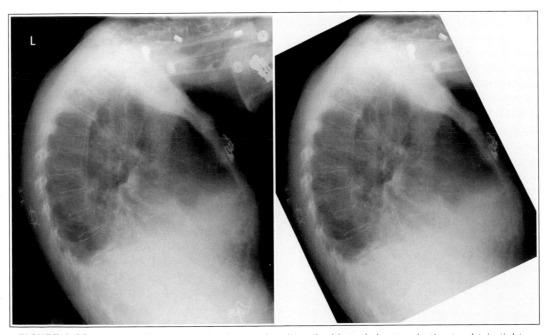

FIGURE 1-33 Nonrotated and rotated collimator head on tilted lateral chest projection to obtain tighter collimation.

radiologist can evaluate the supraspinatus outlet for narrowing caused by variations in the shape (spur) or slope of the acromion or AC joint, which has been found to be the primary cause of shoulder impingements and rotator cuff tears. If instead of being vertical, the patient's upper midcoronal plane was tilted toward the IR, the resulting projection would demonstrate the superior scapular angle positioned above the coracoid tip, preventing clear visualization of the acromion and AC joint

deformities, because their posterior surfaces would no longer be in profile and would narrow or close the supraspinatus outlet (Figure 1-39). Because the reviewer would be unable to diagnose outlet narrowing that results from variations in the shape or slope of the acromion or AC joint, this projection would not be of diagnostic value.

Correlating the Anatomic Relationships and Positioning Procedures. For each projection in the procedural analysis sections of this book, there is a list of image analysis guidelines to use when evaluating the anatomic relationships that are seen on an optimal image of that projection, an explanation that correlates it with the specific positioning procedure(s), and a description of related positioning errors. This information is needed to reposition the patient properly if a poorly positioned

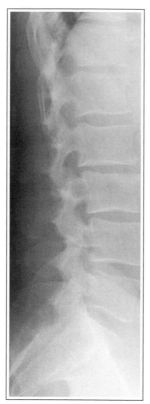

FIGURE 1-34 Overcollimation on a lateral lumbar vertebral projection.

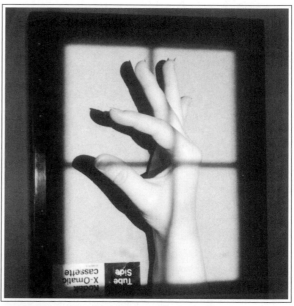

FIGURE 1-35 Viewing the hand's shadow to determine proper collimation.

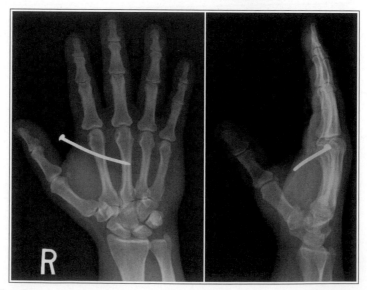

FIGURE 1-36 PA and lateral hand projections to identify location of foreign body (nail).

projection is obtained, because only the aspect of the positioning procedure that was inaccurate should be changed when repeating the projection. For example, a PA chest projection that is demonstrated without foreshortening visualizes the manubrium superimposed by the fourth thoracic vertebra, with approximately 1 inch (2.5 cm) of the apical lung field visible above the clavicles. This analysis guideline is demonstrated on the projection when the patient's midcoronal plane is positioned

vertically. If a PA chest projection demonstrates all the required analysis guidelines, with the exception of the manubrium and fourth thoracic vertebral alignment, the technologist who understands the correlation between the analysis and positioning procedure would know to adjust only the positioning of the patient's midcoronal plane before repeating the projection.

Identifying Anatomic Structures. An optimal projection appears as much like the real object as possible, but because of unavoidable distortion that results from the shape, thickness, and position of the object and beam, part, and IR alignment, this is not always feasible, resulting in some anatomic structures appearing different than the real object. Using skeletal bones positioned in the same manner as the projection will greatly aid in identification of the anatomic structures on a projection. Closely compare the visualization of the anatomic structures on the skeletal scapular bone photograph and tangential shoulder projection shown in Figure 1-38. Note that the superior scapular angle and lateral borders of this surface on the skeletal image are well demonstrated, obscuring the coracoid, but on the tangential projection the superior scapular angle is seen as a thin cortical line, its lateral borders are not demonstrated, and the coracoid can be clearly visualized. Also, note that the superior surface of the spine is visualized on the skeletal bone image between the lateral and medial scapular spine borders but is not seen on the x-ray projection.

When identifying anatomic structures, one must consider how anatomy may appear different from the real object. The following concepts, when understood and

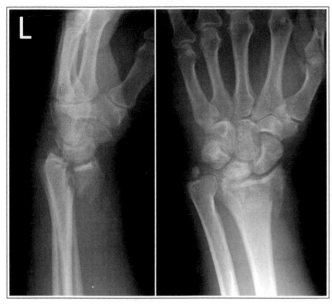

FIGURE 1-37 Lateral and PA wrist projection to demonstrate distal forearm fracture alignment.

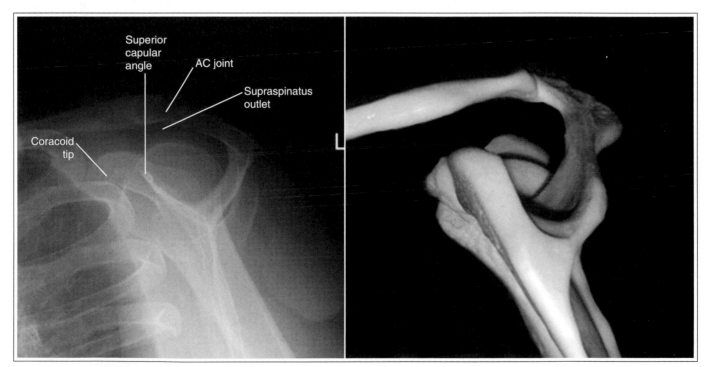

FIGURE 1-38 Properly positioned skeletal bones and shoulder in the tangential (supraspinatus outlet) projection.

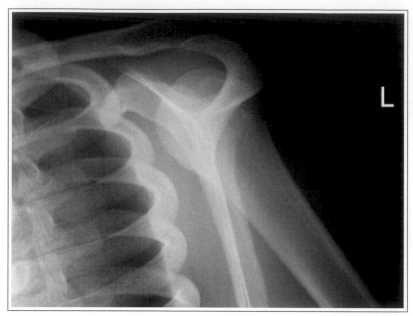

FIGURE 1-39 Poorly positioned tangential (supraspinatus outlet) shoulder projection.

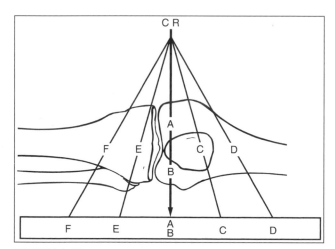

FIGURE 1-40 Effect of CR placement on anatomic alignment.

applied to how the procedure was obtained, can help with identification of the anatomic structures on the projection.

Off-Centering. X-rays used to create an image are emitted from the x-ray tube's focal spot in the form of a fan-shaped beam. The CR is the center of this beam; it is used to center the anatomic structure and IR. It is here that the x-ray beam has the least divergence and the projection of an anatomic structure demonstrates the least amount of distortion. As one moves away from the center of the beam, the x-rays used to record the projection diverge and expose the IR at an angle (Figure 1-40). The farther one moves away from the CR from all sides, the larger is the angle of divergence. Whether straight or angled beams are used to record the anatomic structures, and how those beams traverse the structures, will determine where and how they are visualized on the projection.

Compare the relationship of the symphysis pubis and coccyx, and how differently the sacrum is visualized on accurately positioned AP abdomen and pelvic projections (Figure 1-41). Both projections are taken with a perpendicular CR, but the CR is centered to the midpoint of the abdomen at the level of the iliac crest for the abdomen projection and is centered at the midpoint of the sacrum for the pelvis projection. The symphysis pubis and coccyx on both projections were recorded using diverged beams, but because the CR is centered more superiorly and beams with greater angles of divergence were used to record the symphysis pubis and coccyx on the abdomen projection, the symphysis pubis is moved more inferiorly to the coccyx on this projection when compared with its alignment with the coccyx on the pelvis projection. Also, compare sacral visualization on these two projections. Because of the more inferior centering used in the pelvis projection, the x-rays recording the sacrum are angled cephalically into the curve of the sacrum and those recording the sacrum for the abdomen projection are angled caudally, against the sacral curve. This results in decreased sacral foreshortening on the pelvis projection and increased sacral foreshortening on the abdomen projection. The off-centered diverged beams will affect structures in the same manner that an angled CR will (see preceding section for discussion of angled CR). *According to Q.B. Carroll's* Radiography in the Digital Age *textbook, at a 40-inch SID, the divergence of x-rays is 2 degrees for every inch off-centered in any direction from the CR; at a 72-inch SID, beam divergence is off-centered about 1 degree for every inch.*

It is not uncommon for bilateral (both right and left sides) projections of the hands, feet, or knees to be ordered for a comparison diagnosis. To obtain optimal

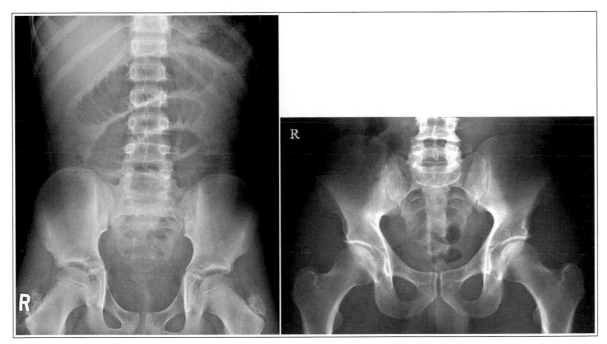

FIGURE 1-41 Properly positioned AP abdomen and pelvis projections demonstrating the effect of CR placement.

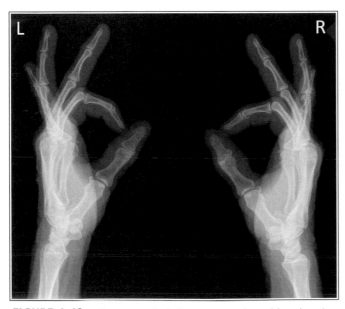

FIGURE 1-42 Poor anatomical alignment on lateral hand projections resulting from poor CR centering.

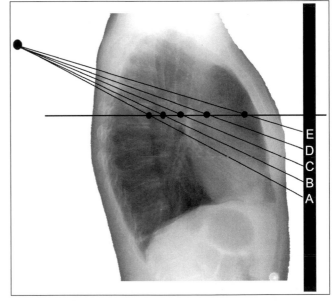

FIGURE 1-43 On angulation, the part farthest from the IR is projected the most.

projections of each side for this order, take separate exposures with the CR centered to each structure. Figure 1-42 demonstrates lateral hand projections obtained with one exposure and the CR centered between the hands. Note that this has caused the second through fourth MC to be projected posterior to the fifth MC on the hands, Producing less than optimal lateral hands because the MCs should be superimposed on lateral hand projections, and they are not on these projections.

Angled Central Ray. When an angled CR or diverged beam is used to record an object, the object will move in the direction in which the beams are traveling. The more the CR is angled, the more the object will move. Also, note that objects positioned on the same plane but at different distances from the IR, which would have been superimposed if a perpendicular CR were used, will be moved different amounts. Figure 1-43 demonstrates this concept. Point A is farther away from the IR than point C. Even though point A is horizontally aligned with point C, an angled CR used to record these two structures would project point A farther inferiorly than point C. If these two structures were closer together (points A and B on Figure 1-43), the amount of separation on the image would be less. If these two structures were farther apart (points A and E on Figure 1-43), the separation on the image would be greater.

Angling the CR can greatly affect how the anatomic structures will appear on a projection. Figure 1-44 demonstrates three AP pelvis projections, one taken with a perpendicular CR, a cephalically angled CR, and a caudally angled CR. Note how the structures situated farther from the IR (symphysis pubis and obturator foramen) have moved the direction that the CR was angled and how the same anatomic structures demonstrate different distortion.

Magnification. Magnification, or size distortion, is present on a projection when all axes of a structure demonstrate an equal percentage of increase in size over the real object. Because of three factors—no projection is taken with the part situated directly on the IR, no anatomic structure imaged is flat, and not all structures are imaged with a perpendicular beam—all projections demonstrate some degree of magnification. The amount of magnification mostly depends on how far each structure is from the IR at a set SID. The farther away the part is situated from the IR, the more magnified the structure will be (Figure 1-45). Magnification also results when the same structure, situated at the same object–image receptor distance (OID), is imaged at a different SID, with the longer SID resulting in the least magnification. *As a general guideline to keep magnification at a minimum, use the shortest possible OID and the longest feasible SID.*

Differences in magnification can be noticed between one side of a structure when compared with the opposite side if they are at significantly different OIDs. This can be seen on an accurately positioned lateral chest projection, which demonstrates about 0.5 inch (1 cm) of space between the right and left posterior ribs, even though both sides of the thorax are of equal size. Because the right lung field and ribs are positioned at a greater OID than the left lung field and ribs on a left lateral projection, the right lung field and ribs are more magnified (Figure 1-46).

Elongation. This is the most common shape distortion and occurs when one of the structure's axes appears

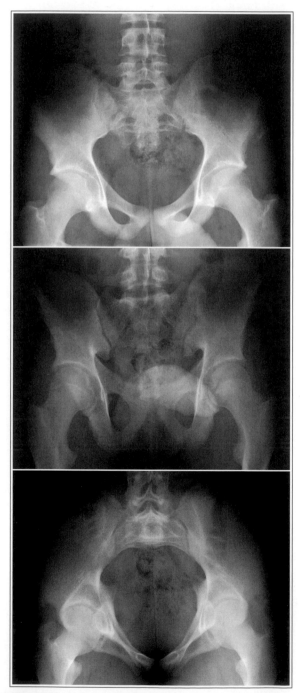

FIGURE 1-44 AP pelvis projections demonstrating the effect of CR angulation. CR perpendicular, CR angled cephalically, CR angled caudally.

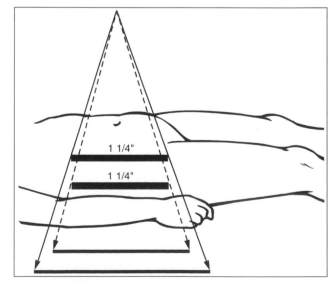

FIGURE 1-45 The part farthest from the IR will be magnified the most.

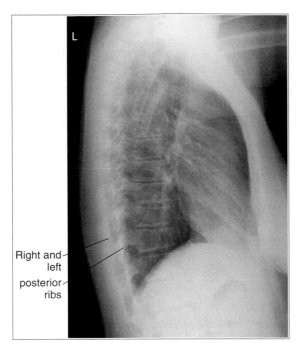

FIGURE 1-46 Left lateral chest projection showing increased magnification of right lung field due to increased OID.

disproportionately longer on the projection than the opposite axis (Figure 1-47). The least amount of elongation occurs when the CR, part, and IR set up is ideal as demonstrated in Figure 1-48*A*, and is most noticeable in the following situations:

- The CR is perpendicular to the part and the IR is parallel with the part (Figure 1-48*B*), but the part is not centered to the CR (off-centered). The greater the off-centering, the greater the elongation.
- The CR is angled and is not aligned perpendicular to the part, but the IR and the part are parallel with each other (Figure 1-48*C*). The greater the CR angulation, the greater the elongation.
- The CR and part are aligned perpendicular to each other, but the IR is not aligned parallel with the part (Figure 1-48*D*). The greater the angle of the IR, the greater the elongation.

Foreshortening. This is another form of shape distortion and is demonstrated when one of the structure's axes appears disproportionately shorter on the projection than the opposite axis (Figure 1-49). Foreshortening occurs when the CR and IR are perpendicular to each other, but the part is inclined (see Figure 1-48 *E*). The greater the incline, the greater will be the foreshortening.

Distinguishing Between Structures of Similar Shape and Size. The most difficult structures to identify are those that are identical in shape and size, such as the talar domes or femoral condyles. For these structures three methods may be used to distinguish the structures from one another.

1. Use structures that surround the structures being identified. For example, if a poorly positioned lateral

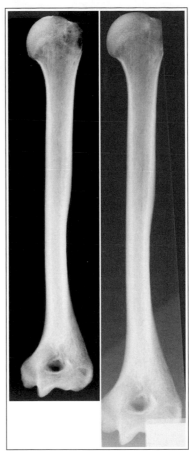

FIGURE 1-47 Humerus bones in AP projection without and with elongation.

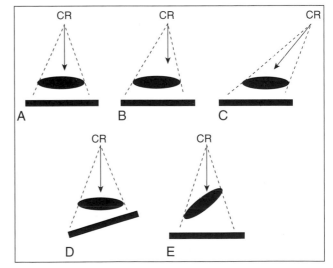

FIGURE 1-48 A-E, Causes of anatomical distortion. See text for details.

ankle projection demonstrates inaccurate anterior alignment of the talar domes and a closed tibiotalar joint space, one cannot view the joint space or distinguish between the talar domes to determine which talar dome is the more anterior, but the relationship of the tibia and fibula can easily be used to deduce

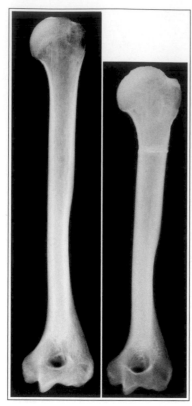

FIGURE 1-49 Humerus bones in AP projection without and with foreshortening.

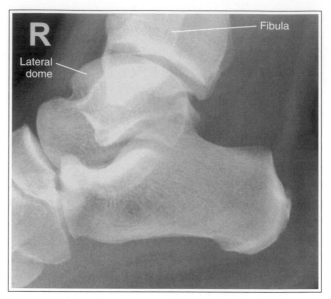

FIGURE 1-50 Poorly positioned right lateral ankle projection with lateral talar dome and fibula shown anteriorly.

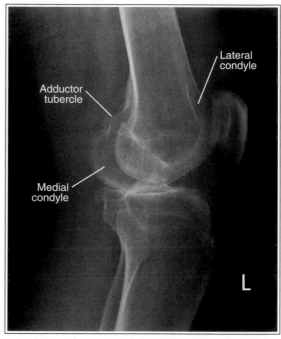

FIGURE 1-51 Poorly positioned left lateral knee projection with the medial condyle shown posteriorly.

this information. An accurately positioned lateral ankle projection demonstrates superimposed talar domes and the fibula demonstrated in the posterior half of the tibia. If a lateral ankle is obtained that demonstrates the talar domes without superimposition and the fibula too anterior on the tibia, the anterior talar dome will be the lateral dome because the lateral dome will move in the same direction as the fibula (Figure 1-50).

2. Use bony projections such as tubercles to identify a similar structure. For example, the medial femoral condyle can be distinguished from the lateral condyle on a lateral knee projection by locating the adductor tubercle situated on the medial condyle (Figure 1-51).

3. Identify the more magnified of the two structures. The anatomic structure situated farthest from the IR is magnified the most (Figure 1-46).

Determining the Degree of Patient Obliquity. To align the anatomic structures correctly, it is necessary to demonstrate precise patient positioning and CR alignment. How accurately the patient is placed in a true AP-PA, lateral, or oblique projection, whether the structure is properly flexed or extended, and how accurately the CR is directed and centered in relation to the structure determines how properly the anatomy is aligned. Because few technologists carry protractors, there must be a method for determining whether the patient is in a true AP-PA or lateral projection, or a specific degree of obliquity. For every projection described, an imaginary

line (e.g., for the midsagittal or midcoronal plane, a line connecting the humeral or femoral epicondyles) is given that can be used to align the patient with the IR or imaging table. When the patient is in an AP-PA projection, the reference line is aligned parallel (0-degree angle) with the IR (Figure 1-52A) and, when the patient is in a lateral projection, the reference line is aligned perpendicular (90-degree angle) to the IR (Figure 1-52B). For a 45-degree AP-PA oblique projection, place the reference line halfway between the AP-PA projection and the lateral projection (Figure 1-52C). For a 68-degree AP-PA

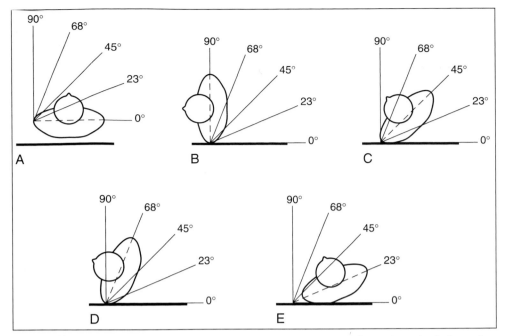

FIGURE 1-52 A-E, Estimating the degree of patient obliquity, viewing the patient's body from the top of the patient's head. See text for details.

oblique projection, place the reference line halfway between the 45- and 90-degree angles (Figure 1-52D). For a 23-degree AP-PA oblique projection, place the reference line halfway between the 0- and 45-degree angles (Figure 1-52E). Even though these five angles are not the only angles used when a patient is positioned for projection, they are easy to locate and can be used to estimate almost any other angle. For example, if a 60-degree AP-PA oblique projection is required, rotate the patient until the reference line is positioned at an angle slightly less than the 68-degree mark. I have used the torso to demonstrate this obliquity principle, but it can also be used for extremities. When an AP-PA oblique projection is required, always use the reference line to determine the amount of obliquity. Do not assume that a sponge will give you the correct angle. A 45-degree sponge may actually turn the patient more than 45 degrees if it is placed too far under the patient or if the patient's posterior or anterior soft tissue is thick.

Determining the Degree of Extremity Flexion. For many examinations a precise degree of structure flexion or extension is required to adequately demonstrate the desired information. Technologists need to estimate the degree to which an extremity is flexed or extended when positioning the patient and when evaluating projections. When an extremity is in full extension, the degree of flexion is 0 (Figure 1-53A), and when the two adjoining bones are aligned perpendicular to each other, the degree of flexion is 90 degrees (Figure 1-53B). As described in the preceding discussion, the angle found halfway between full extension and 90 degrees is 45 degrees (Figure 1-53C). The angle found halfway between the 45- and 90-degree angles is 68 degrees (Figure 1-53D),

and the angle found halfway between full extension and a 45-degree angle is 23 degrees (Figure 1-53E). Because most flexible extremities flex beyond 90 degrees, the 113- and 135-degree angles (Figure 1-53F) should also be known.

Demonstrating Joint Spaces and Fracture Lines. For an open joint space or fracture line to be demonstrated, the CR or diverged rays recording the joint or fracture line must be aligned parallel with it (Figures 1-54 and 1-55). Failure to accomplish this alignment will result in a closed joint or poor fracture visualization because the surrounding structures are projected into the space or over the fracture line (Figures 1-56 and 1-57). This results from poor patient positioning (Figure 1-56) and CR centering (Figure 1-58).

STEPS FOR REPOSITIONING THE PATIENT FOR REPEAT PROJECTIONS

1. Identify the two structures that are mispositioned (e.g., the medial and lateral femoral condyles for a lateral knee projection or the petrous ridges and supraorbital rims for an AP axial [Caldwell method] cranial projection).
2. Determine the number of inches or centimeters that the two mispositioned structures are "off." For example, the anterior surfaces of the medial and lateral femoral condyles should be superimposed on an accurately positioned lateral knee projection, but a 1-inch (2.5-cm) gap is present between them on the produced projection (Figure 1-51). Or consider how the supraorbital margins should be demonstrated 1 inch (2.5 cm) superior to the petrous ridges on an

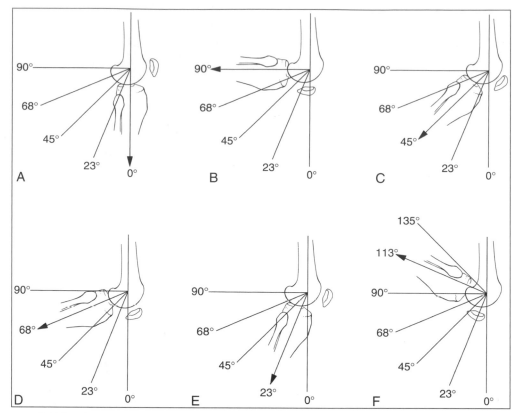

FIGURE 1-53 A-F, Estimating the degree of joint or extremity flexion. See text for details.

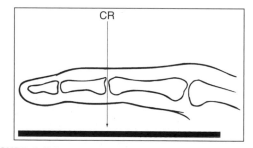

FIGURE 1-54 Accurate alignment of joint space and CR.

accurately positioned AP axial cranial projection, but they are superimposed on the produced projection (Figure 1-59).

3. Determine if the two structures will move toward or away from each other when the main structure is adjusted. For example, when the medial femoral condyle is moved anteriorly, the lateral condyle moves in the opposite direction (posteriorly). Also, when the patient's chin is elevated away from the chest, the supraorbital margins move superiorly, whereas the petrous ridges, being located at the central pivoting point in the cranium, do not move.

4. Begin the repositioning process by first positioning the patient as he or she was positioned for the poorly positioned projection. From this position, move the patient as needed for proper positioning.

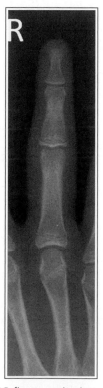

FIGURE 1-55 AP finger projection with open joints.

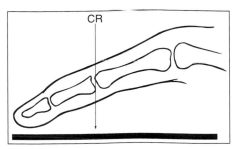

FIGURE 1-56 Poor alignment of joint space and CR.

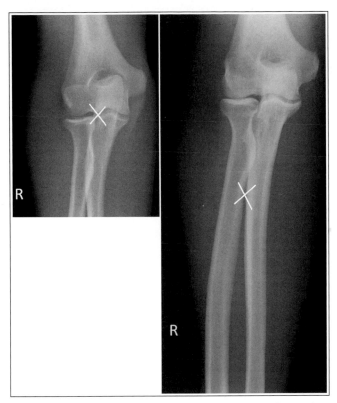

FIGURE 1-58 AP elbow projections comparing the effects of CR centering on joint visualization.

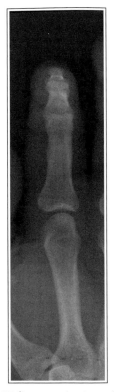

FIGURE 1-57 AP finger projection with closed joints.

5. If the structures move in opposite directions from each other when the patient is repositioned, adjust the patient half the distance that the structures are off. For example, if the anterior surface of the lateral femoral condyle is situated 1 inch (2.5 cm) anterior to the anterior surface of the medial femoral condyle on a poorly positioned lateral knee projection (Figure 1-51), the medial condyle should be rotated anteriorly 0.5 inch (1.25 cm).

6. If only one structure moves when the patient is repositioned, adjust the patient so that the structure that moves is adjusted the full amount. For example, if the petrous ridges should be located 1 inch (2.5 cm) inferior to the supraorbital margins on an accurately positioned AP axial cranial projection but they are superimposed (Figure 1-59), then adjust the patient's chin 1 inch (2.5 cm) away from the chest, moving the supraorbital margins superiorly and 1 inch (2.5 cm) above the petrous ridges.

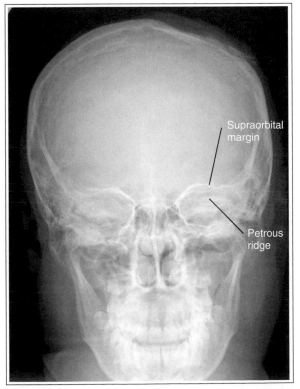

FIGURE 1-59 AP axial (Caldwell method) cranial projection showing poor positioning.

STEPS FOR REPOSITIONING THE CENTRAL RAY FOR REPEAT PROJECTIONS

1. Identify the two structures that are mispositioned—for example, the medial and lateral femoral condyles for a lateral knee projection.
2. Determine which of the identified structures is positioned farthest from the IR. This is the structure that will move the most when the CR angle is adjusted. For example, the medial femoral condyle is positioned farthest from the IR for a lateral knee projection.
3. Determine the direction in which the structure situated farthest from the IR must move to be positioned accurately with respect to the other structure. For example, in Figure 1-51, the medial femoral condyle must be moved anteriorly toward the lateral condyle to obtain accurate positioning.
4. Determine the number of inches or centimeters that the two mispositioned structures are off on the projection. For example, the anterior surfaces of the medial and lateral femoral condyles should be superimposed on an accurately positioned lateral knee projection, but a 1-inch (2.5 cm) gap is present between them on the produced projection (Figure 1-51).
5. Estimate how much the structure situated farthest from the IR will move per 5 degrees of angle adjustment placed on the CR. How much the CR angulation will project two structures away from each other depends on the difference in the physical distance of the structures from each other, as measured on the skeletal bone, and the IR.

Box 1-5 lists guidelines that can be used to determine the degree of CR adjustment required when dealing with different anatomic structures. For example, the physical space between the femoral condyles of the knee, as measured on a skeletal bone, is

| BOX 1-5 | CR Adjustment Guidelines for Structures Situated at the Central Ray |

- If the identified physical structures (actual bone, not as seen on radiographic image) are separated by 0.5 to 1.25 inches, a 5-degree CR angle adjustment will move the structure situated farthest from the IR by about 0.125 inch (0.3 cm).
- If the identified physical structures are separated by 1.5 to 2.25 inches, a 5-degree CR angle adjustment will move the structure situated farthest from the IR about 0.25 inch (0.6 cm).
- If the identified physical structures are separated by 2.5 to 3.25 inches, a 5-degree CR angle adjustment will move the structure situated farthest from the IR about 0.5 inch (1.25 cm).
- If the identified physical structures are separated by 3.5 to 4.5 inches, a 5-degree CR angle adjustment will move the structure situated farthest from the IR about 0.75 inch (1.9 cm).

approximately 2 inches (5 cm). Using the CR adjustment guidelines in Box 1-5, we find that structures that are 2 inches apart will require a 5-degree CR angle adjustment to move the part situated farthest from the IR 0.25 inch (0.6 cm) more than the structure situated closer to the IR.

6. Place the needed angulation on the CR, as determined by steps 4 and 5, and direct the CR in the direction indicated in step 3. For example, if a lateral knee projection demonstrates a separation between the medial and lateral femoral condyle of 1 inch (2.5 cm), then the CR would need to be adjusted 10 degrees and directed toward the part farthest from the IR that needs to be moved to superimpose the condyles on the projection. To obtain an optimal lateral knee projection for Figure 1-51 using the CR only to improve positioning, it should be angled 10 degrees and directed anteriorly. This will move the medial condyle 1 inch (2.5 cm) anteriorly.

Figure 1-59 demonstrates a poorly positioned AP axial projection (Caldwell method). To obtain an optimal AP axial projection using the CR, the technologist will do the following:

- Identify that the petrous ridges and supraorbital margins are superimposed on the projection in Figure 1-59, and the supraorbital margins should be 1 inch (2.5 cm) superior to the petrous ridges on an optimal projection.
- Determine that the supraorbital margins are the farthest from the IR and that they will need to be moved 1 inch (2.5 cm) superiorly to obtain optimal alignment with the petrous ridges.
- Measure the physical distance between the petrous ridges and supraorbital margins on a skeletal structure, which will be found to be about 3 inches (7.5 cm), and then use the chart in Box 1-5 to determine the degree of angulation adjustment that is needed to move the supraorbital margins 1 inch (2.5 cm) superiorly.
- Adjust the CR angulation by 10 degrees cephalically before repeating the projection.

Sharpness of the Recorded Details

The sharpness of the recorded details on a projection refers to the clarity of the anatomic lines that are displayed in the projection and is measured by the degree of blur the details demonstrate. Low blur indicates high detail sharpness and high blur indicates low detail sharpness. The factors that affect the quality of detail sharpness include the geometric factors of focal spot size and distances, motion, and spatial resolution of the IR. The greatest detail sharpness is obtained by using a small focal spot, the longest possible SID, the shortest possible OID, and controlling motion. It is also greatest in computed radiography when the smallest possible IR cassette is chosen.

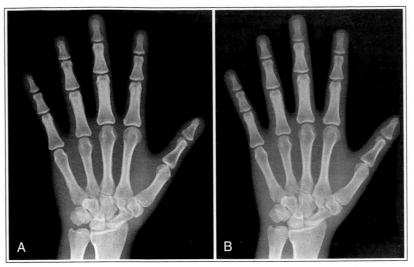

FIGURE 1-60 Comparing sharpness of recorded detail between (**A**) small and (**B**) large focal spot.

Focal Spot Size. The smaller the focal spot size used, the sharper the recorded details will be in the projection. This is because of the increase in outward and inward spread of blur at the edges of the details when a large focal spot is used. A detail that is smaller than the focal spot used to produce the projection will be entirely blurred out and will not be visible. This is why a small focal spot is recommended when fine detail demonstration is important, such as in projections of the extremities. Compare the trabecular patterns and cortical outlines on the hand projections in Figure 1-60. Figure 1-60*A* was taken using a small focal spot and Figure 1-60*B* was taken using a large focal spot. Note how the use of a small focal spot increases the sharpness of the bony trabeculae details.

Using a small focal spot is only feasible when imaging structures that can be obtained using a milliamperage (mA) setting of 300 mA or below. This is because the small area on the anode where the photons are produced cannot hold up to the high heat created when a high mA is used. It is also not recommended that the small focal spot be used when the patient's thickness measurement is large or the patient's ability to hold still is not reliable as it will require a long exposure time to obtain the needed exposure to the IR and patient motion may result. A large focal spot and high mA setting is the better choice in these situations.

Distances. The longer the SID, the sharper the recorded details will be in the projection, because the beams recording the detail edges are nearer to the CR and recorded with straighter x-rays. The shorter the OID, the sharper the recorded details will be because the remnant beam will continue to spread, widening the blurred area, as it diverges to the IR. A long SID and short OID will also keep size distortion at a minimum. *As a general rule the SID is set at the facility's standard to match the facility's technique charts and preprogrammed settings and the OID is kept as low as possible.*

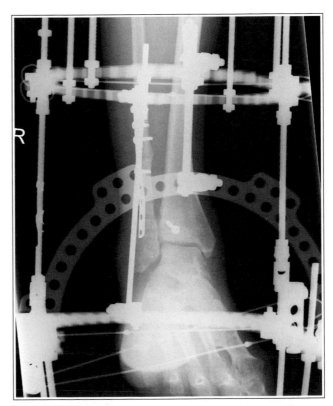

FIGURE 1-61 AP ankle projection obtained at a long OID because of traction device.

In nonroutine clinical situations, the technologist may be unable to get the part as close to the IR as possible. For example, if the patient is unable to straighten the knee for an AP projection or is in traction (Figure 1-61), the part would be at an increased OID that could not be avoided. The technologist can compensate for all or some of this magnification by increasing the SID above the standard used. When doing so, the ratio between the OID and SID must remain the same for equal magnification to result. For example, a projection taken at a 1-inch OID and 40-inch SID would demonstrate the same

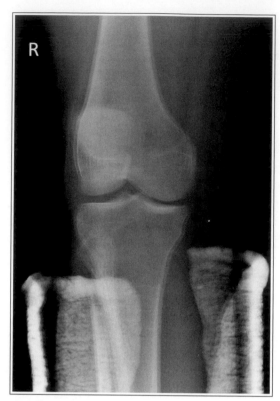

FIGURE 1-62 AP oblique knee projection demonstrating voluntary patient motion.

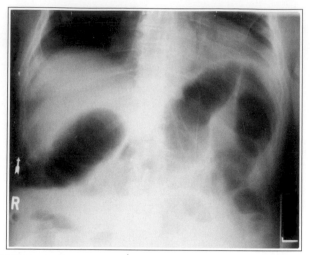

FIGURE 1-63 Involuntary patient motion on AP abdomen projection.

magnification as one taken at a 4-inch OID and 160-inch SID because both have a 1:40 ratio. It is often not feasible to increase the SID the full amount needed to offset the magnification completely because the SID cannot be raised that high. When the SID is increased to offset magnification, it is also necessary to increase the mAs using the exposure maintenance formula *([new mAs]/ [old mAs] = [new distance squared]/[old distance squared])*. This formula is used to adjust the mAs the needed amount to maintain the required exposure to the IR and prevent quantum noise.

Motion. The term *motion unsharpness* refers to lack of detail sharpness in a projection that is caused by patient movement during the exposure. This movement causes the blur at the edges of the details to spread and increase in width. Motion can be voluntary or involuntary. Voluntary motion refers to the patient's breathing or otherwise moving during the exposure. It can be controlled by explaining to the patient the importance of holding still, making the patient as comfortable as possible on the table, using the shortest possible exposure time, and using positioning devices. Voluntary motion can be identified on a projection by blurred details (Figure 1-62). Involuntary motion is movement that the patient cannot control. Its effects will appear the same as those of voluntary motion in most situations, with the exception of within the abdomen. In the abdomen, peristaltic activity of the stomach and small or large intestine can be identified on a projection by sharp bony cortices and blurry

gastric and intestinal gases (Figure 1-63). The only means of decreasing the blur caused by involuntary motion is to use the shortest possible exposure time, which in some cases is not good enough. At times, normal voluntary motions such as breathing or shaking can become involuntary motions. For example, an unconscious patient is unable to control breathing and a patient with severe trauma may be unable to control shivering.

Double Exposure. A double-exposed image may occur with computed radiography when two projections are exposed on the same IR cassette without processing having been done between the exposures. The projections exposed on the IR can be totally different and easy to identify, such as AP and lateral lumbar vertebrae projections (Figure 1-64), or they may be the same projection, with almost identical overlap. Double-exposures of the same projections typically appear blurry and can easily be mistaken for patient motion (Figure 1-65). When evaluating a blurry projection, look at the cortical outlines of bony structures that are lying longitudinally and transversely:

- Is there only one cortical outline to represent each bony structure, or are there two?
- Is one outline lying slightly above or to the side of the other?

If one outline is demonstrated, the patient moved during the exposure, but if two are demonstrated, the projection was exposed twice and the patient was in a slightly different position for the second exposure. A double-exposed computed radiography image will demonstrate adequate brightness because it will be rescaled during processing.

Spatial Resolution. The quality of spatial resolution of a digital imaging system is mainly defined by the matrix size and the size of the pixels within the matrix. Spatial resolution refers to the ability of an imaging system to distinguish small adjacent details from each other in a projection. The closer the details are to each other, with

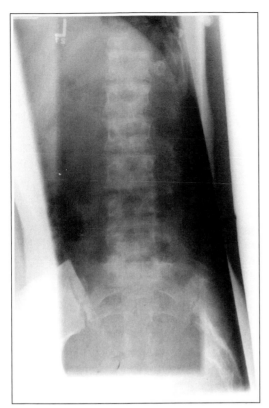

FIGURE 1-64 Double-exposed AP and lateral vertebral projections.

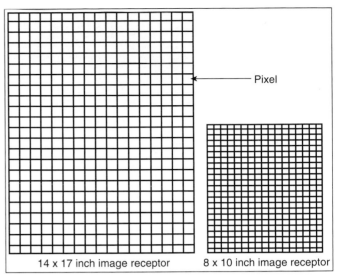

FIGURE 1-66 Image matrix and pixel sizes with different IR sizes.

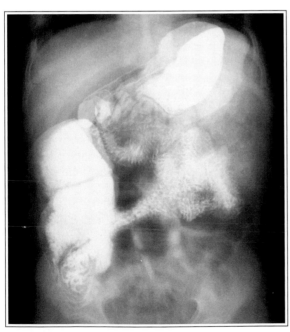

FIGURE 1-65 Double-exposed AP abdomen projections with barium in stomach and intestines.

them still being demonstrated as separate objects, the better the spatial resolution. At the point at which the details are so close together that they blur together and appear as one, spatial resolution is lost. The term *spatial frequency* is used to describe spatial resolution and refers

to the number of details that can clearly be visualized in a set amount of space (distance). This change is not expressed as the size of the object, but in terms of the largest number of line pairs per millimeter (lp/mm) that can be seen when a resolution line pair test tool is imaged using the system. As the spatial frequency number becomes larger, the ability to resolve smaller objects increases. Spatial frequency is directly related to pixel size because each pixel can only visualize one gray shade, distinguishing only one detail, and two pixels are needed to make up a line pair. If the frequency of change in the projection from detail to detail is closer together than the width or height of the pixel, the details will not be resolved.

In the computed radiography system, the pixel size is determined by the image field size relative to the image matrix size. The image matrix refers to the layout of pixels (cells) in rows and columns and is determined by the system's manufacturer. A larger matrix size will provide a higher number of pixels. The size of the pixels in the matrix is determined by the field of view (FOV). The FOV defines the area on the IR from which data is collected. Because the entire IR is scanned during computed radiography processing, the FOV is the entire IR for computed radiography systems, and because different cassette sizes are used, the size of the IR chosen influences the FOV, size of the actual pixels, and resulting spatial resolution. For example, a computed radiography system using a matrix size of 1024 × 1024 will divide the image into 1,048,576 pixels. Spreading this matrix over a 14- × 17-inch FOV (image receptor) will result in larger pixel sizes than spreading the matrix over an 8- × 10-inch FOV (Figure 1-66). Because the 8- × 10-inch IR will contain pixels of smaller size, it will provide superior spatial resolution.

Computed radiography systems have resolution capabilities between 2.55 and 5 lp/mm, with the 14- × 17-inch

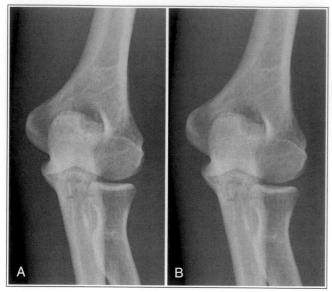

FIGURE 1-67 Comparing spatial resolution between large and small IR sizes using computed radiography. **A,** 8 × 10 inch IR. **B,** 14 × 17 inch IR.

FOV providing about 3 lp/mm and the 8- × 10-inch FOV providing about 5 lp/mm. Choosing the smallest possible IR is important when imaging structures for which small details, such as trabeculae, are needed to make an optimal diagnosis (Figure 1-67).

In DR systems there is an array of detectors electronically linked together to form a matrix, in which the individual detector elements (DELs) form the pixels of the matrix and their size determines the limiting spatial resolution of the system. The DELs contain the electronic components (e.g., conductor, capacitor, thin-film transistor) that store the detected energy and link the detector to the computer. These components take up a fixed amount of the detectors' surfaces, limiting the amount of surface that is used to collect x-ray-forming information. As the DELs become smaller, the spatial resolution capability increases, but the energy-collecting efficiency decreases. The ratio of energy-sensitive surface to the entire surface of each DEL is termed the *fill factor*. A high fill factor is desired, because energy that is not detected does not contribute to the image and an increase in radiation exposure may be required to make up the fill factor difference to prevent obtaining a projection with quantum noise. Hence, this indicates a tradeoff between spatial and contrast resolution and between spatial resolution and radiation dose.

The spatial resolution capability of a DR system is affected by the size of the DELs and the spacing between them. It is not affected by a change in FOV (collimating smaller than the full detector array), because collimation only determines the DELs that will be used in the examination and does not physically change them. DR systems have spatial resolution capabilities of approximately 3.7 lp/mm.

Radiation Protection

Diagnostic imaging professionals have a responsibility to adhere to effective radiation protection practices for the following reasons: (1) to prevent the occurrence of radiation-induced nonstochastic effects by adhering to dose-equivalent limits that are below the threshold dose-equivalent levels and (2) to limit the risk of stochastic effects to a reasonable level compared with nonradiation risks and in relation to society's needs, benefits gained, and economic factors.

More than adults, children are susceptible to low levels of radiation because they possess many rapidly dividing cells and have a longer life expectancy. In rapidly dividing cells, the repair of mutations is less efficient than in resting cells. When radiation causes DNA mutations in a rapidly dividing cell, the cell cannot repair the damaged DNA sufficiently and continue to divide; therefore the DNA remains in disrepair. The risk of cancer from radiologic examinations accumulates over a lifetime, and because children have a longer life expectancy, they have more time to manifest radiation-related cancers. This is particularly concerning because many childhood diseases require follow-up imaging into adulthood.

Continually evaluating one's radiation protection practices is necessary because radiation protection guidelines for diagnostic radiology assume a linear, nonthreshold, dose-risk relationship. Therefore any radiation dose, whether small or large, is expected to produce a response. Even when radiation protection efforts are not demonstrated on the projection, good patient care standards dictate their use. Following are radiation protection practices that should be evaluated to provide projections that can be obtained by following the ALARA (as low as reasonably achievable) philosophy.

Effective Communication. Taking the time to explain the procedure to the patient and giving clear, concise instructions during the procedure will help the patient understand the importance of holding still and maintaining the proper position, reducing the need for repeat radiographic exposures and additional radiation dose.

Immobilization Devices. If the patient moves during a procedure, the resulting projection will be blurred. Such projections have little or no diagnostic value and need to be repeated with additional exposure to the patient. Using appropriate immobilization devices can eliminate or minimize patient motion, which is especially important when imaging children, who may have a limited ability to understand and cooperate.

Source-Skin Distance. Mobile radiography units do not have the SID lock that department equipment is required to have to prevent exposures from being taken at an unsafe SID. When operating mobile radiography units, the technologist must maintain a source-skin distance (SSD) of at least 12 inches (30 cm) to prevent an unacceptable entrance skin dose. The entrance skin dose represents the absorbed dose to the most superficial layers of skin. As the distance between the source of radiation and the person increases, radiation exposure decreases. The amount of exposure decrease can be calculated using the inverse square law *([new mAs]/[old mAs] = [old distance squared]/[new distance squared])*.

Pregnancy. When imaging a female of childbearing age, it is essential that the technologist question the patient regarding the possibility of pregnancy. In some departments this is required of all females older than 11 years. Teenage girls may not admit to being pregnant until they reach the radiology department. If there is hesitancy rather than denial, additional questioning should occur, with follow-up questions such as, "Are you sexually active? If so, are you taking precautions?" If the patient is to have a procedure that requires significant pelvic exposure and there is some doubt as to her pregnancy status, it is recommended that a pregnancy test be performed.

Avoiding unnecessary radiation exposure or limiting it during the embryonic stage of development is essential because it is in this stage that the embryonic cells are dividing and differentiating and they are extremely radiosensitive and easily damaged by ionizing radiation.

Gonadal Shielding. Proper gonadal shielding practices have been proved to reduce radiation exposure of the female and male gonads. Gonadal shielding is recommended in the following situations:

- When the gonads are within 2 inches (5 cm) of the primary x-ray beam
- If the patient is of reproductive age
- If the gonadal shield does not cover the VOI

Professional technologists must always strive to improve skills and develop better ways to ensure good patient care while obtaining optimal images. All projections should be evaluated for the accuracy of gonadal shielding.

Gonadal Shielding in the AP Projection for Female Patients. Shielding the gonads of the female patient for an AP projection of the pelvis, hip, or lumbar vertebrae requires more precise positioning of the shield to prevent the obscuring of pertinent information. The first step in understanding how to shield a woman properly is to know which organs should be shielded and their location. These are the ovaries, uterine (fallopian) tubes, and uterus. The uterus is found at the patient's midline, superior to the bladder. It is approximately 3 inches (7.5 cm) in length; its inferior aspect begins at the level of the symphysis pubis and it extends anterosuperiorly. The uterine tubes are bilateral, beginning at the superolateral angles of the uterus and extending to the lateral sides of the pelvis. Tucked between the lateral side of the pelvis and the uterus and inferior to the uterine tubes are the ovaries. The exact level at which the uterus, uterine tubes, and ovaries are found varies from patient to patient. Figures 1-68 and 1-69 show images from two

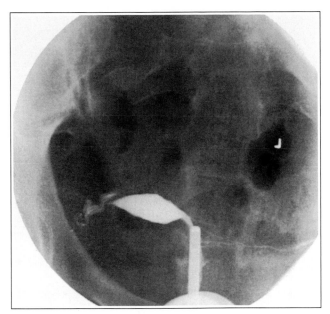

FIGURE 1-68 Hysterosalpingogram.

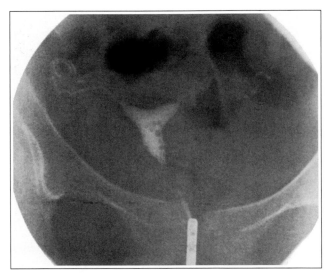

FIGURE 1-69 Hysterosalpingogram.

different hysterosalpingograms. Note the variation in the location of the uterus, uterine tubes, and ovaries in these two patients. Because the location of these organs within the inlet pelvis cannot be determined with certainty, the entire inlet pelvis should be shielded to ensure that all the reproductive organs have been protected.

To shield the female gonads properly, use a flat contact shield made from at least 1 mm of lead and cut to the shape of the inlet pelvis (Figure 1-70). Oddly shaped and male (triangular) shields do not effectively protect the female patient (Figure 1-71). The dimensions of the shield used should be varied according to the amount of magnification that the shield will demonstrate, which is determined by the OID and SID and by the size of the patient's pelvis, which increases from infancy to adulthood. Each department should have different-sized

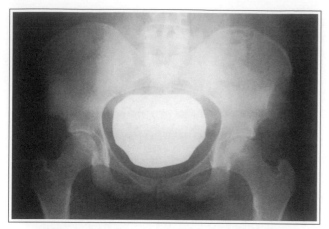

FIGURE 1-70 Proper gonadal shielding in the female.

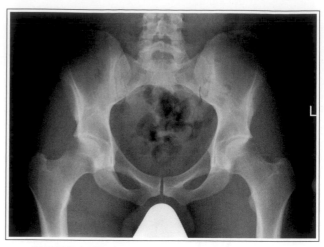

FIGURE 1-72 Proper gonadal shielding in the male.

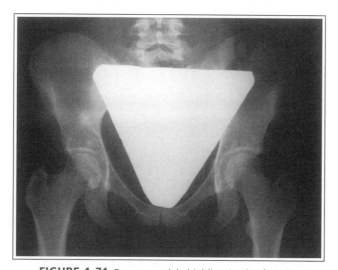

FIGURE 1-71 Poor gonadal shielding in the female.

contact or shadow shields for variations in female pelvic sizes for infants, toddlers, adolescents, and young adults.

Before palpating the anatomic structures used to place the gonadal shield on the patient, explain the reason why you will be palpating for these structures and ask permission to do so. To position the shield on the patient, place the narrower end of the shield just superior to the symphysis pubis and allow the wider end of the shield to lie superiorly over the reproductive organs. Side-to-side centering can be evaluated by placing an index finger just medial to each anterior superior iliac spine (ASIS). The sides of the shield should be placed at equal distances from the index fingers. When imaging children, do not palpate the pubic symphysis because they are taught that no one should touch their "private parts." Instead use the greater trochanters to position the shield because they are at the level of the superior border of the pubic symphysis. It may be wise to tape the shield to the patient. Patient motion such as breathing may cause the shield to shift to one side, inferiorly, or superiorly.

Gonadal Shielding in the AP Projection for Male Patients

The reproductive organs that are to be shielded on the male are the testes, which are found within the scrotal pouch. The testes are located along the midsagittal plane inferior to the symphysis pubis. Shielding the testes of a male patient for an AP projection of the pelvis or hip requires more specific placement of the lead shield to avoid obscuring areas of interest. For these examinations a flat contact shield made from vinyl and 1 mm of lead should be cut out in the shape of a right triangle (one angle should be 90 degrees). Round the 90-degree corner of this triangle. Place the shield on the adult patient with the rounded corner beginning approximately 1 to 1.5 inches (2.5 to 4 cm) inferior to the palpable superior symphysis pubis. When accurately positioned, the shield frames the inferior outlines of the symphysis pubis and inferior ramus and extends inferiorly until the entire scrotum is covered (Figure 1-72). Each department should have different-sized male contact shields for the variations in male pelvic sizes for infants, youths, adolescents, and young adults.

Gonadal Shielding in the Lateral Projection for Male and Female Patients. When male and female patients are imaged in the lateral projection, use gonadal shielding whenever (1) the gonads are within the primary radiation field and (2) shielding will not cover pertinent information. In the lateral projection, male and female patients can be similarly shielded with a large flat contact shield or the straight edge of a lead apron. Begin by palpating the patient's coccyx and elevated ASIS. Next, draw an imaginary line connecting the coccyx with a point 1-inch posterior to the ASIS, and position the longitudinal edge of a large flat contact shield or half-lead apron anteriorly against this imaginary line (Figure 1-73). This shielding method can be safely used on patients being imaged for lateral vertebral, sacral, or coccygeal projections without fear of obscuring areas of interest (Figure 1-74).

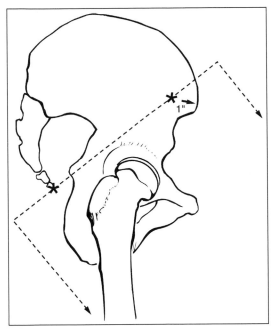

FIGURE 1-73 Gonadal shielding for the lateral projection in both male and female.

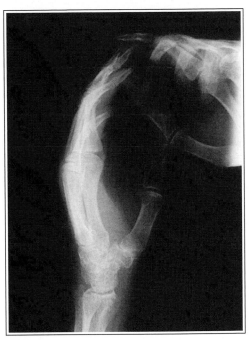

FIGURE 1-75 Anatomic artifact—poor radiation protection.

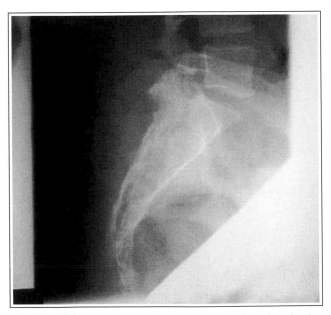

FIGURE 1-74 Proper gonadal shielding in the lateral projection.

Shielding of Radiosensitive Cells Not Within the Primary Beam. Shielding of radiosensitive cells should be done whenever they lie within 2 inches (5 cm) of the primary beam. Radiosensitive cells are the eyes, thyroid, breasts, and gonads. To protect these areas, place a flat contact shield constructed of vinyl and 1 mm of lead or the straight edge of a lead apron over the area to be protected. Because the atomic number of lead is so high, radiation used in the diagnostic range will be readily absorbed in the shield.

Collimation. Tight collimation reduces the radiation exposure of anatomic structures that are not required on the projection. For example, its use on chest projections will reduce exposure of the patient's thyroid; on a cervical vertebral projection, it will reduce exposure of the eyes; on a thoracic vertebrae projection, it will reduce exposure of the breasts; and on a hip projection, it will reduce exposure of the gonads.

Exposure Factors to Minimize Patient Exposure. Selection of appropriate technical exposure factors for a procedure should focus on producing a projection of diagnostic quality with minimal patient dose. This is accomplished by selecting the highest practical kV and the lowest mAs that will produce a projection with sufficient information. Also, when the patient has difficulty holding still or halting respiration, the shortest possible exposure time should be used by selecting a high-mA station.

Automatic Exposure Control Backup Timer. The backup timer is a safety device that prevents overexposure to the patient when the automatic exposure control (AEC) is not properly functioning or the control panel is not set correctly. When using the AEC, set the AEC backup time at 150% to 200% of the expected manual exposure time. Once the backup time is reached, the exposure will automatically terminate.

Avoiding Dose Creep. Digital radiography can reduce exposure to the overall population because repeats for overexposed and poor contrast images are not needed; the image can be adjusted to improve these through automatic rescaling and windowing. It is necessary for the technologist to avoid dose or technique creep, which results when technique values are elevated more than necessary because of fear of producing projections with quantum noise.

Anatomic Artifacts. These are anatomic structures of the patient or x-ray personnel that are demonstrated on the projection but should not be there (Figure 1-75). Note in the figure how the patient's other hand was used to help maintain the position. This is not an acceptable practice. Many sponges and other positioning tools are available to aid in positioning and immobilizing the patient. Whenever the hands of the patient, x-ray personnel, or others must be within the radiation field, they must be properly attired with lead gloves.

Personnel and Family Members in Room During Exposure. Appropriate immobilization devices should be used and all personnel and family members should leave the room before the x-ray exposure is made. If the patient cannot be effectively immobilized or left alone in the room during the exposure, lead protection attire such as aprons, thyroid shields, glasses, and gloves should be worn by the personnel during any x-ray exposure. Anyone remaining in the room should also stand out of the path of the radiation source and as far from it as possible.

Digital Imaging Guidelines

OUTLINE

Digital Radiography, 38
Image (Data) Acquisition, 38
Histogram Formation, 38
Automatic Rescaling, 39
Exposure Indicators, 40
Histogram Analysis Errors, 41
Image Receptor Exposure, 45

Other Exposure-Related
Factors, 50
Contrast Resolution, 56
Post-Processing, 58
Artifacts, 59
Postprocedure Requirements, 66
Special Imaging Situations, 66

Guidelines for Aligning Contrast
Resolution, Part, and Image
Receptor, 69
Pediatric Imaging, 72
Obese Patients, 73

OBJECTIVES

After completion of this chapter, you should be able to do the following:

- Describe the processing steps completed in computed radiography (CR) and direct-indirect digital radiography (DR).
- State why the exposure field recognition process is completed in CR and is not needed in DR.
- Identify the areas of an image histogram and list the guidelines to follow to produce an optimal histogram.
- Explain the relationship between the image histogram and the chosen lookup table in the automatic rescaling process.
- Discuss the causes of a histogram analysis error.
- List the exposure indicator parameters for the digital systems used in your facility and discuss how to use them to evaluate and improve the quality of projections.

- Describe how to identify when a projection has been overexposed and underexposed.
- State the causes of overexposure and underexposure in digital radiography and the effect that each has on image quality.
- Describe the factors that affect contrast resolution.
- List the different artifacts found in radiography and discuss how they can be prevented, when applicable.
- Discuss the difference between an optimal and acceptable projection.
- List the guidelines for obtaining mobile and trauma projections and state how technical factors should be adjusted to adapt for different mobile and trauma-related conditions.
- Describe the differences to consider when performing procedures and evaluating pediatric and obese patient projections.

KEY TERMS

additive condition
algorithm
anode heel effect
artifact
automatic exposure control
automatic rescaling
backup timer
bit depth
brightness
contrast resolution
destructive condition

differential absorption
dynamic range
exposure field recognition
exposure indicator
gray scale
histogram
histogram analysis error
image acquisition
imaging plate
lookup table
moiré grid artifact

phantom image
postprocessing
procedural algorithm
quantum noise
radiopaque
raw data
saturation
scatter radiation
subject contrast
thin-film transistor
windowing

DIGITAL RADIOGRAPHY

Two types of digital imaging systems are used in radiography to acquire and process the radiographic image, the cassette-based system known as computed radiography and the cassette-less detector system known as direct-indirect digital radiography (DR). The systems are unique in the methods that they use to acquire and process the image before sending it to the computer to be analyzed and manipulated. Understanding the acquisition and processing steps of each system will help the technologist to prevent errors that cause poor acquisition and processing and understand the indicators used to analyze the quality and improve the radiographic image.

Image (Data) Acquisition

Computed Radiography. Computed radiography uses cassettes that can be placed in the Bucky or on the table to obtain the projection. During the image acquisition process the radiographic exposure results in the imaging plate (IP) storing trapped electrons in the plate's photostimulable phosphor. The amount of energy trapped in each area of the IP reflects the subject contrast of the body part imaged. Once the IP has been exposed, the examination or body part is selected from the menu choices on the computed radiography workstation and the plate is sent to the reader unit. Selecting the correct examination or body part ensures that the correct lookup table (LUT) is applied when the image is rescaled. The IP is divided into a matrix and the reader unit uses an infrared laser beam to scan back and forth across the plate, releasing the stored energy in the form of visible light. The amount of light produced in each pixel in the matrix is equivalent to the amount of energy that was stored in that area of the IP during the acquisition process. The light is collected and converted to an electrical signal by the photomultiplier tube (PMT) and then sent to the analog-to-digital converter (ADC) to be digitized. During digitization each pixel is assigned a digital number (gray shade value) that represents the amount of light that was emitted from that surface of the IP. Pixels that received greater radiation exposure are assigned values that represent darker gray shades, whereas the pixels receiving less exposure are assigned values that represent lighter gray shades. All the gray shade values together make up what is referred to as the raw or image data.

An exposure recognition field algorithm is then applied to the image data to distinguish the gray shade values that represent the values that are inside the exposure field from those that are outside the exposure field, and ensure that the histogram generated from the image data is shaped correctly and that the volume of interest (VOI) is accurately identified before automatic rescaling of the data occurs.

Direct-Indirect Radiography. Digital radiography uses a cassette-less imaging capture system that is hard-wired to the image processing system and does not require the technologist to physically place the image receptor (IR) into the reader. Because of this the technologist must choose the correct examination from the workstation before the exposure is made to ensure that the correct LUT is applied to the displayed image. The IR contains a matrix of pixel-size detector elements (DELs) that each include a thin-film transistor (TFT) that collects the electric charges produced in the DEL when the remnant radiation strikes it. The subject contrast in the remnant radiation is represented by the TFTs collecting varying intensities. After the exposure the signal from each DEL is sent to the computer in an orderly manner for processing and manipulation where each DEL signal is given a gray shade value. Only the DELs in the TFT that have received radiation, which is determined when the technologist collimates, collect and send electric signals and are included in the image. This eliminates the need for the exposure field recognition process that is completed in computed radiography and the many histogram errors that poor recognition can cause.

Histogram Formation

After the image data have been acquired, a histogram graph is generated that has the pixel gray shade values on the x-axis and the number of pixels with that gray shade values on the y-axis (Figure 2-1). The histogram

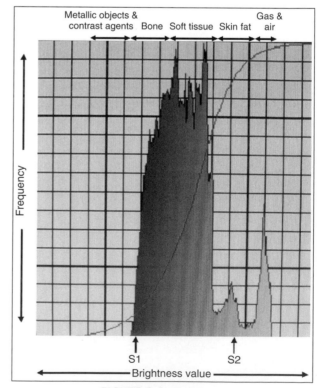

FIGURE 2-1 Histogram.

represents the subject contrast in the remnant radiation and is determined by the total exposure (kV and mAs selected) that is used to create the image. The peaks and valleys of the histogram signify the subject contrast of the structure imaged; the VOI is identified, with S1 representing the minimum useful gray shade value and S2 representing the maximum useful value. Because the subject contrast of a particular anatomic structure (e.g., chest, abdomen, shoulder) is fairly consistent from exposure to exposure, the shape of each structure's histogram should be fairly consistent as well. Gray shade values between white to black are positioned on the histogram from left to right with the metallic objects or contrast agents (light gray) recorded on the left in the graph, followed by bone, soft tissues near the center, fat, and finally gaseous or air values (dark gray) on the right. The tail or high spiked portion on the far right of some histograms represents the background value that is in the exposure field. This background value will be the darkest value because this area is exposed to primary radiation that does not go through any part of the patient, such as with extremity and chest projections that have been collimated close to the skin line (Figure 2-2) but not within it. This spike is not visible on images in which the entire cassette is covered with anatomy, such as abdomen projections or images in which the collimation field is within the skin line, such as for an AP lumbar vertebrae projection.

Poor histogram formation and subsequent histogram analysis errors will occur on both computed radiography and DR systems, as described in the histogram analysis errors section later in the chapter. Box 2-1 lists guidelines for obtaining optimal image histograms.

Automatic Rescaling

Included in the computer software is a LUT, or "ideal" histogram for every radiographic projection. These tables were developed using exposure techniques, positioning, and collimation that produces optimal histograms for

---

BOX 2-1 | Guidelines for Producing Optimal Image Histograms

Computed and Direct-Indirect Radiography
- Set the correct technique factors for the projection.
- Choose the correct body part and projection from the workstation menu.
- Center the CR to the center of the VOI.
- Collimate as closely as possible to the VOI, leaving minimum background in the exposure field.
- Control the amount of scatter reaching the IR (grids, collimation, lead sheets).
- If collimating smaller than the IR, center the VOI and show all four collimation borders.
- Remove unnecessary artifacts from the VOI.

Computed Radiography Only
- Use the smallest possible IR, covering at least 30% of the IR.
- When placing multiple projections on one IR, all of the collimation borders must be parallel and equidistant from the edges of the IR, and at equal distance from each other.
- Do not leave the IR cassette in the imaging room while other exposures are being made and read the IP shortly after the exposure.
- Erase the IP if the IR has not been used within a few days.

IP, Imaging plate; *CR*, central ray; *IR*, image receptor; *VOI*, volume of interest.

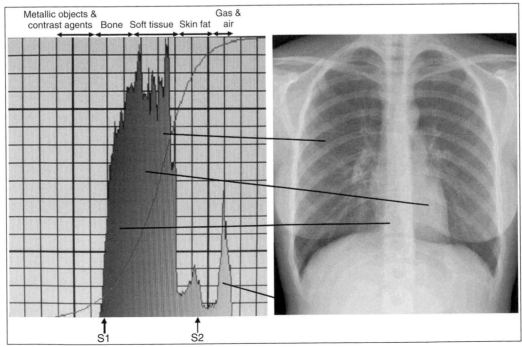

FIGURE 2-2 Histogram of chest projection.

the projection and provides the means for the computer to automatically rescale the obtained image histogram, optimizing the image before it is displayed. During the rescaling process the computer compares the obtained image histogram with the selected LUT and applies algorithms to the image data as needed to align the image histogram with the LUT. The most common rescaling processes are to adjust the brightness and contrast of the image. The position of the image histogram, left to right, is adjusted to change the overall image brightness and the shape of the histogram is adjusted to change the contrast or gray scale.

- If the image histogram was positioned farther to the right than the LUT's histogram, representing an image in which the remnant beam had more intensity than is desired and if displayed, would be at darker gray shade values than desired, the algorithm applied to the data would move the obtained values of each pixel toward the left, aligning them with the values in the LUT and brightening up the image.
- If the image histogram was positioned farther to the left than the LUT's histogram, representing an image in which the remnant beam had less intensity than is desired and would be displayed at lighter gray shade values than desired, the algorithm applied would move the obtained values of each pixel toward the right and decrease the brightness.
- If the image histogram was wider than the LUT's histogram, representing an image in which the remnant beam had lower contrast than desired, the algorithm applied to the data would narrow the histogram, increasing the degree of difference between the gray shades and increasing the contrast.
- If the image histogram was narrower than the LUT's histogram, representing an image in which the remnant beam had high contrast, the algorithm applied to the data would widen the histogram, decreasing the degree of difference between the gray shades and lowering the contrast.

The image that is then displayed on the display monitor is the rescaled image. The computer system is capable of rescaling images that have been overexposed or underexposed by at least a factor of 2 without losing detail visibility.

For optimal rescaling results, the technologist must obtain images that produce histograms that clearly distinguish the subject contrast in the VOI with different gray shades, discern these values from those outside the VOI, and whose shape is similar to that of the LUT chosen. For example, including gray shade values on the histogram that are other than those that are in the VOI will result in a misshapen histogram, which does not accurately represent the anatomic structure imaged and will not match the associated LUT. If the image histogram and selected LUT do not have a somewhat similar shape, the computer software will be unable to align them, resulting in a histogram analysis error that produces a poor-quality image and provides an erroneous exposure indicator value.

Exposure Indicators

Exposure indicators (EIs) are readings that denote the amount of radiation intensity (quantity of photons) that struck the IR. Although they give an indication of the amount of radiation that the patient was exposed to, they are not measures of dose to the patient because they do not take into account the energy level of the x-rays. After the histogram has been developed, the EI reading is read by the computer at the midpoint of the defined VOI (halfway between S1 and S2). This midway point is the median gray shade value, which represents the ideal amount of x-ray exposure at the detectors. The EI is displayed on the digital image. To produce optimal images the technologist's goal is to produce images that result in the EI coming as close to the ideal as possible for the digital system. Images that fall close to the far ends of the EI acceptable range are not repeated but should be evaluated to determine why this has occurred and what changes should be considered in future images to bring the EI closer to the ideal. The EI expression varies from one manufacturer to another, and the technologist should be aware of those in his or her facility. Table 2-1 lists different manufacturers' EIs and ranges for acceptable exposure for many of the CR and DR systems currently on the market. As described in the next section on histogram analysis errors, because the EI value is based on the accuracy of the image histogram,

TABLE 2-1	Exposure Indicator Parameters					
System	Exposure Indicator	Acceptable Range	Ideal Exposure	Insufficient Exposure	Excessive Exposure
CareStream CR	Exposure index (EI)	1700-2300	2000	<1700	>2300
Fuji CR & Konica	Sensitivity (S) number	100-400	200	>400	<100
Phillips CR	Sensitivity (S) number	55-220	110	>220	<55
Agfa CR	Log median value (LgM)	2.2-2.8	2.5	<2.2	>2.8
Phillips DR	Exposure index (EI)	50-200	100	<200	>50
Siemens DR	Exposure index (EI)	500-2000	1000	<500	>2000
CareStream DR	Exposure index (EI)	125-500	250	<125	>500

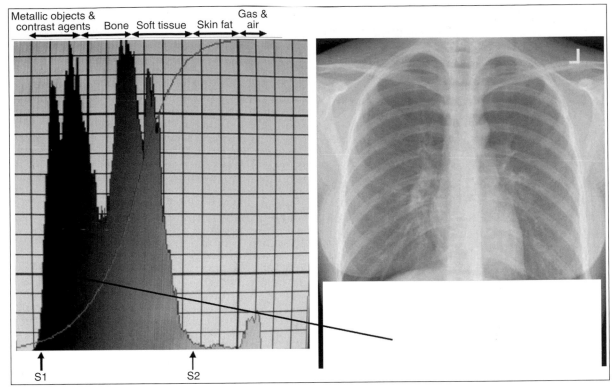

FIGURE 2-3 Computed radiography PA chest projection histogram in which the VOI was not accurately identified.

any factor that affects the accuracy of the histogram will also affect the accuracy of the EI value.

Because the EI is derived from the histogram, anything that causes a histogram analysis error will also cause an erroneous EI value. For example, Figure 2-2 represents a PA chest histogram of a patient for whom the VOI was accurately identified. Figure 2-3 demonstrates the histogram of a PA chest projection in which collimation was such that a portion of the lead apron around the patient's waist was included on the projection. The lead apron produced a digital value that was recorded on the histogram and included as part of the VOI, causing the histogram to widen. Compare the VOI (section between S1 and S2) on the histogram in Figure 2-2 with that in Figure 2-3. Note that the midpoint between the VOIs (where the EI is read) on each of these histograms is different. This difference is caused by the widening of the histogram, not because the exposure to the IR and patient itself was different between the projections, but because of a histogram analysis error. Histogram analysis errors cause the EI to be falsely moved toward a lower or higher value, making its value erroneous and unreliable.

Histogram Analysis Errors

Images with histogram analysis errors may have the same image quality issues as images with exposure errors, but instead of their causes resulting from incorrectly set mAs and kV, they have to do with the accuracy

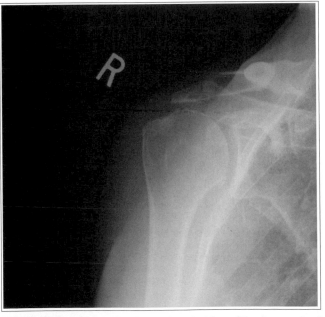

FIGURE 2-4 Computed radiography AP oblique (Grashey method) shoulder projection demonstrating a histogram analysis error.

of the positioning procedures. For example, Figure 2-4 demonstrates an AP shoulder projection that was obtained using the CareStream (previously Kodak) CR system, optimal kV, and the center automatic exposure control (AEC) ionization chamber. The projection demonstrates adequate brightness, low contrast resolution, poor collimation (excessive background included), poor centering beneath the chamber, and quantum mottle, and has an EI of 2410. Even though the EI indicates that excessive exposure was used, the potential for this reading being erroneous is very high. We know that when a portion of the chamber is exposed by part of the beam that does not go through the patient, as is the case with this projection, the exposure terminates early and underexposure results, as indicated by the quantum noise. Also, because the projection was not tightly collimated, excessive background radiation could have been included in the VOI, causing the EI to be read at a midpoint that indicated more exposure to the VOI than was actually delivered. The procedural causes of this low-quality projection clearly conflict with the EI value on the projection. When a poor-quality image is produced, the effect of the positioning procedures on the amount of IR exposure should be considered before deciding if the exposure factors (mAs, kV, AEC) should be adjusted. Begin your evaluation by determining how accurately the positioning procedures listed in Box 2-1 were followed. Only if these are accurate should the mAs or kV be adjusted. Following are common causes of histogram errors.

Part Selection from Workstation Menu. If the wrong body part or projection is selected on the workstation, the image will be rescaled using the wrong LUT. Because each body part has a specific LUT to use for each projection and that LUT has a set gray scale and average brightness level to optimize the projection, rescaling to the incorrect one will cause a histogram analysis error as the computer tries to align the data histogram with the incorrect LUT. This error is easily detected because the study name is noted in the data field underneath each digital image; it may be corrected by reprocessing it under the correct LUT as long as the image has not yet been sent to the PACS system.

Central Ray Centering. If the CR is not centered to the VOI, collimation needs to be expanded to include all the required anatomy. Increasing the collimation field size may result in additional anatomy or excessive background values being included on the image histogram and identified as part of the VOI. This misshapes and widens the histogram, causing a histogram analysis error. Figure 2-5 demonstrates an adult PA chest projection using the CareStream computed radiography system. The projection demonstrates adequate brightness, low subject contrast, and quantum noise, even though the resulting EI is 2300, which indicates excessive exposure. More accurate CR centering and tighter collimation is needed to improve this projection. This problem occurs when excessive abdominal structures are included on chest or lateral lumbar vertebral projections and/or excessive lung structures are included on abdominal projections.

Collimation. Collimating to within 0.5 inch (2.5 cm) of the skin line prevents too much background data from being included within the exposure field. If excessive

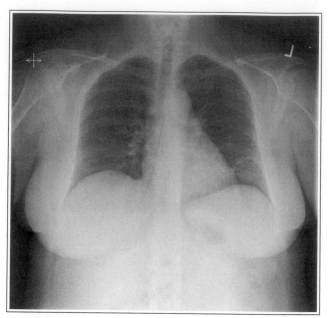

FIGURE 2-5 PA chest projection obtained with Kodak CR system that demonstrates a histogram analysis error caused by poor CR centering and collimation.

background information is inappropriately included in the VOI, a widening of the image histogram results (Figure 2-6). Figure 2-7 demonstrates a PA hand projection taken of a 4-year-old child using the CareStream computed radiography system. The projection demonstrates low contrast resolution and quantum noise, even though the resulting EI is 2430, which indicates excessive exposure. A histogram error resulted because the projection was not tightly collimated and the background information was not excluded from the VOI.

Scatter Radiation Control. Reduce the scatter radiation fog reaching the IR through tight collimation, appropriate grid usage, and by placing a lead sheet along the edge of the exposure field when excessive scatter fogging is expected, such as on the posterior edge of lateral lumbar and thoracic vertebral projections. When the amount of scatter radiation reaching the IR is high and the fog values outside the exposure field are included in the VOI, a widening of the histogram results (Figures 2-8 and 2-9).

Clearly Defining the Volume of Interest (for Computed Radiography Only). Clearly defining the VOI by using an IR size where the VOI will cover the entire IR, eliminating any exposure values from being recorded on the IR that are not of interest, will reduce the chance of histogram analysis errors. When it is necessary to collimate smaller than the IR, make certain to center the VOI in the center of the computed radiography cassette and ideally have all four collimation borders showing and positioned at equal distances from the edges of the cassette (Figure 2-10). When only two collimation borders are present, as with an AP lumbar vertebral projection, they also should be equidistant from the edges of the

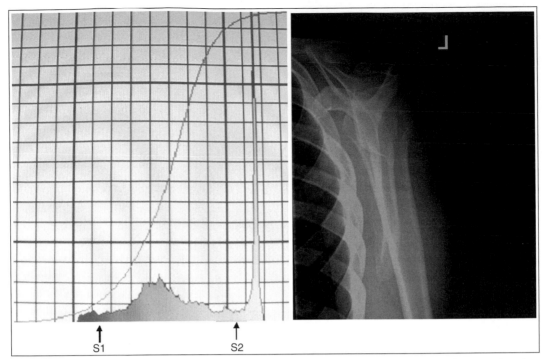

FIGURE 2-6 Computed radiography histogram that includes excessive background radiation values in the VOI.

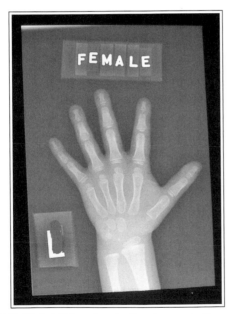

FIGURE 2-7 Digital PA hand projection demonstrating a histogram analysis error caused by poor collimation.

cassette. It is not acceptable to have only one border showing without the opposite border also being present. In the exposure field recognition process, the computer identifies the difference between the gray shade values that are outside from those inside the exposure field. When one of the collimation borders is missing, the computer may not distinguish the collimation border that is present as an actual border, but instead include the area beyond it as part of the VOI, and include it in the histogram. This is especially true if there is fogging present outside the exposure field. When both borders are present, the computer can better identify the value differences at each end of the exposure field as being a collimation border. This often occurs on projections of the axiolateral hip or inferosuperior (axial) shoulder, where the exposure field covers only the bottom two thirds of the cassette, demonstrating the upper collimation border but not the bottom one (Figure 2-11). To prevent this histogram analysis error, either build the patient up enough to collimate on each side equally, or tape a 1-inch lead strip to the bottom of the cassette to serve as the bottom collimation border and build the patient up enough to position the part above this lead strip to prevent clipping needed anatomic structures. Different computed radiography system manufacturers also have suggestions specific to their system that can be used to obtain optimal projections under these circumstances. For example, the projection may be processed under a different scanning mode (Fuji), processed under a different anatomic specifier (CareStream), or you may be told to read only certain portions or sections of the IR.

Coverage of 30% (for Computed Radiography Only). It has been shown that EI errors are likely to occur in computed radiography when less than 30% of the IR is exposed. To ensure that at least 30% of the IR is exposed, the smallest possible IR size should be chosen, and when imaging parts that require tight collimation, such as the fingers or thumbs, it is recommended that two or more projections be taken on one IR.

Multiple Projections on One Image Receptor (for Computed Radiography Only). When multiple

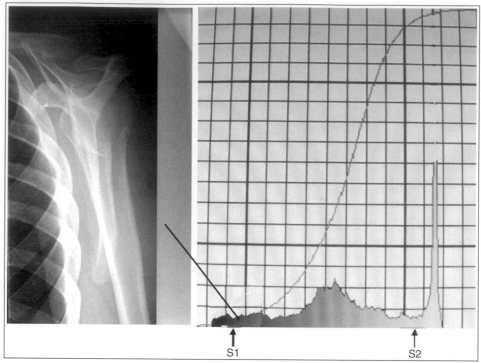

FIGURE 2-8 Computed radiography histogram that includes scatter radiation values from outside the exposure field in the VOI.

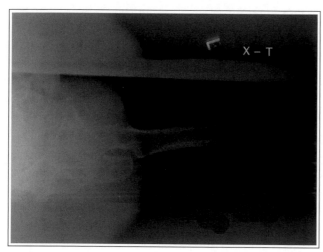

FIGURE 2-9 Computed radiography axiolateral hip projection demonstrating a histogram analysis error caused by including scatter radiation values from outside the exposure field in the VOI.

projections are taken on one IR, it is difficult for the computer to distinguish between the very bright areas between exposure fields and similar very light areas within the VOI when scatter fogging is present between the collimated fields. To assist the exposure field recognition process, the body part is centered within each exposure field, and all collimation borders are parallel and equidistant from the edges of the IR (see Figure 2-10). The farther apart the projections are positioned from each other, the less chance that they will be mistaken for a single projection. Also, use lead sheets over the areas

of the IR that are not being used during exposures to protect them from scatter fogging.

Background Radiation Fogging (for Computed Radiography Only). Computed radiography plates are extra sensitive to scatter radiation. Fogging can accumulate across the plate from IR exposure to scatter radiation when the IR is left in the imaging room while other projections are taken. Fog will decrease the brightness values of the pixels, resulting in histogram analysis errors. Figure 2-12 demonstrates an AP abdomen projection that was exposed and left in the room while a second x-ray was performed. The projection demonstrates low contrast caused by scatter fogging. The brighter streak that runs through the center of the projection is part of the wheelchair that the IR was resting against. The abdominal structures included in the brighter area demonstrate acceptable quality and suggest how the projection would have looked if the scatter fogging had not occurred. Computed radiography plates are also sensitive to accumulated background radiation during long periods of storage. Excessive background radiation fogging will result in decreased pixel brightness values across the image, similar to that demonstrated on the AP abdomen projection in Figure 2-12. Computed radiography cassettes that have been in storage for more than 48 to 72 hours (time frame varies among system manufacturers) are put through the reader's erase process before being used to ensure that background fogging does not affect the subsequent images.

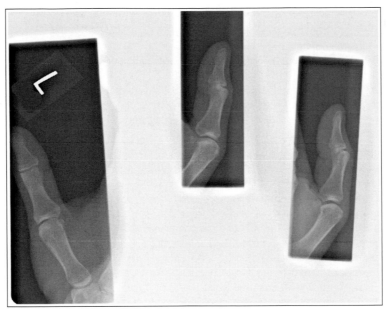

FIGURE 2-10 Computed radiography thumb projections demonstrating poor image alignment when multiple projections are placed on one IR cassette.

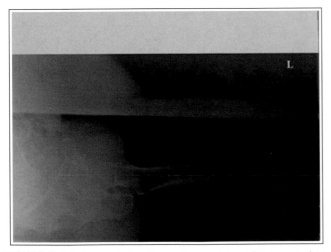

FIGURE 2-11 Computed radiography axiolateral hip image demonstrating a histogram analysis error caused by poor exposure field recognition.

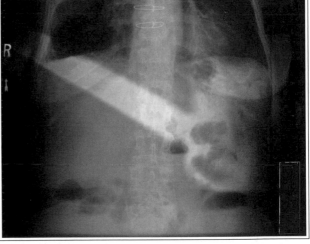

FIGURE 2-12 Computed radiography AP abdomen projection demonstrating a histogram analysis error caused by background radiation fogging.

Image Receptor Exposure

Radiographic exposure refers to the total quantity (intensity) of x-ray photons that expose the patient and image receptor (IR). The controlling factor for exposure is milliampere-seconds (mAs), with factors such as kV, SID, OID, collimation, and grids affecting it in smaller degrees. When these technical factors are set correctly:

- The remnant beam demonstrates the subject contrast in the VOI with a broad range of photon intensities,
- Contrast resolution on the displayed projection distinguishes the subject contrast in the VOI with light gray to dark gray shades, and no part of it is completely white or black, and

- There is no quantum noise or excessive fogging from scatter radiation.
- The EI number is within the acceptable exposure range for the digital system (see Table 2-1).

An advantage of digital images is the wide dynamic range response of the detectors, which allows the IR exposure to be higher or lower than the ideal exposure by a factor of 2 and still create an acceptable image. Tables 2-2 and 2-3 list how overexposure and underexposure may be identified on an image, as well as causes for them.

Identifying Underexposure. Underexposure means that the photon intensity reaching the IR is lower than

TABLE 2-2	Evaluating the Underexposed Projection

Underexposure that requires the projection to be repeated is identified when:
- IE number indicates that the IR received less than needed to put the number within the acceptable exposure range for the digital system, when no histogram analysis error has occurred.
- The VOI demonstrates a loss of contrast resolution, with some or all of the structures demonstrating a white shade (silhouette) and post-processing techniques do not improve their visibility.
- Quantum noise is present, especially in the thicker and denser anatomic structures.

Parameter	Causes of Underexposure and Adjustments
kV	kV too low • Increase kV using the 15% rule to increase IR exposure by a factor of 2.
mAs	mAs too low • Increase mAs by 100% to increase IR exposure by a factor of 2.
AEC	Backup time was shorter than the needed exposure time. • Set backup timer at 150% to 200% of the expected manual exposure time. Density control was left on the minus (−) setting from the previous patient. • Increase density control setting. Ionization chamber(s) was beneath a structure having a lower atomic number or was less dense or thinner than the VOI. • Select ionization chamber(s) centered beneath the VOI. Inadequate collimation caused excessive scatter radiation to reach the ionization chamber(s) and prematurely shut off exposure. • Increase collimation. A small anatomic part was imaged and the activated ionization chamber was not fully covered by VOI or the AEC was used on a peripheral anatomic part and the activated ionization chamber was not fully covered by the VOI. • Do not use AEC. Manually set technique controls.
Grids	Used a nongrid technique but left the grid in or used a low ratio grid technique with a high ratio grid. • Use the grid conversion factor (GCF) in Table 2-4 to determine the mAs adjustment needed. Grid off-level or CR is angled toward the grid's lead strips, demonstrating grid cutoff on the side that the CR is angled toward if parallel grid was used and across the entire image if focused grid was used (see Figure 2-23). • Level the grid, bringing it perpendicular to the CR. If angled CR is needed, change grid directions so CR is angled with the grid's lead strips. SID outside focusing range, demonstrating grid cutoff on each side of the image. • Increase or decrease the SID to bring distance in the grid's focusing range. Focused grid inverted (see Figure 2-24), demonstrating grid cutoff on each side of the image. • Flip grid around. Focused grid off-center, demonstrating grid cutoff across entire image; image will not be in the center of the IR but will be to one side. • Center the CR to the center of the grid.

Underexposure that should not require the projection to be repeated but should be evaluated to determine how to improve IR exposure for future projections is identified when:
- IE number indicates that the IR received less than needed to put the number at the ideal exposure parameter for the digital system, when no histogram analysis error has occurred.

SID and OID	SID was increased without an equivalent increase in mAs • Use the density maintenance formula to adjust mAs for the SID change: old mAs/new mAs = old SID^2/new SID^2 Increased OID without an increase in mAs (Only if procedure would produce a significant amount of scatter radiation that will not reach IR when OID is increased) • Increase the mAs 10% for every 1 inch (2.5 cm) of OID increase.
Collimation	A large decrease in field size was made without an increase in mAs (Only if procedure would produce a significant amount of scatter radiation that will not reach IR when OID is increased.) • 14- × 17-inch field size to a 10- × 12-inch field size: increase mAs by 35%. • 14- × 17-inch field size to a 10- × 12-inch field size: increase mAs by 50%
Additive patient condition	Patient had an additive condition that caused the tissues to have increased mass density or thickness, and require an increase in exposure. • Adjust the mAs or kVp as indicated for the additive condition as listed in Table 2-6.

TABLE 2-3	**Evaluating the Overexposed Projection**

Overexposure that requires the projection to be repeated is identified when:
- IE number indicates that the IR received more exposure than needed to put the number within the acceptable exposure range for the digital system, when no histogram analysis error has occurred.
- The VOI demonstrates a loss of contrast resolution, with some or all of the structures demonstrating a black shade (saturation), and post-processing techniques do not improve their visibility.
- An overall graying is demonstrated because of excessive scatter radiation fogging.

Parameter	Causes of Overexposure and Adjustments
kV	kV too high • Decrease kV using the 15% rule to increase IR exposure by a factor of 2.
mAs	mAs too high • Decrease mAs by 100% to increase IR exposure by a factor of 2.
AEC	Wrong IR was activated and the backup timer shut the exposure off. • Activate correct IR. Exposure time needed was less than the minimum response time. • Reduce mA station until time needed for exposure is above minimum response time. Density control was left on the plus (+) setting from the previous patient. • Decrease density control setting. Ionization chamber(s) was beneath a structure having a higher atomic number or was denser or thicker than the VOI. • Select ionization chamber(s) centered beneath the VOI. A radiopaque artifact or appliance is included within or over the VOI. • Do not use AEC. Manually set technique controls.
Grids	Used a grid technique without a grid or used a high ratio grid technique with a low ratio grid. • Use the grid conversion factor (GCF) in Table 2-4 to determine the mAs adjustment needed.

Overexposure that does not require the projection to be repeated but should be evaluated to determine how to improve IR exposure for future projections is identified when:
- IE number indicates that the IR received more than needed to put the number at the ideal exposure parameter for the digital system, when no histogram analysis error has occurred.

SID	SID was decreased without an equivalent increase in mAs • Use the density maintenance formula to adjust mAs for the SID change: old mAs/new mAs = old SID^2/new SID^2
Additive patient condition	Patient had a destructive condition that caused the tissues to have decreased mass density or thickness, and require a decrease in exposure. • Adjust the mAs or kVp as indicated for the destructive condition as listed in Table 2-6.

that required to produce an acceptable projection. Underexposure is identified on the projection when:

1. The IE number indicates that the IR received less exposure than needed to put the number within the acceptable exposure range for the digital system, when no histogram analysis error has occurred.
2. The VOI demonstrates a loss of contrast resolution, with some or all of the structures demonstrating a white shade (silhouette) and postprocessing techniques (e.g., windowing, processing under alternate procedural algorithms) do not improve their visibility.
3. Quantum noise is present, especially in the thicker and denser anatomic structures.

The EI number that is displayed for a projection can be compared with the ideal and acceptable range for the digital system used to determine if underexposure has occurred as long as a histogram analysis error has not occurred. The more that this obtained number is outside the system's EI range, the lower is the IR exposure and the more rescaling that occurs, resulting in the projection presented. Projections produced at EI numbers that specify values that are lower than the acceptable range

for the system necessitate repeating because of the quantum noise and a loss of contrast resolution. Quantum noise is characterized by graininess or a random pattern superimposed on the projection. It can obscure borders, affecting edge discrimination, and can obscure underlying differences in shading, affecting contrast resolution. It is the most common noise seen in digital radiography and is present when photon flux (number of photons striking a specific area per unit of time) is insufficient. The postprocessing technique of windowing that is used to adjust brightness levels will only make the quantum noise more visible. The only way to decrease quantum noise is to increase the IR exposure by increasing the kV or mAs. Whether the IR exposure is increased using kV, mAs, or a combination of the two, will depend on whether all of the structures in the VOI are demonstrated on the displayed projection. If quantum mottle is present and the densest and thickest structures in the VOI are not all distinguishable, then a kV change is indicated. If quantum mottle is present and all of the structures in the VOI are distinguishable, then a mAs change is indicated.

Determining the Technical Adjustment for Underexposure

Step 1. Determine if a histogram analysis error has occurred (see Box 2-1). If no error is identified, proceed to step 2.

Step 2. Determine if the projection differentiates the densest and thickest structures in the VOI. If there are structures that have not been distinguished, then a kV adjustment should be made. If all of the structures can be distinguished, then a mAs adjustment should be made.

Step 3. Determine how much the kV and/or mAs needs to be adjusted to move the EI number to the ideal value (see Table 2-1) and eliminate quantum noise.

Subject Contrast. Subject contrast is the difference in radiation intensity in the remnant beam that demonstrates the degree of differential absorption resulting from the differing absorption characteristics of the body structures (atomic density, atomic number, and part thickness). It is demonstrated on the displayed projection with differing gray shades. Kilovoltage (kV) is the technical factor that determines the energy and penetrating ability of the x-ray photons produced and is the controlling factor for differential absorption and hence, subject contrast in the remnant beam and contrast resolution on the displayed projection. Optimal kV is chosen to provide at least partial penetration of all the tissues in the VOI. Without some degree of penetration and differing degrees of penetration in the tissues, subject contrast will not exist. Subject contrast cannot be recovered or manipulated with postprocessing; it must be in the remnant beam or it will not be seen on the displayed image. The optimal kV to use to create the best subject contrast for each projection is provided in the following procedure chapters.

A bony structure that has been adequately penetrated demonstrates the cortical outlines of the densest and thickest bony structures of interest, whereas an inadequately penetrated bony structure would not demonstrate all of the bony structures of interest. Note that if a transparency were laid over the bottom pelvis in Figure 2-13 and an outline of the bony structures drawn on the transparency, with lines made only where the cortical outlines of the bone were clearly visible, the cortical outlines of the sacroiliac joints and the acetabulum would not be drawn. If the cortical outlines of the structure of interest are not seen an increase in kV is required. When an organ with contrast medium is not adequately penetrated (Figure 2-14), the information is limited to the edges of the anatomy and does not visualize information within the organ. It should be noted that no amount of adjustment in mAs will ever compensate for insufficient kV and that subject contrast that is not demonstrated in the remnant beam cannot be restored through postprocessing techniques.

Adjusting kV for Inadequate Contrast Resolution. If a projection is to be repeated because it does not

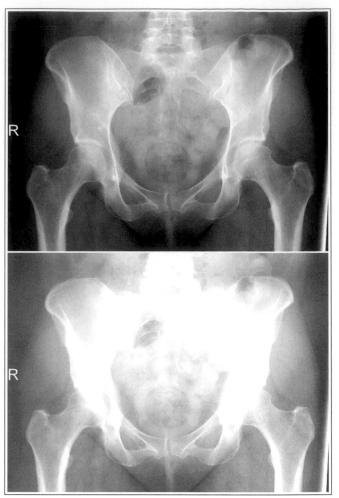

FIGURE 2-13 Accurately penetrated (*top*) and underpenetrated (*bottom*) AP pelvic projection.

demonstrate adequate contrast resolution of the VOI use the 15% rule and the EI number (see Table 2-1) to determine the amount of needed change. *The 15% rule indicates that for every 15% change in kV the exposure to the IR is changed by a factor of 2.* For the AP chest projection in Figure 2-15 with the EI number of 1600, a 15% increase in kV would increase the EI the 300 points needed to bring the number closer to the ideal EI number of 2000, improve contrast resolution and eliminate quantum noise. A 15% kV change is calculated by multiplying the original kV used by 0.15 and adding the results to the original kV. If 60 kV were used for the original projection, a 15% change would make the new kV 69.

If a projection demonstrates poor contrast resolution and the EI number indicates that a four times IR exposure adjustment is needed, a combination of kV and mAs change should be made. *As a general rule, no more than a 15% increase (two times) above optimum should be made with kV in this situation because an increase too far above optimum may result in saturation of the thinnest and less dense structures and will cause an*

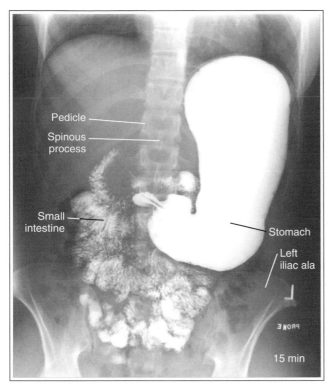

FIGURE 2-14 PA small intestinal projection demonstrating contrast media in the stomach that has not been fully penetrated.

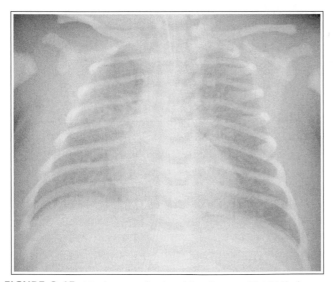

FIGURE 2-15 AP chest projection (CareStream EI 1600) demonstrating quantum noise caused by underexposure.

increase in scatter radiation being directed toward the IR, which will decrease the subject contrast due to scatter fogging. The additional exposure adjustment (two times) should be made with mAs.

Adjusting for Quantum Noise. Quantum noise is decreased by increasing the IR exposure by increasing the kV or mAs. If the kV is increased for inadequate contrast resolution using the 15% rule, the IR exposure will have also been increased by a factor of 2, reducing

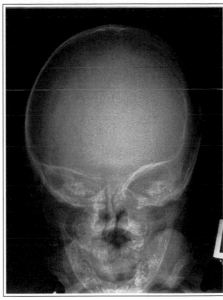

FIGURE 2-16 AP skull projection (CareStream EI 1600) demonstrating quantum noise caused by underexposure.

quantum noise. If contrast resolution is adequate, mAs should be adjusted to offset quantum noise. mAs is the controlling factor for the intensity (quantity) of photons in the x-ray beam. An increase in mAs will cause a direct increase in IR exposure and decrease in quantum noise. *To calculate a two times increase in IR exposure using mAs, multiply the original mAs by 2 and add the results to the original mAs.* If the original mAs were 20, the new mAs would be 40. The mAs was increased by a factor of 2 to raise the EI by 300 points to 1900 for the PA cranium projection in Figure 2-16.

Identifying Overexposure. Overexposure means that the photon intensity reaching the IR is higher than that required to produce an acceptable projection, and an excessive radiation dose was delivered to the patient. Overexposure is identified on the projection when:

1. The IE number indicates that the IR received more exposure than needed to put the number within the acceptable exposure parameters for the digital system, when no histogram analysis error has occurred.
2. The VOI demonstrates a loss of contrast resolution, with some or all of the structures demonstrating a black shade (saturation); postprocessing techniques do not improve their visibility.
3. An overall graying is demonstrated because of excessive scatter radiation fogging.

Exposure indicator numbers that specify higher than ideal exposure values typically do not require repeating because of image quality unless saturation or excessive scatter radiation fogging impairs contrast resolution. Figure 2-17 displays an AP femur projection that was obtained using the CareStream computed radiography system. The projection has an EI of 2490, which indicates overexposure, but the structures in the VOI are all distinguishable even though they are gray because of

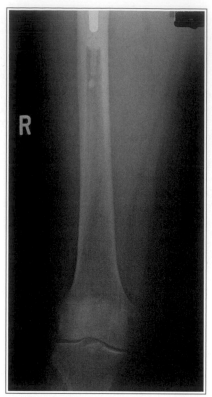

FIGURE 2-17 Overexposed AP femur projection demonstrating proper procedure, and poor contrast resolution because of scatter radiation fogging (CareStream EI 2490).

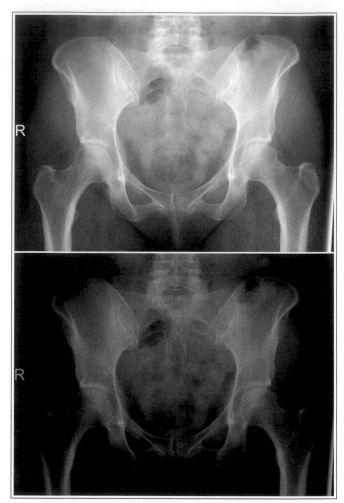

FIGURE 2-18 Accurately exposed (*top*) and overexposed (*bottom*) AP pelvic projections.

scattered fogging. As long as contrast resolution is such that all aspects of the anatomic structure can be evaluated, it is not necessary to repeat this projection because the postprocessing technique of windowing can be used to adjust the brightness and contrast levels and reveal the hidden details. It should be noted though that when exposures are excessive, the reason for the overexposure requires researching to reduce exposure and radiation doses for the next similar examination.

The projection should be repeated for overexposure if any of the details in the VOI demonstrate a pitch black shade that cannot be made distinguishable through windowing and indicates saturation. Saturation occurs when the pixels representing structures have reached the point where they have collected as much exposure as possible and the subject contrast is no longer visible. *A portion of the VOI may be saturated if the IR exposure is four or five times the ideal (Figure 2-18) and total saturation is seen when eight to ten times of the ideal IR exposure is reached.* Windowing to lighter brightness levels will not repair the subject contrast that has been lost.

Other Exposure-Related Factors

A projection will seldom need repeating because of failure to make adjustments from the procedural routine for the following exposure related factors, unless the change has caused significant overexposure or

underexposure or a procedural error occurred. Projections that do require repeating will demonstrate the same characteristics as described for identifying overexposure and underexposure. In most cases, the exposure adjustments should be made for these changes before the projection is obtained, with the goal being to keep the EI number as close to the ideal as possible.

Scatter Radiation. Scatter radiation is created when primary photons interact with the tissue's atomic structure and are scattered in a direction that differs from the primary photon's original path. They are destructive to the projection because they add an evenly distributed blanket of exposure, also referred to as fog, over the IR, lowering contrast resolution as the individual and distinct gray shades of adjacent details on the projection blend with each other. The amount of scatter radiation that is directed toward the IR is determined by the kV, field size, and patient thickness. As the amount of scatter radiation reaching the IR increases, the greater is the decrease in contrast resolution and detail visibility.

Technologists can control the amount of scatter that reaches the IR and improve contrast resolution by reducing the amount of tissue irradiated through increasing

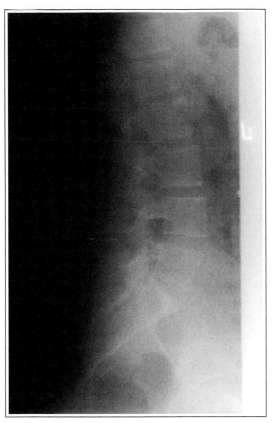

FIGURE 2-19 Contact shield was not used along posterior collimated border.

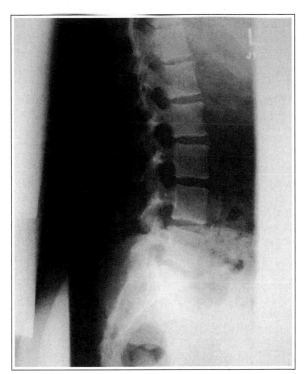

FIGURE 2-20 Contact shield was used along posterior collimated border.

collimation and by using a grid. The more collimation is increased and the higher the grid ratio that is used, the greater will be the scatter cleanup and the contrast resolution. Flat contact shields made of lead can also be used to control the amount of scatter radiation that reaches the IR by eliminating scatter produced in the table from being scattered toward the VOI on the IR. When the anatomic structures being examined demonstrate an excessive amount of scatter fogging along the outside of the collimated borders (e.g., the lateral lumbar vertebrae), place a large flat contact shield or the straight edge of a lead apron along the appropriate border. This greatly improves the contrast resolution. Compare the lateral lumbar vertebral projections in Figures 2-19 and 2-20. Figure 2-20 was taken with a lead contact shield placed against the posterior edge of the collimator's light field, but a contact shield was not used for Figure 2-19. Note the improvement in visualization of the lumbar structures using a contact shield.

Grids. When a grid is added or the technologist changes from one grid ratio to another, IR exposure will be inadequate and a repeat will be necessary unless the mAs is adjusted (Table 2-4) to compensate for the resulting change in scatter radiation cleanup and primary radiation absorption that takes place in the grid. When changing to a higher grid ratio, an increase in mAs is needed or insufficient IR exposure will result; when changing to

TABLE 2-4	Grid Conversion Factor
Grid Ratio	**Grid Conversion Factor**
5:1	2
6:1	3
8:1	4
12:1	5
16:1	6

Nongrid to Grid: New GCF × old mAs = new mAs with new grid ratio

Grid to grid: mAs (old) = GCF(old)

mAs (new) GCF (new)

a lower grid ratio, a decrease in mAs is needed or excessive IR exposure to the IR and patient will result.

Insufficient IR exposure will also result when the grid and CR are misaligned, causing a decrease in the number of remnant photons from reaching the IR and grid cutoff. The exposure decrease caused by grid cutoff can be distinguished from other underexposure problems by the additional appearance of grid lines (small white lines) on the projection where the cutoff is demonstrated (Figure 2-21).

Source-Image Receptor Distance. Increasing the source-image receptor distance (SID) will decrease IR exposure and decreasing the SID will increase IR exposure by the inverse square law because the area through which the x-rays are distributed is spread out or condensed, respectively, with distance changes. *To keep the EI number at the ideal, any change in SID of greater*

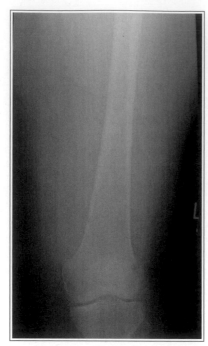

FIGURE 2-21 Digital AP femur projection demonstrating grid line artifacts.

than 10 percent should be compensated for by adjusting the mAs by the exposure maintenance formula ([new mAs]/[old mAs] = [new distance squared]/[old distance squared]).

Object-Image Receptor Distance. Although it is standard to maintain the lowest possible object-image receptor distance (OID), there are situations in which increasing the OID is unavoidable, such as when the patient is in traction and the device extends beyond the anatomic structure being imaged (see Figure 1-61). Increasing the OID may result in a noticeable decrease in IR exposure because of the reduction in the amount of scatter radiation detected by the IR when a portion of the scattered x-rays generated in the patient are scattered away from the IR. The amount of exposure loss will depend on the degree of OID increase and the amount of scatter that would typically reach the IR for such a procedure, which is determined by the kV selected, field size, and patient thickness. As tube potentials are raised above 60 kV, scatter radiation is directed in an increasingly forward direction, so the image will demonstrate significant exposure loss as the OID is increased and scatter misses the IR. With tube potentials below 60 kV, there is a decrease in the number of scatter photons that are scattered in a forward direction, so an increase in OID will not result in a significant change in the amount of scatter or exposure reaching the IR. A larger field size and body part thickness affects the amount of scatter produced, with more production resulting in increased reduction of scatter reaching the IR as the OID increases. *When an OID increase causes significant scatter radiation to be diverted from the IR, the mAs should be increased by about 10% for every*

centimeter of OID to compensate and to keep the EI number at the ideal.

Collimation. A decrease in the area exposed on the patient, as determined by collimation, changes the amount of scatter radiation produced and hence the amount of scatter reaching the IR and the overall IR exposure. The amount of exposure change will depend on the field size and the amount of scatter that would typically reach the IR for such a procedure, which is determined by the kV selected and patient thickness (see object-IR distance). The mAs needs to be increased to compensate for the exposure that is lost, when the field size is significantly reduced on a procedure that produces significant scatter radiation. This mAs adjustment will keep the EI number at the ideal. *A 35% mAs adjustment is needed for a field size change from a 14- × 17-inch to a 10- × 12-inch and a 50% mAs change is needed for a field size change from a 14- × 17-inch to an 8- × 10-inch.*

Anode Heel Effect. The anode heel effect should be considered when a 17-inch (43-cm) or longer field length is used to accommodate the structure, as with long bones and the vertebral column. When this field length is used, a noticeable intensity variation occurs across the entire field size that is significant enough between the ends of the field that when they are compared, it can be seen. This intensity variation is a result of the greater photon absorption that occurs at the thicker "heel" portion of the anode compared with the thinner "toe" portion when a long field is used. Consequently, intensity at the anode end of the tube is lower because fewer photons emerge from that end of the tube than at the cathode end. Using this knowledge to our advantage can help produce images of long bones and vertebral columns that demonstrate uniform brightness at both ends. Position the thinner side of the structure at the anode end of the tube and the thicker side of the structure at the cathode end. Set an exposure (mAs) that will adequately demonstrate the midpoint of the structure (where the CR is centered). Because the anode will absorb some of the photons aimed at the anode end of the IR and the thinnest structure, but not as many of the photons aimed at the cathode end and the thickest structure, a more uniform brightness across that part will be demonstrated (Figure 2-22). Table 2-5 provides guidelines for positioning structures to take advantage of the anode heel effect. Because the intensity variation between the ends of the IR is only approximately 30%, the anode heel effect will not adequately adjust for large thickness differences but will help improve projections of the structures as listed in Table 2-5.

Most imaging rooms are designed so that the patient's head is positioned on the technologist's left side (when facing the imaging table), placing the anode end of the x-ray tube at the head end of the patient. The placement of the anode end of the tube may vary in reference to the patient as the tube is moved into the horizontal

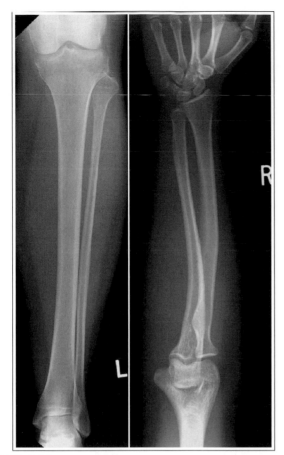

FIGURE 2-22 AP lower leg projection where anode heel effect was used properly (knee positioned at cathode end) and AP forearm projection where the anode heel effect was not used properly (wrist positioned at cathode end).

TABLE 2-5	Guidelines for Positioning to Incorporate Anode Heel Effect	
Projection(s)	Placement of Anode	Placement of Cathode
AP and lateral forearm	Wrist	Elbow
AP and lateral humerus	Elbow	Shoulder
AP and lateral lower leg	Ankle	Knee
AP and lateral femur	Knee	Hip
AP thoracic vertebrae	1st thoracic vertebrae	12th thoracic vertebrae
AP lumbar vertebrae	1st lumbar vertebrae	5th lumbar vertebrae

position. To identify the anode and cathode ends of the x-ray tube, locate the + and − symbols attached to the tube housing where the electrical supply enters. The + symbol is used to identify the anode end of the tube and the − symbol indicates the cathode end (Figure 2-23). Although this factor will not require a kV or mAs adjustment if done incorrectly, it may demonstrate signs of

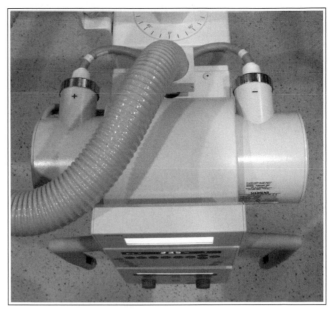

FIGURE 2-23 Top of the x-ray tube housing identifying anode (+) and cathode (−) ends of the x-ray tube.

underexposure or overexposure of the structure at most proximal and distal aspects.

Additive and Destructive Patient Conditions. Additive and destructive patient conditions that result in change to the normal bony structures, soft tissues, or air or fluid content of the patient require technical adjustments to compensate for the exposure change that the condition causes over the routinely used. Additive diseases cause tissues to increase in mass density or thickness, resulting in them being more radiopaque, whereas destructive diseases cause tissues to break down, resulting in them being more radiolucent. Table 2-6 lists common additive and destructive diseases that require technique adjustments and provides a starting point for adjusting technical factors for the condition.

Automatic Exposure Control. The AEC allows the mAs to be automatically determined by controlling the exposure time, but it is the technologist's responsibility to set an optimum kV and mA manually. Optimum mA refers to using a high enough mA at a given focal spot size to minimize motion, but not so high that the exposure times are shorter than the AEC's minimum response time. The minimum response time is the time that it takes for the circuit to detect and react to the radiation received; this is determined by the AEC manufacturer. The factors in the following and in Box 2-2 are best practice guidelines to consider when setting the AEC for optimal IR exposure.

- Set optimum kV for body part being imaged to obtain adequate subject contrast.

  (See earlier discussions on subject contrast.)
- Set mA at the highest station for the focal spot size needed, but not so high that the exposure time required for proper IR exposure is less than the minimum response time.

TABLE 2-6	Adjusting Technical Factors for Patient Conditions		
Additive Diseases		**Destructive Diseases**	
Condition	Amount to Increase	Condition	Amount to Decrease
Acromegaly	8%-10% kV	Aseptic necrosis	8% kV
Ascites	50% mAs	Blastomycosis	8% kV
Cardiomegaly	50% mAs	Bowel obstruction	8% kV
Fibrous carcinomas	50% mAs	Emphysema	8% kV
Hydrocephalus	50%-75% mAs	Ewing's tumor	8% kV
Hydropneumothorax	50%	Exostosis	8% kV
Osteoarthritis	50% mAs	Gout	8% kV
Osteochondroma	8% kV	Hodgkin's disease	8% kV
Osteopetrosis	8% kV	Hyperparathyroidism	8% kV
Paget's disease	8% kV	Osteolytic cancer	8% kV
Pleural effusion	35% mAs	Osteomalacia	8% kV
Pneumonia	50% mAs	Osteoporosis	8% kV
Pulmonary edema	50% mAs	Pneumothorax	8% kV
Pulmonary tuberculosis	50% mAs	Rheumatoid arthritis	8% kV

From Carroll QB: *Practical radiographic imaging*, ed 8, Springfield, IL, 2007, Charles C Thomas.

BOX 2-2	Best Practice Guidelines for Automatic Exposure Control Use

- Set optimum kV for body part being imaged.
- Set mA at the highest statin for the focal spot size needed, but not so high that the exposure time required for proper IR exposure is less than the minimum response time.
- Set backup time at 150% to 200% of the expected manual exposure time.
- Select and activate the ionization chamber(s) that will be centered beneath the VOI.
- Do not use AEC on peripheral or very small anatomy where the activated chamber(s) is not completely covered by the anatomy.
- Tightly collimate to the VOI.
- Do not use the AEC when the VOI is in close proximity to thicker structures and both will be situated above the activated ionization chamber.
- Never use the AEC when any type of radiopaque hardware or prosthetic device will be positioned above the activated chamber(s).
- Make certain that no external radiopaque artifacts, such as lead sheets or sandbags, are positioned over the activated chamber(s).
- Exposure (density) controls can temporarily be used when AEC equipment is out of calibration and to fine tune IR exposure when the VOI and activated chamber(s) are only slightly misaligned.

Images taken with an exposure time that is less than the minimum response time will result in overexposure. This is because the AEC circuit does not have enough time to detect and react to the radiation received to shut the exposure off in the time needed to produce the ideal image. The mA station should be decreased until exposure times are sufficient to produce the desired IR exposure.

- Set backup time at 150% to 200% of the expected manual exposure time. As a general guideline, use 0.2 seconds for all chest and proximal extremities, 1 second for abdominal and skull projections, and 2 to 4 seconds for very large torso projections.

The backup timer is the maximum time that the x-ray exposure will be allowed to continue. Once the backup time is met the exposure will automatically terminate. If the set backup time is too short the exposure will prematurely stop before adequate exposure has reached the ionization chamber(s), resulting in underexposure. If the set backup time is too long because the AEC is not functioning properly or the control panel is not correctly set, the exposure will continue much longer than needed and result in overexposure.

- Select and activate the ionization chamber(s) that will be centered beneath the VOI.

Recommendations for ionization chamber selection can be found in the table at the beginning of each procedural analysis chapter of the book. Failure to properly activate the correct ionization chamber(s) and center the VOI beneath them will result in projections that are overexposed or underexposed. An overexposed image results when the ionization chamber chosen is located beneath a structure that has a higher atomic number or is thicker or denser than the VOI. For example, when an AP abdomen projection is taken, the outside ionization chambers should be chosen and situated within the soft tissue, away from the lumbar vertebrae, to yield the desired abdominal soft tissue density. If the chamber situated under the lumbar vertebrae is used instead, the capacitor (device that stores energy) requires a longer exposure time to reach its maximum filling level and terminate the exposure. This occurs because of

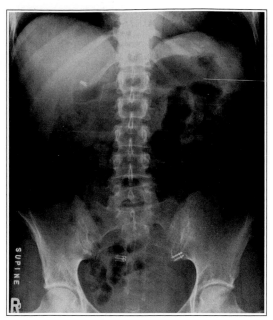

FIGURE 2-24 AP abdomen projection that was exposed using the center AEC chamber.

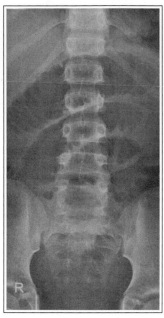

FIGURE 2-25 AP lumbar vertebrae projection exposed using the two outside AEC chambers.

the high atomic number of bone and the higher number of photons that bone absorbs compared with soft tissue. The result will be a projection with high bone contrast resolution but overexposed soft tissue structures with the potential of saturation (Figure 2-24).

An underexposed image results, however, when the ionization chamber chosen is located beneath a structure that has a lower atomic number or is thinner or less dense than the VOI. When an AP lumbar vertebral projection is taken, the center ionization chamber is chosen and centered directly beneath the lumbar vertebrae. If instead, one or both of the outside chambers are used or the center ionization chamber is off-centered, because the soft tissue, which has a lower atomic number than bone, is above the activated chamber, the projection will demonstrate poor contrast resolution of the vertebral structures and possible quantum noise (Figure 2-25).

- Do not use AEC on peripheral or very small anatomy where the activated chamber(s) is not completely covered by the anatomy, resulting in a portion of the chamber(s) being exposed with a part of the x-ray beam that does not go through the patient.

Each activated ionization chamber measures the average amount of radiation striking the area it covers. The part of the chamber not covered with tissue will collect radiation so quickly that it will charge the capacitor to its maximum level, terminating the exposure before proper IR exposure has been reached and may result in an underexposure that demonstrates poor contrast resolution and possible quantum noise (Figure 2-26).

- Tightly collimate to the VOI to reduce scatter radiation from the table or body that may cause the AEC to shut off prematurely.

An AP thoracic vertebrae projection that has inadequate side-to-side collimation will demonstrate too much scatter through the lungs, hitting the AEC before the vertebrae can be adequately exposed.

- Do not use the AEC when the VOI is in close proximity to thicker structures and both will be situated above the activated ionization chamber.

For example, it is best not to use the AEC on an AP atlas and axis (open-mouthed) projection of the dens. With this examination, the upper incisors, occipital cranial base, and mandible add thickness to the areas superior and inferior to the dens and atlantoaxial joint. This added thickness causes the VOI to be overexposed, because more time is needed for the capacitor to reach its maximum level as photons are absorbed in the thicker areas, and the projection demonstrates poor contrast resolution and possible saturation (Figure 2-27).

- Never use the AEC when any type of radiopaque hardware or prosthetic device will be positioned above the activated chamber(s). For these situations, use a manual technique.
- Make certain that no external radiopaque artifacts such as lead sheets or sandbags are positioned over the activated chamber(s).

Radiopaque materials, such as metal, lead sheets, or sandbags, have a much higher atomic number than that of the bony and soft tissue structures of the body. When a radiopaque material is situated within the activated chamber(s), the AEC will attempt to expose

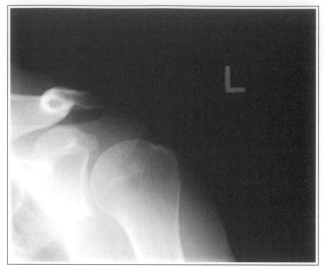

FIGURE 2-26 AP oblique (Grashey method) shoulder projection that was exposed with the center AEC chamber positioned too peripherally.

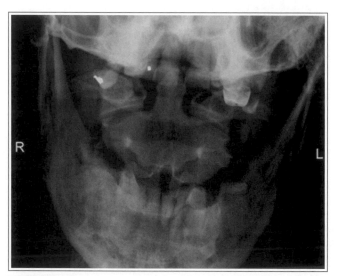

FIGURE 2-27 AP atlas and axis (open-mouthed) projection that was exposed using the center AEC chamber.

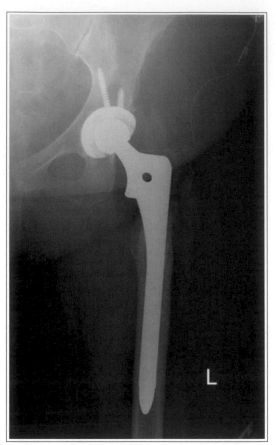

FIGURE 2-28 AP hip projection with radiopaque prosthesis exposed using the center AEC chamber.

the radiopaque structure adequately, resulting in the anatomic structures being overexposed and that demonstrates poor contrast resolution and possible saturation (Figure 2-28).

• Exposure (density) controls can temporarily be used when AEC equipment is out of calibration and to fine tune IR exposure when the VOI and activated chamber(s) are only slightly misaligned.

The exposure (density) controls change the preset exposure halt signals, increasing or decreasing the amount of IR exposure needed before the signal is sent to terminate the exposure, adjusting IR exposure by the control setting amount. Typical exposure control settings change the exposure level by increments of 25%, with the +1 and +2 buttons increasing the exposure and the −1 and −2 buttons decreasing the exposure. The 1 buttons will result in a 25%

exposure change and the 2 buttons in a 50% exposure change. Some facilities have the AEC exposure controls set to obtain a 100% exposure increase and a 50% exposure decrease.

Correcting Poor Automatic Exposure Control Images. When an unacceptable AEC image is produced, the technologist needs to consider each potential cause to determine the correct adjustment to make before repeating the image. Many imaging units include a mAs readout display, on which the amount of mAs used for the image is shown after the exposure. In situations in which it is not advisable to repeat an unacceptable image using the AEC, the technologist can revert to a manual technique by using this readout to adjust the mAs to the value needed.

Contrast Resolution

Contrast resolution refers to the degree of difference in brightness (gray shade) levels between adjacent tissues on the displayed image. The higher the contrast resolution, the greater the gray shade differences (Figure 2-29) and the lower the contrast resolution, the lower the gray shade differences (Figure 2-30). Digital radiography provides superior contrast resolution because of the ability of the IR to discern a 1% difference in subject contrast

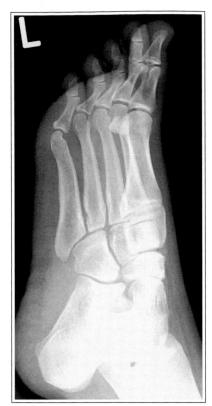

FIGURE 2-29 AP oblique foot projection with high contrast.

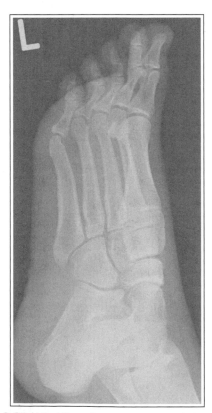

FIGURE 2-30 AP oblique foot projection with low contrast.

and because of the extensive dynamic range (gray levels) that is available to display the image. The degree of contrast resolution presented on images is determined by the quality of the subject contrast in the remnant beam, the dynamic range available, and the processing algorithm applied to the image data before they are displayed. Box 2-3 describes the contrast differences that are demonstrated for common conditions.

Bit Depth and Dynamic Range. The maximum range of pixel values that a digital system can store is expressed as the bit depth of the pixels. Digital systems currently manufactured have pixels that are 14-bit (2^{14}) deep, allowing 16,384 potential values to be stored for each

| BOX 2-3 | Contrast Differences Demonstrated on Common Conditions |

- Patients who are in good physical shape, with strong muscles, low fat content, and dense bones usually display the highest subject contrast (Figure 2-31).
- Patients whose bodies have deteriorated because of disease or age and obese patients ordinarily display less subject contrast because their muscles have lost strength and have become the consistency of fat. On an image of this patient, subject contrast is low because the densities representing fat and muscle are more alike (Figure 2-32).
- Images of bony structures that have lost minerals and are less dense because of disease appear darker gray on images rather than lighter gray, blending in more with the surrounding structures and demonstrating lower subject contrast (Figure 2-33).
- Patients who have retained fluid because of disease or injury display lower subject contrast because the fluid surrounds the body tissues and causes their tissue densities to become more alike (Figure 2-34).
- The bones of infants and children are less dense and more porous than adult bones, resulting in lower subject contrast being demonstrated between the bone and soft tissue in children's images compared with adults' images (Figure 2-35).

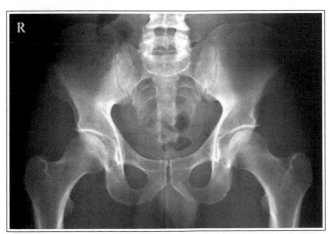

FIGURE 2-31 AP pelvic projection on patient with high subject contrast.

pixel. These values are used to define the gray shades that are displayed on the display monitor. Because the remnant beam contains only about 1024 different gray levels and the human eyes are only capable of distinguishing about 32 (2^5) different gray shades, the full information obtained by the system during an exposure (raw data) does not need to be displayed. Instead, the predetermined system software indicates the range of values that will be made available to display images. This system range is called the dynamic range (gray scale) of the digital system. For each procedure there is a procedural algorithm that indicates the dynamic range and average brightness levels for the computer to use when displaying the procedure. These are embedded in the

LUTs that are used when the histogram is automatically rescaled to optimize the anatomic structures for that procedure.

Post-Processing

Windowing. Digital radiography also allows for post-processing manipulation of the image's brightness and

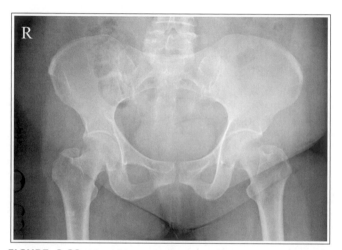

FIGURE 2-32 AP pelvic projection on obese patient with low subject contrast.

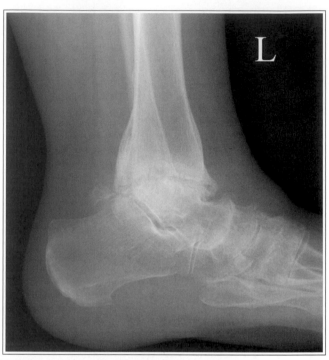

FIGURE 2-33 Lateral ankle projection demonstrating low subject contrast caused by a destructive disease.

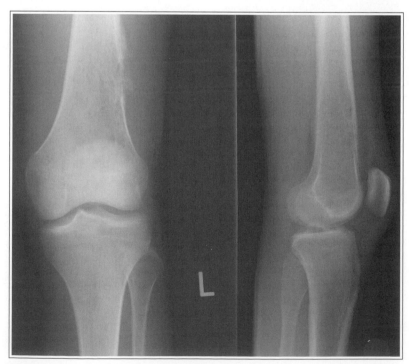

FIGURE 2-34 AP and lateral knee projections that demonstrate fluid around the knee joint that affects subject contrast.

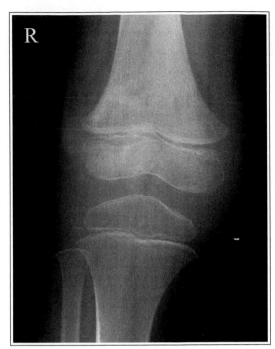

FIGURE 2-35 AP knee projection on pediatric patient that demonstrates low subject contrast.

contrast to demonstrate the VOI more accurately. This process, called windowing, occurs after the image is displayed on the monitor. Adjusting the window level allows the viewer to change the average gray level (center gray shade on the dynamic range) for the image toward lighter or darker shades, increasing or decreasing the overall image brightness. Adjusting the window width changes the length of the dynamic range (total number of different gray shades) used for the image by adding or subtracting gray shades, which increases or decreases the difference between adjacent shades and contrast. When contrast is changed by adjusting the window width there is often a perceived difference in image brightness, with decreased width (shorter gray scale) appearing brighter and increased width appearing less bright. This is a result of additional structures being given lighter and darker gray values, respectively. As long as the window level does not change the average brightness level remains unchanged.

To provide the latitude for image brightness to be adjusted for underexposures and overexposures by a factor of 2 and the long gray scale to adjust contrast, the original image data need to be maintained. Technologists should avoid adjusting the window width and level to improve image quality and then saving the new window settings to the PACS. Once windowing has been done and the image saved, the total data from the original histogram are lost, leaving only the range that was saved. The radiologist is then left with a narrower dynamic range of settings to use when evaluating different aspects of the image, which may lead to misdiagnosis and potential legal issues.

Contrast Masking. Contrast resolution on an image can demonstrate a perceived improvement by adding a contrast mask to the outside of the exposure field. When adding the mask it should only be added around the outside of the exposure field and not be added within the exposure field. Masking must not take the place of good collimation practices (see Figure 1-13).

Choosing Alternative Procedural Algorithms (Lookup Table) to Modify Image. An image can also be modified by selecting a different preset algorithm for processing. One way of doing this is to process the image under a different procedural algorithm. For example, if a chest projection demonstrates low contrast, it can be reprocessed by the computer under the knee procedure. The computer then rescales the chest histogram using the knee LUT, and because the knee LUT is set to create a higher-contrast image than the chest LUT, the reprocessed chest projection will be display with higher contrast.

As with windowing, if an alternate algorithm is used and the image is saved to the PACS the original histogram data set is permanently lost. Routinely needing to use alternate processing algorithms indicates a problem with the equipment or with the procedural practices.

Artifacts

An artifact is any undesirable structure or substance recorded on an image. Before an image is taken, it may be wise to have the patient change into a hospital gown and to ask whether any patient belongings are in or around the area being imaged. Patients are often nervous and may forget to remove articles of clothing or, for sentimental reasons they may not remove jewelry, so you should recheck the VOI, even after the patient has changed into a gown. Once the patient is positioned and the IR is ready to be exposed, take a last look to make sure that all hospital possessions that can be moved out of the imaging field have been moved. Check that those items that must remain in the field, such as heart monitoring leads, have been shifted so that they will superimpose the least amount of information. It would be impossible to delineate in this book all the possible artifacts that can appear on an image, but it is important for technologists to familiarize themselves with as many artifacts as possible.

Most possession-related artifacts are demonstrated on the image at brightness levels that are lighter gray than the anatomic structures that surround them. The following discussion concerns different categories of image artifacts and common examples of each.

Anatomic Artifact. An anatomic artifact is any anatomic structure that is within the image that could have been removed. These include those that are superimposed over the VOI, as well as those that are not superimposed over the VOI but are still located within the collimated field and could easily have been excluded. A

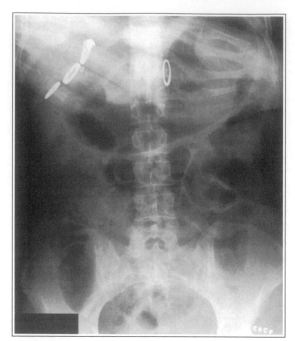

FIGURE 2-36 Anatomic artifact—patient's hands superimposed on AP abdomen projection.

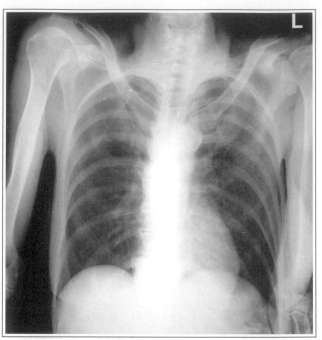

FIGURE 2-37 Anatomic artifact—patient's arms included in AP chest projection.

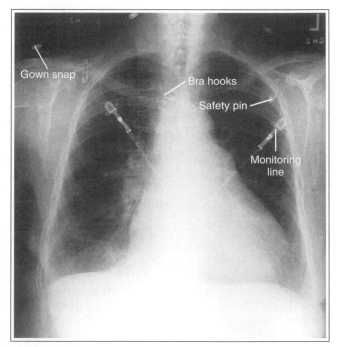

FIGURE 2-38 AP chest projection showing external artifacts from patient clothing and hospital monitoring equipment.

common anatomic artifact is the patient's own hands or arm. Figure 2-36 shows an AP abdomen projection obtained in the supine position in which the patient's hands are superimposed over the upper abdominal region. More than likely the patient was not positioned in this manner when the technologist left the room. After the technologist positioned the patient and before the exposure was taken, however, the patient found a more comfortable position. This example stresses the importance of explaining examinations to patients so that they understand how important it is for them to remain in the position in which the technologist placed them. This also shows the importance of rechecking each patient's position before the exposure is taken if much time has elapsed between positioning the patient and exposing the image. It is also not uncommon for a patient who is experiencing hip or lower back pain from lying on the table to place a hand beneath an affected hip. This will result in superimposition of the hip and hand on the image. Remember, the patient does not know that repositioning because of discomfort is not acceptable. Figure 2-37 shows an AP chest projection produced with a mobile x-ray machine, which was taken with the patient's arms positioned tightly against the sides. Because humeri are not evaluated on a chest projection, there is no reason for them to be included, and they could easily have been shifted out of the exposure field.

External Artifact. An external artifact is found outside the patient's body, such as a patient's possession that remained in a pocket or a hospital possession (e.g., needle cap, ice bag) that was lying on top of or beneath the patient. Common external artifacts include earrings, rings, necklaces, bra hooks, dental structures, hairpins, heart monitoring lines, and gown snaps (Figure 2-38). Two external artifacts that are not as common but that do occasionally appear are caused by pillows (Figure 2-39) and by the imprinted designs on shirts and pants (Figure 2-40). Most of these artifacts can easily be avoided with proper patient preparation and positioning. Being aware of as many objects as possible that can create artifacts on the image is the best way of preventing

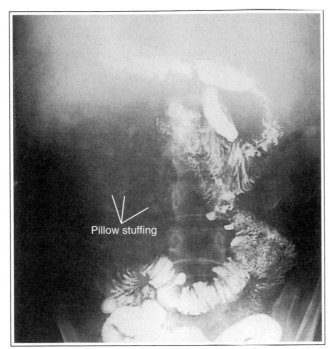

FIGURE 2-39 AP abdomen projection showing an external artifact from a pillow.

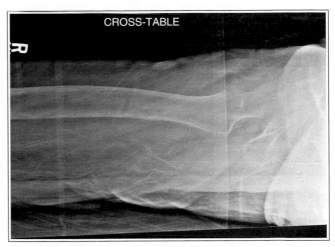

FIGURE 2-41 Lateral femur projection demonstrating clothing artifact.

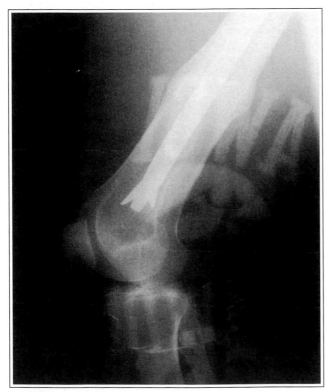

FIGURE 2-40 Lateral knee projection showing external and internal artifacts caused by imprint of patient clothing and leg prosthesis.

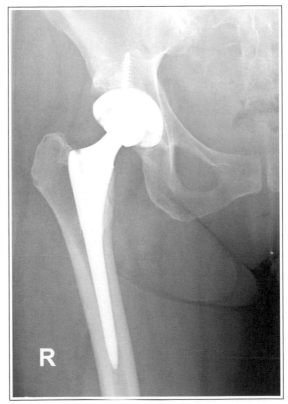

FIGURE 2-42 AP hip projection showing an internal artifact caused by prosthesis.

them. Clothing that has been bunched or folded are often demonstrated if not removed (Figure 2-41).

Internal Artifact. Internal artifacts are found within the patient. They cannot be removed and must be accepted. Examples of commonly seen internal artifacts are the prosthesis (Figures 2-40 and 2-42), pacemaker (see Figure 3-16), central venous catheter (see Figures 3-12 and 3-13), pleural drainage tube (see Figures 3-10 and 3-11), and endotracheal tube (see Figure 3-9). If an artifact that is normally not found within the body is identified on an image, it is the technologist's duty to discretely search and interview the patient or to consult the ordering physician to determine whether the artifact can be located outside the patient's body. If it is not found, it may have been introduced into the patient through one of the body orifices. Your search and interview

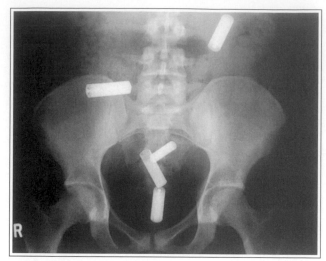

FIGURE 2-43 AP pelvis projection showing an internal artifact (five swallowed batteries).

BOX 2-4	**Causes of Grid Cutoff**

- If a parallel grid was tilted (off level) or the CR was angled toward the grid's lead strips, the image demonstrates grid cutoff on the side toward which the CR was angled (Figures 2-44A and 2-45).
- If a parallel or focused grid was off focus (taken at an SID outside focusing range), the image demonstrates grid cutoff on each side of the image (Figure 2-46; see Figure 2-44*B*).
- If a focused grid was tilted (off level) or the CR was angled toward the grid's lead strips, the image demonstrates grid cutoff across the entire image (Figure 2-47; see Figure 2-44*C*).
- If a focused grid was upside down, the image demonstrates grid cutoff on each side of the image (Figure 2-48; see Figure 2-44*D*).
- If a focused grid was off-center (CR not centered on the center of the grid), the image demonstrates grid cutoff across the entire image (Figure 2-49; see Figure 2-44*E*).

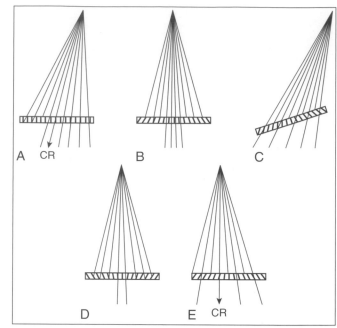

FIGURE 2-44 Causes of grid cutoff. A, CR angled against grid's lead lines. **B,** Off focus. **C,** Off level. **D,** Inverted. **E,** Off center.

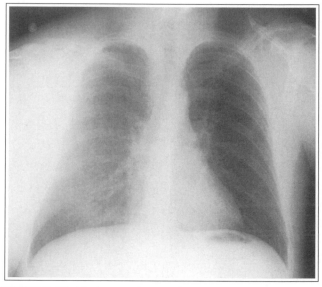

FIGURE 2-45 AP chest projection showing an equipment-related artifact. Parallel grid was tilted or the CR was angled toward the grid's lead strips.

discoveries should be recorded as part of the patient's history. Figure 2-43 shows a pelvic projection of a patient who had swallowed several batteries.

Grid Cutoff Artifact. Grid cutoff artifacts refer to the grid lines that result from poor alignment of the grid and x-ray beam. They occur because the grid's lead strips absorb primary radiation, are visible as small white lines on the image, and are more noticeable with higher ratio grids. They can be avoided by choosing a moving grid whenever possible and by properly aligning the CR and grid. Box 2-4 lists the causes of grid cutoff.

Images demonstrating grid cutoff across the entire image will demonstrate grid lines and signs of underexposure across the entire image. Images where grid cutoff is demonstrated only on portions of the image, such as when a focused grid is inverted or the SID is out of the grid's focusing range, will demonstrate grid lines and underexposure only in the areas where grid cutoff occurred. Lower contrast will also be seen on the areas in the image where there is grid cutoff because the grid's lead lines will work like a filter to increase the uniformity of the exposure.

Aliasing or Moiré Artifact. The CR moiré grid artifact occurs when a stationary grid is used and the IP is placed in the plate reader so that the grid's lead strips are aligned parallel with the scanning direction, resulting in a wavy line pattern on the image (Figure 2-50). It is more common with grids that have a frequency below 60 lines/cm. The moiré grid artifact can be eliminated by using

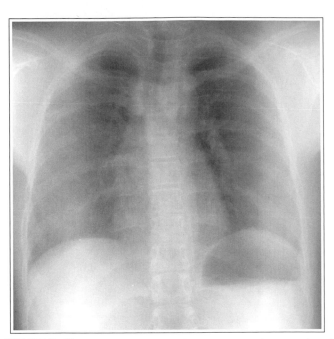

FIGURE 2-46 AP chest projection showing an equipment-related artifact. Off-focused grid cutoff.

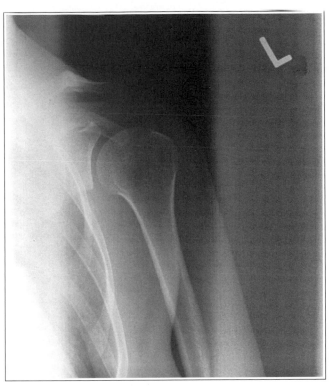

FIGURE 2-48 AP oblique (Grashey method) shoulder projection demonstrating an inverted grid artifact.

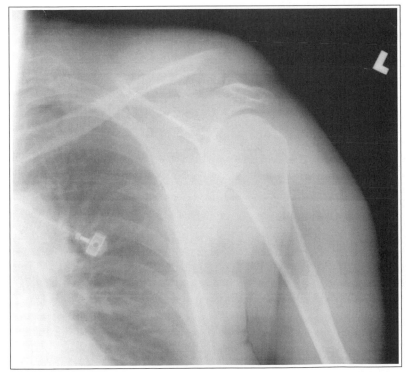

FIGURE 2-47 AP shoulder projection showing an equipment-related artifact. Focused grid was tilted or the CR was angled toward the grid's lead strips.

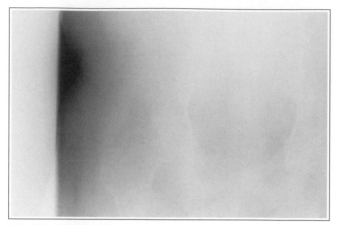

FIGURE 2-49 AP pelvis projection showing an equipment-related artifact. Off-centered grid cutoff.

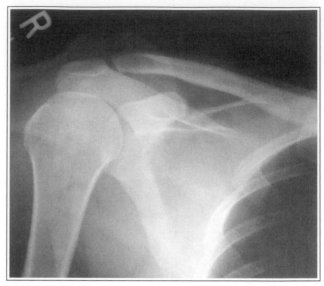

FIGURE 2-51 Computed radiography AP shoulder projection demonstrating a phantom image artifact.

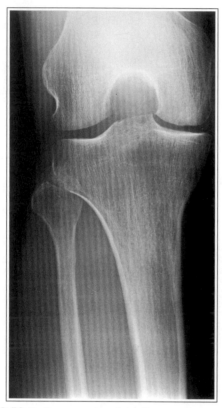

FIGURE 2-50 Equipment-related artifact—moiré grid artifact. *(Courtesy Cesar LJ, Schueler BA, Zink FE, et al. Artefacts found in computed radiography, Br J Radiol 74:195–202, 2001.)*

a moving grid to blur lines and a grid frequency of 60 lines/cm or higher and by processing the image so that the grid's lead strips are aligned perpendicular to the plate reader's laser scanning direction. When you scan a 10- × 12-inch or 14- × 17-inch IP, it is scanned across its short axis. To position the grid's lead strips perpendicular to the scanning direction, the grid's lead strips should be placed with the long axis of the IP. An 8- × 10-inch IP is scanned across its long axis. To position the grid's lead strips perpendicular to the scanning direction, the

grid's lead strips should be aligned with the short axis of the IP.

Phantom Image Artifact. Phantom images are artifacts in computed radiography that occur when the IP is not adequately erased before the next image is exposed on it. The resulting image is a shadow of the image that was previously exposed onto the phosphors on the plate. These images resemble a double exposure (Figure 2-51). After the exposure the IP is placed into the reader for processing. Information stored on the plate is released when it is exposed to a red laser light and then the plate goes to the erasing block, where it is exposed to a high-intensity light to release any remaining stored energy. The erasure block system is capable of erasing a phosphor plate that has received up to five times the normal exposure. If an exposure is more than this, stored energy in the form of a phantom image will remain on the plate and when reexposed and read may be seen on the new image, appearing similar to a double-exposed image. For this artifact to be prevented, the phosphor plate should be sent back to the erasure block for a second erasing when the exposure indicator indicates that an excessive exposure was used to create the image.

Scatter and Background Fogging. Phantom images may also be produced when the computed radiography IR is accidentally exposed to scatter radiation when left in the room during other exposures (see Figure 2-12) or has not been used for 48 to 72 hours and has collected a sufficient exposure from natural background radiation. Storing exposed and unexposed IR outside the x-ray room before and after exposures will prevent fogging caused by scatter radiation that occurs when an exposure is made. Completing a secondary erasure before using a phosphor plate that has not been used for some time will prevent background radiation fogging.

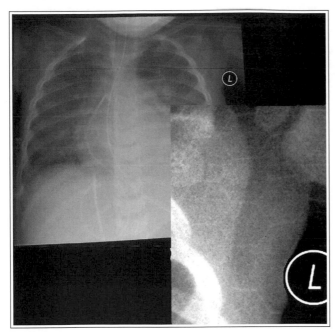

FIGURE 2-52 Computed radiography AP chest projection demonstrating honeycomb pattern overlying the image. This was caused by the back of the cassette being positioned toward the radiation source for the exposure.

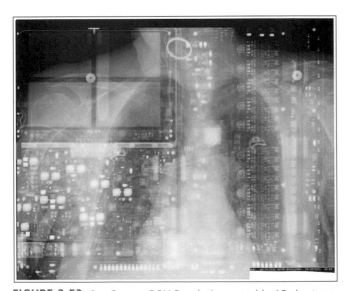

FIGURE 2-53 CareStream DRX-Revolution portable AP chest projection taken with the IR reversed.

Back of Cassette Toward Source During Exposure. If the computed radiography cassette is exposed with its back positioned toward the x-ray source, a faint white grid-type, honeycomb or square pattern will be overlaying the image (Figure 2-52). There will also be white areas that correspond to the hinges if they are included within the exposure field. Figure 2-53 demonstrates an AP chest projection obtained using the CareStream DRX-Revolution portable where the IR was reversed when placed beneath the patient.

Phosphor Plate–Handling Artifact. Dust or dirt particles and scratches on the surface of the phosphor

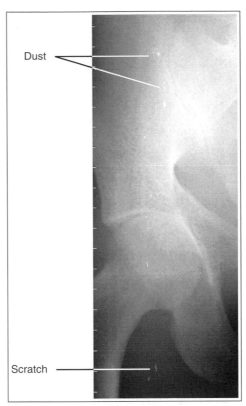

FIGURE 2-54 Equipment-handling artifact. Computed radiography phosphor plate with scratches and dust on AP hip projection.

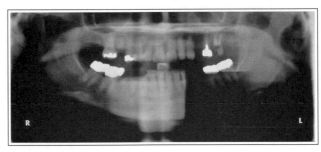

FIGURE 2-55 Orthopantomogram image with dark rectangular box in the lower left jaw from unknown cause.

plate produce small white dots or curved white lines, respectively (Figure 2-54). Dust or dirt artifacts can be corrected by cleaning the screen. Scratches are permanent, and replacement of the plate is required to eliminate them.

Digital System Artifact. Occasionally, there are artifacts that appear on images that cannot be explained from a technologist's perspective and require the system expert. Figure 2-55 has an orthopantomogram image that demonstrates a dark rectangular box in the lower left jaw area. Figure 2-56 shows an AP knee projection with bright spots in the knee joint. Both of these artifacts were caused by problems with the digital system and were not a result of a technologist's error.

If an artifact that can be eliminated obscures any portion of the VOI, the image needs to be repeated. A gown snap superimposed on an area of the lungs on a

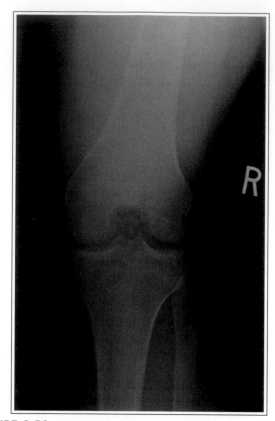

FIGURE 2-56 AP knee projection with bright spots in the knee joint caused by poor detector elements.

chest projection can easily obscure a small lesion. A ring can easily obscure a hairline finger fracture. If the artifact is located outside the field of interest, the image does not need to be repeated.

Postprocedure Requirements

Defining Image Acceptability. When a projection meets all the necessary requirements, it is considered optimal and is ready to be sent to PACS. When a projection is not optimal but may be acceptable, the question arises as to whether it is poor enough to repeat or whether the information needed can be obtained without exposing the patient to further radiation. Factors that should be considered when making this decision include the following:

- Your facility's standards
- The age and condition of the patient
- The conditions under which the patient was imaged
- Whether obvious pathology is evident
- Whether the indications for the examination have been fulfilled
- Whether windowing or modifying the projection by processing it with a different procedural algorithm will display the needed information

Each facility has its own standards that will determine whether a projection needs to be repeated. If standards are low, improving imaging skills can raise them, thereby

increasing the accuracy of diagnosis. The age and condition of the patient, as well as the conditions under which the patient was imaged, are most important in the decision to repeat a projection. Sometimes a less than optimal projection must be accepted because repeating the projection is impossible, as in a surgery case; at other times, the patient cannot or will not cooperate. Whenever a projection is accepted that does not meet optimal standards, record in the patient's history any information about the patient's condition or situation that resulted in acceptance of this projection. A less than optimal projection may also be accepted when the indication for the examination is clearly fulfilled by the projections obtained; for example, a lateral lower leg projection was obtained to evaluate the healing of a distal fibular fracture and the knee joint was not included. In this case, the patient's knee is not being evaluated. As long as the distal fibula and ankle joint were included in their entirety and accurately positioned, the projection would not need to be repeated.

It is important that all unacceptable projections and those less than optimal projections that have been accepted are studied carefully to determine whether the situation(s) that caused them could be eliminated on future examinations. When a projection is repeated, the overall radiation dose to the patient increases and the cost of patient care rises because reimaging requires more technologist time, supplies, and equipment use.

Fulfillment of Exam Indication. One of the last steps to take before deciding whether a projection is acceptable is to make sure that you have taken all the projections that are recommended by your facility for the body part being imaged. For example, many facilities require that AP and lateral projections are taken whenever projections of the knee are requested. This series of projections provides the reviewer with the needed information to accurately evaluate the patient's knee. Not only should the entire series be taken, but the technologist should also evaluate whether the indication for the examination has been fulfilled to the best of their knowledge. If an elbow examination is ordered and the indication for the examination was to evaluate or rule out a radial head fracture, an additional external AP oblique or axiolateral (Coyle method) projection of the elbow may be needed to rule out this fracture definitively. In these situations, consulting with the reviewer before allowing the patient to leave the imaging department can be very beneficial.

Special Imaging Situations

Mobile and Trauma Imaging. The goal of mobile and trauma imaging is to produce optimal images without causing further patient injury and with minimal patient discomfort. The following are general guidelines for obtaining this goal.

1. Based on the requested order, determine the projections that will be needed and the order in which they

will be completed. First, obtain the projections that will provide information about the most life-threatening condition (cross-table lateral cervical vertebrae projection if a cervical fracture is questioned or when obtaining an AP chest projection for a patient having difficulty breathing). Speed is of the essence in many mobile and trauma situations, because the patient can be quite ill. Having a thought-out plan of action before starting allows the technologist to work in an organized and speedy manner. As a general rule, after the initial projections associated with life-threatening conditions have been exposed and checked by the radiologist or physician, the remaining projections are exposed in an order that will require the least amount of CR adjustment. All AP projections are exposed, and then the CR is moved horizontally for the lateral projections. It is important that projections be obtained that are at 90-degree angles from each other (AP-PA and lateral) when fractures and foreign bodies are suspected to determine the degree of bone displacement (Figure 2-57) and depth location.

2. Gather and organize the supplies (e.g., positioning aides, disposable gloves, radiation protection supplies) that will be needed, and determine the starting technical factors (kV, mAs, AEC) for the needed projections. Cover the positioning aids and IRs to protect them from contamination.

3. Determine the degree of patient mobility, alertness, and ability to follow requests. Can the patient be placed in a seated position or be rotated to one side? Can the arm or leg fully extend or flex? When the patient is asked to breathe deeply, can he or she follow the request? Can the patient control movement?

4. Assess the site of interest for physical signs of injury (swelling, bruising, deformity, pain). Understanding the degree of injury will help the technologist prevent further injury during the positioning process.

5. Determine whether positioning devices (e.g., slings, backboards, casts) and artifacts (e.g., heart leads, clothing, jewelry) may be removed and, if not, whether they will obscure the VOI on the ordered projections. If positioning devices or artifacts will obscure the area, consult with the radiologist or ordering physician about possible alternatives (e.g., taking a slight oblique instead of a true projection).

6. Set an optimal kV and mAs or AEC for the anatomic structure and projection being imaged. Technical adjustments may also be needed due to the increased photon absorption that may occur because of positioning devices, artifacts, additive or destructive patient conditions, or the SID or OID not being set at the routine settings. Table 2-7 lists common technical adjustments needed when imaging trauma patients. Either increase (+) or decrease (−) the kV or mAs from the routine amount for the patient thickness measurement, as indicated in Table 2-7.

7. Obtain the requested projections. The technologist should use the routine positioning guidelines such as for patient positioning, CR centering, IR and part orientation, and collimation when obtaining mobile

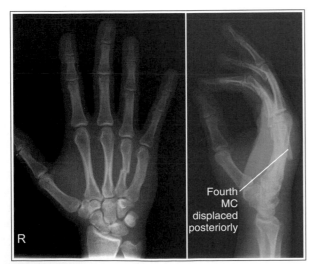

FIGURE 2-57 PA and lateral hand projections showing posterior displacement of the fourth metacarpal *(MC)* caused by a fracture.

Fourth MC displaced posteriorly

TABLE 2-7	Technical Adjustments for Trauma Patients	
Immobilization Devices or Patient Condition	**kV Adjustment**	**mAs Adjustment**
Small to medium plaster cast	+5-7 kV	+50%-60%
Large plaster cast	+8-10 KV	+100%
Fiberglass cast (Figure 2-58)	No adjustment	No adjustment
Inflated air splint	No adjustment	No adjustment
Wood backboard (Figure 2-59)	+5 kV	+25%-30%
Ascites (accumulation of fluid) (Figure 2-34)		+50%-75%
Pleural effusion (fluid in pleural cavity)		+35%
Pneumothorax (air or gas in pleural cavity)	−8% kV	
Postmortem imaging of head, thorax, and abdomen (because of pooling of blood and fluid)		+35%-50%
Soft tissue injury (used for foreign objects, such as slivers of wood, glass, or metal, embedding in the soft tissue and to demonstrate the upper airway)	−15% to 20% kV	

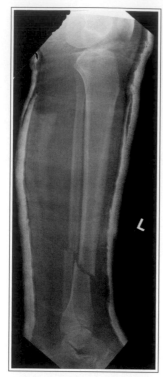

FIGURE 2-58 Lateral lower leg projection with fiberglass cast.

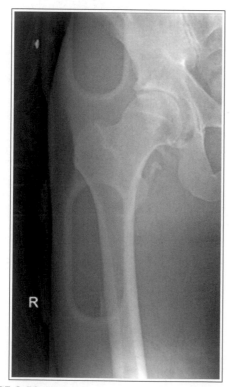

FIGURE 2-59 AP hip projection taken through backboard.

and trauma projections. For patients who are unable to follow the routine positioning requirements, adaptations to this setup can be made. Never force the patient into a position. Instead, adjust the CR and IR. As long as the CR, part, and IR form the

same alignments that are indicated for routine positioning, identical projections will result.

8. Use the smallest possible OID and increase the SID to compensate if a longer than routine OID is needed.

9. Use a grid if the patient part thickness is over 4 inches (10 cm) and over 60 kV is used. When positioning latitude is narrow because of the patient's condition or when the mobile unit is used, choose a linear low-ratio grid to allow for the greatest positioning error latitude. Evaluate the alignment of the CR and grid:

   • Is the CR aligned accurately with the center of the grid?
   • If a CR angle is used, is it angled with the grid lines?
   • Is the grid level?
   • Is the SID within the grid's focusing range?
   • Is the correct side of the grid facing the CR?

10. Use good radiation protection practices. Ask female patients if there is any chance they could be pregnant. Never assume that other staff members have asked. Use gonadal shielding whenever possible, collimate tightly, and provide those assisting with patient holding during the exposure with aprons and lead gloves. On recumbent patients, projections of the extremity should not be taken by placing the IR and part on the patient's torso unless it is the only means of obtaining accurate positioning. If this is the case, always place a lead apron between the IR and torso. Not all the radiation directed toward the IR is absorbed; high-energy beams will exit through the back of the IR, exposing structures beneath.

11. Never leave a confused patient or a trauma patient unattended in the imaging room.

12. Process the projections and evaluate them for positioning and technical accuracy. Determine whether repeat projections are needed and how much adjustment will be required. When the trauma is severe, all the evaluating guidelines listed in the procedural sections of this textbook may not be evident. This is one of the reasons why I have often described more than one anatomic relationship to indicate accurate positioning in the evaluating guidelines. For example, on the lateral ankle projection in Figure 2-60, the tibial-fibular relationship cannot be used to determine accuracy of the positioning, but the domes of the talus are well visualized and indicate that the ankle was well positioned.

13. Repeat any necessary projections.

14. Return the patient to the emergency room or, if the projections were taken with the mobile unit, replace the bed, monitoring devices, and personal items to the positions they occupied when you entered the room or to positions that make the patient most comfortable.

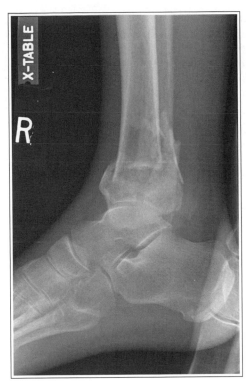

FIGURE 2-60 Trauma lateral ankle projection.

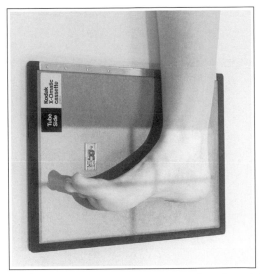

FIGURE 2-61 Accurate tabletop positioning for a lateral (mediolateral) foot projection.

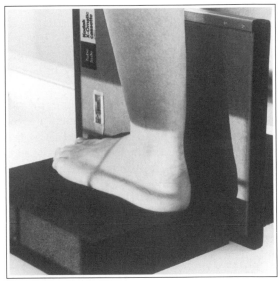

FIGURE 2-62 Accurate standing positioning for a lateral (lateromedial) foot projection.

15. Disinfect all equipment and devices used during the procedures.

Guidelines for Aligning Contrast Resolution, Part, and Image Receptor

Whenever possible, set up the routinely used CR, part, and IR alignments as you would for the routine projections. The word *part* with regard to alignment refers to the specific plane, imaginary line, or anatomic structure used to position the patient with the CR and IR in routine positioning.

Lateral Projections. Routine lateral foot projections require that the foot's lateral surface be aligned parallel to the IR and the CR be aligned perpendicular to the part and the IR. In this situation the lateral foot surface is the part, because this is what is used to position the foot in relation to the CR and IR. If the lateral foot projection is taken on the imaging table, the patient will externally rotate his or her leg until the lateral foot surface is parallel to the IR, and the CR will be aligned perpendicular to the IR and part (Figure 2-61). If the lateral foot projection is taken in a standing position, the IR will be positioned vertically and the CR horizontally. Even though the setup appears different, the CR, part, and IR alignments are the same as in the previous setup. The lateral foot surface is positioned parallel to the IR, and the CR is perpendicular to the IR and lateral foot surface. Often, when a cross-table projection is created, the path that the CR takes is opposite. For a routine tabletop lateral foot projection, a mediolateral projection is performed, whereas a lateromedial projection is used for cross-table projections. To obtain identical projections for both pathways, the CR, part, and IR must maintain the same alignment. This means that the lateral surface of the foot must still be positioned parallel to the IR for a lateromedial projection, even if this surface is not placed directly adjacent to the IR. For a lateral foot projection, this will require the medial aspect of the heel to be positioned slightly away from the IR (Figure 2-62).

If a patient arrives in the radiology department in a wheelchair and is unable to move to the imaging table for the lateral foot projection, the projection can be obtained with the patient remaining in the wheelchair. First, align the lateral foot surface with the IR and then align the CR perpendicular to the IR and

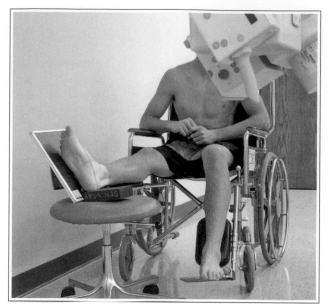

FIGURE 2-63 Accurate wheelchair positioning for a lateral (mediolateral) foot projection.

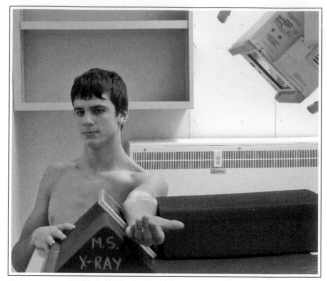

FIGURE 2-64 Accurate trauma positioning for an internal AP oblique elbow projection.

lateral foot surface. Again, because the relationships between the CR, IR, and part are the same as in the two previous setups, the resulting projection will be identical (Figure 2-63).

Oblique Projections. For trauma oblique projections, begin by aligning the CR with the plane, line, or anatomic structure that is used for an AP projection of the part being imaged. Next, adjust the CR in the direction needed to set up the correct alignment between the CR and structure. Because the degree of angulation in which patients are rotated for oblique projections is always referenced from the AP-PA projection, the amount of angle adjustment would be the same as the required degree of obliquity. For a routine internal AP oblique elbow projection, the CR is aligned at a 45-degree angle with an imaginary line connecting the humeral epicondyles (the medial epicondyle is placed farther from the tube than the lateral). To obtain the same projection in a patient who is unable to rotate his or her arm, the technologist first positions the CR perpendicular to the line connecting the epicondyles and then adjusts the angle 45 degrees medially, positioning the medial epicondyle farther from the x-ray tube than the lateral epicondyle. The IR would then be aligned as close to perpendicular to the CR as possible (Figure 2-64).

Alignment of Contrast Resolution and Part versus Contrast Resolution and Image Receptor. To obtain open joint spaces, clearly see fracture lines, or obtain specific anatomic relationships, the alignment of the CR with the part must be accurate. Although IR alignment with the CR and part is important to prevent elongation distortion, it does not have an effect on the anatomic relationships that are demonstrated. After the CR and part are accurately aligned, the IR should be positioned as close to perpendicular to the CR as possible. If the CR is not positioned perpendicular to the IR, the resulting projection will demonstrate elongation in the direction toward which the CR was angled, but the anatomic alignment of the structures are demonstrated as required for the projection. The more acute the CR and IR angle, the greater will be the elongation. In this situation, the IR will need to be offset in the direction toward which the CR is angled more than what would occur if the IR were positioned perpendicular to the CR. Because of this offset, careful attention should be given to centering the center of the IR to the CR.

Imaging Long Bones. To demonstrate long bones with the least amount of distortion and obtain optimal anatomical alignment, the CR is aligned perpendicular and the IR parallel with the bone's long axis (Figures 1-48A and 2-65A). When imaging a long bone where the patient is unable to position the bone so its long axis is parallel with the IR, the alignments created between the CR, IR, and bone determines the degree and type of distortion and the anatomical relationships demonstrated on the resulting projection. Figure 2-65B was obtained with the distal forearm in a PA projection and elevated so the forearm's long axis was at a 20-degree tilt with the IR and the CR aligned perpendicular with the IR. This setup is the least desired because it will produce the greatest foreshortening and poorest anatomic alignment at the joints. Compare the forearm length and the anatomic alignments of the elbow bones between Figures 2-65A and B. The forearm image in Figure 2-65C was obtained using the law of isometry (Figure 2-66). The law of isometry indicates that the CR should be set at half of the angle formed between the object and IR to minimize foreshortening. For example, if the patient's knee cannot be fully extended for an AP femur projection, causing the femur to be at a 30-degree angle with the IR and the distal femur positioned at a larger OID than the

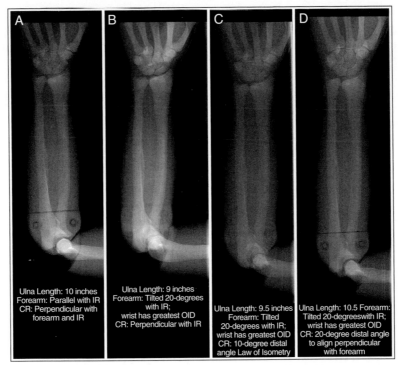

FIGURE 2-65 Creating optimal projections of long bones.

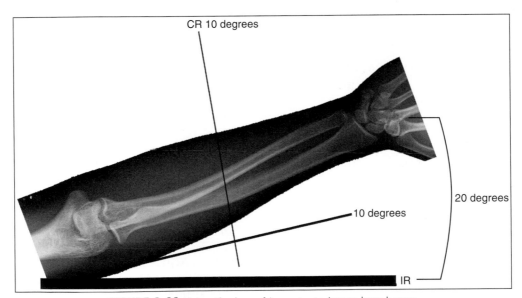

FIGURE 2-66 Using the law of isometry to image long bones.

proximal femur, the CR should be angled 15 degrees toward the proximal femur. This setup provides a projection with reduced foreshortening and improved, although not optimal, anatomic alignment of the joints. Compare the anatomic alignment of the elbow joints in Figures 2-65*A*-*C*. Note that elbow joint is open in Figure 2-65*A* and is closed in Figures 2-65*B* and *C*. The joints will not demonstrate optimal anatomical alignment when the law of isometry is used because the CR is not perpendicular with the long bone for this setup and the diverged x-rays recording the joints are not at the same angles as they are when the CR is perpendicular. Figure 2-65*D* was

obtained with the forearm aligned at a 20-degree tilt with the IR and the CR aligned perpendicular to the forearm (see Figure 1-48*D*). This setup produces the same anatomic alignments of the bones at the elbow joint as was obtained for the ideal setup in Figure 2-65*A*, but because the wrist was positioned at a greater OID than the elbow (20-degree forearm to IR tilt) the forearm demonstrates elongation.

Whether the ideal setup for a long bone that cannot be positioned with its long axis parallel with the IR is obtained using the law of isometry (Figure 2-65*C*) or a perpendicular CR (Figure 2-65*D*) is best decided by using the setup that will optimally demonstrated the VOI. The law of isometry demonstrates the least foreshortening and a perpendicular CR best demonstrates the anatomic relationships at the joints.

When imaging long bones that require both joints to be included on the same projection, but the joints cannot be positioned in the true projection simultaneously because of a fracture, the joint closest to the fracture should be positioned in the true projection (Figure 2-67).

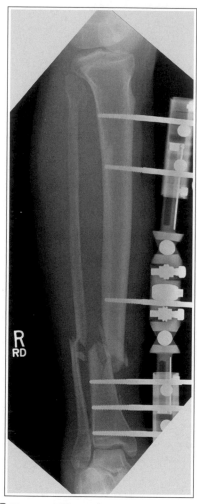

FIGURE 2-67 Trauma AP lower leg projection with joint closest to fracture demonstrating accurate positioning.

Pediatric Imaging

The images of pediatric patients are very different from those of adults and from each other during the various stages of bone growth and development (Figure 2-68). Bones throughout the body enlarge through the deposits of bone at cartilaginous growth regions, and long bones lengthen by the addition of bone material at the epiphyseal plate. Cartilaginous spaces and epiphyseal plates exist throughout the skeletal structure. They appear as darker shaded spaces and lines on projections and may look similar to an irregular fracture or joint space to those unfamiliar with pediatric imaging. The appearances of these spaces and lines are reduced as the child develops, until early adulthood, when they are replaced by bone and are no longer are visible on the projection. Round bones, such as the carpal and tarsal bones, are rarely formed at birth and therefore are not demonstrated on projections of neonatal and very young pediatric patients. Because of this continual state of development, some anatomic relationships described in the imaging analysis sections may not be useful for determining accurate positioning for the pediatric patient. It is beyond our scope here to explain all the differences that could be demonstrated at different growth stages for each projection included in this text. When evaluating pediatric projections for proper anatomic alignment, use only the analysis guidelines that describe bony structures that are developed enough to use. For example, the section on PA wrist projection analysis describes the alignment of the carpal bones and metacarpals to determine accurate positioning. The carpal bone alignment cannot be used to evaluate young pediatric wrists, because all the carpal bones are not formed, but the metacarpals can be used to determine positioning accuracy.

Technical Considerations. Pediatric imaging requires lower technical values (kV and mAs) when compared with those for adults. Box 2-5 lists guidelines to follow when selecting technical values for pediatric patients.

Clothing Artifacts. Because lower kV is used in pediatrics, clothing artifacts may be problematic in neonates and smaller children (Figure 2-69). The kV used may not

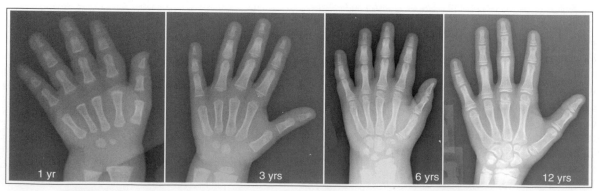

FIGURE 2-68 Pediatric PA hand and wrist projections at different ages of skeletal development.

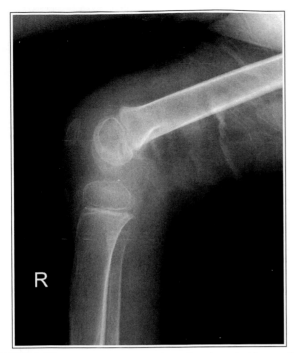

FIGURE 2-69 Lateral knee projection showing clothing artifacts around the distal femur on pediatric patient.

BOX 2-5	**Guidelines for Setting Technical Factors for Pediatric Patients**

- Choose a high mA and short exposure times to prevent patient motion.
- Only use a grid if the part thickness measures over 4 to 5 inches (10-12 cm).
- Follow the best practices guidelines for AEC usage listed in Box 2-2 very closely, as fast enough exposure times and chamber coverage may limit use, or use a thickness measurement driven manual technique.
- Lower IR exposure by adjusting kV and mAs over that used for adults to maintain ideal EI levels.

be high enough to obscure creases or folds, particularly in unlaundered material or flame-resistant clothing. It is best to image children without upper clothing or with a tee shirt when modesty is an issue. Skinfolds of neonates may also cause artifacts when they overlie the chest.

Obese Patients

According to the U.S. Centers for Disease Control and Prevention (CDC), approximately 64% of Americans are overweight. This has a direct impact on the health care system and imaging departments because these individuals have an increased incidence of diabetes, heart disease, and certain types of cancer and there is increasing popularity of bariatric surgery to help manage this condition. The challenges facing technologists as they image obese patients include transporting and accommodating larger

patients on the current equipment, and difficulties in acquiring quality projections.[1] The following are considerations for imaging this population.

1. Obese patients often feel unwelcome in medical settings, where they encounter negative attitudes, discriminatory behavior, and a challenging physical environment. The emotional needs of these patients must be considered when they are imaged. Avoid making remarks about their size, being mindful of terms used such as "big" when referring to special equipment needs or requests for "lots of help" when transferring the patient.
2. Patient weight and body diameter are factors that should be evaluated before transporting the patient to the department or performing the examination. Use this information to determine whether the patient's weight exceeds any of the equipment weight limits, including waiting room chairs or support structures, or his or her diameter exceeds the wheelchair or cart dimensions.
3. Avoid injury to the patient and personnel by making certain that enough people are available to assist if the patient requires moving before or during the procedure. Use moving devices, such as table sliders and lifts, whenever possible.
4. Determine how the positioning procedure (IR cassette size, CW-LW position of IR) will need to be adjusted from the routine to accommodate the increased structure size. For example, to include the entire abdomen on a morbidly obese patient may require a separate IR for each of the four abdominal quadrants, instead of one for the top and bottom.
5. Obese patients have inherently low subject contrast because their muscles have lost strength and have become the consistency of fat, so technical values must be set to enhance subject contrast while producing the lowest possible patient dose to produce an image with sufficient image contrast.

Technical Considerations. Thicker patients attenuate more of the primary x-ray photons than thin patients, requiring the technologist to increase mAs and/or kV to compensate for the exposure loss that would result if a change were not made. Thicker patients also demonstrate a higher signal-to-noise ratio (SNR) reaching the IR, causing a loss in contrast resolution. For example, a typical abdominal projection taken on a patient measuring 20 cm will demonstrate a SNR of 3:1, meaning that 75% of the photons striking the IR are scattered photons that carry little or no useful information. For larger patients, the ratio in the abdomen can approach 5:1 or 6:1 (83%-86%).

When determining how to adjust the technique for a thicker patient, the technologist must consider the effect that the change will have on patient dose and contrast resolution. As long as the kV is set to provide adequate demonstration of subject contrast throughout the part, increasing the mAs will generate enough x-rays to provide more IR exposure. *As a general rule, for every 4 cm of added tissue thickness, the mAs should be doubled to maintain IR exposure.* This technique adjustment will have a significant increase on patient dose because the increase in dose is directly proportional to the mAs increase. It will also demonstrate lower contrast because the amount of scatter radiation produced will increase with increased thickness.

Another technique adjustment option is to increase the kV. This will increase the penetration ability of the photons, resulting in more of them reaching the IR and increasing IR exposure. *As a general rule, for every centimeter of added tissue thickness, the kV is adjusted by 2 kV.* This option will increase patient dosage, but not directly or nearly as much, as with mAs. The drawback with using kV is that it will increase the amount of scatter radiation that will be directed toward the IR and lower contrast resolution.

For best results when adjusting technique for a thick patient, the kV should be set as high as possible (to reduce radiation dose), but should not exceed a kV value that will result in the scatter fogging being detrimental to the quality of the projection. After kV value maximum has been attained, additional adjustments should be made with mAs.

Scatter Radiation Control. One of the biggest obstacles when imaging the obese patient is controlling scatter radiation enough to provide a projection that has sufficient contrast resolution. This is accomplished by using very aggressive, tight collimation, using a high-ratio grid, or using an air-gap technique.

1. Tight collimation is often difficult when imaging obese patients because the collimator's light field demonstrated on the patient does not represent the true width and length of the field set on the collimator. The thicker the part being imaged, the smaller the collimator's light field that appears on the patient's skin surface. On a very thick patient, it is difficult to collimate the needed amount when the light field appears so small, but on these patients, tight collimation demonstrates the largest improvement in the visibility

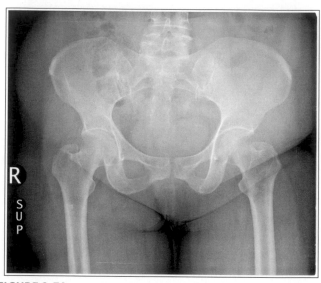

FIGURE 2-70 AP pelvis projection showing overlapping soft tissue, preventing uniform density of hip joints and proximal femurs.

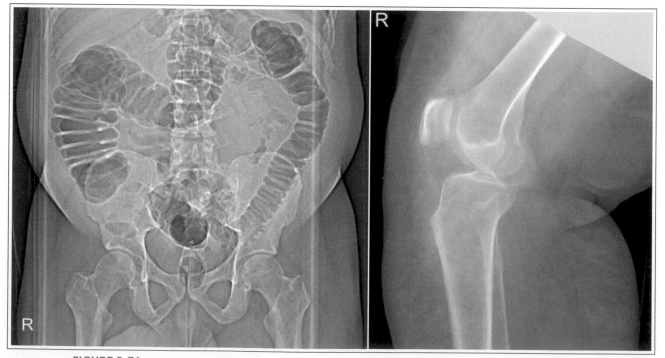

FIGURE 2-71 AP abdomen and lateral knee projections on an obese patient to show placement of skeletal structure within surrounding soft tissue.

of recorded details. Learn to use the collimator guide (see Figure 1-20) to determine the actual IR coverage.

2. Many projections, such as the inferosuperior (axial) shoulder projection, which do not require a grid on the typical patient, will need to be performed using a grid. Measure all structures and use a grid when the part thickness is more than 10 cm.

Focal Spot Size. When using a small focal spot, the mA is typically limited to 300 mA or less. Using such a small focal spot may not be feasible when imaging an obese patient because it would require a long exposure time to achieve the needed IR exposure and motion may result.

Automatic Exposure Control. Select a high mA to avoid long exposure times and the potential motion it causes. Also, adjust the backup timer to 150% to 200% of the expected manual exposure time.

1. When possible, remove overlapping soft tissue from the area being imaged to decrease the thickness of the tissue being penetrated. Figure 2-70 demonstrates an AP pelvis projection in which the soft tissue overlapping the hips could have been pulled superiorly and held with tape or by the patient, decreasing the soft tissue over the hips and allowing them to be demonstrated more effectively. Overlapping breast and arm tissue can also be held away from the shoulder during inferosuperior (axial) shoulder projections to decrease thickness and improve detail visibility.

2. Use palpable bony structures to position the patient and to collimate whenever possible. Remember, the skeletal structure does not increase in size with an increase in the soft tissue surrounding it. Figure 2-71 shows a bone scan on an obese patient that clearly illustrates this point. Using palpable bony structures to determine where structures are located whenever possible will help you to position accurately and collimate more specifically to the structures of interest.

When the soft tissue thickness prevents palpation of bony structures, use signs such as depressions or dimples in the soft tissue that suggest where the bony structures are located. Observe closely how the patient is positioned for each projection so if a repeat is needed, you can adjust the amount needed from the original positioning.

REFERENCE

1. Upport RN, Sahani DV, Hahn PF, et al: *Impact of obesity on medical imaging*, ed 2, Philadelphia, 2002, Lippincott Williams & Wilkins.

Chest and Abdomen

OUTLINE

Chest, 77
Chest: PA Projection, 84
  PA Chest Analysis
    Practice, 91
Chest: Lateral Projection
  (Left Lateral Position), 91
  Lateral Chest Analysis
    Practice, 97
Chest: AP Projection (Supine or with
  Mobile X-Ray Unit), 98
  AP Chest (Portable) Analysis
    Practice, 103
Chest: AP or PA Projection
  (Right or Left Lateral Decubitus
  Position), 104
  Decubitus Chest Analysis
    Practice, 107
Chest: AP Axial Projection
  (Lordotic Position), 107
  AP Lordotic Chest Analysis
    Practice, 109
Chest: PA Oblique Projection
  (Right Anterior Oblique and Left
  Anterior Oblique Positions), 110
  PA Oblique Chest Analysis
    Practice, 112
Neonate and Infant Chest:
  AP Projection, 113
  Neonate and Infant AP Chest
    Analysis Practice, 116

Child Chest: PA and AP (Portable)
  Projections, 117
  Child Chest PA and AP
    (Portable) Chest Analysis
    Practice, 117
Neonate and Infant Chest:
  Cross-Table Lateral Projection
  (Left Lateral Position), 120
Child Chest: Lateral Projection
  (Left Lateral Position), 122
  Child Lateral Chest Analysis
    Practice, 122
Neonate and Infant Chest: AP
  Projection (Right or Left Lateral
  Decubitus Position), 124
  Neonate and Infant AP
    Decubitus Chest Analysis
    Practice, 127
Child Chest: AP and PA Projection
  (Right or Left Lateral Decubitus
  Position), 127
  Child AP-PA (Lateral
    Decubitus) Chest Analysis
    Practice, 128
Abdomen: AP Projection (Supine
  and Upright), 132
  AP Abdomen Analysis
    Practice, 138
Abdomen: AP Projection (Left
  Lateral Decubitus Position), 139

AP (Left Lateral Decubitus)
  Abdomen Analysis
    Practice, 141
Neonate and Infant Abdomen:
  AP Projection (Supine), 141
  Neonate and Infant: AP
    Abdominal Analysis
    Practice, 142
Child Abdomen: AP Projection
  (Supine and Upright), 143
  Child AP Abdominal
    Analysis Practice, 143
Neonate and Infant Abdomen:
  AP Projection (Left Lateral
  Decubitus Position), 143
  Neonate and Infant AP
    (Left Lateral Decubitus)
    Abdominal Analysis
    Practice, 145
Child Abdomen: AP Projection
  (Left Lateral Decubitus
  Position), 145
  Child AP (Left Lateral
    Decubitus) Abdomen
    Analysis Practice, 148

OBJECTIVES

After completion of this chapter, you should be able to do the following:

- Identify the required anatomy on all chest and abdominal projections.
- Describe how to position the patient, image receptor (IR), and central ray (CR) properly for adult and pediatric chest and abdominal projections.
- State the technical data used in chest and abdominal projections.
- List the image analysis guidelines for accurately positioned adult and pediatric chest and abdominal projections.
- State how to reposition the patient when chest and abdominal projections with poor positioning are produced.

- Discuss how to determine the amount of patient or CR adjustment required to improve poor positioning on chest and abdominal projections.
- State how the patient and CR are positioned to demonstrate air and fluid levels best within the pleural cavity. Explain how this detection is affected on an AP-PA chest projection if the patient is placed in a supine or partial upright position.
- State the purpose and proper location of the internal devices, tubes, and catheters demonstrated on adult and pediatric AP chest and abdominal projections.
- Explain why a 72-inch (183-cm) source–image receptor distance (SID) is routinely used for chest projections.
- List the chest dimensions that expand when the patient inhales and the conditions that prevent full lung expansion.

- Describe scoliosis, and identify a chest projection of a patient with this condition.
- Describe methods of identifying the right and left hemidiaphragms on lateral chest projections.
- Explain the location of the liver and discuss how its location affects the height of the right hemidiaphragm.
- Discuss how the patient is positioned for a lateral decubitus chest projection to rule out pneumothorax and pleural effusion.
- Explain the difference in the degree of patient obliquity needed to see the heart shadow without spinal column superimposition for right anterior oblique (RAO) and left anterior oblique (LAO) chest projections.
- Explain how neonates' lungs develop and change as they grow and how CR centering is adjusted because of these changes.

- Describe the location of the psoas muscles and kidneys.
- Discuss how technique is adjusted for chest and abdomen projections of patients with additive and destructive conditions. Explain why this adjustment is required.
- Explain why a patient is positioned in the upright or lateral decubitus position for at least 10 to 20 minutes before the abdominal projection is taken.
- Describe why it is necessary to center differently for female and male patients when positioning for an AP abdominal projection.
- State why it is necessary for the diaphragm to be included in all upright and lateral decubitus abdominal projections.

KEY TERMS

automatic implantable cardioverter defibrillator (ICD)
body habitus
central venous catheter (CVC)
cortical outline
endotracheal tube (ETT)
intraperitoneal air

kyphosis
mammary line
pacemaker
pleural drainage tube
pleural effusion
pneumectomy
pneumothorax

pulmonary arterial catheter
scoliosis
umbilical artery catheter (UAC)
umbilical vein catheter (UVC)
vascular lung markings

IMAGE ANALYSIS GUIDELINES

CHEST

Technical Data. When the technical data in Table 3-1 are followed, or adjusted as needed for additive and destructive patient conditions (see Table 2-6), along with the best practices discussed in Chapters 1 and 2, all chest projections will demonstrate the image analysis guidelines listed in Box 3-1 unless otherwise indicated.

Source-to-IR Distance (SID). Because the heart is situated at a large object–image receptor distance (OID) for chest projections, a 72-inch (183-cm) source–image receptor distance (SID) is used to decrease the magnification of the heart and lung details.

Vascular Lung Markings. Vascular lung markings are scattered throughout the lungs and are evaluated for changes that may indicate pathology. To visualize these markings on chest projections, the lungs must be fully expanded. To obtain maximum lung aeration in a patient who is able to follow instructions, take the exposure after the second full inspiration. For the unconscious patient, observe the chest moving and take the exposure after the patient takes a deep breath.

Ventilated Patient. For the patient who is being ventilated with a conventional ventilator, observe the ventilator's pressure manometer to determine when full lung aeration has occurred. The exposure should be taken when the manometer digital bar or analog needle moves to its highest position. If a high-frequency ventilator is

being used, the exposure may be made at any time, because this ventilator maintains the lung expansion at a steady mean pressure without the bulk gas exchange of the conventional type.

Lung Conditions Affecting Vascular Lung Marking Visualization

Pneumothorax and Pneumectomy. A pneumothorax (Figure 3-1) or pneumectomy (Figure 3-2) may be indicated if no lung markings are present, whereas excessive lung markings may suggest conditions such as fibrosis, interstitial or alveolar edema, or compression of the lung tissue. When selecting the technical factors (mAs and kV) to be used for chest projections, if a pneumothorax is suspected, decrease the kV 8% from the routinely used setting (Table 3-1). When a pneumectomy is indicated, do not select the AEC chamber that is positioned beneath the removed lung or saturation of the opposite lung may be present (Figure 3-3).

Pleural Effusion. To demonstrate precise fluid levels when a pleural effusion is suspected, chest projections are taken with the patient upright and the x-ray beam horizontal. With this setup the air rises and the fluid gravitates to the lowest position, creating an air-fluid line or separation. This separation can be identified as an increase in brightness and an absence of lung markings on the projection wherever the denser fluid is present in the lung field (Figures 3-4).

If the patient is positioned only partially upright, the fluid line will slant, like water in a tilted jar. To demonstrate the true fluid line in this position, the CR must

Projection	kV*	Grid	AEC	mAs	SID
TABLE 3-1	**Chest Technical Data**				
Adult Chest Technical Data					
PA	110-125	Grid	Both outside		72 inches (183 cm)
Lateral	110-125	Grid	Center		72 inches (183 cm)
AP mobile	110-125			3	50-60 inches (125-150 cm)
AP supine in Bucky	80-100	Grid	Both outside		50-60 inches (125-150 cm)
AP-PA (lateral decubitus)	110-125	Grid	Center	3	72 inches (183 cm)
AP axial (lordotic)	110-125	Grid	Both outside		72 inches (183 cm)
AP-PA oblique	110-125	Grid	Over lung of interest		72 inches (183 cm)
Pediatric Chest Technical Data					
Neonate: AP	70-80			1	50-60 inches (125-150 cm)
Infant: AP	75-85			1.5	50-60 inches (125-150 cm)
Child: AP	75-85			2	50-60 inches (125-150 cm)
Child: PA	75-80	Grid**	Both outside		72 inches (183 cm)
Neonate: Cross-table lateral	75-85			2	50-60 inches (125-150 cm)
Infant: Cross-table lateral	80-90			3	50-60 inches (125-150 cm)
Child: Lateral	85-110	Grid**	Center		72 inches (180 cm)
Neonate: AP (lateral decubitus)	70-80			1	50-60 inches (125-150 cm)
Infant: AP (lateral decubitus)	75-85			1.5	50-60 inches (125-150 cm)
Child: AP (lateral decubitus)	85-110	Grid**	Center		72 inches (183 cm)

*kV listed is for digital radiography systems
**Use grid if patient part thickness measures 4 inches (10 cm) or more.

BOX 3-1	Chest Technical Data Imaging Analysis Guidelines

- The facility's identification requirements are visible.
- A right or left marker identifying the correct side of the patient is present on the projection and is not superimposed over the VOI.
- Good radiation protection practices are evident.
- Lung markings, diaphragm, heart borders, hilum, greater vessels, and bony cortical outlines are sharply defined.
- Contrast resolution is adequate to demonstrate the thoracic vertebrae, mediastinal structures, vascular lung markings throughout the lung field, fluid-air levels, and internal monitoring apparatus, when present.
- No quantum mottle or saturation is present.
- Scatter radiation has been kept to a minimum.
- There is no evidence of preventable artifacts, such as undergarments, necklaces, gown snaps, or removable external monitoring tubes or lines.

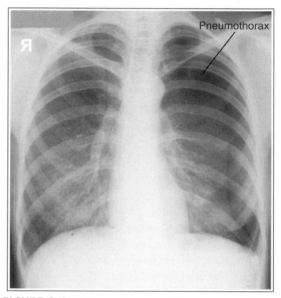

FIGURE 3-1 PA chest demonstrating a pneumothorax.

remain horizontal even though it will result in foreshortening of the chest structures in the AP and PA projections. When the patient is supine, the fluid is evenly spread throughout the lung field, preventing visualization of fluid levels in the AP projection because a horizontal beam cannot be used.

If pleural effusion is suspected, increase the mAs by 35% over the routinely used setting (Table 3-1).

Free Intraperitoneal Air. Along with the AP and AP lateral decubitus abdomen projections, the erect chest projection is also an excellent method of discerning the presence of free intraperitoneal (within abdominal cavity) air because it will closely outline the diaphragm (Figure 3-5). To demonstrate the air, when present, the exam must be taken with the patient upright and the CR horizontal.

Chest Devices, Tubes, Lines and Catheters. Familiarizing yourself with the accurate placement of the devices, lines, and catheters that are seen on chest projections will provide the information needed to understand when special care must be taken during positioning, and to identify when proper technique was used to visualize them and when poor placement is suspected (Table 3-2). Figure 3-6 demonstrates poor placement of the pulmonary arterial line, because it was not advanced to the pulmonary artery. When a chest projection is taken to determine the accuracy of line placement, it is within the technologist's scope of practice to inform the radiologist or attending physician immediately when a mispositioned device, line, or catheter is suspected.

Tracheostomy. The tracheotomy is a surgical procedure that creates an opening into the trachea to provide an airway. The distal tip of the tracheostomy tube should be positioned 1 to 2 inches (2.5-7 cm) from the tracheal bifurcation (carina). Projections are not taken

for placement of the tube, but it should be noted that when the patient has a tracheostomy special care needs to be taken when moving the patient so it does not come loose (Figure 3-7).

Endotracheal Tube. The endotracheal tube (ETT) is a large, stiff plastic, thick-walled tube inserted through the patient's nose or mouth into the trachea. It is used to manage the patient's airway, for mechanical

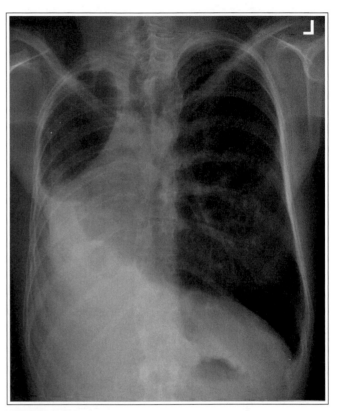

FIGURE 3-3 PA chest with right-sided pneumectomy taken with right AEC chamber activated.

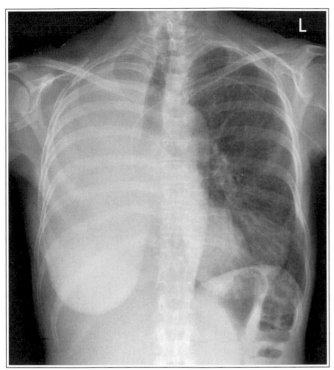

FIGURE 3-2 AP chest on patient with right-sided pneumectomy.

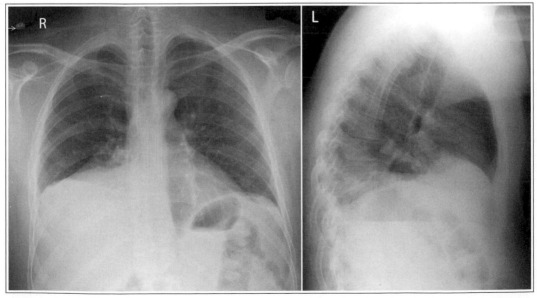

FIGURE 3-4 PA and lateral chest on patient with right-sided pleural effusion.

TABLE 3-2	Chest Devices, Tubes, Lines, and Catheters	
Device, Tube, or Catheter	**Desired Location**	**Brightness and Subject Contrast to Visualize:**
Tracheostomy	Distal tip is placed 1-2 inches superior to carina	Upper mediastinal region.
Endotracheal tube (ETT)	Distal tip is placed 1-2 inches superior to carina when patient's neck is in neutral position	Upper mediastinal region
Pleural drainage tube (chest tube)	Fluid drainage—located laterally within pleural space at level of the fifth or six intercostal space Air drainage—located anteriorly within pleural space at level of midclavicle	Radiopaque identification line and side hole interruption
Central venous catheter (CVC)	Inserted into subclavian or jugular vein and extends to superior vena cava, about 2.5 cm above right atrial junction	CVC within heart shadow
Umbilical artery catheter (umbilical artery catheter [UAC])	Inserted into umbilicus and coursed to midthoracic aorta (T6 to T9) or below level of renal arteries, at approximately L1 to L2	UAC on lateral chest projection adjacent to vertebral bodies
Umbilical vein catheter (UVC)	Inserted into umbilicus and advanced to junction of right atrium and inferior vena cava	UVC from umbilicus to heart
Pulmonary arterial catheter	Inserted into subclavian, internal or external jugular, or femoral vein and advanced through right atrium into pulmonary artery	Catheter within heart shadow
Pacemaker	Internal pacemaker implanted in subcutaneous fat in anterior chest wall and catheter tip(s) directed to right atrium or right ventricle	Pacemaker in lateral thorax and catheter tip(s) within heart shadow
Automatic implantable cardioverter defibrillator (ICD)	ICD is implanted in subcutaneous fat in anterior chest wall and catheter tip(s) directed to right atrium or right ventricle	ICD in lateral thorax and catheter tip(s) within heart shadow

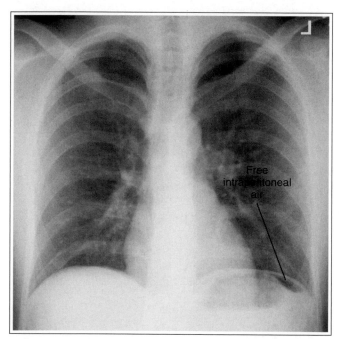

FIGURE 3-5 PA chest demonstrating free intraperitoneal air.

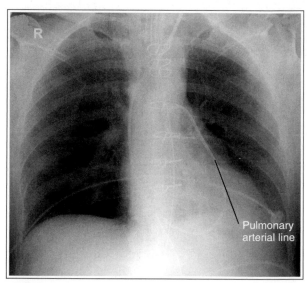

FIGURE 3-6 AP chest demonstrating poor pulmonary arterial line placement.

ventilation, and for suctioning. For adults, the distal tip of the ETT should be positioned 1 to 2 inches (2.5-7 cm) superior to the carina (Figure 3-8). For neonates, the distal tip of the ETT should reside between the thoracic inlet and carina, which is at the level of T4 on the neonate (Figure 3-9). With the distance from the thoracic inlet to the carina being minimal on a neonate, the position of this tube is critical to within a few millimeters.

When imaging for ETT placement, the patient's face should be facing forward and the cervical vertebrae in a neutral position. With head rotation and cervical vertebrae flexion and extension, the ETT tip can move superiorly and inferiorly about 2 cm, respectively, making it more uncertain whether the tube is positioned in the correct location. Too superior positioning of the tube

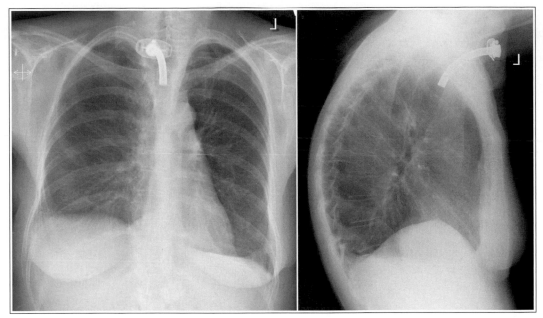

FIGURE 3-7 PA and lateral chest demonstrating tracheostomy placement.

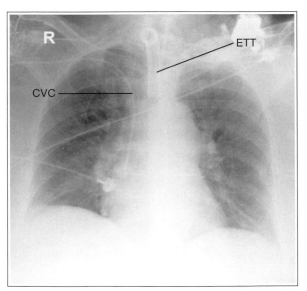

FIGURE 3-8 AP chest demonstrating accurate placement of an endotracheal tube (*ETT*) and central venous catheter (*CVC*).

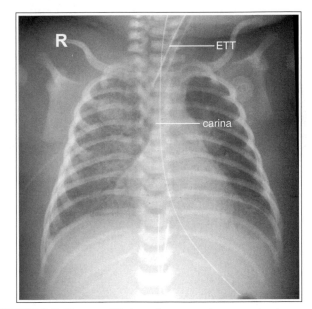

FIGURE 3-9 Neonate AP chest demonstrating accurate placement of an endotracheal tube (*ETT*).

may place it in the esophagus, and too inferior placement may place the tube in the right main bronchus, causing hyperinflation of the right lung and collapse of the left lung. Projections taken for ETT placement should demonstrate penetration of the upper mediastinal region, and the longitudinal collimation should remain open to the bottom of the lip to include the upper airway.

Pleural Drainage Tube. The pleural drainage tube is a 1.25-cm diameter thick-walled tube used to remove fluid or air from the pleural space that could result in atelectasis (collapse of the lung). For drainage of air (e.g., pneumothorax), the tube is placed anteriorly within the pleural space at the level of the midclavicle (Figures 3-10

and 3-11). For drainage of fluid (e.g., hemothorax or pleural effusion), the tube is placed laterally within the pleural space at the level of the fifth or six intercostal space. The side hole of the tube is marked by an interruption of the radiopaque identification line. Projections taken for pleural drainage tube placement should visualize the radiopaque identification line interruption at the side hole.

Central Venous Catheter. The central venous catheter (CVC) is a small (2- to 3-mm) radiopaque catheter used to allow infusion of substances that are too toxic for peripheral infusion, such as for chemotherapy, total parenteral nutrition, dialysis, or blood transfusions, and

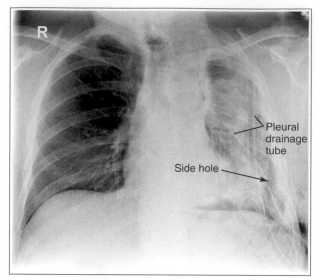

FIGURE 3-10 AP chest projection demonstrating accurate placement of two pleural drainage tubes.

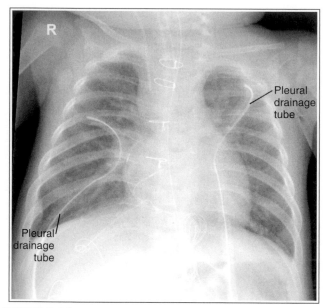

FIGURE 3-11 Infant AP chest demonstrating accurate placement of a pleural drainage tube in each lung.

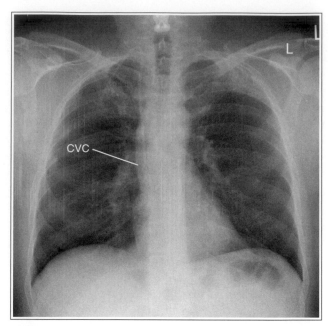

FIGURE 3-12 AP chest demonstrating accurate placement of a central venous catheter (*CVC*).

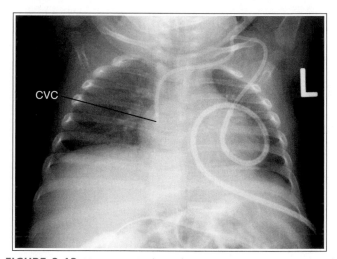

FIGURE 3-13 Neonate AP chest demonstrating accurate central venous catheter (*CVC*) placement.

to measure central venous pressure. The CVC is commonly inserted into the subclavian or jugular vein and extends to the superior vena cava, about 2.5 cm above the right atrial junction (Figures 3-12 and 3-13). Projections taken for CVC placement should visualize the CVC and any lung condition that might result if tissue perforation occurred during line insertion, such as pneumothorax or hemothorax.

Pulmonary Arterial Catheter (Swan-Ganz Catheter). The pulmonary arterial catheter is similar to the CVC catheter but it is longer. It is used to measure atrial pressures, pulmonary artery pressure, and cardiac output. The measurements obtained are used to diagnose ventricular failure and monitor the effects of specific medication, exercise, and stress on heart function. The pulmonary arterial catheter is inserted into the subclavian, internal or external jugular, or femoral vein and is advanced through the right atrium into the pulmonary artery (Figure 3-14). Projections taken for pulmonary arterial catheter placement should visualize the catheter and mediastinal structures to determine adequate placement.

Umbilical Artery Catheter. The umbilical artery catheter (UAC) is only seen in neonates because the cord has dried up and fallen off in older infants. The UAC is used to measure oxygen saturation. Optimal location for the UAC is in the midthoracic aorta (T6 to T9) or below the level of the renal arteries, at approximately L1 to L2.

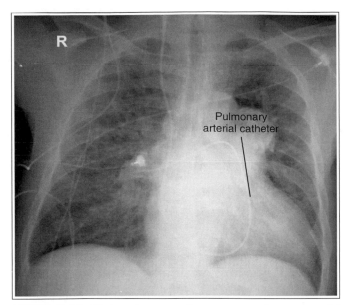

FIGURE 3-14 AP chest demonstrating accurate pulmonary arterial catheter placement.

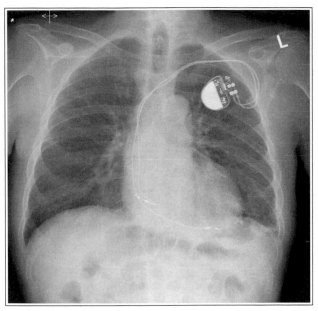

FIGURE 3-16 AP chest demonstrating accurate pacemaker placement, with optimal heart penetration.

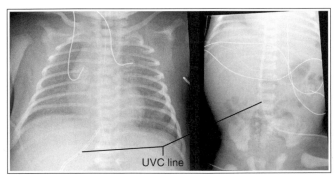

FIGURE 3-15 Neonate AP chest and abdomen demonstrating accurate placement of an umbilical vein catheter (*UVC*).

On a lateral chest projection, the UAC is seen to lie posteriorly adjacent to the vertebral bodies because it courses in the aorta.

Umbilical Vein Catheter. The umbilical vein catheter (UVC) is only seen in neonates, because the cord has dried up and fallen off in older infants. The UVC is used to deliver fluids and medications. The UVC courses anteriorly and superiorly to the level of the heart. The ideal location of the UVC is at the junction of the right atrium and inferior vena cava (Figure 3-15).

Pacemaker. The pacemaker is used to regulate the heart rate by supplying electrical stimulation to the heart. This electrical signal will stimulate the heart the needed amount to maintain an effective rate and rhythm. The internal pacemaker is surgically implanted in the subcutaneous fat in the patient's anterior chest wall below the clavicle and the catheter tip(s) directed to the right atrium or the right ventricle. On a PA or AP chest projection the pacemaker is typically seen laterally and the catheter tip(s) is seen in the heart shadow (Figure 3-16). Projections taken for pacemaker placement should

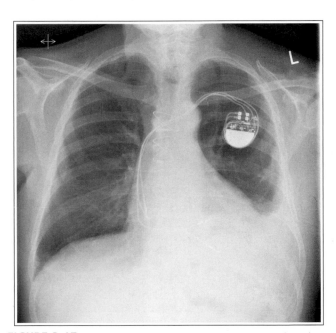

FIGURE 3-17 AP chest demonstrating accurate pacemaker placement, with poor heart penetration.

visualize the catheter tips through the mediastinal structures. Compare the difference in heart penetration and catheter tips visualization between the PA chests in Figures 3-16 and 3-17. Figure 3-16 is optimal. Because the pacemaker is inserted in the patient's upper thorax, care should be taken when lifting the arm of a patient whose pacemaker was inserted within 24 hours of the examination, because elevation may dislodge the pacemaker and catheter (Figure 3-18).

Automatic Implantable Cardioverter Defibrillator. The implantable cardioverter defibrillator (ICD) is implanted in the anterior chest wall, as with the

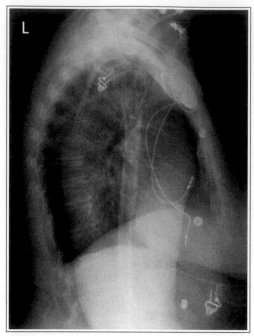

FIGURE 3-18 Lateral chest demonstrating accurate pacemaker placement and arm in chest.

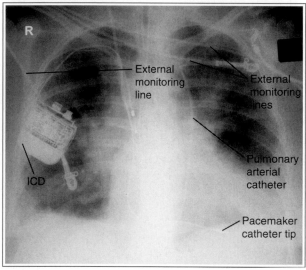

FIGURE 3-19 AP chest demonstrating accurate placement of implanted cardioverter defibrillator (*ICD*) and pulmonary arterial catheter.

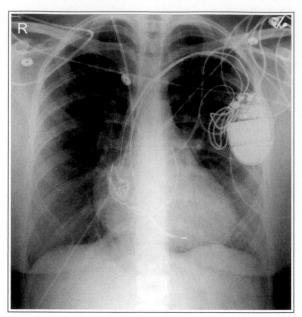

FIGURE 3-20 AP chest demonstrating removable external monitoring lines obscuring lung details.

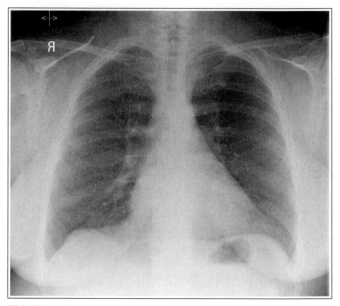

FIGURE 3-21 PA chest on patient with large pendulous breasts.

pacemaker, and the catheter tip(s) directed to the right atrium or the right ventricle. It is used to detect heart arrhythmias and then deliver an electrical shock to the heart to convert it to a normal rhythm. On a PA or AP chest projection the ICD is typically seen laterally and the catheter tip(s) is seen in the heart shadow (Figure 3-19).

External Monitoring Tubes and Lines. All external monitoring tubes or lines that can be removed or shifted out of the lung field should be. This includes oxygen tubing, electrocardiographic leads, external portions of nasogastric tubes, enteral feeding tubes, temporary pacemakers, and telemetry devices. Leaving these tubes and lines overlaying the lung field may result in obscuring important lung details (Figure 3-20).

CHEST: PA PROJECTION

See Table 3-3, (Figures 3-32 and 3-33).

Special Positioning Situations Dealing With Breasts

Large Pendulous Breasts. Large pendulous breasts may obscure the lung bases, as they add a dense thickness to this region of the lungs (Figure 3-21). This density is reduced by elevating and separating the breasts before resting the patient against the upright IR.

Nipple Shadows. The nipples on male and female patients can appear to be soft tissue masses. When in question the projection is repeated after attaching small lead markers on the nipples. These markers will identify the nipples from the overlapping lung tissue.

Singular Mastectomy. Special attention should be given to female patients who have had one breast removed. The side of the patient on which the breast was removed may need to be placed at a greater object–image receptor distance (OID) than the opposite side to prevent rotation (Figure 3-22).

Augmentation Mammoplasty. Augmentation mammoplasty (breast implants) is a surgical procedure to enhance the size and shape of a woman's breast. Women get breast implants for reconstructive purposes or cosmetic reasons. They are medical devices with a solid silicone, rubber shell that is filled with either saline solution or elastic silicone gel. Breast implants vary by filler, size, shape, diameter, and position on the chest and they are inserted directly under the breast tissue or beneath the chest wall muscle. On chest projections the breast implant may obscure the lung region that they are over, as they add a dense thickness to this region of the lungs (Figure 3-23).

Body Habitus and IR Placement. There are four types of body habitus to consider when determining the direction, crosswise (CW) or lengthwise (LW), that the IR cassette is positioned for a PA chest projection when using the computed radiography system—hypersthenic, sthenic, hyposthenic, and asthenic. The hypersthenic patient has a wide, short thorax, with a high diaphragm (Figure 3-24). This body habitus requires the IR to be placed CW for the PA chest projections to include the entire lung field. The asthenic patient has a long, narrow thoracic cavity, with a lower diaphragm (Figure 3-25). The sthenic and hyposthenic types of body habitus have thoracic cavities, with lengths and widths that are between those of the hypersthenic and asthenic body habitus (Figures 3-26 and 3-27). The sthenic, hyposthenic, and asthenic types of body habitus require the IR to be placed LW for the PA chest projections to include the entire lung field. This is not a consideration when using the digital radiography (DR) system because it uses a 17 × 17 inch (42.5 × 42.5 cm) IR, though it is useful information to use when determining how to more tightly collimate for the different body habitus.

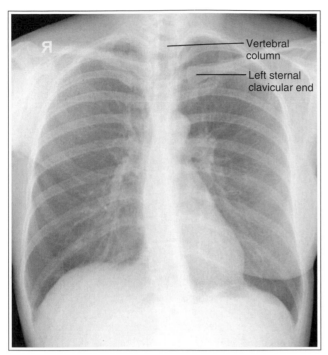

FIGURE 3-22 PA chest on patient with a right-sided mastectomy, with right side of chest rotated closer to IR than left side.

Vertebral column
Left sternal clavicular end

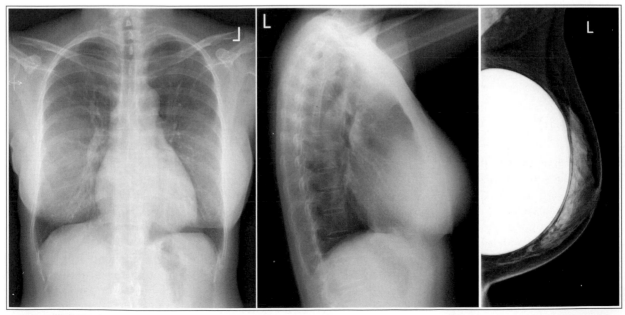

FIGURE 3-23 PA and lateral chest, and mammogram on same patient after augmentation mammoplasty.

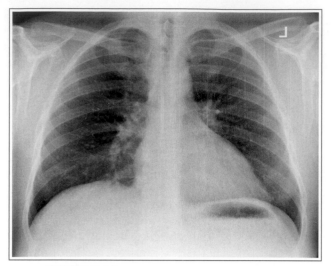

FIGURE 3-24 PA chest of hypersthenic patient.

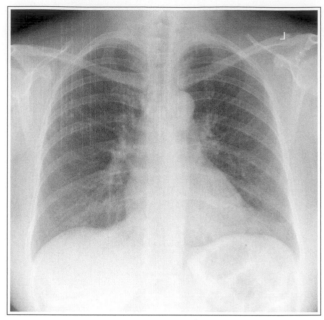

FIGURE 3-26 PA chest of sthenic patient.

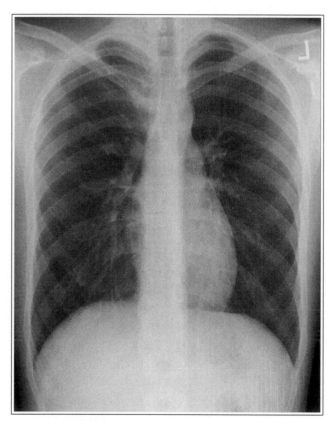

FIGURE 3-25 PA chest of asthenic patient.

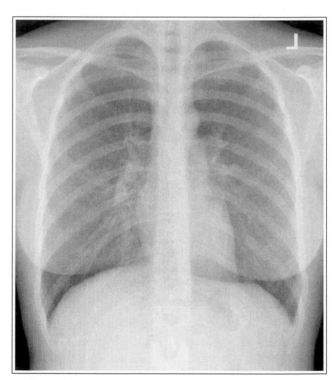

FIGURE 3-27 PA chest of hyposthenic patient.

Midcoronal Plane Positioning and Rotation. Positioning the midcoronal plane parallel with the IR prevents chest rotation in a PA Chest and demonstrates a projection with symmetrical lung fields, clavicles, and posterior ribs. A rotated chest demonstrates distorted mediastinal structures and creates an uneven brightness between the lateral borders of the chest. This brightness difference occurs because the x-ray beam traveled through less tissue on the chest side positioned away from the IR than on the side positioned closer to the IR. It may be detected when the chest has been rotated as little as 2 or 3 degrees. Because any variation in structural relationships or image brightness may represent a pathologic condition, the importance of providing nonrotated PA chest projections cannot be overemphasized.

Identifying Rotation. Rotation is readily detected on a PA chest by evaluating the distances between the vertebral column and the sternal ends of the clavicles and by comparing the lengths of the posterior ribs. On a nonrotated PA chest, these distances and lengths are

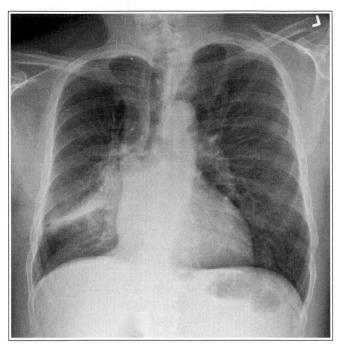

FIGURE 3-28 PA chest taken with left side of chest rotated closer to IR than right side.

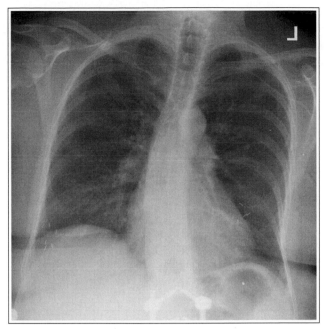

FIGURE 3-29 PA chest on patient with scoliosis.

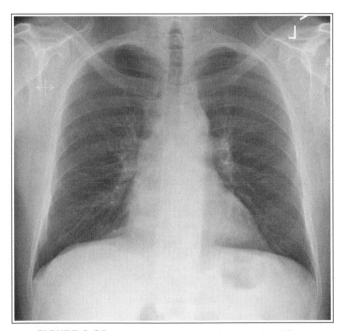

FIGURE 3-30 PA chest taken with elevated shoulders.

equal, respectively. On a rotated PA chest, the sternal clavicular end that demonstrates the least vertebral column superimposition and the side of the chest with the greatest posterior rib length represents the side of the chest positioned farthest from the IR (see Figures 3-22 and 3-28).

Distinguishing Scoliosis from Rotation. Scoliosis is a condition of the spine that results in the vertebral column curving laterally instead of remaining straight. Scoliosis can be distinguished from rotation by comparing the distance from the vertebral column to the lateral lung edges down the length of the lungs. On projections of a rotated patient, the distances are uniform down the length of the lung field, although when both lungs are compared, the distance is shorter on one side. If the patient has scoliosis, the vertebral column to lateral lung edge distances vary down the length of each lung and between each lung (Figure 3-29). The amount of distance variation increases with the severity of the scoliosis.

Clavicles. The lateral ends of the clavicles are positioned on the same horizontal plane as the medial clavicle ends by depressing the patient's shoulders. Accurate clavicle positioning lowers the lateral clavicles, positioning the middle and lateral clavicles away from the apical chest region and providing better visualization of the apical lung field. When a PA chest projection is taken without depression of the shoulders, the lateral ends of the clavicles are elevated, causing the middle and lateral clavicles to be demonstrated within the apical chest region (Figure 3-30).

Scapulae. When the scapulae are accurately positioned outside the lung field by rolling the elbows and shoulders anteriorly, the superolateral portion of the lungs is better visualized. If a chest projection is taken without shoulder protraction, the scapulae are seen superimposing the superolateral lung field (Figure 3-31). Scapular densities may prevent detection of abnormalities in the periphery of the lungs.

Many dedicated chest units provide holding bars for the patient's arms. When using these units, make certain that the shoulders are protracted. If the patient is unable to protract the shoulders while using the bars, position the patient's arms as described in Table 3-3.

Midcoronal Plane Tilting. The tilt of the superior midcoronal plane with the IR determines the relationship of the manubrium to the thoracic vertebrae level, the amount of apical lung field seen above the clavicles, and the degree of lung and heart foreshortening. When the

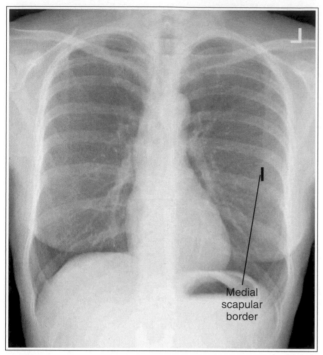

FIGURE 3-31 PA chest taken without shoulder protraction.

midcoronal plane is positioned parallel to the IR without tilting, the manubrium is positioned at the level of the fourth thoracic vertebra, approximately 1 inch (2.5 cm) of the apices is visible above the clavicles, and the lungs and heart are demonstrated without foreshortening.

Identifying Midcoronal Plane Tilting. If the superior midcoronal plane is tilted anteriorly (forward), as demonstrated in Figure 3-34, the lungs and heart are foreshortened, the manubrium is situated at the level of the fifth thoracic vertebra or lower, and more than 1 inch (2.5 cm) of the apices is demonstrated above the clavicles (Figure 3-35). This positioning error often occurs during imaging of women with pendulous breasts (see Figure 3-21) and patients with protruding abdomens. Conversely, if the superior midcoronal plane is tilted posteriorly (backward), as demonstrated in Figure 3-36, the lungs and heart are foreshortened, the manubrium is situated at a level between the first and third thoracic vertebrae, and less than 1 inch (2.5 cm) of the apices is demonstrated above the clavicles (Figure 3-37).

Distinguishing Midcoronal Plane Tilting from Poor Shoulder Depression. When a PA chest projection is taken with the patient's superior midcoronal plane tilted toward the IR, the clavicles are not always demonstrated horizontally but may be seen vertically, as seen on a projection that demonstrates poor shoulder depression. Distinguish poor shoulder depression from poor midcoronal plane positioning by measuring the amount of lung field visualized superior to the clavicles and

TABLE 3-3	PA Chest Projection	
Image Analysis Guidelines (Figure 3-32)		**Related Positioning Procedures (Figure 3-33)**
• Thoracic vertebrae and posterior ribs are seen through the heart and mediastinal structures.		• Appropriate technical data have been set.
• Lung fields demonstrate symmetry. • Distances from the vertebral column to the sternal clavicular ends are equal. • Lengths of the right and left corresponding posterior ribs are equal.		• *Computed radiography:* Use a 14 × 17 inch (35 × 43 cm) IR cassette, positioned CW/LW to fit the body habitus. • Center the chest to the upright IR in a PA projection. • Align the shoulders, the posterior ribs, and the ASISs at equal distances from the IR, aligning the midcoronal plane parallel with IR • Equally distribute the weight between feet.
• Mandible is not in the exposure field. • Clavicles are positioned on the same horizontal plane. • Scapulae are located outside the lung field.		• Elevate the chin, positioning it outside the collimated field. • Depress the shoulders. • Protract the shoulders by placing the back of the hands low enough on the hips that they are not in the collimated field and rotating the elbows and shoulders anteriorly, or use the imaging equipment holding bars.
• Chest is demonstrated without foreshortening. • Manubrium is superimposed by the fourth thoracic vertebra. • 1 inch (2.5 cm) of apical lung field is visible above the clavicles.		• Align the midcoronal plane vertical and parallel with the IR.
• Seventh thoracic vertebra is at the center of the exposure field.		• Center a horizontal CR to the midsagittal plane, at a level 7.5 inches (18 cm) inferior to the vertebra prominens.
• Both lungs, from apices to costophrenic angles, are included within the exposure field.		• Center the IR and grid to the CR. • Open the longitudinal collimation to include the inferior ribs. • Transversely collimate to within 0.5 inch (2.5 cm) of the patient's lateral skin line.
• At least 10 posterior ribs are visualized above the diaphragm.		• Take the exposure after the second full suspended inspiration.

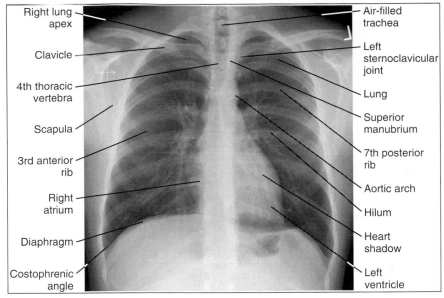

Right lung apex — Air-filled trachea

Clavicle — Left sternoclavicular joint

4th thoracic vertebra — Lung

Scapula — Superior manubrium

3rd anterior rib — 7th posterior rib

Right atrium — Aortic arch

— Hilum

Diaphragm — Heart shadow

Costophrenic angle — Left ventricle

FIGURE 3-32 PA chest projection with accurate positioning.

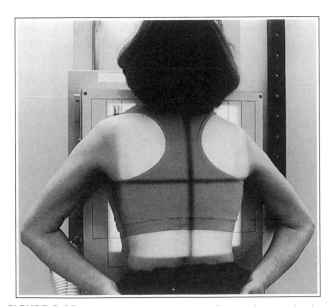

FIGURE 3-33 Proper patient positioning for PA chest projection.

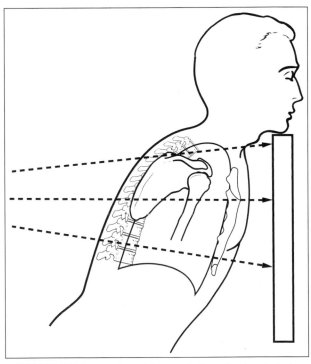

FIGURE 3-34 Superior midcoronal plane tilted anteriorly.

determining which vertebrae are superimposed over the manubrium. A projection with poor shoulder depression demonstrates decreased lung field superior to the clavicles and the manubrium at the level of the fourth vertebra (see Figure 3-30). A projection with the superior midcoronal plane tilting anteriorly demonstrates increased lung field superior to the clavicles and the manubrium at a level inferior to the fourth vertebra (see Figure 3-35).

Lung Aeration. On deep inspiration the lungs expand in three dimensions—transversely, anteroposteriorly, and vertically. It is the vertical dimension that will demonstrate the greatest expansion. During normal quiet breathing, the vertical dimension increases about 0.4 inches (1 cm). In high levels of breathing, as when we coax a patient into deep inspiration for a chest

projection, the vertical dimension can increase by as much as 4 inches (10 cm). This full vertical lung expansion is necessary to demonstrate the entire lung field. Imaging the patient in an upright position and encouraging a deep inspiration by taking the exposure at the end of the second full inspiration allow demonstration of the greatest amount of vertical lung field.

Maximum lung aeration is demonstrated on a PA chest projection when at least 10 posterior ribs are demonstrated above the diaphragm. Circumstances that may prevent full lung expansion include disease processes,

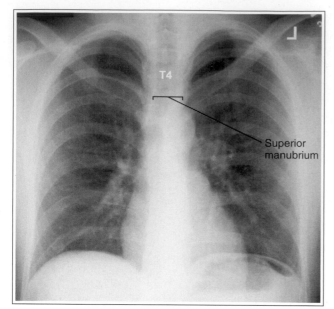

FIGURE 3-35 PA chest taken with superior midcoronal plane tilted anteriorly.

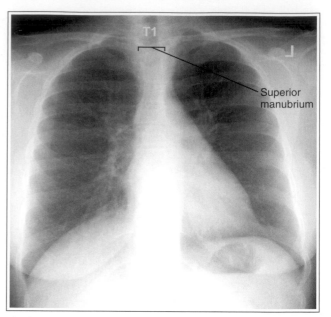

FIGURE 3-37 PA chest taken with superior midcoronal plane tilted posteriorly.

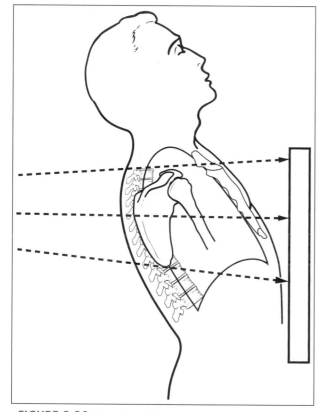

FIGURE 3-36 Superior midcoronal plane tilted posteriorly.

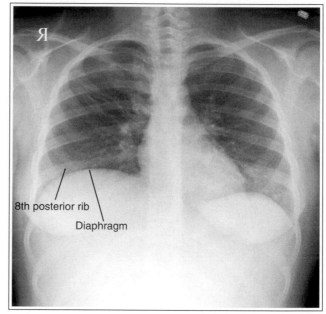

FIGURE 3-38 PA chest taken without full lung aeration.

advanced pregnancy, excessive obesity, being seated in a slouching position, and confining abdominal clothing.

Identifying Poor Lung Aeration. If fewer than 10 posterior ribs are demonstrated, the lungs were not fully inflated. Before repeating the procedure, attempt to obtain a deeper inspiration and determine whether a patient's condition might have caused the poor inhalation. Chest projections that are taken with inadequate

inspiration also demonstrate a wider appearing heart shadow and an increase in lung tissue brightness, because the decrease in air volume increases the concentration of pulmonary tissues (Figure 3-38).

Expiration Chest. Abnormalities such as a pneumothorax or foreign body may indicate the need for an expiration PA chest. For such a projection, all of the image analysis guidelines listed for an inspiration PA chest should be met except for the number of ribs demonstrated above the diaphragm. On an expiration PA chest, as few as nine posterior ribs may be demonstrated, the lungs are denser, and the heart shadow is broader and shorter. When manually setting technique, because of the increased lung tissue density it may be necessary to increase the exposure (mAs) when a PA chest is taken on expiration and lung details are of interest.

PA Chest Analysis Practice

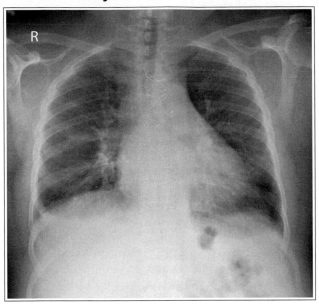

IMAGE 3-1

Analysis. The manubrium is situated at the level of the third thoracic vertebra, and less than 1 inch (2.5 cm) of the apices is demonstrated superior to the clavicles. The upper midcoronal plane was tilted posteriorly. Fewer than 10 posterior ribs are demonstrated above the diaphragm.

Correction. Move the patient's upper thorax toward the IR until the midcoronal plane is parallel with the IR and coax patient into a deeper inspiration by making the exposure after the second full inspiration.

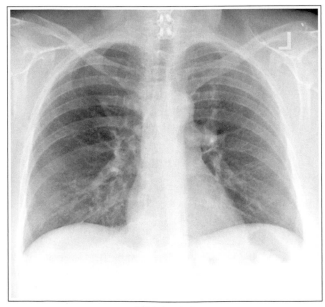

IMAGE 3-2

Analysis. The manubrium is situated at the level of the fifth thoracic vertebra, and more than 1 inch (2.5 cm) of

the apices is demonstrated superior to the clavicles. The upper midcoronal plane was tilted anteriorly.

Correction. Move the patient's upper thorax away from the IR until the midcoronal plane is vertical.

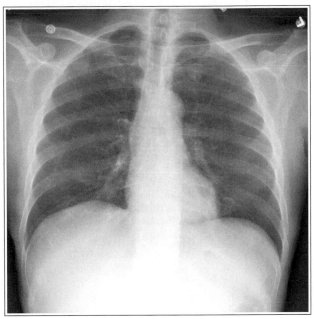

IMAGE 3-3

Analysis. The right sternal clavicular end is demonstrated farther from the vertebral column than the left. The right side of the chest was situated farther from the IR than the left side. The scapulae are in the lung fields. Fewer than 10 posterior ribs are demonstrated above the diaphragm.

Correction. Rotate the right side of the chest toward the IR until the midcoronal plane is parallel with the IR. Protract the shoulders by placing the back of the patient's hand on the hips and rotating the elbows and shoulders anteriorly, and coax patient into a deeper inspiration by making the exposure after the second full inspiration.

CHEST: LATERAL PROJECTION (LEFT LATERAL POSITION)

See Table 3-4, (Figures 3-39 and 3-40).

Anteroinferior Lung and Heart Visualization. The anteroinferior lung and heart region is most clearly defined when the patient is imaged in a standing position. If the patient is seated and leaning forward, the anterior abdominal tissue is compressed, obscuring the anteroinferior lung and the heart shadow; this is especially true in an obese patient (Figure 3-41). To best demonstrate this region on the seated patient, have the patient lean back slightly, allowing the anterior abdominal tissue to stretch out. Do not lean the patient so far back, however, that the posterior lungs are not on the projection. Consideration of patient condition dictates how the projection will be taken.

TABLE 3-4	Lateral Chest Projection
Image Analysis Guidelines (Figure 3-39)	**Related Positioning Procedures (Figure 3-40)**
• Anteroinferior lung and heart are well defined.	• *Computed radiography*: Use a 14 × 17 inch (35 × 43 cm) IR cassette, positioned LW. • Center the chest to the upright IR in a left lateral position.
• Right and left posterior ribs are nearly superimposed, demonstrating no more than a 0.5 inch (1 cm) of space between them. • Sternum is in profile. • Mandible is not in the exposure field. • Lungs are demonstrated without foreshortening, with nearly superimposed hemidiaphragms.	• Place the shoulders, the posterior ribs, and the ASISs directly in line with each other, with the midcoronal plane aligned perpendicular to the IR. • Elevate the chin, positioning it outside the collimated field. • Align the midsagittal plane parallel with the IR.
• No humeral soft tissue is seen superimposing the anterior lung apices.	• Place the humeri in an upright vertical position, with forearms crossed and resting on the patient's head, or use the imaging equipment holding bars.
• Midcoronal plane, at the level of the eighth thoracic vertebra, is at the center of the exposure field. • Entire lung field, including apices, costophrenic angles, and posterior ribs, is included within the exposure field.	• Center a horizontal CR to the midcoronal plane, at a level 8.5 inches (21.25 cm) inferior to the vertebra prominens. • Center the IR and grid to the CR. • Open the longitudinal collimation to include the inferior ribs. • Transversely collimate to within 0.5 inch (2.5 cm) of the patient's lateral skin line.
• Hemidiaphragms demonstrate a gentle, superiorly bowed contour and are inferior to the eleventh thoracic vertebra.	• Take the exposure after the second full suspended inspiration.

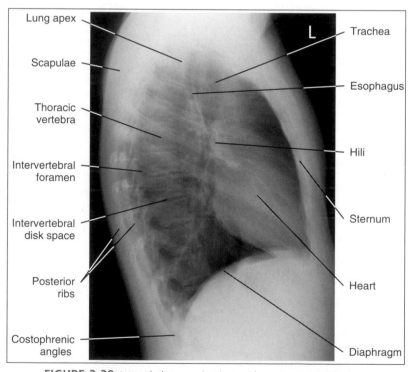

FIGURE 3-39 Lateral chest projection with accurate positioning.

Midcoronal Plane Positioning and Rotation. Placing the midcoronal plane perpendicular with the IR prevents patient rotation. In this position, because the right lung field and ribs are positioned at a greater OID than the left lung field and ribs, the right lung field and ribs are more magnified. This magnification prevents the right and left ribs from being directly superimposed on a lateral chest projection. Approximately a 0.5 inch (1 cm) separation is demonstrated between the right and left posterior ribs, with the right posterior ribs projecting behind the left (see Figure 3-39). When the posterior ribs are directly superimposed, this separation is demonstrated between the anterior ribs, but it is more difficult to distinguish.

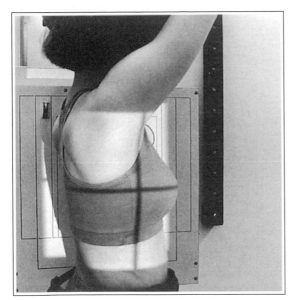

FIGURE 3-40 Proper patient positioning for lateral chest projection.

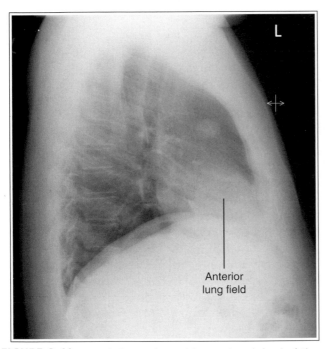

FIGURE 3-41 Lateral chest taken with anterior abdominal tissue compressing anteroinferior lungs.

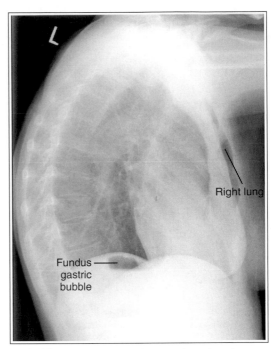

FIGURE 3-42 Lateral chest taken with right thorax rotated anteriorly.

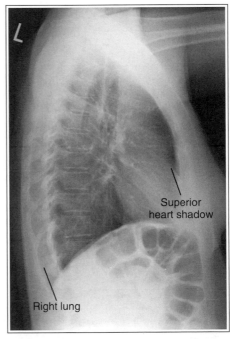

FIGURE 3-43 Lateral chest taken with right thorax rotated posteriorly.

Distinguishing the Right and Left Lungs. The first method of discerning the hemidiaphragm is to identify the gastric air bubble. On an upright patient, gas in the stomach rises to the fundus (superior section of stomach), which is located just beneath the left hemidiaphragm (Figure 3-42). If this gastric bubble is visible on the projection, you know that the left hemidiaphragm is located directly above it. The second method of distinguishing the lungs is to look for lung tissue that is anterior to the sternum (see Figure 3-42). This lung tissue shows when the right lung is rotated anteriorly, and is not

demonstrated when the left lung is rotated anteriorly (Figure 3-43). The reason for this is that the right lung is more magnified than the left because it is at a greater OID and it takes less rotation for the lung tissue to be seen anteriorly. The amount of rotation it would take to see the left lung tissue anterior to the sternum would be great enough that it would be identified during positioning. The third method of distinguishing one lung from

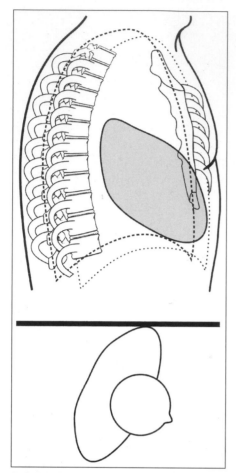

FIGURE 3-44 Rotation—left lung anterior.

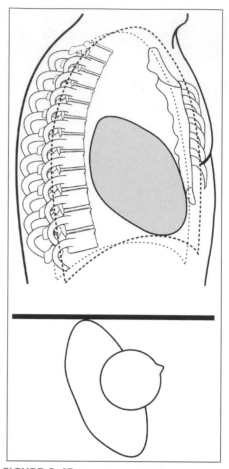

FIGURE 3-45 Rotation—right lung anterior.

the other uses the heart shadow. Because the heart shadow is located in the left chest cavity and extends anteroinferiorly to the left hemidiaphragm, outlining the superior heart shadow enables you to recognize the left lung. As demonstrated in Figure 3-44, if the left lung is positioned anteriorly, the outline of the superior heart shadow continues beyond the sternum and into the anterior lung (see Figure 3-43). Figure 3-45 demonstrates the opposite rotation; the right lung is positioned anteriorly. Note how the superior heart shadow does not extend into the anterior situated lung but ends at the sternum (see Figure 3-42). It is most common on rotated lateral chest projections for the left lung to be rotated anteriorly and the right lung to be rotated posteriorly.

Identifying Rotation. Chest rotation is effectively detected on a lateral chest by evaluating the degree of superimposition of the posterior ribs and anterior ribs. When more than 0.5 inch (1.25 cm) of space exists between the right and left posterior ribs, the chest was rotated for the projection. A rotated lateral chest obscures portions of the lung field and distorts the heart and hilum shadows. When a rotated lateral chest has been obtained, determine how to reposition the patient by identifying the hemidiaphragms and therefore the lungs.

Once the lungs have been identified, reposition the patient by rotating the thorax. When the left lung was anteriorly positioned on the original projection, rotate the left thorax posteriorly, and when the right lung was anteriorly positioned, rotate the right thorax posteriorly. Because both lungs move simultaneously, the amount of adjustment should be only half of the distance demonstrated between the posterior ribs.

Distinguishing Scoliosis from Rotation. On lateral chests of patients with spinal scoliosis, the lung field may appear rotated because of the lateral deviation of the vertebral column (Figure 3-46). The anterior ribs are superimposed, but the posterior ribs demonstrate differing degrees of separation, depending on the severity of scoliosis. View the accompanying PA chest projection to confirm this patient condition. Although the separation between the posterior ribs is not acceptable beyond 0.5 inch (1.25 cm) on a patient without scoliosis, it is acceptable on a patient with the condition.

Midsagittal Plane Positioning and Hemidiaphragm Visualization. To obtain a lateral chest without lung foreshortening, align the midsagittal plane parallel with the IR. When imaging a patient with broad shoulders and narrow hips, it may be necessary to place the hips

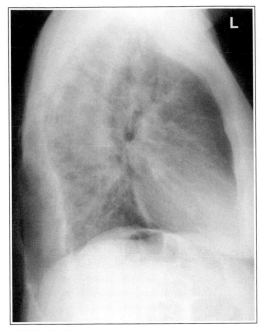

FIGURE 3-46 Lateral chest on patient with scoliosis.

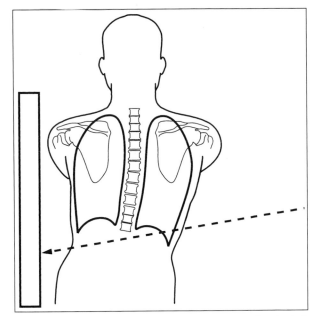

FIGURE 3-47 Lateral chest positioning with poor midsagittal plane and IR alignment.

away from the IR to maintain a parallel midsagittal plane. In 90% of persons the right lung and diaphragm are situated at a slightly higher elevation than the left lung and diaphragm. This elevation is caused by the liver, which is situated directly below the right diaphragm and prevents the right hemidiaphragm from lowering as far as the left hemidiaphragm. Because the right diaphragm is elevated, one might expect it to be demonstrated above the left diaphragm when the patient is imaged in a left lateral position, but this is not true when the midsagittal plane is correctly positioned. Because the anatomic part positioned farthest from the IR diverges and magnifies the most, the right lung will be projected and magnified more than the left lung, resulting in near superimposition of the two hemidiaphragms. When the midsagittal plane has not been positioned parallel with the IR, lung foreshortening and poor hemidiaphragm positioning occur.

Figure 3-47 demonstrates lateral chest positioning in which the patient's shoulders and hips were both resting against the IR, causing the inferior midsagittal plane to tilt toward the IR. This positioning projects the right hemidiaphragm inferior to the left (Figure 3-48). When a projection has been obtained that demonstrates the right hemidiaphragm situated inferior to the left, determine how the patient was mispositioned by using one of the methods described earlier to distinguish the right lung from the left lung. Before retaking a lateral chest because of this, scrutinize the patient's accompanying PA projection to determine whether the patient is one of the 10% of those whose hemidiaphragms are at the same height or whether a pathologic condition is causing

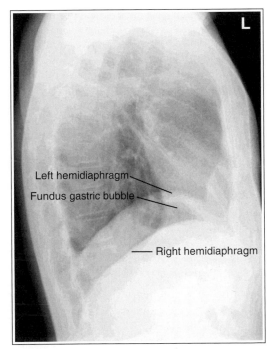

FIGURE 3-48 Lateral chest taken with inferior midsagittal plane tilted toward IR.

the left hemidiaphragm to be projected above the right (Figure 3-49).

Right Versus Left Lateral Chest Projection. A left lateral chest and right lateral chest have two distinct differences, the size of the heart shadow and the superimposition of the hemidiaphragms. Both differences are a result of a change in OID and magnification. For a right

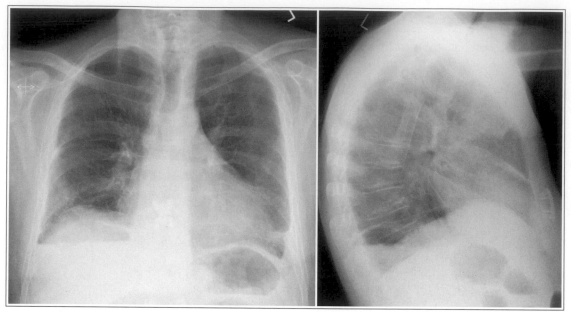

FIGURE 3-49 PA and lateral chest with accurate positioning that demonstrates hemidiaphragms at different levels due to a pathological condition.

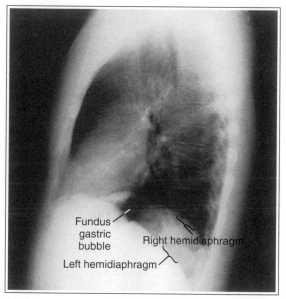

FIGURE 3-50 Right lateral chest projection with accurate positioning.

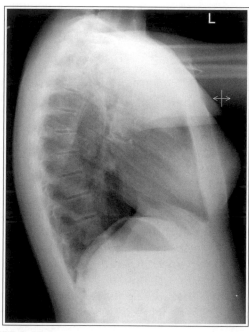

FIGURE 3-51 Lateral chest taken with humeri not elevated.

lateral, the right thorax is positioned closer to the IR. In this position, any anatomic structures located in the right thorax are magnified less than structures located in the left thorax because of the difference in OID. Radiographically, the heart shadow is more magnified and the left hemidiaphragm projects lower than the right hemidiaphragm (Figure 3-50). One advantage of obtaining a right rather than a left lateral chest is the increase in right lung radiographic detail that results from positioning of the right lung closer to the IR.

Arm Positioning and Anterior Lung Visualization. Accurate arm positioning prevents superimposition of the humeral soft tissue over the anterior lung apices (Figure 3-51). Many dedicated chest units provide holding bars for the patient's arms. When they are used, make sure that the humeri are placed high enough to

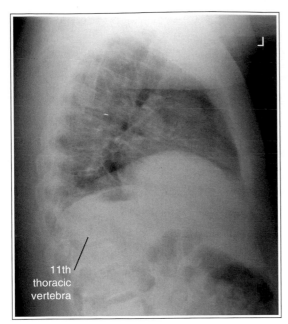

FIGURE 3-52 Lateral chest without full lung aeration.

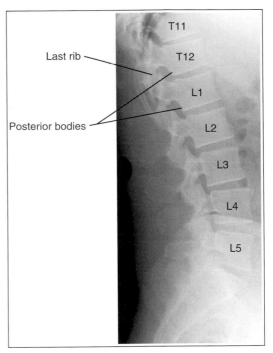

FIGURE 3-53 Identifying the twelfth thoracic vertebra.

prevent this soft tissue overlap. If the holding bars cannot be raised high enough and the patient is able to prevent motion, position the patient's humeri in an upright vertical position with the forearms crossed and resting on the patient's head.

Maximum Lung Aeration. Full lung aeration has been accomplished when the hemidiaphragms are inferior to the eleventh thoracic vertebra. When a lateral chest demonstrates the hemidiaphragms with an exaggerated cephalic bow, in addition to a portion of the eleventh thoracic vertebra inferior to the hemidiaphragms in a patient with no condition to have caused such a projection, full lung aeration has not been accomplished (Figure 3-52). Repeat the procedure with a deeper patient inspiration. The lungs must be fully inflated for lung markings to be evaluated. Chest projections taken on expiration may also demonstrate an increase in brightness, because a decrease in air volume increases the concentration of pulmonary tissues.

Identifying the Eleventh Thoracic Vertebra. The eleventh thoracic vertebra can be identified by locating the twelfth thoracic vertebra, which has the last rib attached to it, and counting up one. To confirm this finding, evaluate the curvature of the posterior aspect of the thoracic and lumbar bodies. The thoracic curvature is kyphotic (forward curvature) and the lumbar curvature is lordotic (backward curvature). Follow the posterior vertebral bodies of the lower thoracic and upper lumbar vertebrae, watching for the subtle change in curvature from kyphotic to lordotic. The twelfth thoracic vertebra is located just above this change (Figure 3-53). On most fully aerated adult lateral chest projections, the diaphragms are demonstrated dividing the body of the twelfth thoracic vertebra.

Lateral Chest Analysis Practice

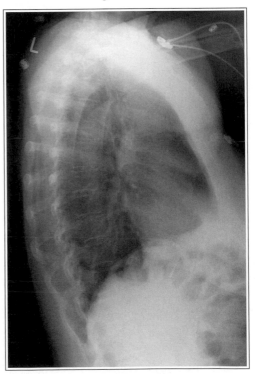

IMAGE 3-4

Analysis. The right and left posterior ribs are separated by more than 0.5 inch (1.25 cm), indicating that the chest was rotated. Lung tissue is not demonstrated anterior to the sternum. The patient was positioned with the left thorax rotated anteriorly and the right thorax rotated posteriorly. The humeral soft tissue shadows are obscuring the anterior lung apices.

Correction. Position the right thorax anteriorly. The amount of movement should be only half the distance between the posterior ribs. Have the patient raise the arms until the humeri are vertical, removing them from the exposure field.

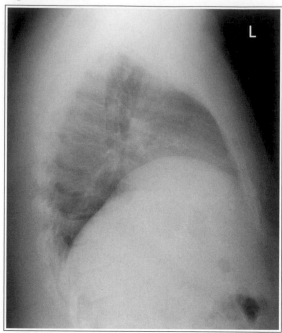

IMAGE 3-5

Analysis. The eleventh thoracic vertebra is demonstrated inferior to the hemidiaphragms. The projection was not taken after full inspiration.

Correction. Coax patient into a deeper inspiration by making the exposure after the second full inspiration.

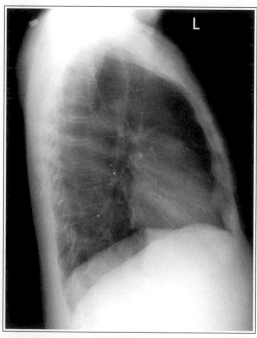

IMAGE 3-6

Analysis. The hemidiaphragms are not superimposed.
Correction. Scrutinize the patient's accompanying PA projection carefully. Determine whether the diaphragms

are at the same height or whether a pathologic condition might have caused one diaphragm to be projected above the other. If no such condition is evident, shift the patient's hips away from the IR until the midsagittal plane is parallel with the IR before repeating the projection.

CHEST: AP PROJECTION (SUPINE OR WITH PORTABLE X-RAY UNIT)

See Table 3-5, (Figures 3-54 and 3-55).
Demographic and Positioning Data. Patients in intensive care units often have mobile chest projections taken on a daily basis that are compared for subtle changes. Consistent positioning is important to ensure that the subtle changes are not caused by poor positioning or technical factors, but is difficult to obtain when follow-up projections are performed by multiple technologists. Consistency can best be accomplished through proper documentation. To do this, radiology departments have ways to electronically annotate the information on the projection or in the patient's records. At a minimum, the information should include the date and time of examination, the SID used, the degree of patient elevation, and the technical factors used. The technologists should review this information prior to obtaining a subsequent chest projection.

Heart Magnification and SID. The 48- to 50-inch (120- to 125-cm) SID used for AP chest projections, compared to the 72-inch (180-cm) used for routine PA chest projections, results in projections that demonstrate greater heart magnification owing to the increase in x-ray divergence caused by using the shorter SID. The SID is often estimated during mobile procedures, but if available, a tape measure should be used to maintain appropriate SID, providing consistency in magnification and reducing the need to adjust technical factors.

AP Versus PA Projection. The AP projection will also demonstrate increased heart magnification compared to a PA projection because the heart is positioned closer to the IR.
Body Habitus and IR Placement. The hypersthenic patient has a wide, short thorax with a high diaphragm (see Figure 3-24) and requires the IR to be placed CW for the AP chest projections to include the entire lung field. The sthenic, hyposthenic, and asthenic types have longer and narrower thoracic cavities with lower diaphragms and require the IR to be placed LW to include the entire lung field (see Figures 3-25, 3-26, and 3-27).
Side-to-Side CR Alignment. In the AP chest projection chest rotation is caused by poor IR balance or poor side to side (lateral) CR alignment. To prevent chest rotation, align the IR and the midcoronal plane parallel with the bed (Figure 3-55). On beds with special padding, it may be necessary to place positioning aids (sponges) beneath different aspects of the IR to level it and place it parallel in both the transverse and longitudinal axes. Then angle

TABLE 3-5	AP Chest Projection (Supine or Portable)
Image Analysis Guidelines (Figure 3-54)	**Related Positioning Procedures (Figure 3-55)**
• Universal precautions where followed.	• Clean x-ray machine before exiting patient room. • Use appropriate personal coverings. • Cover IR with plastic bag or pillow case.
• Thoracic vertebrae and posterior ribs are faintly seen through the heart and mediastinal structures.	• Appropriate technical data have been set.
• Date and time of examination, SID used, degree of patient elevation, and technical factors used are recorded on the projection.	• Record the required data.
• Lung fields demonstrate symmetry. • Distances from the vertebral column to the sternal clavicular ends are equal. • Lengths of the right and left corresponding posterior ribs are equal.	• Position the patient in an upright, seated AP projection. • Center a 14 × 17 inch (35 × 43 cm) IR cassette or digital plate, CW/LW beneath the chest to fit the body habitus. • Align the IR and midcoronal plane parallel with the bed. • Align the front face of the collimator parallel with the IR.
• Chest is demonstrated without foreshortening. • Manubrium is superimposed by the fourth thoracic vertebra. • 1 inch (2.5 cm) of apical lung field visible above the clavicles. • Posterior ribs demonstrate a gentle superiorly bowed contour.	• Align the CR perpendicular to the IR.
• Mandible is not in the exposure field. • Clavicles are positioned on the same horizontal plane. • Scapulae are located outside the lung field, when possible.	• Elevate the chin out of collimated field. • Depress the shoulders. • Place the back of the hands on the hips and rotate the elbows and shoulders anteriorly if possible.
• Seventh thoracic vertebra is at the center of the exposure field.	• Center the CR to the midsagittal plane at a level 4 inches (10 cm) inferior to the jugular notch.

• Both lungs, from apices to costophrenic angles, are included within the exposure field.	• Longitudinally collimate:
	  • *LW IR:* to include the inferior ribs.
	  • *CW IR:* to within 0.5 inch (2.5 cm) of the lateral skin line.
	• Transversely collimate:
	  • *LW IR:* to within 0.5 inch (2.5 cm) of the lateral skin line.
	  • *CW IR:* to include the inferior ribs.

• No anatomical artifacts or removable lead wires are seen.	• Move the arms and any movable lead wires outside the collimation field (Figure 3-63).
• At least 9 posterior ribs are visualized above the diaphragm	• Take the exposure after the second full suspended inspiration.

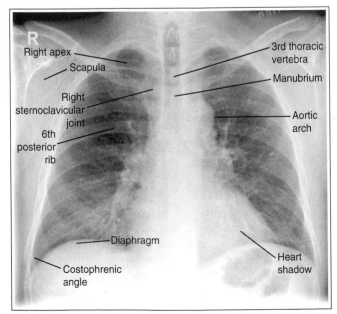

FIGURE 3-54 AP chest projection with accurate positioning.

Right apex
Scapula
Right sternoclavicular joint
6th posterior rib
Diaphragm
Costophrenic angle
3rd thoracic vertebra
Manubrium
Aortic arch
Heart shadow

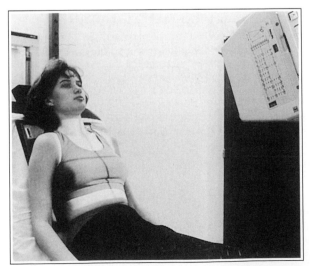

FIGURE 3-55 Proper patient positioning for AP chest projection.

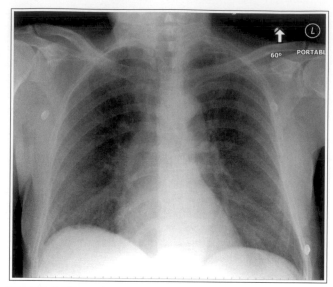

FIGURE 3-56 AP chest taken with right side positioned too close to bed and too far from collimator.

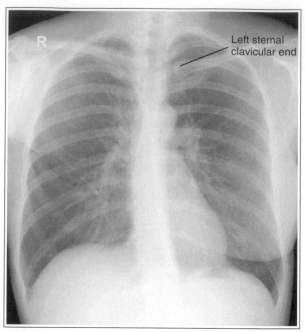

FIGURE 3-57 AP chest taken with left side positioned too close to bed and too far from collimator.

the CR until it is perpendicular to the IR. Once the procedure has been set up, the technologist needs to evaluate whether the collimator's face is parallel with the IR and midcoronal plane to make certain that the CR is not angled laterally. This is best judged by observing from behind the x-ray tube, looking straight at the patient.

Identifying Side-to-Side CR Alignment with IR. Rotation is identified on an AP chest by evaluating the distances between the vertebral column and the sternal ends of the clavicles and by comparing the lengths of the posterior ribs. When the right sternal clavicular end demonstrates no superimposition of the vertebral column and the right posterior ribs demonstrate greater length than the left, the patient's right side was placed closer to the bed and farther from the collimator's face than the left side (Figure 3-56). When the right sternal clavicular end is seen superimposing the vertebral column and the right side demonstrates less posterior rib length than the left, the patient's right side was placed farther from the bed and closer to the collimator's face than the left (Figure 3-57).

Cephalic-Caudal CR Alignment. The cephalic-caudal alignment of the CR with respect to the patient determines the relationship of the manubrium to the thoracic vertebrae, the amount of apical lung field seen above the clavicles, and the contour of the posterior ribs. For accurate alignment of this anatomy, position the CR perpendicular to the patient's midcoronal plane. Inaccurate CR angulation misaligns this anatomy and distorts the heart and lung structures.

Identifying Poor CR and Midcoronal Plane Alignment. The anatomic structures positioned farthest from the IR will move the greatest distance when the CR is angled, so angling the CR caudally for an AP chest projection moves the manubrium inferior to the fourth thoracic vertebra, demonstrating more than 1 inch (2.5 cm)

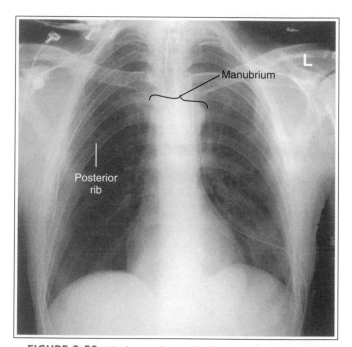

FIGURE 3-58 AP chest taken with CR angled too caudally.

of lung apices superior to the clavicles, and changes the posterior rib contour to vertical. A caudal angle also elongates the heart and lung structures (Figure 3-58). Angling the CR cephalically projects the manubrium superior to the fourth thoracic vertebra, demonstrating less than 1 inch (2.5 cm) of lung apices superior to the clavicles, and changes the posterior rib contour to horizontal. A cephalic angle also foreshortens the heart and lung structures (Figure 3-59). The more the angulation is mispositioned, either caudally or cephalically, the more distorted the anatomy.

Spinal Kyphosis. The thoracic spine demonstrates kyphosis (convex curves, posteriorly). This curve can become exaggerated to get the impression of rounded shoulders (expression for mild kyphosis) or a rounded back or hunchback (expressions for severe kyphosis). This condition can be caused by poor posture and ergonomics, an injury, collapsed vertebra, and degenerative changes. The kyphotic patient's increase in spinal convexity prevents the upper midcoronal plane from being straightened and positioned parallel with the IR and the patient from extending the neck enough to position parts of the mandible and face superior to the apices and outside of the collimated field. As a result, AP/PA chest projections obtained with the patient positioned as close to the routine for the projection as the patient can accommodate will demonstrate the manubrium situated inferior to the fourth thoracic vertebrae and the chin and apices superimposing (Figure 3-60). There are alternative positioning methods to better demonstrate the apices on a kyphotic patient. One method keeps the midcoronal plane parallel with the IR and uses a 5- to 10-degree cephalic CR angulation. This angle will project the chin and manubrium cephalically and demonstrate the posterior ribs similar to those on a nonkyphotic chest projection. The second method is to lean the patient's shoulders and upper thoracic vertebrae back to place the midcoronal plane at an angle with the IR and use a horizontal CR (Figure 3-61). Do note that the chest demonstrates foreshortening with these methods.

Supine Patient. For the supine AP chest projection, the patient's kyphotic thoracic vertebrae are forced to extend slightly, straightening because of the body weight and gravitational pull on them. This straightening causes the anterior thoracic cage, with the manubrium and clavicles, to move superiorly and results in the projection demonstrating less than 1 inch (2.5 cm) of apical lung field superior to the clavicles (Figure 3-62). Placing a 5-degree caudal angle on the CR can offset this.

Clavicle. When the patient's condition allows, position the lateral ends of the clavicles on the same horizontal plane as the medial ends by depressing the shoulders. Accurate positioning of the clavicles lowers the lateral ends of the clavicles, positioning the middle and lateral clavicles away from the apical chest region and improving visualization of the apical lung field. If the patient is unable to depress his or her shoulders, the middle and lateral ends of the clavicles will be seen in the apical chest region (Figure 3-63).

Scapulae. To position most of the scapulae outside the lung field, place the back of the hands low enough on

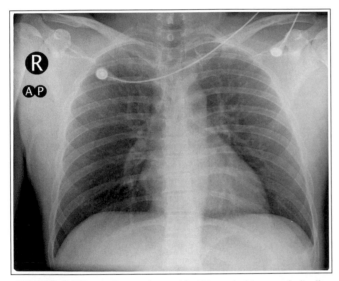

FIGURE 3-59 AP chest taken with CR angled too cephalically.

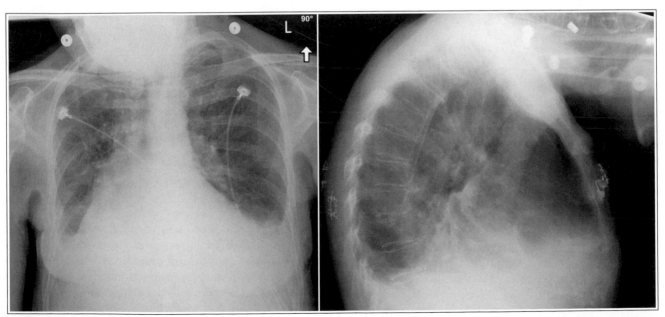

FIGURE 3-60 AP and lateral chest on patient with spinal kyphosis taken with midcoronal plane parallel with IR and CR perpendicular.

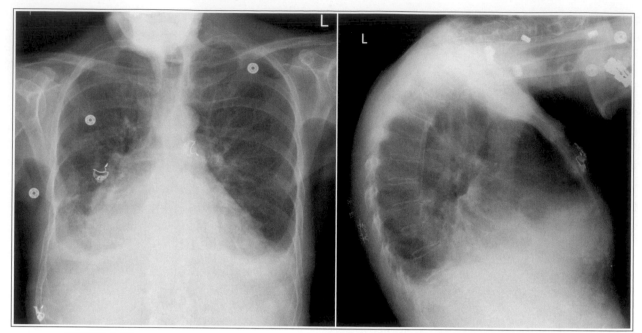

FIGURE 3-61 AP and lateral chest on patient with spinal kyphosis taken with midcoronal plane tilted with IR and CR perpendicular.

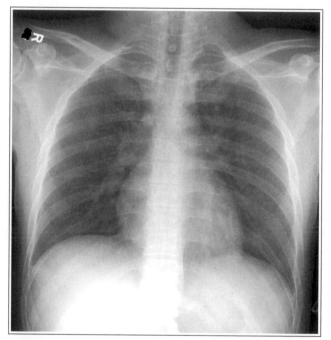

FIGURE 3-62 Supine AP chest projection with accurate positioning.

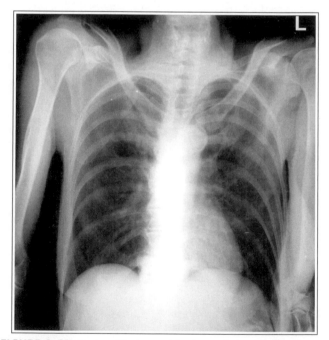

FIGURE 3-63 Supine AP chest with elevated shoulders and arms in the exposure field.

the hips so they are not in the collimated field and rotate the elbows and shoulders anteriorly. Most patients who require mobile or supine chest projections are incapable of positioning their arms in this manner, resulting in a projection with the scapulae positioned in the lung field. In such a situation, abduct the patient's arms until they are placed outside the imaging field to prevent unnecessary exposure to them (see Figure 3-62).

Lung Aeration. In a supine or seated patient the diaphragm is unable to shift to its lowest position because the abdominal organs are compressed and push against the diaphragm. As a result, adequate lung aeration for an AP chest has resulted when at least 9 posterior ribs are demonstrated above the diaphragm. If fewer than nine posterior ribs are demonstrated, lung expansion is not acceptable (Figure 3-64).

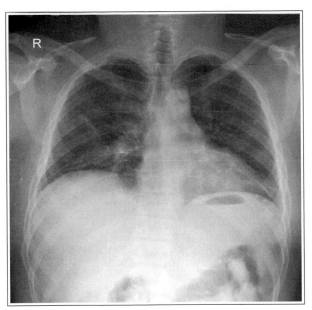

FIGURE 3-64 AP chest without full lung aeration.

AP Chest (Portable) Analysis Practice

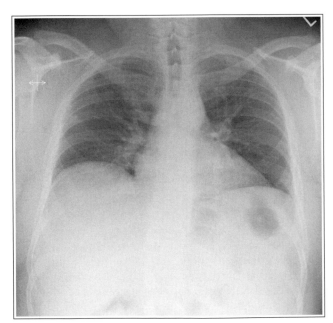

IMAGE 3-7

Analysis. Only eight posterior ribs are demonstrated above the diaphragm. The clavicles are not horizontal.
Correction. If the patient's condition allows, take the exposure after coaxing the patient into a deeper inspiration or at the point at which the ventilator indicates the greatest lung expansion. Depress the shoulders.

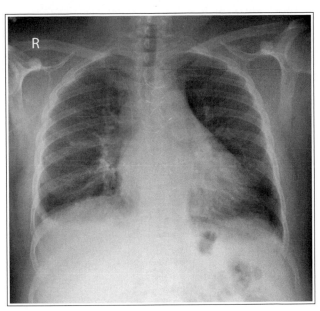

IMAGE 3-8

Analysis. The manubrium is superimposed over the third thoracic vertebra, and less than 1 inch (2.5 cm) of apical lung field is visible above the clavicles. The posterior ribs demonstrate a horizontal contour. The CR was angled cephalically.
Correction. Adjust the CR angulation caudally until it is aligned perpendicular to the midcoronal plane.

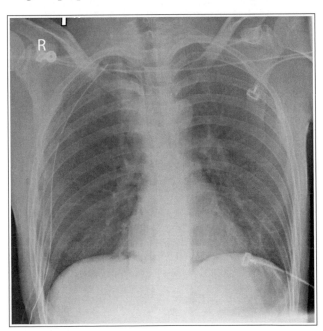

IMAGE 3-9

Analysis. The manubrium is inferior to the fourth thoracic vertebra, more than 1 inch (2.5 cm) of lung apices is demonstrated superior to the clavicles, and the posterior rib contour is vertical. The CR was angled too caudally.
Correction. Adjust the CR angulation cephalically until it is aligned perpendicular to the midcoronal plane.

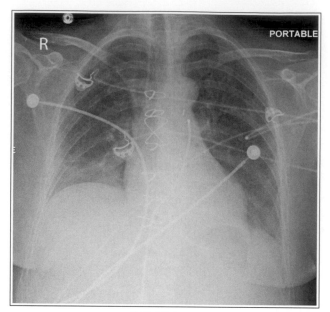

IMAGE 3-10

Analysis. The right sternal clavicular end demonstrated farther from the vertebral column than the left. The right side of the patient and IR were placed closer to the bed and farther from the collimator's face than the left side. The manubrium is inferior to the fourth thoracic vertebra, more than 1 inch (2.5 cm) of lung apices is demonstrated superior to the clavicles, and the posterior rib contour is vertical. The CR was angled too caudally.

Correction. Elevate the right side of the patient and IR or adjust the CR angle toward the left side of the patient until the collimator's face is parallel with the IR and CR is perpendicular to the IR. Adjust the CR angulation cephalically until it is aligned perpendicular to the mid-coronal plane.

CHEST: AP OR PA PROJECTION (RIGHT OR LEFT LATERAL DECUBITUS POSITION)

See Table 3-6, (Figures 3-65 and 3-66).

Positioning to Demonstrate Air or Fluid Levels. The lateral decubitus position is primarily used to confirm the presence of a pneumothorax or pleural effusion in the pleural cavity.

To best demonstrate the presence of a pneumothorax, position the affected side of the thorax away from the table or cart so that the air rises to the highest level in the pleural cavity. If the affected side were placed against the table or cart, the air might be obscured by the mediastinal structures.

TABLE 3-6	AP-PA (Lateral Decubitus) Chest Projection
Image Analysis Guidelines (Figure 3-65)	**Related Positioning Procedures (Figure 3-66)**
• Thoracic vertebrae and posterior ribs are seen through the heart and mediastinal structures.	• Appropriate technical data have been set.
• An arrow or "word" marker identifies the side of the patient positioned up and away from the imaging table or cart.	• Place proper marker on IR.
• Lung field adjacent to the table or cart is demonstrated without superimposition of pad.	• Position the side of the patient that best demonstrates the suspected condition closest to the table or cart, on a radiolucent sponge or a hard surface in a lateral recumbent position.
• Lung field demonstrates symmetry. • Distances from the vertebral column to the sternal clavicular ends are equal. • Lengths of the right and left corresponding posterior ribs are equal.	• *Computed radiography:* Use a 14 × 17 inch (35 × 43 cm) IR cassette, positioned CW/LW to fit the body habitus. • Center chest to the upright IR in an AP or PA projection. • Align the shoulders, the posterior ribs, and the ASISs at equal distances with the IR, aligning the midcoronal plane parallel with the IR. • Flex knees and place a pillow between them to help maintain position.
• Chest is demonstrated without foreshortening. • Manubrium is superimposed by the fourth thoracic vertebra.	• Align the midcoronal plane parallel with the IR.
• Arms, lateral borders of the scapulae, and mandible are situated outside the lung field. • Lateral aspects of the clavicles are projected upward.	• Reach the patient's arms above the head. • Elevate the chin.
• Seventh thoracic vertebra is at the center of the exposure field.	• *AP:* Center a horizontal CR to the midsagittal plane at a level 4 inches (10 cm) inferior to the jugular notch. • *PA:* Center a horizontal CR to the midsagittal plane at a level 7.5 inches (18 cm) inferior to the vertebra prominens.
• Both lungs, from apices to costophrenic angles, are included within the exposure field.	• Center IR and grid to CR. • Open the collimation to include the inferior ribs and to within 0.5 inch (2.5 cm) of the patient's lateral skin line.
• At least 9 posterior ribs are visualized above the diaphragm.	• Take the exposure after the second full suspended inspiration. The patient's recumbent position will prevent full lung aeration.

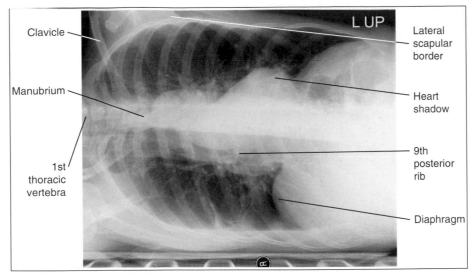

FIGURE 3-65 AP (right lateral decubitus) chest projection with accurate positioning.

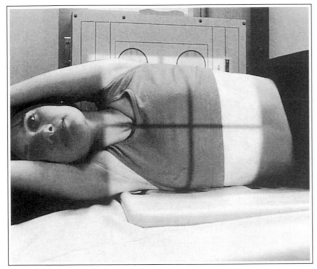

FIGURE 3-66 Proper patient positioning for AP (right lateral decubitus) chest projection.

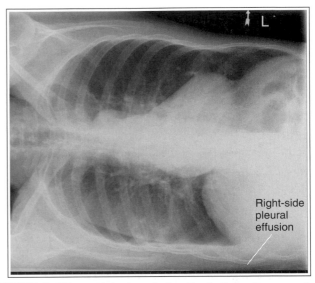

FIGURE 3-67 AP (right lateral decubitus) chest demonstrating right-sided pleural effusion.

To best demonstrate pleural effusion, position the affected side against the table or cart. This positioning allows the fluid to gravitate to the lowest level of the pleural cavity, away from the mediastinal structures (Figure 3-67).

Cart Pad Artifact. Elevating the patient on a radiolucent sponge or on a hard surface, such as a cardiac board, prevents the chest from sinking into the table or cart pad. When the patient's thorax is allowed to sink into the pad, artifact lines are seen superimposed over the lateral lung field of the side placed against the pad. Because fluid in the pleural cavity gravitates to the lowest level, superimposition of the cart pad and the lower lung field may obscure fluid that has settled in the lowest position.

Body Habitus and IR Cassette Placement. When using the computed radiography system, place the IR cassette LW for patients with the hypersthenic and sthenic body habitus and place the IR cassette CW for patients with the asthenic and hyposthenic body habitus.

This is not a consideration when using the DR system because it uses a 17 × 17 inch (42.5 × 42.5 cm) IR, though it is useful information to use when determining how to adjust collimation for the different body habitus.

Midcoronal Plane Positioning and Rotation

Using the Cervical Vertebrae to Distinguish between the AP and PA Projections. Whether the lateral decubitus chest is obtained in the AP or PA projection is not a concern, because the projection is not obtained to evaluate the heart size. But to be able to determine how to improve a rotated projection, it is necessary to be able to tell the difference. To determine whether a chest projection was taken in an AP or PA projection, analyze the appearance of the sixth and seventh cervical vertebrae and the first thoracic vertebra. In the AP projection these vertebral bodies and their intervertebral disk spaces are demonstrated without distortion (Figure 3-68). In the PA projection, the vertebral bodies are distorted, the intervertebral disk spaces are

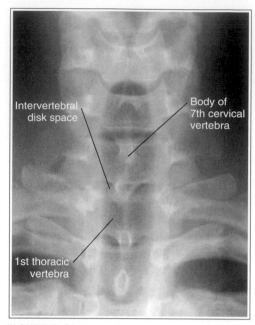

FIGURE 3-68 AP projection of cervical vertebrae.

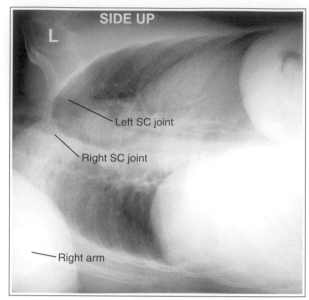

FIGURE 3-70 AP (right lateral decubitus) chest with left side rotated closer to IR than right side.

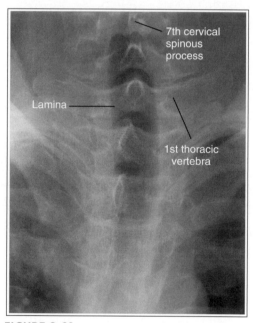

FIGURE 3-69 PA projection of cervical vertebrae.

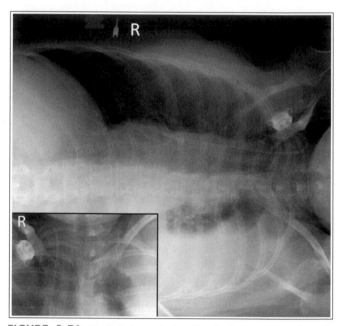

FIGURE 3-71 AP (left lateral decubitus) chest with right side rotated closer to IR than left side.

closed, and the spinous processes and laminae of these three vertebrae are well demonstrated (Figure 3-69). The reason for these variations is related to the divergence of the x-ray beam used to image these three vertebrae and the anterior convexity of the cervical and upper thoracic vertebrae.

Identifying Rotation. Rotation is readily detected on an AP or PA (lateral decubitus) chest by evaluating the distances between the vertebral column and the sternal ends of the clavicles and by comparing the lengths of the posterior ribs. On a nonrotated AP/PA (lateral decubitus) chest, the distances and lengths, respectively, on each side of the patient should be equal. On a rotated

AP projection the sternal clavicular end that demonstrates the least vertebral column superimposition, and the side on which the posterior ribs demonstrate the greatest length, is the side of the chest positioned closer to the IR (Figures 3-70 and 3-71). The opposite is true for a PA projection. For this projection, the sternal clavicular end that demonstrates the least amount of the vertebral column and the posterior ribs that demonstrate the greatest length represent the side of the chest positioned farther from the IR. In the AP projection it is easier for the patient to maintain a nonrotated projection, because the knees can be flexed and a pillow placed between them to stabilize the patient.

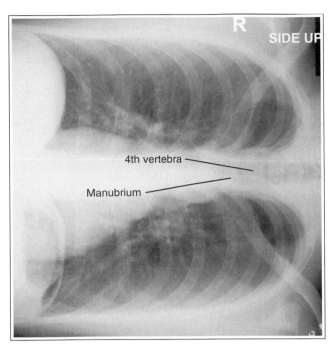

FIGURE 3-72 AP (left lateral decubitus) chest with superior mid-coronal plane tilted away from IR.

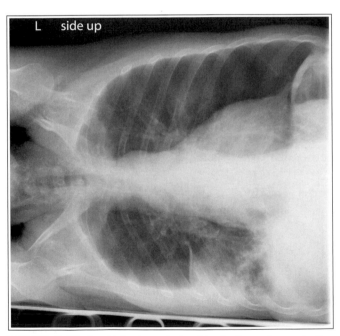

FIGURE 3-73 AP (right lateral decubitus) chest demonstrating accurate arm and scapulae positioning, with superior mid-coronal plane tilted toward the IR.

Midcoronal Plane Tilting. The tilt of the midcoronal plane determines the degree of lung and heart foreshortening and the transverse level at which the manubrium is situated in comparison to the fourth thoracic vertebra. If an AP projection is taken and the superior midcoronal plane is tilted anteriorly (forward), the manubrium will move inferior to the fourth thoracic vertebra (Figure 3-72). Conversely, if the superior midcoronal plane is tilted posteriorly (backward), the manubrium will move superior to the fourth thoracic vertebra (Figure 3-73). If a PA projection is taken and the superior midcoronal plane

is tilted anteriorly, the manubrium will move inferior to the fourth thoracic vertebra. Conversely, if the superior midcoronal plane is tilted posteriorly, the manubrium will move superior to the fourth thoracic vertebra.

Scapulae. The lateral borders of the scapulae are drawn away from the lung field when the patient's arms are positioned above the head. This positioning also draws the lateral ends of the clavicles superiorly. If the arms are not positioned in this manner, the arms and the lateral borders of the scapulae are demonstrated within the upper lung field (see Figure 3-73).

Lung Aeration. In the recumbent position the diaphragm is unable to shift to its lowest position because of pressure from the peritoneal cavity. As a result, adequate lung aeration for an AP/PA (lateral decubitus) chest has resulted when at least 9 posterior ribs are demonstrated above the diaphragm. If fewer than nine posterior ribs are demonstrated, lung expansion is not acceptable.

Decubitus Chest Analysis Practice

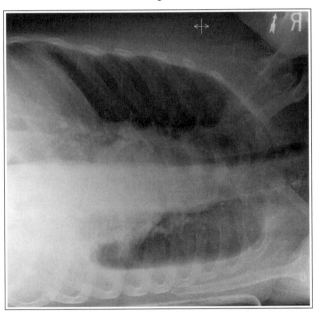

IMAGE 3-11 PA (left lateral decubitus) projection.

Analysis. The right sternal clavicular end is situated farther from the vertebral column than the left and the posterior ribs on the right side demonstrate the greater length. The patient's right thorax was rotated away from the IR.

Correction. Rotate the patient's right side toward the IR until the midcoronal plane is aligned parallel with the IR.

CHEST: AP AXIAL PROJECTION (LORDOTIC POSITION)

See Table 3-7, (Figures 3-74, 3-75, and 3-76).

Overlying soft tissues, clavicles, and upper ribs often obscure the apical lung markings on a PA projection of the chest. The anterior ends of the first ribs may also

TABLE 3-7	AP Axial (Lordotic) Chest Projection
Image Analysis Guidelines (Figure 3-74)	**Related Positioning Procedures (Figures 3-75 and 3-76)**

• Sternal clavicular ends are projected superior to the lung apices.
• Posterior and anterior aspects of the first through fourth ribs lie horizontally and are superimposed.
	• *Computed radiography:* Use a 14 × 17 inch (35 × 43 cm) IR cassette, positioned LW.
	• Center the chest to the upright IR in an upright AP projection.
	• Method 1:
	  • Move patient 12 inches (30 cm) away from the IR.
	  • Have patient arch back, leaning the upper thorax and shoulders against the IR, until the midcoronal plane and IR form a 45-degree angle.
	  • Align the CR horizontally.
	• Method 2:
	  • Position patient as close to method 1 as possible.
	  • Angle the CR cephalically the amount necessary to create a 45-degree angle between the midcoronal plane and CR.
	• Method 3:
	  • Position the midcoronal plane parallel to the IR.
	  • Angle the CR 45 degrees cephalad.

• Distances from the vertebral column to sternal clavicular ends are equal.	• Position the patient's shoulders at equal distances from the IR.
• Lateral borders of the scapulae are drawn away from the lung field. • Superior angles of the scapulae are demonstrated away from lung apices.	• Place back of hands on iliac crests and rotate the shoulders and elbows anteriorly.
• Superior lung field is at the center of the exposure field. • Clavicles, apices, and two thirds of the lungs are included within the exposure field.	• Center the CR to the midsagittal plane halfway between the manubrium and the xiphoid. • Center the IR and grid to the CR. • Longitudinally and transversely collimate to within 0.5 inches (1.25 cm) of the top of the shoulders and the lateral skin line, respectively.
• Lungs demonstrate aeration.	• Take the exposure after the second full suspended inspiration.

SC, Sternoclavicular.

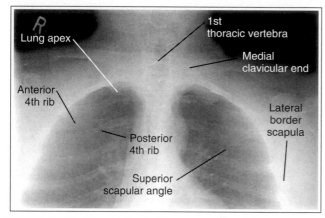

FIGURE 3-74 AP axial (lordotic) chest projection with accurate positioning.

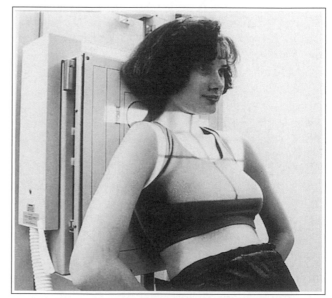

FIGURE 3-75 Proper patient positioning for AP axial (lordotic) chest projection—no CR angle.

project a suspicious-looking shadow in the apices. The AP axial projection is taken to demonstrate areas of the apical lungs obscured on the PA projection and to provide a different anatomic perspective that can be used to evaluate suspicious areas.

Clavicle and Ribs. The midcoronal plane and CR have formed a 45-degree angle for an AP axial chest projection when the sternoclavicular ends of the clavicles are projected superior to the apices and the posterior and anterior first through fourth ribs lie horizontally and are superimposed. Depending on the patient condition, this can be accomplished by adjusting the patient and/or

the CR until a 45-degree angle is created between the midcoronal plane and the CR as described in Table 3-7. Of the three methods described, method 1 is the most preferred because it presents the least CR to IR angulation and will result in the least amount of elongation distortion.

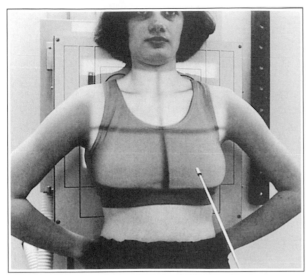

FIGURE 3-76 Proper patient positioning for AP axial (lordotic) chest projection—CR angled.

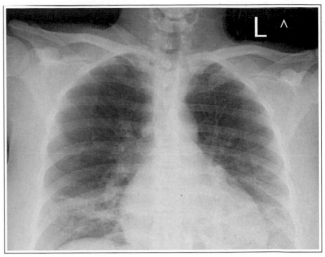

FIGURE 3-77 AP axial (lordotic) chest taken with less than a 45-degree midcoronal plane to CR angulation and demonstrating the scapulae in the lung field.

Determining the Degree of CR Angulation for Method 2. In method 2 the patient is unable to arch the back enough to bring the midcoronal plane at a 45-degree angle with the IR, so it requires the CR to be angled cephalically to obtain the needed 45-degree angle between the midcoronal plane and CR. The required angulation is determined by estimating the degree of midcoronal plane and IR angle and subtracting that angle from 45 degrees. For example, if the midcoronal plane is placed at a 30-degree angle with the IR, the needed CR angle would be 15 degrees cephalically.

Identifying Inadequate Midcoronal Plane and CR Angulation. Inadequate back extension or CR angulation is identified on an AP axial chest when the clavicles are not adequately projected superior to the lung apices and when the anterior and posterior ribs are not superimposed. If the patient's back is not arched enough or when more cephalic angulation is needed, the clavicles superimpose the lung apices, and the anterior ribs are demonstrated inferior to their corresponding posterior rib (Figure 3-77). If a projection is obtained that demonstrates the lung fields with so much foreshortening that the apices are obscured and the posterior ribs are superimposed and cannot be distinguished, the patient's back was arched too much or the cephalic angle was too extreme (Figure 3-78).

Rotation. Chest rotation can be identified on an AP axial projection by evaluating the distance between the vertebral column and the sternal clavicular ends. When the distances between the sternal clavicular ends and the vertebral column are unequal, the clavicular end that is superimposed over the greatest amount of the vertebral column is the side of the chest that was positioned farthest from the IR.

Scapulae. When the elbows and shoulders are not rotated anteriorly, the lateral borders of the scapulae are demonstrated in the lung fields, and the superior

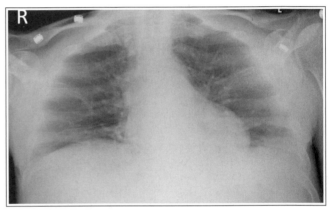

FIGURE 3-78 AP axial (lordotic) chest taken with more than a 45-degree midcoronal plane to CR angulation.

scapular angles are projected into the lung apices (see Figure 3-77).

AP Lordotic Chest Analysis Practice

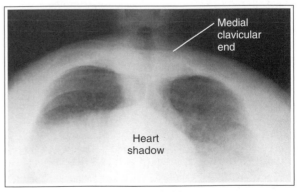

IMAGE 3-12

Analysis. The lung fields demonstrate excessive foreshortening, and the individual ribs cannot be identified.

Correction. If the patient's back was arched to obtain this projection, decrease the amount of arch until the midcoronal plane and CR form a 45-degree angle. If this examination was obtained with a cephalic CR angulation, decrease the degree of angulation until the midcoronal plane and CR form a 45-degree angle.

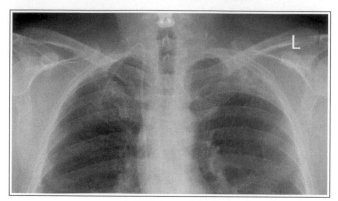

IMAGE 3-13

Analysis. The clavicles are superimposed over the lung apices, and the anterior ribs are demonstrated inferior to their corresponding posterior rib.

Correction. If the patient's back was arched to obtain this projection and a perpendicular CR was used, increase the amount of arch or angle the CR cephalically until it forms a 45-degree angle with the midcoronal plane.

CHEST: PA OBLIQUE PROJECTION (RIGHT AND LEFT ANTERIOR OBLIQUE POSITIONS)

See Table 3-8, (Figures 3-79, 3-80, and 3-81).

Accuracy of Obliquity. When evaluating a PA oblique chest, you can be certain that a 45-degree obliquity has been obtained if (1) twice as much lung field is demonstrated on one side of the thoracic vertebrae as on the other side, and (2) the sternoclavicular (SC) joints, air-filled trachea, and principal bronchi are demonstrated without spinal superimposition. The heart shadow is also demonstrated without spinal superimposition on an RAO position, whereas a portion of the heart shadow is superimposed over the thoracic vertebrae on an LAO chest position.

Obliquity to Visualize the Heart. Because the heart is located more to the left of the thoracic vertebrae, a 60-degree patient obliquity is necessary to demonstrate the heart shadow without spinal superimposition on the LAO. Figure 3-80 demonstrates a 45-degree LAO chest position. Note that the lung field on one side is twice as large as on the other and that slight superimposition of the thoracic vertebrae and heart shadow is present. Compare this projection with the 60-degree LAO chest position shown in Figure 3-82. Note that more than twice as much lung field is present on one side of the thoracic vertebrae as on the other in Figure 3-82, and that the heart shadow and thoracic vertebrae are not superimposed. How much obliquity should be obtained when an LAO chest projection is requested depends on the examination indications. When the examination is being performed to evaluate the lung field, a 45-degree oblique is required; when the outline of the heart is of interest, a 60-degree oblique is required.

Repositioning for Improper Patient Obliquity. If the desired 45-degree obliquity is not obtained on a PA oblique chest, compare the amount of lung field demonstrated on both sides of the thoracic vertebrae. If the projection demonstrates more than twice the lung field on one side of the thoracic vertebrae as on the other side, the patient was rotated more than 45 degrees (see Figure 3-82). If less than twice the lung field is demonstrated on one side of the thoracic vertebrae as on the

TABLE 3-8	PA Oblique Chest Projection	
Image Analysis Guidelines (Figures 3-79 and 3-80)	**Related Positioning Procedures (Figure 3-81)**	
• Sternoclavicular (SC) joints are demonstrated without spinal superimposition. • Twice as much lung field is demonstrated on one side of the thoracic vertebrae as on the other side.	• *Computed radiography:* Use a 14 × 17 inch (35 × 43 cm) IR cassette, positioned LW. • Center chest to the upright IR in a PA projection. • Rotate patient the direction to demonstrate the lung of interest, aligning the midcoronal plane 45 degrees to the IR.	
• Manubrium is superimposed by the fourth thoracic vertebra. • 1 inch (2.5 cm) of apical lung field visible above the clavicles.	• Align the midcoronal plane vertically.	
• Humeri or their soft tissue do not superimpose the lung field.	• Flex and position arm closest to the IR so the back of the hand is on the hip. • Raise the opposite arm and rest on head or upright IR.	
• Right and left principal bronchi are at the center of the exposure field. • Both lungs, from the apices to costophrenic angles, are included within the exposure field.	• Center a horizontal CR at a level 7.5 inches (18 cm) inferior to the vertebra prominens. • Center the IR and grid to the CR. • Longitudinally collimate to include the inferior ribs. • Transversely collimate to within 0.5 inch (2.5 cm) of the lateral skin line.	
• At least 10 posterior ribs are visualized above the diaphragm.	• Take the exposure after the second full suspended inspiration.	

SC, Sternoclavicular.

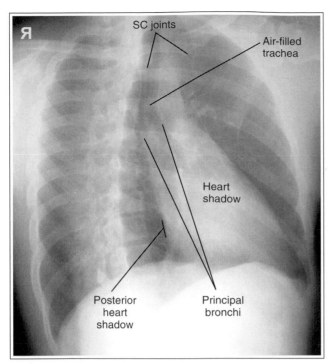

FIGURE 3-79 45-degree PA oblique (RAO) chest projection with accurate positioning.

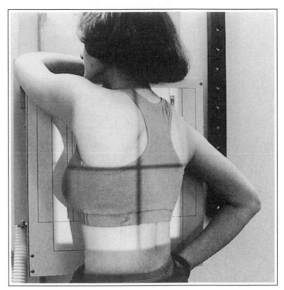

FIGURE 3-81 Proper patient positioning for PA oblique (RAO) chest projection.

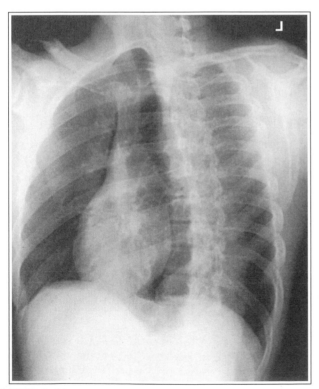

FIGURE 3-80 45-degree PA oblique (LAO) chest projection with proper positioning.

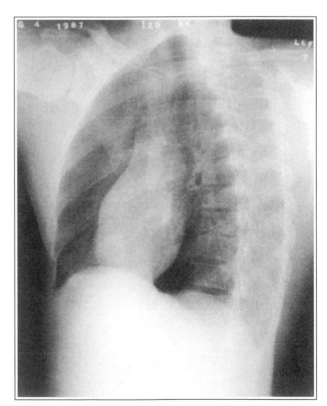

FIGURE 3-82 60-degree PA oblique (LAO) chest projection with proper positioning.

opposite side, the patient was not rotated enough (Figure 3-83). To determine repositioning movements for the 60-degree LAO position, evaluate the heart shadow and thoracic vertebrae superimposition. With adequate obliquity, the heart shadow is positioned just to the right

of the thoracic vertebrae (see Figure 3-82). If the LAO position is less than 60 degrees, the heart shadow is superimposed over the thoracic vertebrae, as on a 45-degree LAO position (see Figure 3-80). Excess obliquity produces a projection similar to a rotated lateral chest projection.

AP Oblique Chest Projections. A PA versus an AP oblique projection is routinely performed because it

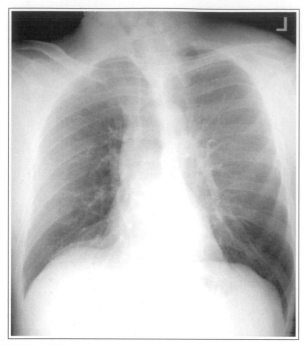

FIGURE 3-83 45-degree PA oblique (LAO) chest taken with less than 45 degrees of rotation.

positions the heart closer to the IR. When AP oblique projections (RPO and LPO positions) are taken, however, the preceding image analysis guidelines correspond in the following way. The LPO position demonstrates the lung situated closer to the IR, which is the left lung. To review this position, use the RAO evaluation previously described. For the RPO position, the right lung is of interest and the LAO evaluation should be followed. A 45-degree obliquity is required in the LPO position to rotate the heart away from the thoracic vertebrae, but a 60-degree obliquity is needed for the RPO position.

Midcoronal Plane Tilting. The tilt of the superior midcoronal plane determines the relationship of the manubrium to the thoracic vertebrae, the amount of apical lung field seen superior to the clavicles, and the degree of lung and heart foreshortening. In PA oblique projections, if the superior midcoronal plane is tilted anteriorly, as demonstrated in Figure 3-34, the lungs and heart are foreshortened, the manubrium is situated at a transverse level inferior to the fourth thoracic vertebra or lower, and more than 1 inch (2.5 cm) of apices is demonstrated above the clavicles (see Figure 3-35). Conversely, if the superior midcoronal plane is tilted posteriorly, as demonstrated in Figure 3-36, the lungs and heart are foreshortened, the manubrium is situated at a transverse level above the fourth thoracic vertebrae, and less than 1 inch (2.5 cm) of apices is demonstrated superior to the clavicles (Figure 3-84). The opposite is true for AP oblique projections. Anterior tilt of the superior midcoronal plane will result in the manubrium projecting inferior to the fourth thoracic vertebra, and posterior tilt of the superior midcoronal plane will result in the manubrium projecting superior to the fourth thoracic vertebra.

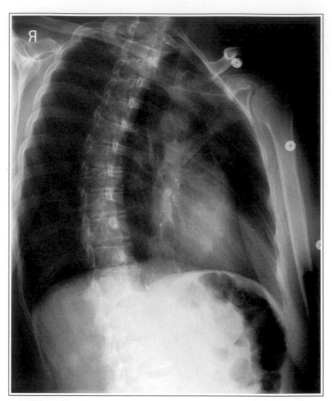

FIGURE 3-84 45-degree PA oblique (RAO) chest taken with superior midcoronal plane tilted posteriorly and arms poorly positioned.

Arm Position. Accurate arm positioning moves the humeri and their soft tissue away from the thorax, preventing lung field superimposition (see Figure 3-84).

PA Oblique Chest Analysis Practice

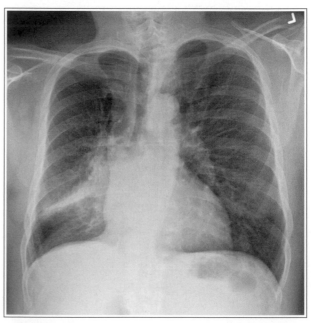

IMAGE 3-14 45-Degree PA Oblique (LAO) Projection.

Analysis. More than twice as much lung field is demonstrated on the right side of the chest than the left side;

the vertebral column superimposes the left SC joint, trachea, principle bronchi, and heart shadow. The patient was rotated less than 45 degrees.

Correction. Increase the degree of rotation until the midcoronal plane forms a 45-degree angle with the IR.

PEDIATRIC CHEST

Lung Development. The lungs of the neonate continue to grow for at least 8 years after birth. The growth results mainly from an increase in the number of respiratory bronchioles and alveoli. Only from one eighth to one sixth of the number of alveoli in adults are present in newborn infants, causing the lungs to be denser. Therefore, on neonate/infant chest projections, the lungs demonstrate less contrast within them and between them and the surrounding soft tissue than on child/adult chest projections.

Chest Shape and Size. As the lungs grow, the shape of the thoracic cavity changes from the neonate/infant's short, wide shape to the older child/adult's longer, narrower shape. To accommodate these changes, the CR will require a more inferior centering and the degree of collimation will need to be reduced as the infant grows to adulthood. For computed radiography systems, this also requires larger IR cassettes to be chosen as the infant grows. For best spatial resolution, choose the smallest possible IR cassette that will accommodate the required structures.

NEONATE AND INFANT CHEST: AP PROJECTION

See Table 3-9, (Figure 3-85 and 3-86).

Chest Rotation

Positioning Patient to Prevent Rotation. To accurately position the infant without rotation, immobilize the child using the appropriate immobilization equipment (see Figure 3-86). The head should be turned so the face is forward. Head rotation is the most common cause of chest rotation in neonates and infants. The chest will rotate in the same direction in which the head is rotated.

TABLE 3-9	Neonate and Infant AP Chest Projection	
Image Analysis Guidelines (Figure 3-85)		**Related Positioning Procedures (Figure 3-86)**
• Universal precautions where followed.		• Clean x-ray machine before exiting patient room. • Use appropriate personal coverings. • Cover IR with plastic bag or pillow case.
• *Neonate:* Lungs demonstrate a fluffy appearance, with linear-appearing connecting tissue • *Infant:* Thoracic vertebrae and posterior ribs are seen through the heart and mediastinal structures.		• Set the appropriate technical data for patient size.
• Lung fields demonstrate symmetry. • Distances from the vertebral column to the sternal clavicular ends are equal. • Lengths of the right and left corresponding posterior ribs are equal.		• Center the chest to the IR in a supine AP projection. • Position the shoulders and the ASISs at equal distances from the IR, aligning the midcoronal plane parallel with the IR. • Place the face in a forward position.

• Each upper anterior rib is demonstrated above its corresponding posterior rib and each lower anterior rib is demonstrated below its corresponding posterior rib.
• Posterior ribs are horizontal.
• *Alternate:*
  • Each anterior rib is demonstrated below its corresponding posterior rib.
  • Posterior ribs demonstrate a gentle, superiorly bowed contour.
		• Use a perpendicular CR.
		• *Alternate:* Angle the CR 5 degrees caudally or tilt the foot end of the bed or table 5 degrees lower than the head end.

• Sixth thoracic vertebra is at the center of the exposure field.		• *Neonate and Small Infant:* Center CR to the midsagittal plane at the level of the mammary line (imaginary line connecting the nipples). • *Larger Infant:* Center inferior to the mammary line.
• Mandible does not obscure the airway or apical lung field. • Arms do not obscure lung field • Upper airway, lungs, mediastinal structures, and costophrenic angles are included within the exposure field.		• Elevate the chin, placing the neck in a neutral position. • Position the arms away from the chest. • Longitudinally collimate to include the upper airway (infant's bottom lip) and inferior ribs. • Transversely collimate to within 0.5 inches (2.5 cm) of the lateral skin line.
• *Neonate:* 8 posterior ribs are demonstrated above the diaphragm. • *Infant:* 9 posterior ribs are demonstrated above the diaphragm.		• Observe the chest movement and take x-ray exposure after the infant takes a deep breath.

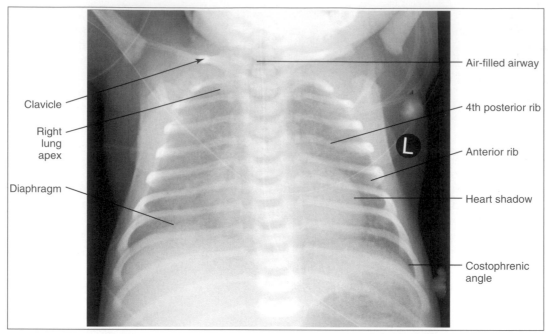

FIGURE 3-85 Neonate AP chest projection with accurate positioning.

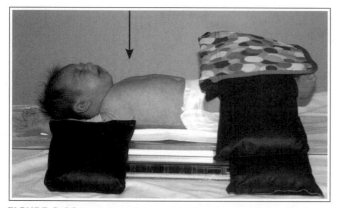

FIGURE 3-86 Proper patient positioning for AP infant chest projection using immobilization equipment.

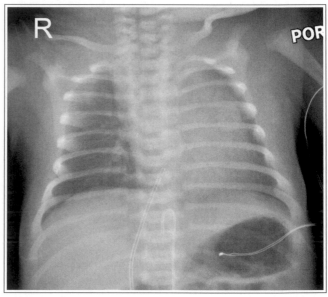

FIGURE 3-87 Neonate AP chest taken with left side of chest rotated closer to IR than right side.

Identifying Chest Rotation Caused by Poor Patient Positioning. Chest rotation is detected by evaluating the distance between the vertebral column and the sternal ends of the clavicles and by comparing the length of the right and left inferior posterior ribs. Both should be equal on each side. When this is not the case, the sternal clavicular end that is demonstrated farther from the vertebral column and the side of the chest that demonstrates the longer posterior ribs represents the side of the chest toward which the infant is rotated (Figures 3-87, 3-88, and 3-89).

Side-to-Side CR Alignment to Prevent Rotation. To avoid rotation caused by poor side-to-side (lateral) CR alignment during mobile imaging, make certain that the CR is not off-angled toward the right or left lateral side of the infant instead of being perpendicular to the IR. This can be accomplished by evaluating the collimator face's parallelism with the IR and midcoronal plane.

Identifying Chest Rotation Caused by Poor IR or Side-to-Side CR Alignment. When the right sternal clavicular end demonstrates no superimposition of the vertebral column and the right posterior ribs demonstrate greater length than the left, the patient's right side was placed farther from the collimator's face than the left side or the CR was angled toward the right side of the chest (see Figures 3-88 and 89). When the right sternal clavicular end is seen superimposing the vertebral column and the right side demonstrates less posterior rib

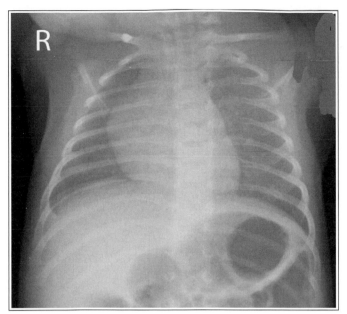

FIGURE 3-88 Neonate AP chest taken with right side of chest rotated closer to IR than left side and a 5-degree caudal CR angle.

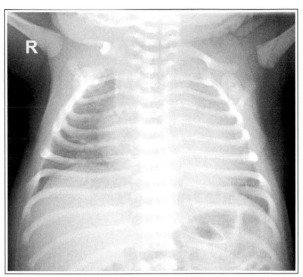

FIGURE 3-90 Neonate AP chest obtained without a caudal CR angle and low CR centering.

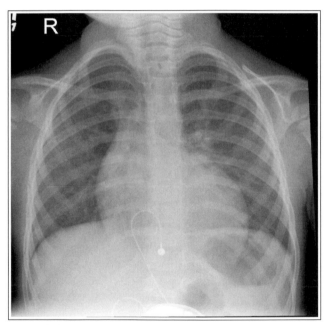

FIGURE 3-89 Infant AP chest taken with right side of chest rotated closer to IR than left side.

length than the left, the patient's right side was placed closer to the collimator's face than the left or the CR was angled toward the left side of the chest (see Figure 3-87).

CR and IR Alignment (Perpendicular or Cephalic Angle). The neonate/infant lacks the kyphotic curvature in the thoracic vertebrae that the child and adult display. As a result, the supine AP chest tends to have a lordotic appearance when compared to that of a child or adult. The lordotic appearance is demonstrated on AP chest projection when an anterior rib is demonstrated superior to its corresponding posterior rib. When the CR and IR are aligned perpendicular, the AP chest demonstrates each upper anterior rib superior to its corresponding posterior rib, whereas each lower anterior rib is demonstrated below its corresponding posterior rib (see Figure 3-85). The dividing point for this appearance change is at where the CR was centered. Because the chest in neonates/infants is shorter than in children and adults, a common error is to center the CR too inferiorly. This inferior CR centering only results in an increase in the lordotic appearance, because additional ribs demonstrate the anterior rib superior to its corresponding posterior rib (Figure 3-90). Such distortion foreshortens the lungs and mediastinal structures, causing the cardiac apex to appear uptilted and the main pulmonary artery to be concealed beneath the cardiac silhouette.

Alternate CR and IR Alignment. To produce an AP chest without the lordotic appearance, a 5-degree caudal angle can be placed on the CR or the foot end of the bed can be tilted 5 degrees lower than the head end. This CR and IR alignment will place each anterior rib below its corresponding posterior rib and demonstrate the posterior ribs with a gentle, superiorly bowed contour (see Figures 3-88 and 3-91).

Chin Position. To prevent the chin from being superimposed on the airway and apical lung field, lift the neonate or infant's chin until the neck is in a neutral position. When the chin is superimposed on the airway and apical lung field, ETT placement cannot be evaluated (Figure 3-91).

Appearance of Lungs and Aeration. The appearance of the neonate's lungs may change with even one rib's difference in inflation. With dense substances such as blood, pus, protein, and cells filling the alveoli, it is the addition of the less dense air that will give the projection the fluffy appearance, because the air is demonstrated on the projection with less brightness when compared with the blood, pus, protein, and cells. A lung that demonstrates a white-out appearance, even though the

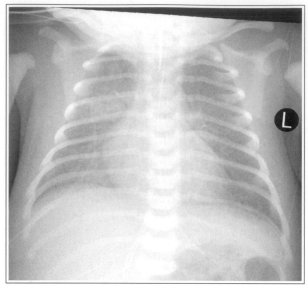

FIGURE 3-91 Neonate AP chest obtained with a 5-degree caudal CR angle and chin not elevated.

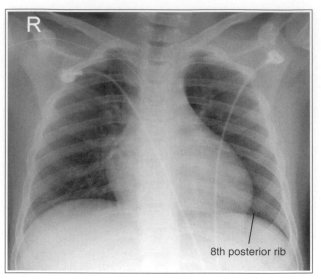

8th posterior rib

FIGURE 3-93 Infant AP chest without full lung aeration.

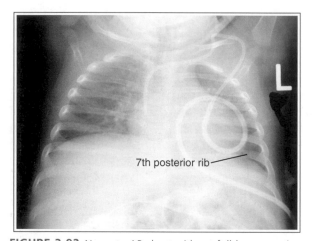

7th posterior rib

FIGURE 3-92 Neonate AP chest without full lung aeration.

previous projections to determine whether a patient's condition might have caused the poor inhalation.

Neonate and Infant AP Chest Analysis Practice

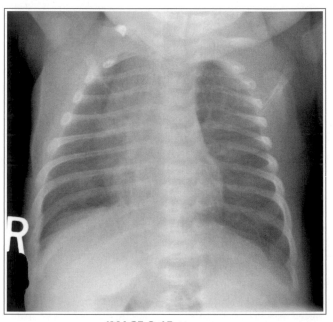

IMAGE 3-15 Neonate.

diaphragm is below the eighth rib, is filled with dense substances that do not allow air to fill the alveoli. The high-frequency ventilator is most commonly used on neonates/infants. This ventilator allows the exposure to be made at any time because it maintains the lung expansion at a steady mean pressure. For neonates and infants breathing without a respirator, observe the chest movement and expose the projection after the infant takes a deep breath.

Identifying Poor Lung Aeration. If fewer than 8 posterior ribs are demonstrated above the diaphragm for the neonate and nine for the infant, the lungs were not fully inflated. Chest projections that are taken with inadequate inspiration demonstrate a wider-appearing heart shadow and an increase in lung tissue brightness, because the decrease in air volume increases the concentration of pulmonary tissues (Figures 3-92 and 3-93). Before repeating the procedure, observe the patient or evaluate

Analysis. The right sternal clavicular end is demonstrated further from the vertebral column than the left, and the right lower posterior ribs are longer than the left. The right side of the chest is rotated toward the IR.
Correction. Rotate the right side of the chest away from the IR until the midcoronal plane is parallel with the IR and perpendicular to the CR.

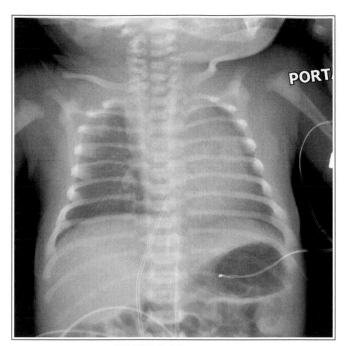

IMAGE 3-16 Neonate.

Analysis. The left sternal clavicular end is demonstrated further from the vertebral column than the right and the left-side posterior ribs are longer than the right. The head is turned so the face is toward the left side. The left side of the chest is rotated toward the IR.

Correction. Rotate the left side of the chest away from the IR until the midcoronal plane is parallel with the IR and perpendicular to the CR. Turn the head so the face is forward.

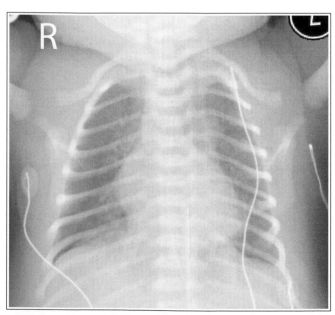

IMAGE 3-17 Neonate.

Analysis. Each of the upper anterior ribs is demonstrated above its corresponding posterior rib. The chest is lordotic. The CR was aligned too cephalically or centered too caudally.

Correction. Decrease the cephalic angulation until the CR and IR are perpendicular or lower the foot end of the bed until the midcoronal plane and CR are perpendicular.

CHILD CHEST: PA AND AP (PORTABLE) PROJECTIONS

See Table 3-10, (Figure 3-94 and 3-95).

The image analysis guidelines of the child PA and AP chest are similar to that for the infant or adult PA or AP chest, already discussed. The size of the child determines which of the guidelines best meets the situation. For a discussion on topics needed to analyze the following images, refer to the PA-AP (portable) adult or infant chest discussions earlier in this chapter.

Child Chest PA and AP (Portable) Chest Analysis Practice

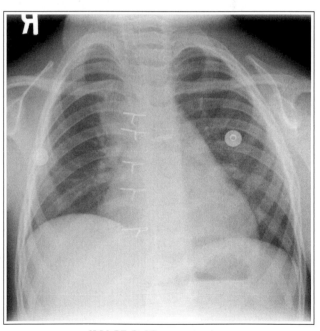

IMAGE 3-18 PA projection.

Analysis. The right sternal clavicular end is situated farther from the vertebral column than the left. The right side of the chest was rotated away from the IR. The manubrium is situated at the level of the fifth thoracic vertebra. The upper midcoronal plane was tilted anteriorly.

Correction. Rotate the right side of the patient's thorax toward the IR and move the patient's upper thorax away from the IR until the midcoronal plane is parallel with the IR.

TABLE 3-10	Child PA and AP (Portable) Chest Projection
Image Analysis Guidelines (Figure 3-94)	**Related Positioning Procedures (Figure 3-95)**
• Thoracic vertebrae and posterior ribs are seen through the heart and mediastinal structures.	• Appropriate technical data have been set.
• Lung fields demonstrate symmetry. • Distances from the vertebral column to the sternal clavicular ends are equal. • Lengths of the right and left corresponding posterior ribs are equal. • Mandible is not in exposure field.	• *Method 1:* Center the chest to the upright IR in a PA projection. • *Method 2:* Center the chest on the IR in a supine AP projection. • Position the shoulders, the posterior ribs, and the ASISs at equal distances from the IR, aligning the midcoronal plane parallel with the IR. • Place the face in a forward position and elevate the chin, positioning it outside the collimation field.
• Clavicles are positioned on the same horizontal plane. • Scapulae are located outside the lung field.	• Depress the shoulders. • Protract the shoulders by placing the back of the patient's hands on the hips and rotating the elbows and shoulders anteriorly or use the imaging equipment holding bars.
• Manubrium is superimposed by the fourth thoracic vertebra. • Sixth or seventh thoracic vertebra is at the center of the exposure field.	• Align the midcoronal plane parallel with the IR. • Center a perpendicular CR at or slightly inferior to the mammary line.
• Upper airway, lungs, mediastinal structures, and costophrenic angles are included within the exposure field.	• Longitudinally collimate to include the shoulder top and inferior ribs. • Transversely collimate to within 0.5 inches (2.5 cm) of the lateral skin line.
• At least 9 posterior ribs are visualized above the diaphragm.	• Take the exposure after the second full suspended inspiration.

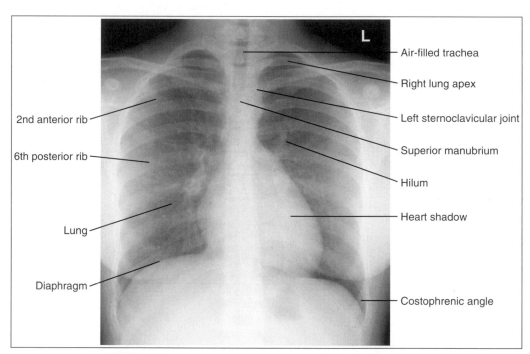

FIGURE 3-94 Child AP chest projection with proper positioning.

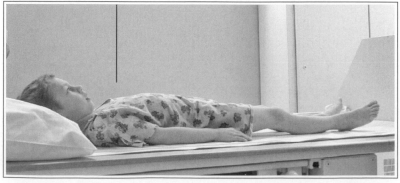

FIGURE 3-95 Proper patient positioning for a child AP chest projection.

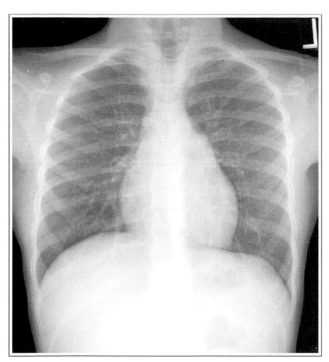

IMAGE 3-19 PA projection.

Analysis. The manubrium is at the level of the second thoracic vertebra. The patient's upper midcoronal plane was tilted posteriorly.

Correction. Anteriorly tilt the upper midcoronal plane until it is aligned parallel with the IR.

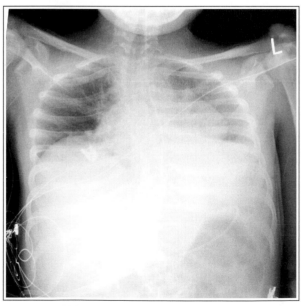

IMAGE 3-20 AP (mobile) projection.

Analysis. Only six posterior ribs are demonstrated above the diaphragm. The manubrium is superimposed over the second thoracic vertebra and the posterior ribs demonstrate a horizontal contour. The projection was taken on expiration, and the CR was angled too cephalically.

Correction. If the patient's condition allows, take the exposure after coaxing the patient into a deeper inspiration and adjust the CR caudally until it is aligned perpendicular to the patient's midcoronal plane.

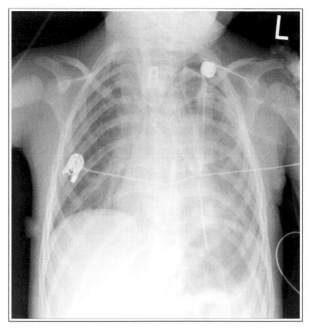

IMAGE 3-21 AP (mobile) projection.

Analysis. The manubrium is superimposed over the fifth thoracic vertebra and the posterior ribs demonstrate a vertical contour. The CR was angled too caudally.

Correction. Adjust the CR cephalically until it is aligned perpendicular to the midcoronal plane.

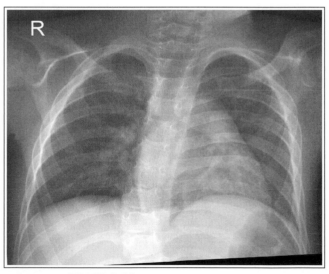

IMAGE 3-22 AP (portable) projection.

Analysis. The left sternal clavicular end is situated farther from the vertebral column than the right. The left side of the patient and IR were placed closer to the bed and farther from the collimator's face than the right side. Only eight posterior ribs are demonstrated above the diaphragm.

Correction. Elevate the left side of the patient and IR or adjust the CR angulation toward the right side of the chest until the collimator's face is parallel with the IR and CR is perpendicular. Coax the patient into a deeper inspiration.

NEONATE AND INFANT CHEST: CROSS-TABLE LATERAL PROJECTION (LEFT LATERAL POSITION)

See Table 3-11, (Figures 3-96 and 3-97).

The lateral chest projection is useful for assessing the degree of inflation, permits confident recognition of cardiomegaly, and provides the clearest view of the thoracic vertebrae and sternum.

Cross-Table Versus Overhead Lateral. Neonates are very sensitive. Performing a cross-table lateral projection on the neonate instead of an overhead lateral projection will reduce the amount of disturbance. Also, on overhead lateral projections, the lung adjacent to the IR tends to collapse from the body weight, whereas the superior lung tends to overinflate.

Posterior Rib Superimposition. Because the OID difference between the right and left lung fields is minimal on neonates and small infants, the posterior ribs on lateral chest do not demonstrate the 0.5-inch (1.25-cm) separation that is seen on adult lateral chest when they are accurately positioned. Instead, the ribs are directly

TABLE 3-11	Neonate and Infant Lateral Chest Projection
Image Analysis Guidelines (Figure 3-96)	**Related Positioning Procedures (Figure 3-97)**
• Posterior ribs are superimposed. • Sternum is in profile. • Mandible is not in exposure field.	• *Cross-table*: Elevate the patient on a radiolucent sponge or immobilization board in the supine position. Center the chest to the upright IR in a left lateral position. • *Overhead*: Center the patient to the IR in a left lateral position. • Position the shoulders, the posterior ribs, and the ASISs directly in line with one another, aligning midcoronal plane perpendicular to IR. • Turn head to bring face forward and elevate chin, positioning it outside the collimation field.
• Humeral soft tissue is not superimposed over the anterior lung apices.	• Position the humeri upward, near the head.
• Chin is not in the exposure field.	• Elevate the chin, bringing the neck neutral.
• Midcoronal plane, at the level of the sixth thoracic vertebra, is at the center of the exposure field.	• *Cross-table:* Center a horizontal CR to the midcoronal plane at the mammary line. • *Overhead:* Center a perpendicular CR to the midcoronal plane at the mammary line.
• Both lung fields, including the apices and costophrenic angles, and the posterior ribs and airway are demonstrated within the exposure field. • Hemidiaphragms form a gentle cephalic curve.	• Longitudinally collimate to include the fifth through seventh cervical vertebrae and the inferior ribs. • Transversely collimate to within 0.5 inch (1.25 cm) of the skin line. • Observe the chest movement and expose the projection after the infant takes a deep breath.

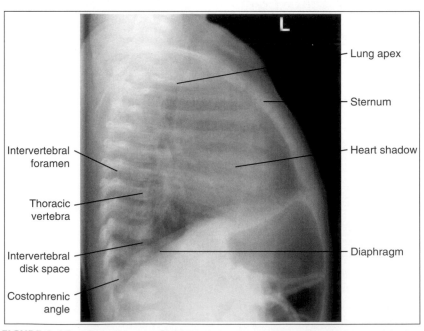

FIGURE 3-96 Neonatal cross-table lateral chest projection with accurate positioning.

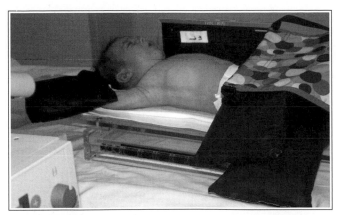

FIGURE 3-97 Proper patient positioning for a cross-table lateral infant chest projection using immobilization equipment.

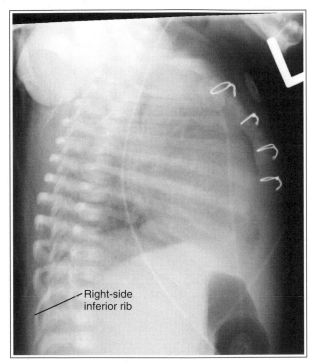

FIGURE 3-98 Neonate lateral chest taken with right lung rotated posteriorly.

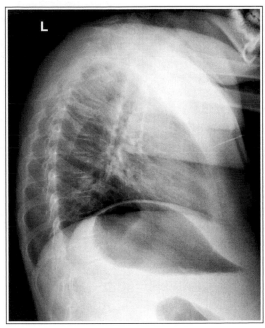

FIGURE 3-99 Infant lateral chest taken with right lung rotated posteriorly and humeri not elevated.

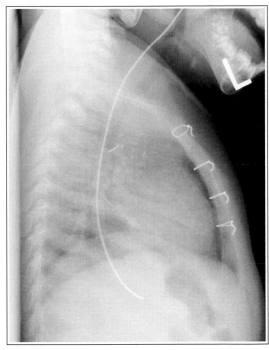

FIGURE 3-100 Infant lateral chest taken with chin in exposure field.

superimposed. To detect rotation on neonate and infant lateral chest projections, evaluate the degree of superimposition of the posterior ribs. When the posterior ribs are demonstrated without superimposition, the chest was rotated for the projection (Figures 3-98 and 3-99).

Identifying Right and Left Lungs. One means of identifying the lung that is positioned posteriorly on a rotated lateral chest is to locate the most inferiorly demonstrated right and left corresponding ribs. The rib on the right side will be projected slightly more inferiorly than the rib on the left side because it is positioned farthest from the IR. The heart shadow and gastric bubble may also be used, as described in the earlier discussion of the adult lateral chest projections.

Arms. Positioning the humeri upward, near the patient's head, prevents superimposition of the humeral soft tissue over the anterior lung apices (see Figure 3-99).

Chin. Good radiation protection practices dictate that anatomic structures that are not evaluated on a projection should not be included, whenever possible. To prevent the chin from being included in the exposure field, lift it upward above the collimation field (Figure 3-100).

Respiration. For neonates and infants breathing without a respirator, observe the chest movement and take the exposure after the infant takes a deep breath. Chest

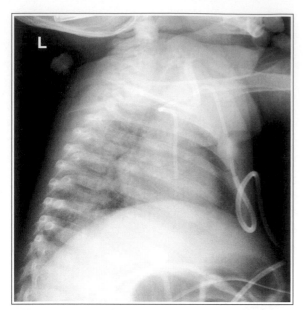

FIGURE 3-101 Neonate lateral chest without full lung aeration.

projections that are taken on expiration may demonstrate an increase in image brightness because the decrease in air volume increases the concentration of pulmonary tissues. With underaeration, the cephalic curve of the hemidiaphragms is exaggerated and their position is higher in the thorax (Figure 3-101).

CHILD CHEST: LATERAL PROJECTION (LEFT LATERAL POSITION)

See Table 3-12, (Figures 3-102 and 3-103).

The analysis of the child lateral chest projection (Table 3-12) is the same as that of the infant or adult lateral chest projection (see earlier). The size of the child determines which image analysis guidelines best meets the

situation. For a discussion on the topics needed to analyze the following images, see the lateral adult or infant chest discussions earlier in this chapter.

Child Lateral Chest Analysis Practice

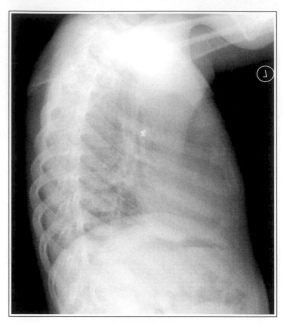

IMAGE 3-23

Analysis. More than 0.5 inch (1.25 cm) of separation is demonstrated between the posterior ribs. The right lung is anterior. The mandible is within the exposure field, and the humeral soft tissue is superimposed over the superior lung field. The chin and the humeri were not adequately elevated.

Correction. Rotate the left side of the thorax anteriorly and the right side posteriorly until the midcoronal plane is aligned perpendicular to the IR. Elevate the chin

TABLE 3-12	Child Lateral Chest Projection	
Image Analysis Guidelines (Figure 3-102)	**Related Positioning Procedures (Figure 3-103)**
• Lung fields demonstrate symmetry. • Distances from the vertebral column to the sternal clavicular ends are equal. • Lengths of the right and left corresponding posterior ribs are equal. • Mandible is not in exposure field.	• Center the chest to the upright IR in a left lateral position. • Place the shoulders, the posterior ribs, and the ASISs directly in line with each other, aligning midcoronal plane perpendicular to IR. • Turn head until face is forward and elevate the chin, positioning it outside the collimation field.
• Lungs are demonstrated without foreshortening, with almost superimposed hemidiaphragms.	• Align the midsagittal plane parallel with the IR.
• No humeral soft tissue is seen superimposing the anterior lung apices.	• Place the humeri in an upright vertical position, with forearms crossed and resting on the patient's head, or use the imaging equipment holding bars.
• Sixth or seventh thoracic vertebra is at the center of the exposure field.	• Center a horizontal CR to the midcoronal plane at or slightly inferior to the mammary line.
• Both lung fields, including the apices and costophrenic angles, and the posterior ribs and airway are demonstrated within the exposure field.	• Center the IR to the CR. • Longitudinally collimate to include the shoulder top and inferior ribs. • Transversely collimate to within 0.5 inches (2.5 cm) of the lateral skin line.
• Hemidiaphragms demonstrate a gentle cephalic curve.	• Take the exposure after the second full suspended inspiration.

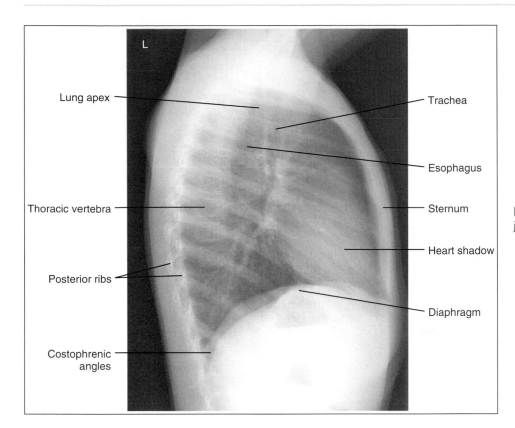

FIGURE 3-102 Child lateral chest projection with accurate positioning.

Labels: Lung apex, Trachea, Esophagus, Thoracic vertebra, Sternum, Heart shadow, Posterior ribs, Diaphragm, Costophrenic angles

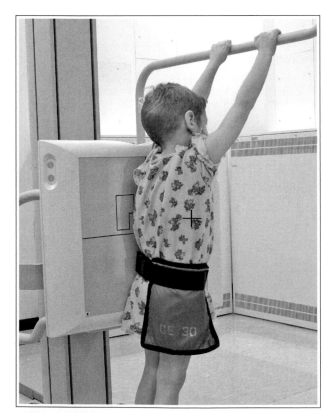

FIGURE 3-103 Proper positioning for a child lateral chest projection.

outside the collimated field, and raise the humeri next to the patient's head.

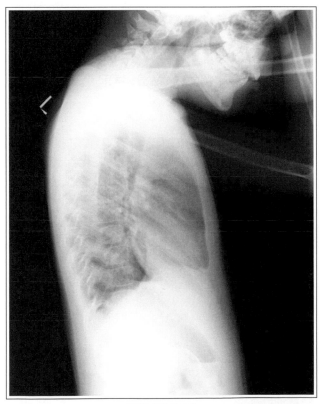

IMAGE 3-24

Analysis. The patient's arms and mandible are demonstrated in the exposure field. Poor collimation is demonstrated.

Correction. Increase the longitudinal collimation to the shoulder top and inferior ribs and transverse collimation to within 0.5 inch (1.25 cm) of thorax skin line. Raise the patient's chin and humeri out the collimated field.

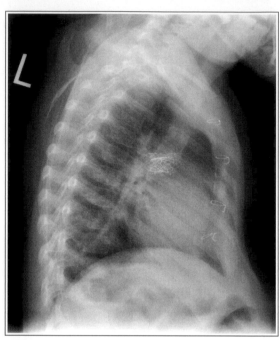

IMAGE 3-25

Analysis. More than 0.5 inch (1.25 cm) of separation is demonstrated between the posterior ribs. The left lung is anterior. The mandible is within the exposure field. The chin was not adequately elevated.

Correction. Rotate the right side of the thorax anteriorly and the left side posteriorly until the midcoronal plane is aligned perpendicular to the IR. Elevate the chin outside the collimated field.

NEONATE AND INFANT CHEST: AP PROJECTION (RIGHT OR LEFT LATERAL DECUBITUS POSITION)

See Table 3-13, (Figures 3-104 and 3-105).

Midcoronal Plane Positioning and Rotation. Chest rotation is detected on a lateral decubitus position by evaluating the distance between the vertebral column and the sternal ends of the clavicles and by comparing the length of the right and left inferior posterior ribs. The sternal clavicular end that is superimposed over the least amount of the vertebral column, along with the side of the chest that demonstrates the longest inferior posterior ribs, represents the side of the chest toward which the infant is rotated (Figures 3-106 and 3-107).

Preventing Artifact Lines in Lung Field. Elevating the neonate or infant on a radiolucent sponge prevents the chest from sinking into the pad. When the body is allowed to sink into the pad, artifact lines are seen superimposed over the lateral lung field of the side adjacent to the cart (Figure 3-108). Because fluid in the pleural cavity gravitates to the lowest level, it is in this area that the fluid will be demonstrated, and superimposition of the pad and lower lung field may obscure fluid that has settled in the lowest level.

Midsagittal Plane Tilting. If the neonate or infant's entire body is placed on the radiolucent sponge the midsagittal plane can be aligned parallel with the bed or cart, preventing lateral tilting (see Figure 3-108).

Chin and Arm Positioning. To prevent the chin from being superimposed over the lung apices on the projection, elevate the chin until the neck is in a neutral position (see Figure 3-107). Placing the arms upward toward the patient's head positions them away from the lung

TABLE 3-13	Neonate and Infant AP (Lateral Decubitus) Chest Projection
Image Analysis Guidelines (Figure 3-104)	**Related Positioning Procedures (Figure 3-105)**
• *Neonate:* Lungs demonstrate a fluffy appearance, with linear-appearing connecting tissue • *Infant:* Thoracic vertebrae and posterior ribs are seen through the heart and mediastinal structures.	• Appropriate technical data have been set.
• An arrow or "word" marker identifies the side of the patient positioned up and away from the bed or table.	• Place proper marker on IR.
• Lung field adjacent to the bed or table is demonstrated without superimposition of the pad.	• Place patient on a radiolucent sponge or a hard surface in a lateral recumbent position. • Position the affected side of chest up if a pneumothorax is suspected and down if pleural effusion is suspected.
• Vertebral column is seen without lateral tilting. • Lung fields demonstrate symmetry. • Distances from the vertebral column to the sternal clavicular ends are equal. • Lengths of the right and left corresponding posterior ribs are equal.	• Align midsagittal plane with IR long axis. • Center the chest to the upright IR, in an AP projection. • Position the shoulders, the posterior ribs, and the ASISs at equal distances to the IR, aligning the midcoronal plane parallel with the IR. • Turn head until face is forward.
• Chin and arms are not demonstrated in the lung field.	• Elevate the chin, bringing the neck neutral. • Position the humeri upward, near the head.

TABLE 3-13	Neonate and Infant AP (Lateral Decubitus) Chest Projection—cont'd	
Image Analysis Guidelines (Figure 3-104)	**Related Positioning Procedures (Figure 3-105)**	

• Each upper anterior rib is demonstrated above its corresponding posterior rib and each lower anterior rib is demonstrated below its corresponding posterior rib.
• Posterior ribs are horizontal.
• *Alternate:*
  • Each anterior rib is demonstrated below its corresponding posterior rib.
  • Posterior ribs demonstrate a gentle, superiorly bowed contour.
	• With posterior surface resting against the IR, use a perpendicular CR.
	• *Alternate:* Move the upper chest and shoulders approximately 5 degrees away from the IR and use a perpendicular CR.	

• Sixth thoracic vertebra is at the center of the exposure field.	• *Neonate and Small Infant:* Center a perpendicular CR to the midsagittal plane at the level of the mammary line. • *Larger Infant:* Center a perpendicular CR to the midsagittal plane at a level inferior to the mammary line.	
• Upper airway, lungs, mediastinal structures, and costophrenic angles are included within the exposure field.	• Longitudinally collimate to include the upper airway (infant's bottom lip) and inferior ribs. • Transversely collimate to within 0.5 inch (1.25 cm) of the lateral skin line.	
• At least 8 posterior ribs are demonstrated above the diaphragm.	• Observe the chest movement and expose the projection after the infant takes a deep breath.	

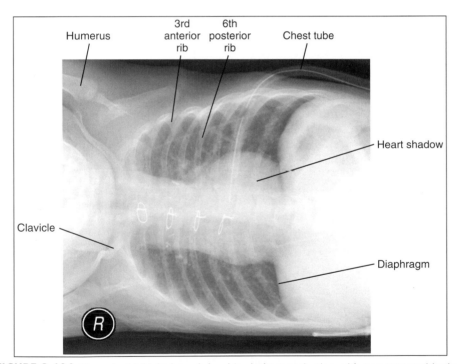

FIGURE 3-104 Neonate AP (right lateral decubitus) chest projection with accurate positioning.

field and projects the lateral clavicles in an upward position (Figures 3-108 and 3-109).

CR and IR Alignment. As discussed in the AP neonate/infant chest projection previously, because of the lack of thoracic kyphotic curvature, the resulting image can take on an excessive lordotic appearance without appropriately centering the CR or adjusting the CR and IR alignment. When the neonate/infant's posterior surface rests against the IR and a perpendicular CR is used, the AP

decubitus chest will demonstrate each upper anterior rib superior to its corresponding posterior rib, whereas each lower anterior rib is demonstrated below its corresponding posterior rib (Figures 3-107 and 3-110). The dividing point for this appearance change is where the CR was centered.

Alternate Patient and IR Alignment. To produce a neonate/infant AP decubitus chest with a reduced lordotic appearance, move the upper chest and shoulders

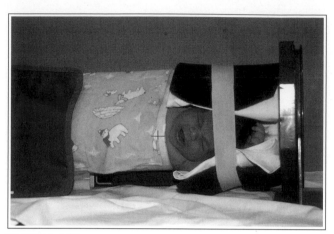

FIGURE 3-105 Proper patient positioning for AP (left lateral decubitus) neonate and infant chest projection.

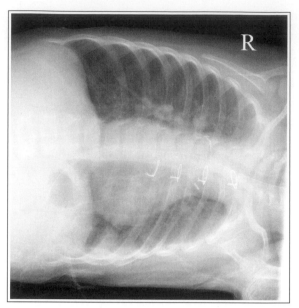

FIGURE 3-107 Neonate AP (left lateral decubitus) chest taken with right side rotated closer to IR than left side and the chin not elevated. Chest has lordotic appearance.

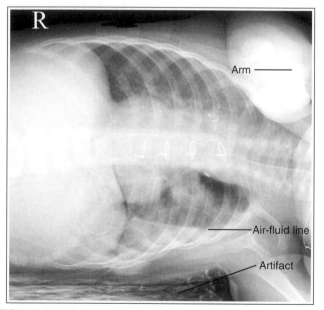

FIGURE 3-106 Neonate AP (left lateral decubitus) chest taken with left side rotated closer to IR than right side and with upper chest positioned slightly away from IR.

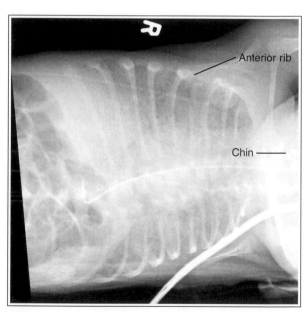

FIGURE 3-108 Neonate AP (left lateral decubitus) chest demonstrating left side pleural effusion, a pad artifact, lateral tilting of the midsagittal plane, and right arm not elevated.

approximately 5 degrees away from the IR, instead of having its posterior surface against it. This will create a small OID, but not enough to result in a significant loss of detail sharpness. The CR remains perpendicular to the IR. The resulting projection will place each anterior rib below its corresponding posterior rib and demonstrate the posterior ribs with a gentle, superiorly bowed contour (Figures 3-106 and 3-111). This could also be accomplished by leaving the posterior chest against the IR and angling the CR 5 degrees caudally.

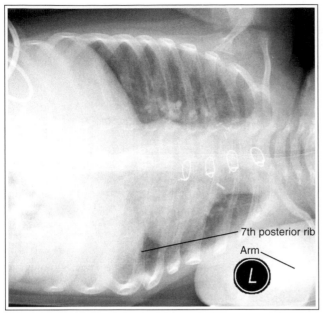

FIGURE 3-109 Neonate AP (left lateral decubitus) chest taken with left arm not elevated.

Neonate and Infant AP Decubitus Chest Analysis Practice

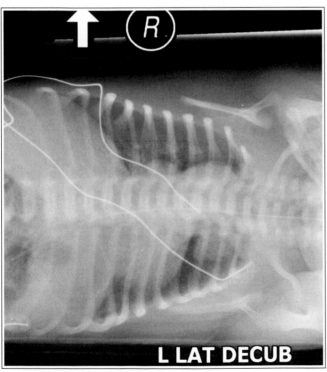

IMAGE 3-26

Analysis. The chest demonstrates a lordotic appearance. Each upper anterior rib is superior to its corresponding posterior rib, whereas each lower anterior rib is demonstrated below its corresponding posterior rib. The upper midcoronal plane is too close to the IR and the CR is centered too inferiorly. The left sternal clavicular end is demonstrated further from the vertebral column

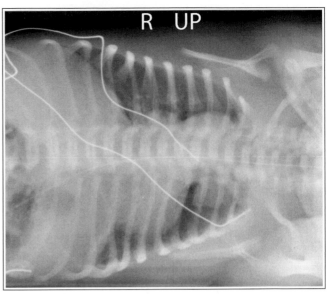

FIGURE 3-110 Neonate AP (left lateral decubitus) chest with lordotic appearance.

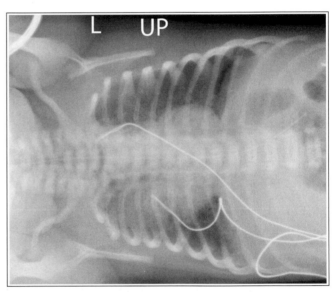

FIGURE 3-111 Neonate AP (right lateral decubitus) chest taken with upper chest positioned slightly away from IR.

than the right and the left posterior ribs are longer than the right.

Correction. Angle the CR 5 degrees caudally or move the superior chest and shoulders 5 degrees away from the IR. Rotate the left side of the chest away from the IR until the midcoronal plane is parallel with the IR.

CHILD CHEST: AP AND PA PROJECTION (RIGHT OR LEFT LATERAL DECUBITUS POSITION)

See Table 3-14, (Figures 3-112 and 3-113).

The image analysis guidelines for AP/PA decubitus chest projections in children are the same as those of infant or adult AP/PA decubitus chest. The size of the

TABLE 3-14	Child AP-PA (Lateral Decubitus) Chest Projection
Image Analysis Guidelines (Figure 3-112)	**Related Positioning Procedures (Figure 3-113)**
• Thoracic vertebrae and posterior ribs are seen through the heart and mediastinal structures.	• Appropriate technical data have been set.
• An arrow or "word" marker identifies the side of the patient positioned up and away from the imaging table or cart.	• Place proper marker on IR.
• Lung field adjacent to the table or cart is demonstrated without superimposition of the pad.	• Position the side of the child that will best demonstrate the suspected condition closest to the table or cart, on a radiolucent sponge or a hard surface in a lateral recumbent position.
• Lung fields demonstrate symmetry. • Distances from the vertebral column to the sternal clavicular ends are equal. • Lengths of the right and left corresponding posterior ribs are equal.	• Center the chest to the upright IR in an AP or PA projection. • Align the shoulders, the posterior ribs, and the ASISs at equal distances with the IR, aligning the midcoronal plane parallel with the IR. • Flex knees and place a pillow between them.
• Arms, mandible, lateral borders of the scapulae and chin are situated outside the lung field.	• Reach the arms above the head. • Elevate the chin.
• Manubrium is superimposed by the fourth thoracic vertebra. • 1 inch (2.5 cm) of apical lung field visible above the clavicles.	• Align the midcoronal plane parallel with the IR.
• Sixth or seventh thoracic vertebra is at the center of the exposure field.	• Center a perpendicular CR at or slightly inferior to the mammary line.
• Both lungs, from apices to costophrenic angles, are included within the exposure field.	• Center the IR to the CR. • Longitudinally collimate to include the shoulder top and inferior ribs. • Transversely collimate to within 0.5 inches (2.5 cm) of the lateral skin line.
• At least 9 posterior ribs are visualized above the diaphragm.	• Take the exposure after the second full suspended inspiration.

child determines the guidelines that best meet the situation. For a discussion on the topics needed to analyze the following image, refer to the discussion of AP-PA (lateral decubitus) chest projections earlier in this chapter.

Child AP-PA (Lateral Decubitus) Chest Analysis Practice

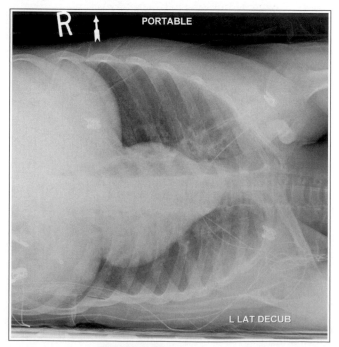

IMAGE 3-27 AP projection.

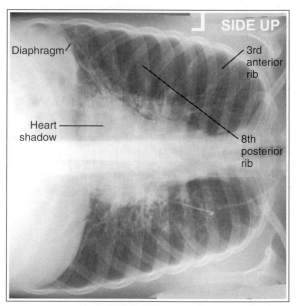

FIGURE 3-112 Child PA (right lateral decubitus) chest projection with accurate positioning.

Analysis. The right sternal clavicular end is situated farther from the vertebral column than the left side and the posterior ribs on the right side demonstrate the greater length. The patient was rotated toward the right side. The manubrium is situated at the level of the second thoracic vertebrae. The upper midcoronal plane was tilted toward the IR.

Correction. Rotate the patient's right side away from the IR and tilt the upper thorax away from the IR until the midcoronal plane is parallel with the IR.

ABDOMEN

Technical Data. When the technical data in Table 3-15 are followed, or adjusted as needed for additive and destructive patient conditions (see Table 2-6), along with the best practices discussed in Chapters 1 and 2, the abdominal projections will demonstrate the image analysis guidelines listed in Box 3-2 unless otherwise indicated.

Subject Contrast and Brightness. The subject contrast and image brightness are adequate on adult abdominal projections when the collections of fat that outline the psoas major muscles and kidney as well as the bony structures of the inferior ribs and transverse processes of the lumbar vertebrae are visualized. Because soft tissue abdominal structures are similar in atomic number and tissue density, whether two soft tissue structures that border each other are visible or not depends on their arrangement with respect to the gas and fat collections that lie next to them, around them, or within them. These same gas and fat collections are used to identify

diseases and masses within the abdomen. The presence or absence of gas, as well as its amount and location within the intestinal system, may indicate a functional, metabolic, or mechanical disease, whereas routinely seen collections of fat may be displaced or obscured with organ enlargement or mass invasion.

Locating the Psoas Major Muscles and Kidneys. The psoas major muscles are located laterally to the lumbar vertebrae. They originate at the first lumbar vertebra on each side and extend to the corresponding lesser trochanter. On an AP abdominal projection, the psoas major muscles are visible as long, triangular, soft tissue shadows on each side of the vertebral bodies. The kidneys are found in the posterior abdomen and are identified on abdominal projections as bean-shaped densities located on each side of the vertebral column 3 inches (7.5 cm) from the midline. The upper poles of the kidney lie on the same transverse level as the spinous process of the eleventh thoracic vertebra, and the lower poles lie on the

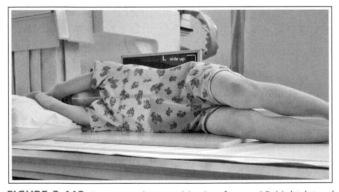

FIGURE 3-113 Proper patient positioning for an AP (right lateral decubitus) chest projection.

BOX 3-2	Abdomen Technical Data Imaging Analysis Guidelines

- The facility's identification requirements are visible.
- A right and left marker identifying the correct side of the patient is present on the projection and is not superimposed over the VOI.
- Good radiation protection practices are evident.
- Cortical outlines of the posterior ribs, lumbar vertebrae, and pelvis and the gases within the stomach and intestine lines are sharply defined.
- Adult: Contrast resolution is adequate to demonstrate the collections of fat that outline the psoas major muscles and kidneys, and the bony structures of the inferior ribs and transverse processes of the lumbar vertebrae.
- Children: Contrast resolution is adequate to demonstrate the diaphragm, bowel gas pattern, and faint outline of bony structures.
- No quantum mottle or saturation is present.
- Scattered radiation has been kept to a minimum.
- There is no evidence of removable artifacts.

TABLE 3-15	Abdomen Technical Data				
Adult Abdomen Technical Data					
Projection	kV	Grid	AEC	mAs	SID
AP, supine and upright	70-80	Grid	All three		40-48 inches (100-120 cm)
AP (lateral decubitus)	70-80	Grid	Center		40-48 inches (100-120 cm)
Pediatric Abdomen Technical Data					
Neonate: AP	70-80			3	40-48 inches (100-120 cm)
Infant: AP	70-80			5	40-48 inches (100-120 cm)
Child: AP	70-80	Grid*	All three		40-inches (100-120 cm)
Neonate: AP (lateral decubitus)	70-80			3	40-48 inches (100-120 cm)
Infant: AP (lateral decubitus)	70-80			5	40-48 inches (100-120 cm)
Child: AP (lateral decubitus)	70-80	Grid*	Center		40-48 inches (100-120 cm)

*Use grid if part thickness measures 4 inches (10 cm) or more.

same transverse level as the spinous process of the third lumbar vertebra. The right kidney is usually demonstrated approximately 1 inch (2.5 cm) inferior to the left kidney because of its location beneath the liver. Occasionally a kidney may be displaced inferiorly (nephroptosis) to this location, because it is not held in place by adjacent organs or its fat covering; this condition is most often seen in thin patients.

Adjusting Technical Data for Patient Conditions

Bowel Gas. The routinely set technical factors obtained from the AP body measurement of patients with suspected large amounts of bowel gas may cause IR overexposure and saturation in areas of the abdomen that are overlaid with gas (Figure 3-114). (The patient

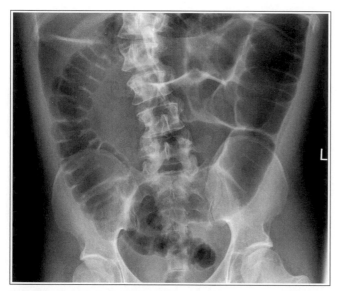

FIGURE 3-114 Supine AP abdomen demonstrating excessive bowel gas.

measures the same whether gas or dense soft tissue causes the thickness.) This decreased brightness results from the low tissue density characteristic of gas. As the radiation passes through the patient's body, fewer photons are absorbed where gas is located than where dense soft tissue is present. To compensate for this situation, decrease the exposure (mAs) 30% to 50% or the kV 5% to 8% from the routinely used manual technique before the projection is taken.

Ascites, Obesity, Bowel Obstruction, or Soft Tissue Masses. An underexposed projection may result when patients have ascites, obesity, bowel obstructions, or soft tissue masses. This is because sections of the abdomen that normally contain gas or fat do not, resulting in an increase in the tissue density of the soft tissue. To compensate for this situation, increase the exposure (mAs) 30% to 50% or the kV 5% to 8% from the routinely used technique before the projection is taken.

Pendulous Breasts. Large pendulous breasts may obscure the upper abdominal area on the upright AP abdomen projection, as they add a thicker, dense region to this area. To reduce this tissue density and provide more uniform brightness across the abdomen, have the patient elevate and shift the breasts laterally for the projection (Figure 3-115).

Abdominal Lines, Devices, Tubes, and Catheters.
Familiarizing yourself with the accurate placement of the devices, lines, and catheters that are seen on abdominal projections will provide the information needed to identify when proper technique was used to visualize them and when poor placement is suspected.

Nasogastric Tubes. The nasogastric (NG) tube passes through the nose and extends to the stomach. The NG tube is used for feeding, when the patient is unable to swallow normally because of trauma or disease, for

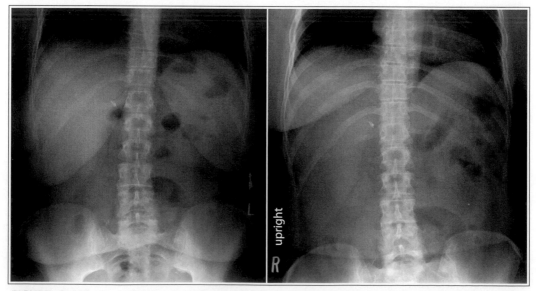

FIGURE 3-115 AP abdomens comparing brightness change when pendulous breasts are moved laterally.

the removal of gas and secretions by suction (decompression), and for radiographic examinations of the stomach. Projections taken that demonstrate the NG tube should demonstrate adequate subject contrast to visualize the upper left abdominal region (Figure 3-116).

Spinal Stimulator Implant. The spinal stimulator implant is used to treat chronic pain. The stimulator is implanted under the skin in the abdomen, and the leads are inserted under the skin to where they are inserted into the spinal canal. Projections taken that demonstrate

the spinal stimulator should demonstrate adequate subject contrast to visualize the abdominal and spinal structures (Figure 3-117).

Free Intraperitoneal Air. The upright AP abdomen is most often used to evaluate the peritoneal cavity for intraperitoneal air. For intraperitoneal air to be demonstrated best, the patient should be positioned upright for 5 to 20 minutes before the projection is taken. This allows enough time for the air to move away from the soft tissue abdominal structures and rise to the level of the diaphragms (Figure 3-118). If a patient has come to the imaging department for a supine and upright abdominal series, begin with the upright projection if the patient is ambulatory (able to walk) or transported by wheelchair. An ambulatory or wheelchair-using patient has been upright long enough for the air to rise, so it is not necessary to wait to take the projection.

Variations in Positioning Procedure Due to Body Habitus. Because the abdominal cavity varies in size and length owing to differences in body habitus and because the abdomen carries much of the fat tissue on the obese patient, there is not a standard protocol that can be followed for all patients for the number of IRs that are needed, the IR size and direction to use, or where the CR is centered. These are chosen so that when all the projections obtained for the exam are combined they together include all of the required image analysis guidelines. Failing to choose correctly results in clipped structures and an incomplete picture of the peritoneal cavity (Figure 3-119). The guidelines in Tables 3-16 and 3-17 are for the routine sthenic, hyposthenic, and asthenic, nonobese patient with descriptions for other body habitus to follow. The sthenic and hyposthenic patients make up about 85% of the population.

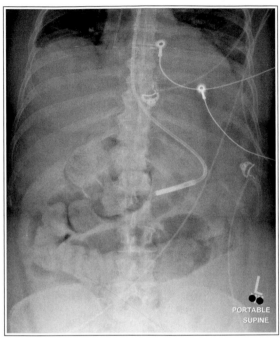

FIGURE 3-116 Supine AP abdomen with accurate nasogastric tube placement.

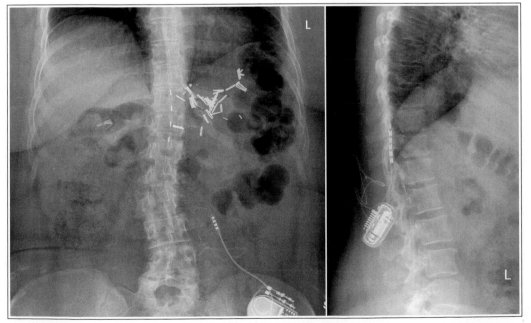

FIGURE 3-117 AP abdomen and lateral vertebrae demonstrating spinal stimulator implant.

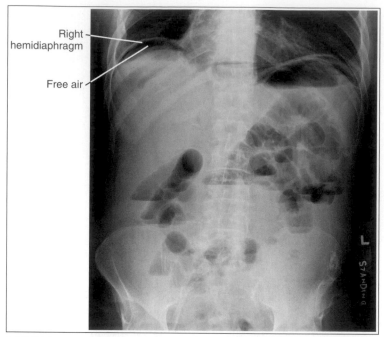

FIGURE 3-118 Upright AP abdomen demonstrating free intraperitoneal air.

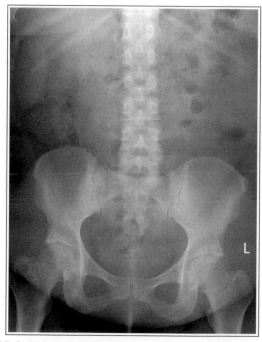

FIGURE 3-119 Supine AP abdomen that does not include all of the required abdominal tissue.

ABDOMEN: AP PROJECTION (SUPINE AND UPRIGHT)

See Tables 3-16 and 3-17, (Figures 3-120, 3-121, 3-122, and 3-123).

Abdominal Body Habitus

Hypersthenic. The hypersthenic patient's abdomen is broad across the lower thorax (lateral rib to lateral rib) and the torso is short (less distance between lower rib cage and the symphysis pubis) in comparison to the other body types (Figure 12-2). The widest part of the abdominal cavity is at the upper abdomen.

Asthenic. The asthenic patient's abdomen is generally narrow across the lower thorax and the torso is long in comparison to the other body types (Figure 12-3). The widest part of the abdominal cavity is at the lower abdomen.

Sthenic. The sthenic habitus is the most common, being between the hypersthenic and asthenic body types, and is considered to have the average torso width and length (Figure 12-4).

Obese. The obese patient can have the bony architect of any of the above body habitus. In these patients the peritoneal cavity and the soft tissue that surrounds it increases in size outside the bony structures that are used to define these habitus (Figure 3-125).

Body Habitus and IR Size and Placement Variations. For the supine AP abdomen, including the twelfth thoracic vertebra ensures that the kidneys, tip of liver, and spleen, all of which lie inferior to it, will be present on the projection. Including the symphysis pubis ensures that the inferior border of the peritoneal cavity is present on the projection (see Figure 3-120). For intraperitoneal air to be demonstrated on the upright AP abdomen, the diaphragm must be included in its entirety, because the air would be located directly inferior to the domes of the diaphragm (see Figure 3-118). When the projection is taken on expiration, including the eighth thoracic vertebra will ensure demonstration of the right and the left diaphragm domes. To include these needed anatomic

TABLE 3-16	**Supine AP Abdomen Projection**
	For Sthenic, Hyposthenic, and Asthenic, Nonobese Patient

Image Analysis Guidelines (Figure 3-120)	Related Positioning Procedures (Figure 3-121)
• Spinous processes are aligned with the midline of the vertebral bodies, with pedicles at equal distances from them. • Iliac wings are symmetrical. • Sacrum is centered within the inlet of pelvis and is aligned with the symphysis pubis.	• *Computed radiography:* Use a 14 × 17 inch (35 × 43 cm) IR cassette, positioned LW. • Position the patient on the table in a supine AP projection. • Place the shoulders, the posterior ribs, and the ASISs at equal distanced from the table, aligning the midcoronal plane parallel with table.
• Long axis of the vertebral column is centered on projection. • Fourth lumbar vertebra is at the center of the exposure field.	• Align the midsagittal plane to the center of the IR and grid. • Center a perpendicular CR to the midsagittal plane at the level of the iliac crest for female patients and at a level of 1 inch (2.5 cm) inferior to the iliac crest for male patients. • Center IR and grid to CR.
• Twelfth thoracic vertebra, the lateral body soft tissues, the iliac wings, and the symphysis pubis are included within the exposure field. • Diaphragm domes are located superior to the ninth posterior ribs.	• Open the longitudinal collimation to a 17 inch (43 cm) field size. • Transversely collimate to within 0.5 inch (2.5 cm) of the lateral skin line. • Take the exposure after full suspended expiration.

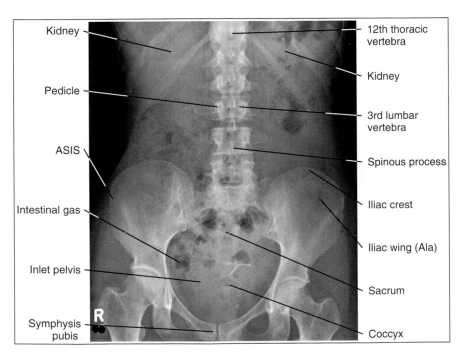

FIGURE 3-120 Supine AP abdomen projection with accurate positioning.

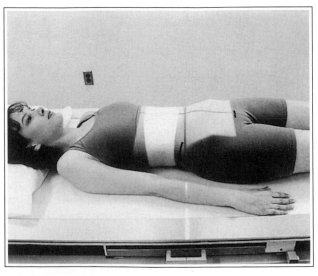

FIGURE 3-121 Proper patient positioning for supine AP abdomen projection.

TABLE 3-17	**Upright AP Abdomen Projection**
	For Sthenic, Hyposthenic, and Asthenic, Nonobese Patient

Image Analysis Guidelines (Figure 3-122)	Related Positioning Procedures (Figure 3-123)
• An arrow or "word" marker, indicating that the patient was in an upright position, is present. • Spinous processes are aligned with the midline of the vertebral bodies, with pedicles at equal distances from them. • Iliac wings are symmetrical. • Sacrum is centered within the inlet of pelvis and is aligned with the symphysis pubis.	• Add arrow or "word" marker to indicate that the patient was in an upright position. • *Computed radiography:* Use a 14 × 17 inch (35 × 43 cm) IR cassette, positioned LW. • Position the patient against the upright table or IR in an AP projection. • Place the shoulders, the posterior ribs, and the ASISs at equal distances from the table or upright IR, aligning the midcoronal plane parallel with IR.
• Long axis of the vertebral column is centered on projection. • Third lumbar vertebra is at the center of the exposure field.	• Center the midsagittal plane to IR and grid. • Place the top of the IR at a level of the axilla (not the top of the collimator light field). • Center a horizontal CR to the grid and IR.
• Eighth thoracic vertebra, lateral body soft tissue, and iliac wings are included within the exposure field.	• Open the longitudinal collimation to a 17 inch (43 cm) field size. • Transversely collimate to within 0.5 inch (2.5 cm) of the lateral skin line.
• Diaphragm domes are located superior to the ninth posterior ribs.	• Take the exposure after full suspended expiration.

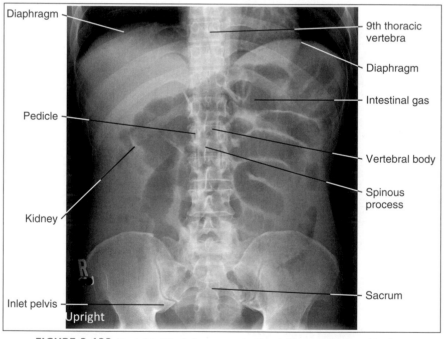

Diaphragm — 9th thoracic vertebra — Diaphragm — Intestinal gas — Pedicle — Vertebral body — Spinous process — Kidney — Inlet pelvis — Sacrum — Upright — R

FIGURE 3-122 Upright AP abdomen projection with accurate positioning.

structures, the number and sizes of IRs that are required, the IR placement, and the CR centering will need to be varied as follows for the differing body habitus and patient sizes.

Supine Hypersthenic Patient. If using the computed radiography system, two 14 × 17 inch (35 × 43 cm) crosswise IRs are needed to include the required anatomic structures as long as the transverse abdominal measurement is less than 17 inches (43 cm) (Figure 3-124). Take the first projection with the CR centered to the midsagittal plane at a level halfway between the symphysis pubis and ASIS. Position the bottom of the second IR so that it includes 2 to 3 inches (5-7.5 cm) of the same transverse section of the peritoneal cavity imaged on the first projection to ensure that no middle peritoneal information has been excluded. The top of the

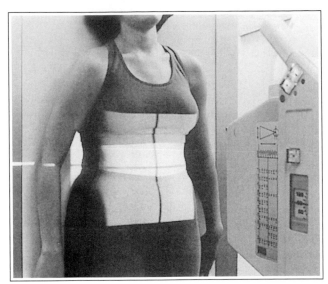

FIGURE 3-123 Proper patient positioning for upright AP abdomen projection.

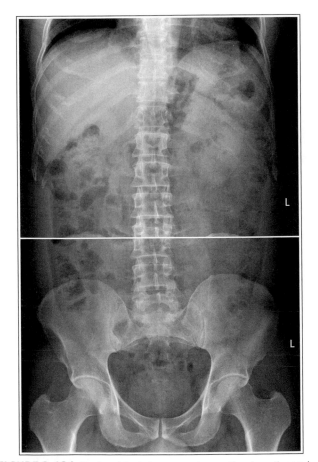

FIGURE 3-124 Supine AP abdomen on hypersthenic patient taken using to crosswise IR cassettes.

IR should extend to the patient's xiphoid, to make sure that the twelfth thoracic vertebra is included.

If using the DR system, open the longitudinal collimation the full 17 inches (43 cm) and transversely collimate to within 0.5 inches (2.5 cm) of the lateral skin line as

needed to the full 17 inches (43 cm) available. If more than 17 inches (43 cm) of transverse width is needed for either of these systems, follow the obese procedure following.

Upright Hypersthenic Patient. Follow the same general procedure explained for the supine hypersthenic patient with the exception that the first projection is taken with the top of the IR positioned just a bit higher than the axilla and the second projection includes 2 to 3 inches (5-7.5 cm) of the same transverse section of the peritoneal cavity imaged on the first projection.

Supine Obese Patient. It may be necessary to obtain three or four images to demonstrate all of the abdominal structures for the obese patient. Figure 3-125 demonstrates a supine AP abdomen procedure on an obese patient that required three projections to include all of the required abdominal tissue. If using the computed radiography system, take the first projection with the IR crosswise and the CR centered to the midsagittal plane at a level halfway between the symphysis pubis and ASIS. To obtain the second projection, place the IR lengthwise and positioned so the bottom of the IR includes 2 to 3 inches (5-7.5 cm) of the same transverse section of peritoneal cavity imaged on the first projection, center the CR to the IR, and then move the patient (and tabletop) laterally until the CR is centered on the right side half-way between the midsagittal plane and lateral soft tissue. For the third projection, repeat the procedure for the left side of the patient. The second and third projections should include 2 to 3 inches (5-7.5 cm) of overlapping peritoneal tissue at the midsagittal plane.

If using the DR system, follow that used for the computed radiography system with the exception that collimation will need to be increased below the full 17 inches (43 cm) for the projections or more than 2 to 3 inches (5-7.5 cm) of overlap will result.

Upright Obese Patient. Follow the same general procedure explained for the supine obese patient with the exception that the two lengthwise projections should be obtained first, with the top of the IRs positioned at the axilla, and then the third crosswise projection is obtained of the lower peritoneal cavity. Each projection should include 2 to 3 inches (5-7.5 cm) of the same tissue that is included in the adjacent projection.

Midcoronal Plane Positioning and Rotation. Failing to position the midcoronal plane parallel with the IR for an AP abdomen decreases the visualization of fat lines that surround abdominal structures. For example, the psoas major muscles are outlined on the projection because of the fat that lies next to them. When the patient is rotated to one side, this fat shifts from lateral to anterior or posterior with respect to the muscle. The shift eliminates the subject contrast difference that exists when the muscle and fat are separated, hindering the usefulness of the psoas major muscles as diagnostic indicators.

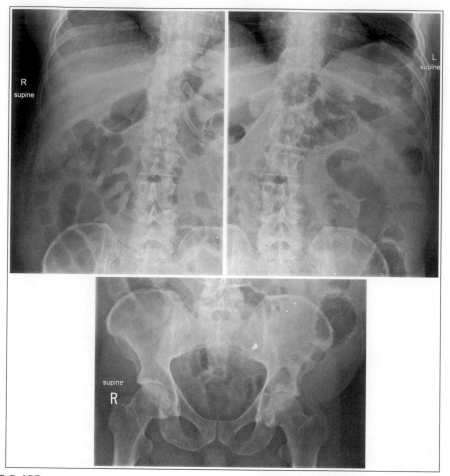

FIGURE 3-125 Supine AP abdomen on obese patient taken using two lengthwise and one crosswise IR cassettes.

The upper and lower lumbar vertebrae can demonstrate rotation independently or simultaneously, depending on which section of the body is rotated. If the patient's thorax was rotated but the pelvis remained in an AP projection, the upper lumbar vertebrae and abdominal cavity demonstrate rotation. If the patient's pelvis was rotated but the thorax remained in an AP projection, the lower vertebrae and abdominal cavity demonstrate rotation. If the patient's thorax and pelvis were rotated simultaneously, the entire lumbar column and abdominal cavity demonstrate rotation. Rotation is effectively detected on an AP abdomen projection by comparing the distance from the pedicles to the spinous processes on each side, by comparing the widths of the iliac wings, and by evaluating the centering of the sacrum within the inlet pelvis. If the distance from the pedicles to the spinous processes is greater on one side of the vertebrae than on the other, one iliac wing is narrower than the other, or if the sacrum is rotated toward one side of the inlet, pelvic rotation is present (Figures 3-126 and 3-127). The side with the smaller distance between the pedicles and spinous processes, the narrower iliac wing, and the side toward which the sacrum is rotated is the side of the patient positioned farther from the table and IR.

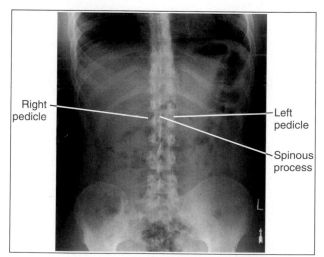

FIGURE 3-126 Upright AP abdomen taken with left side of abdomen rotated closer to IR than right side.

Distinguishing Abdominal Rotation from Scoliosis. In patients with scoliosis, the lumbar bodies may appear rotated because of the lateral twisting of the vertebrae. Scoliosis of the vertebral column can be very severe, demonstrating a large degree of lateral deviation,

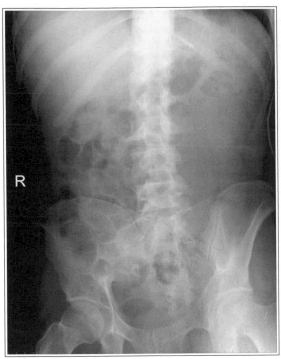

FIGURE 3-127 Supine AP abdomen taken with right side of abdomen rotated closer to IR than left side.

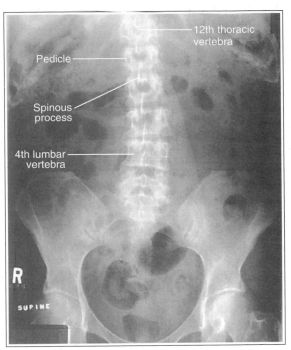

FIGURE 3-129 Supine AP abdomen taken on patient with subtle scoliosis.

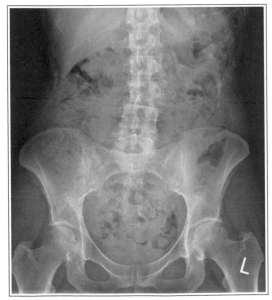

FIGURE 3-128 Supine AP abdomen taken on patient with scoliosis.

or it can be subtle, demonstrating only a small degree of deviation. Severe scoliosis is very obvious and is seldom mistaken for patient rotation, whereas subtle scoliotic changes can be easily mistaken for patient rotation (Figures 3-128 and 3-129). Although both demonstrate unequal distances between the pedicles and spinous processes, clues that can be used to distinguish subtle

scoliosis from rotation are present. The long axis of a rotated vertebral column remains straight, whereas the scoliotic vertebral column demonstrates lateral deviation. When the lumbar vertebrae demonstrate rotation, it has been caused by the rotation of the upper or lower torso. The middle lumbar vertebrae (L3 and L4) cannot rotate unless the lower thoracic vertebrae or upper or lower lumbar vertebrae are also rotated. On the scoliotic projection, the middle lumbar vertebrae may demonstrate rotation without corresponding upper or lower vertebral rotation. This constitutes an acceptable projection for a patient with this condition.

Respiration. From full inspiration to expiration, the diaphragm position moves in the vertical dimension as much as 4 inches (10 cm). This movement also changes the pressure placed on the abdominal structures. On full expiration, the right side of the diaphragm dome is at the same transverse level as the eighth or ninth thoracic vertebra, whereas on inspiration, it may be found at a transverse level as low as the twelfth thoracic vertebra (Figure 3-130). Expiration is preferred for the AP abdominal projection, because it places less diaphragm pressure on the abdominal organs, resulting in more space in the peritoneal cavity and less abdominal density.

AEC Chamber and Respiration. Quantum mottle may also result in AP upper projections that are obtained with full inspiration when the three AEC chambers are chosen, because the outside AEC chambers will be positioned beneath the lungs instead of abdominal structures.

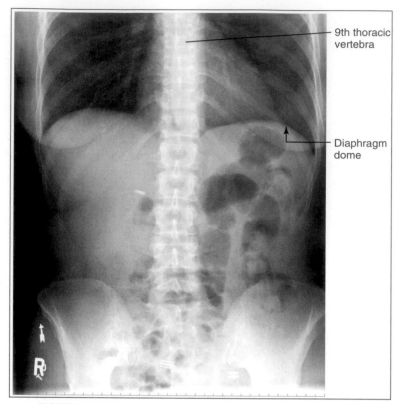

FIGURE 3-130 Upright AP abdomen taken after full inspiration.

AP Abdomen Analysis Practice

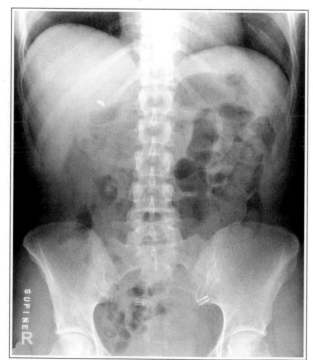

IMAGE 3-28 Supine abdomen.

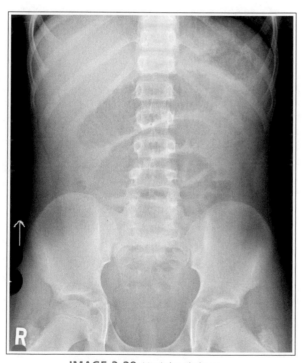

IMAGE 3-29 Upright abdomen.

Analysis. The symphysis pubis is not included on the projection. The CR was centered too superiorly.
Correction. Because this is a male patient, center the CR 1 inch (2.5 cm) inferior to the iliac crest.

Analysis. The domes of the diaphragm are not included on the projection. The CR was centered too inferiorly.
Correction. Center the CR and IR approximately 2 inches (5 cm) superiorly.

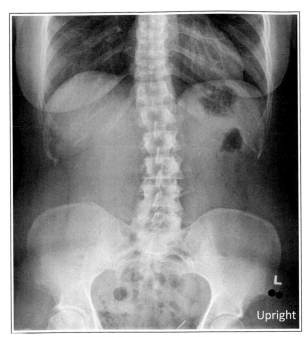

IMAGE 3-30 Upright abdomen.

Analysis. The diaphragm is at the level of the eleventh thoracic vertebra. The projection was taken on inspiration.

Correction. Take the exposure after full expiration.

ABDOMEN: AP PROJECTION (LEFT LATERAL DECUBITUS POSITION)

See Table 3-18, (Figures 3-131 and 3-132).

IR Size and Direction

Hypersthenic and Obese Patient. When using the computed radiography system, position two IRs crosswise with respect to the patient to include all the necessary anatomic structures in the hypersthenic patient. Take the first projection with the side of the IR placed at a level 2.5 inches (6.25 cm) superior to the xiphoid. Position the top of the second IR such that it includes approximately 2 to 3 inches (5-7.5 cm) of the same transverse section of the peritoneal cavity imaged on the

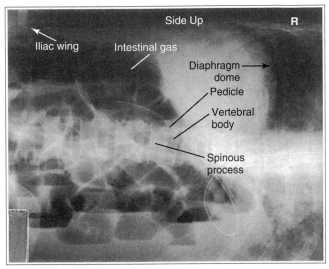

FIGURE 3-131 AP (left lateral decubitus) abdomen with accurate positioning.

TABLE 3-18	AP (Lateral Decubitus) Abdomen Projection *For Sthenic, Hyposthenic, and Asthenic, Nonobese Patient*
Image Analysis Guidelines (Figure 3-131)	**Related Positioning Procedures (Figure 3-132)**
• An arrow or "word" marker, indicating that the right side of the patient was positioned up and away from the table or cart, is present.	• Add right marker and arrow or "word" marker next to the right side to indicate that the side was positioned up, away from table or cart.
• Spinous processes are aligned with the midline of the vertebral bodies, with pedicles at equal distances from them. • Iliac wings are symmetrical.	• *Computed radiography:* Use a 14 × 17 inch (35 × 43 cm) IR cassette, positioned LW. • Position the patient on the table or cart in a left lateral recumbent position. • Place the abdomen against the IR in an AP projection. • Position the shoulders, the posterior ribs, and the ASISs directly on top of each other and at equal distances from the IR, aligning the midcoronal plane parallel with IR. • Flex knees and place a pillow between them.
• Third lumbar vertebra is at the center of the exposure field.	• Place the top of the IR at a level 2.5 inches (6.25 cm) superior to the xiphoid. • Center the midsagittal plane to the IR. • Center a horizontal CR to the grid and IR.
• Right hemidiaphragm, eighth thoracic vertebra, right lateral body soft tissue, and iliac wings are included within the exposure field. • Density is uniform across the abdomen.	• Open the longitudinal collimation to a 17 inch (43 cm) field size. • Transversely collimate to within 0.5 inch (2.5 cm) of the lateral skin line. • Use a wedge compensation filter for patients with excessive abdominal soft tissue that drops toward the table or cart.
• Diaphragm domes are located superior to the ninth posterior rib.	• Take the exposure after full suspended expiration.

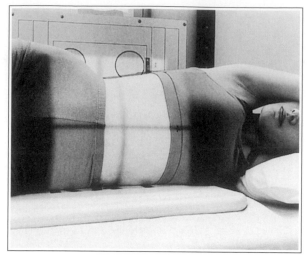

FIGURE 3-132 Proper patient positioning for AP (left lateral decubitus) abdomen projection.

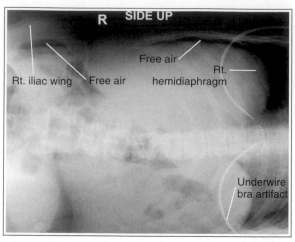

FIGURE 3-133 AP (left lateral decubitus) abdomen demonstrating free intraperitoneal air under right hemidiaphragm and right iliac wing.

first projection to ensure that no middle peritoneal information has been excluded. For the obese patient the IR and the CR centering may need to be offset from the midsagittal plane toward the side up and away from the table or cart to include the required hemidiaphragm and iliac wing.

Demonstrating Intraperitoneal Air. The AP (decubitus) projection is primarily used to confirm the presence of intraperitoneal air. In the AP decubitus position, intraperitoneal air will rise to the highest level, which in most patients means it moves to the right upper quadrant just below the elevated hemidiaphragm, between the liver and abdominal wall. The left over the right lateral decubitus position is chosen to place the gastric bubble away from the elevated hemidiaphragm, preventing it from being mistaken for intraperitoneal air. For intraperitoneal air to be demonstrated best, the patient should be left in the lateral decubitus position for 5 to 20 minutes before the projection is taken, allowing enough time for the air to move away from the soft-tissue abdominal structures and rise (Figure 3-133). To eliminate long waiting periods for patients who are scheduled to have a decubitus abdomen, have them transported to the imaging department in the left lateral recumbent position.

Patients with Wide Hips. In women with wide hips the right hemidiaphragm and iliac wing should be included on the projection, as the highest level within the peritoneal cavity in such a patient is just over the iliac bone (see Figure 3-133).

Midcoronal Plane Positioning and Rotation

Detecting Abdominal Rotation. Rotation is effectively detected on an AP abdominal (decubitus) projection by comparing the distance from the pedicles to the spinous processes on each side and the symmetry of the iliac wings. If the distance from the pedicles to the spinous processes is greater on one side of the vertebrae

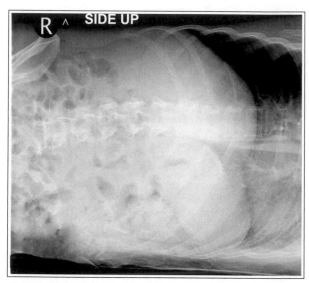

FIGURE 3-134 AP (left lateral decubitus) abdomen taken with left side of abdomen rotated closer to IR than right side.

than on the other side, the side with the smaller distance between the pedicles and spinous processes was the side of the patient positioned farther from the IR. If the iliac wings are not symmetrical, the narrower is on the side of the patient positioned farther from the IR (Figure 3-134).

Using a Wedge-Compensating Filter to Obtain Uniform Density. When an AP (decubitus) abdominal projection from a patient with excessive abdominal soft tissue is taken, the belly soft tissue often drops toward the table or cart. This movement results in a smaller AP measurement at the elevated right side than at the left side, which is positioned closer to the table or cart. To compensate for this thickness difference, a wedge-compensating filter may be used. When a wedge-compensating filter is used, attach it to the x-ray collimator head, with the thick end positioned toward the patient's right side and the thin end toward the left side. The collimator light projects a shadow of the compensating filter onto the patient. Position the shadow of the thin end at the level of the thickest part of the abdomen, allowing the thick end to extend toward the right side. Then use a technique that will accurately expose the thickest abdominal region. The wedge-compensating filter should absorb the needed photons to prevent too much exposure reaching the IR behind the thinner abdominal region. When the filter has been accurately positioned, brightness is uniform throughout the abdominal structures.

Respiration. See the discussion on supine AP abdomen projection.

AP (Left Lateral Decubitus) Abdomen Analysis Practice

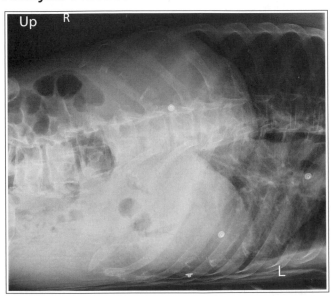

IMAGE 3-31

Analysis. The distances from the left pedicles to the spinous processes are greater than the distances from the right pedicles to the spinous process, and the right iliac

wing is narrower than the left iliac wing. The right side of the patient was positioned further from the IR than the left side.

Correction. Rotate the right side of the patient toward the IR until the midcoronal plane is aligned parallel with the IR. Place a pillow between the knees to help patient holds accurate positioning.

PEDIATRIC ABDOMEN

In infants and young children, it is difficult to differentiate between the small and large bowels. The gas loops tend to look the same. The abdominal organs (such as kidneys) are also not well defined because little intrinsic fat is present to outline them.

NEONATE AND INFANT ABDOMEN: AP PROJECTION (SUPINE)

See Table 3-19, (Figures 3-135 and 3-136).

Lumbar Vertebrae Alignment with IR. Aligning the long axis of the lumbar vertebral column with the long axis of the collimated field allows for tighter transverse collimation (Figure 3-137).

Midcoronal Plane and Rotation. The upper and lower lumbar vertebrae can demonstrate rotation independently or simultaneously, depending on which section of the body is rotated. Rotation is effectively detected on an AP abdomen projection by comparing the symmetry of the inferior posterior ribs and the iliac wings (Figure 3-138). The ribs that demonstrate the longer length and the iliac wing demonstrating the greater width are on the side toward which the patient is rotated.

Respiration. On full expiration the diaphragm dome is demonstrated above the eighth posterior rib. If the AP projection is taken on inspiration, the inferior placement of the diaphragm puts pressure on the abdominal organs, resulting in less space in the peritoneal cavity and greater abdominal density (see Figure 3-138).

TABLE 3-19	Neonate and Infant AP Abdomen Projection
Image Analysis Guidelines (Figure 3-135)	**Related Positioning Procedures (Figure 3-136)**
• Long axis of the vertebral column is centered on projection.	• Center the abdomen on the IR in a supine position. • Align the midsagittal plane to the center of the IR.
• Right and left inferior posterior ribs and iliac wings are symmetrical.	• Position the shoulders and the ASISs at equal distances from the IR, aligning the midcoronal plane parallel with the IR.
• Fourth lumbar vertebra is at the center of the exposure field.	• Center a perpendicular CR to the midsagittal plane at a transverse level 2 inches (5 cm) superior to the iliac crest. Slightly inferior centering may be needed for larger infants.
• Diaphragm, abdominal structures, and symphysis pubis are included in the exposure field.	• Longitudinal collimation to include the diaphragm (1 inch inferior to the mammary line) and symphysis pubis. • Transversely collimate to within 0.5 inch (1.25 cm) of the lateral skin line.
• Diaphragm domes are superior to the 8th posterior rib.	• Observe the chest movement and expose the image on expiration.

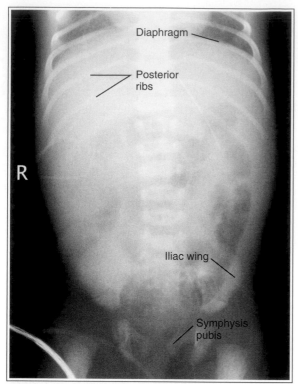

FIGURE 3-135 Neonatal AP abdomen projection with accurate positioning.

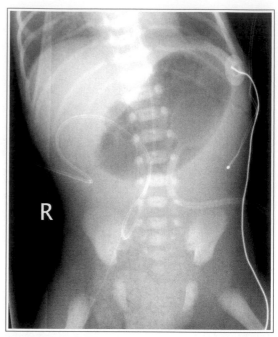

FIGURE 3-137 Neonate AP abdomen taken without alignment of the long axis of the vertebral column and the collimator light field.

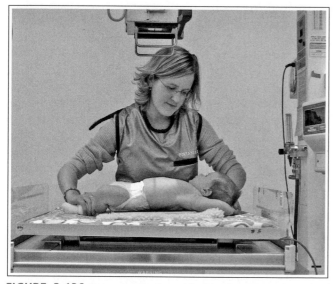

FIGURE 3-136 Proper patient positioning for AP neonate and infant abdomen projection.

Neonate and Infant: AP Abdominal Analysis

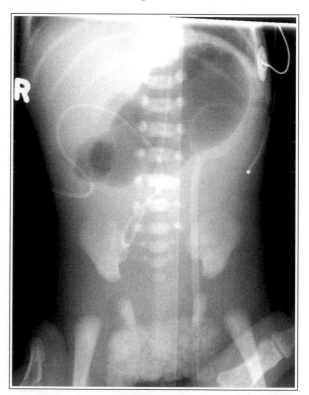

IMAGE 3-32

Ventilated Patient. If a high-frequency ventilator is being used, the exposure may be made at any time, but because this ventilator maintains the lung expansion at a steady mean pressure the projection will not be able to be taken on expiration. This will result in an acceptable projection demonstrating the diaphragm domes below the eighth posterior rib.

Analysis. The diaphragm is not included on the projection, and anatomic artifacts (positioning attendant's fingers) are demonstrated in the exposure field.

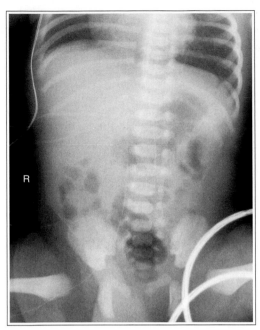

FIGURE 3-138 Neonate AP abdomen taken with right side of abdomen rotated closer to IR than left side and with full lung aeration.

Correction. Move the CR and IR 1 inch (2.5 cm) superiorly, and move the attendant's hands inferiorly outside of the collimated field.

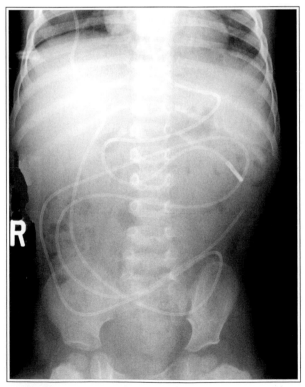

IMAGE 3-33

Analysis. The right posterior ribs are longer than the left, and the right iliac wing is wider than the left, indicating that the patient was rotated toward the right side.

Correction. Rotate the left side of the patient toward the IR until the midcoronal plane is aligned parallel with the IR.

CHILD ABDOMEN: AP PROJECTION (SUPINE AND UPRIGHT)

(Table 3-20), (Figures 3-139, 3-140, 3-141, and 3-142).

The analysis of child AP abdomen projections is the same as that of infant or adult AP abdomen projections (see earlier). The size of the child determines which guidelines best meet the situation. For a discussion on topics needed to analyze the following image, refer to the adult or infant abdominal discussion earlier in this chapter.

Child AP Abdominal Analysis Practice

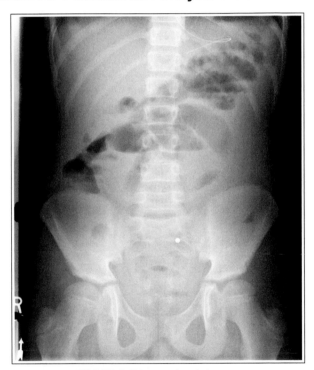

IMAGE 3-34 Upright abdomen.

Analysis. The diaphragm is not included on this projection. The CR and IR are positioned too inferiorly.
Correction. Move the CR and IR 2 inches (5 cm) superiorly.

NEONATE AND INFANT ABDOMEN: AP PROJECTION (LEFT LATERAL DECUBITUS POSITION)

See Table 3-21, (Figures 3-143 and 3-144).
Demonstrating Intraperitoneal Air. To demonstrate intraperitoneal air best, the patient should be left in this position for a few minutes to allow enough time for the air to move away from the soft tissue abdominal structures and rise to the level of the right diaphragm. With

TABLE 3-20	Child AP Abdomen Projection	
Image Analysis Guidelines (Figure 3-139)	**Related Positioning Procedures (Figures 3-140, 141, 142)**	
• Spinous processes are aligned with the midline of the vertebral bodies, with pedicles at equal distances from them. • Iliac wings are symmetrical. • Sacrum is centered within the inlet of pelvis and is aligned with the symphysis pubis. • *Supine:* fourth lumbar vertebra is at the center of the exposure field. • *Upright:* third lumbar vertebra is at the center of the exposure field. • *Supine:* eleventh thoracic vertebra, the lateral body soft tissues, the iliac wings, and the symphysis pubis are included within the exposure field. • *Upright:* ninth thoracic vertebra, lateral body soft tissue, and iliac wings are included within the exposure field. • Diaphragm domes are located superior to the ninth posterior ribs.	• *Supine:* Center the abdomen to the IR in a supine AP projection. • *Upright:* Center the abdomen to the upright IR in an AP projection. • Position the shoulders, the posterior ribs, and the ASISs at equal distances from the table or upright IR, aligning the midcoronal plane parallel with the IR. • *Supine:* Center a perpendicular CR to the patient's midsagittal plane at the level of the iliac crest. Center IR and CR. • *Upright:* Place the top of the IR at a level of the axilla. Center a horizontal CR to the midsagittal plane and IR. • Longitudinally collimate to include the diaphragm (1 inch inferior to the mammary line) and symphysis pubis. • Transversely collimate to within 0.5 inch (1.25 cm) of the lateral skin line. • Take the exposure after full suspended expiration.	

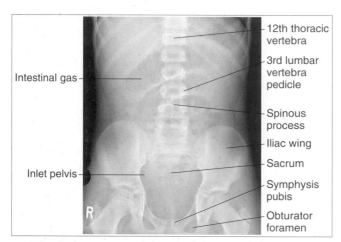

Intestinal gas

Inlet pelvis

R

12th thoracic vertebra

3rd lumbar vertebra pedicle

Spinous process

Iliac wing

Sacrum

Symphysis pubis

Obturator foramen

FIGURE 3-139 Child supine AP abdomen projection with accurate positioning.

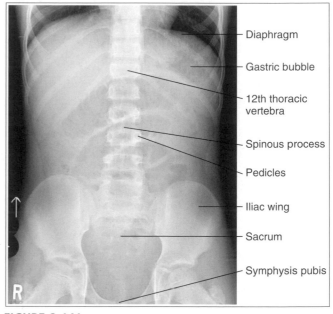

Diaphragm

Gastric bubble

12th thoracic vertebra

Spinous process

Pedicles

Iliac wing

Sacrum

Symphysis pubis

R

FIGURE 3-141 Child upright AP abdomen projection with accurate positioning.

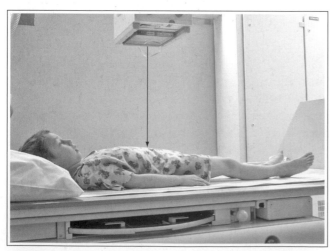

FIGURE 3-140 Proper positioning for a child supine AP abdomen projection.

the AP (decubitus) projection, intraperitoneal air will rise to the highest level of the right hemidiaphragm, so it must be included (Figure 3-145).

Midcoronal Plane Positioning and Rotation. Rotation is effectively detected on an AP (decubitus) abdominal projection by comparing the symmetry of the posterior ribs and the iliac wings (see Figure 3-146). The ribs that demonstrate the longer length and the ilium demonstrating the greater width are present on the side toward which the patient is rotated.

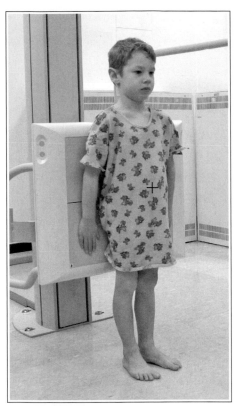

FIGURE 3-142 Proper positioning for a child upright AP abdomen projection.

Neonate and Infant AP (Left Lateral Decubitus) Abdominal Analysis Practice

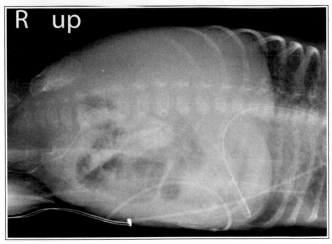

IMAGE 3-35

Analysis. The left-side posterior ribs are longer than the right side, and the right iliac wing is wider than the left, indicating that the patient was rotated toward the left side.

Correction. Rotate the right side of patient toward the IR until the midcoronal plane is aligned parallel with the IR.

CHILD ABDOMEN: AP PROJECTION (LEFT LATERAL DECUBITUS POSITION)

See Table 3-22, (Figures 3-146, 3-147, and 3-148).

The analysis of the child AP (left lateral decubitus) abdominal projection is the same as that of the infant or adult AP (left lateral decubitus) abdomen (see earlier). The size of the child determines which guidelines

TABLE 3-21	Neonate and Infant AP (Left Lateral Decubitus) Abdomen Projection
Imaging Analysis Guidelines (Figure 3-143)	**Related Positioning Procedures (Figure 3-144)**
• An arrow or "word" marker, indicating that the right side of the patient was positioned up and away from the imaging table or cart, is present.	• Add right marker and arrow or "word" that indicates that the right side was positioned up.
• Right and left inferior posterior ribs and the iliac wings are symmetrical.	• Position the infant in the immobilization device in a left lateral recumbent position. • Place the abdomen against the IR in an AP projection. • Position the shoulders, the posterior ribs, and the ASISs at equal distances with the IR, aligning the midcoronal plane parallel with the IR.
• Fourth lumbar vertebra is at the center of the exposure field.	• Center a horizontal CR to the midsagittal plane at a transverse level 2 inches (5 cm) superior to the iliac crest.
• Diaphragm and abdominal structures are included within the exposure field.	• Longitudinally collimate to include the diaphragm (1 inch inferior to the mammary line). • Transversely collimate to within 0.5 inch (1.25 cm) of the lateral skin line.
• Diaphragm domes are superior to the eighth posterior rib.	• Observe the chest movement and expose the image on expiration.

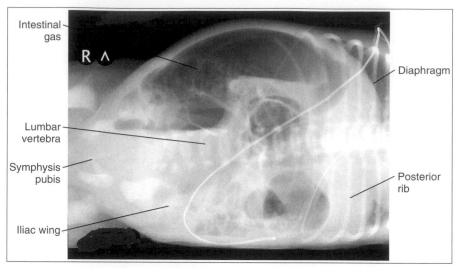

FIGURE 3-143 Neonatal AP (left lateral decubitus) abdomen projection with accurate positioning.

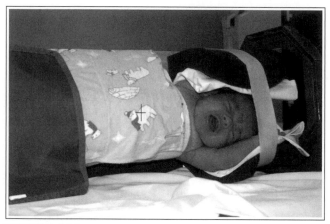

FIGURE 3-144 Proper patient positioning for AP (left lateral decubitus) neonate and infant abdomen projection.

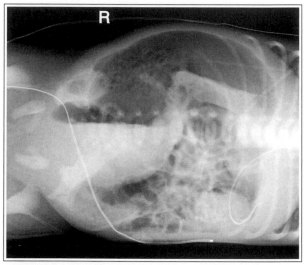

FIGURE 3-145 AP (left lateral decubitus) neonate abdomen demonstrating intraperitoneal air.

TABLE 3-22	**Child AP (Left Lateral Decubitus) Abdomen Projection**
Image Analysis Guidelines (Figures 3-146 and 3-147)	**Related Positioning Procedures (Figure 3-148)**
• An arrow or "word" marker, indicating that the right side of the patient was positioned up and away from the table or cart, is present.	• Add right marker and arrow or "word" marker next to the right side to indicate that the side was positioned up, away from table or cart.
• Right and left inferior posterior ribs and iliac wings are symmetrical. • Sacrum is centered within the inlet of pelvis and is aligned with the symphysis pubis.	• Position the patient on the table or cart in a left lateral recumbent position. • Place the patient against the IR in an AP projection. • Position the shoulders, the posterior ribs, and the ASISs directly on top of each other and at equal distances from the IR, aligning the midcoronal plane parallel with IR. • Flex knees and place a pillow between them.
• Third lumbar vertebra is at the center of the exposure field.	• Place the top of the IR at the axilla. • Center the midsagittal plane to the IR. • Center a horizontal CR to the IR.
• Right hemidiaphragm, ninth thoracic vertebra, right lateral body soft tissue, and iliac wings are included within the exposure field.	• Longitudinally collimate to include the diaphragm (1 inch inferior to the mammary line) and symphysis pubis. • Transversely collimate to within 0.5 inch (1.25 cm) of the lateral skin line.
• Diaphragm domes are located superior to the ninth posterior ribs.	• Take the exposure after full suspended expiration.

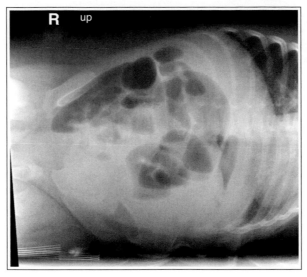

FIGURE 3-146 AP (left lateral decubitus) neonate abdomen taken with left side of abdomen rotated closer to IR than right side.

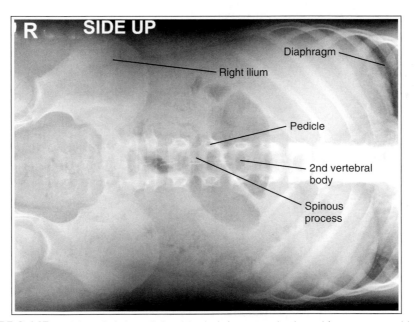

FIGURE 3-147 Child AP (left lateral decubitus) abdomen projection with accurate positioning.

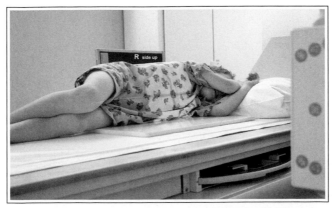

FIGURE 3-148 Proper positioning for a child AP (left lateral decubitus) abdomen projection.

best meet the situation. For discussion on topics needed to analyze the following image, refer to the earlier discussion of adult or infant AP (decubitus) abdomen projections.

Child AP (Left Lateral Decubitus) Abdomen Analysis Practice

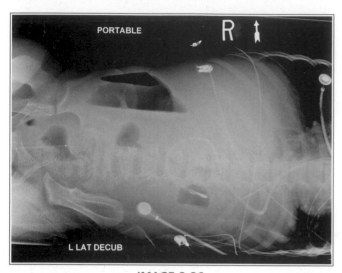

IMAGE 3-36

Analysis. The right-side posterior ribs are longer than the left side, and the right iliac wing is wider than the left, indicating that the patient was rotated toward the right side.

Correction. Rotate the right side of the patient away from the IR until the midcoronal plane is aligned parallel with the IR.

4

Upper Extremity

OUTLINE

Finger: PA Projection, 150
  PA Finger Analysis Practice, 154
Finger: PA Oblique Projection, 154
  PA Oblique Finger Analysis
    Practice, 157
Finger: Lateral Projection, 157
  Lateral Finger Analysis
    Practice, 159
Thumb: AP Projection, 159
  AP Thumb Analysis Practice, 162
Thumb: Lateral Projection, 162
  Lateral Thumb Analysis
    Practice, 164
Thumb: PA Oblique Projection, 164
  PA Oblique Thumb Analysis
    Practice, 167
Hand: PA Projection, 167
  PA Hand Analysis Practice, 170
Hand: PA Oblique Projection
  (Lateral Rotation), 170
  PA Oblique Hand Analysis
    Practice, 173
Hand: "Fan" Lateral Projection
  (Lateromedial), 173
  Lateral Hand Analysis
    Practice, 176

Wrist: PA Projection, 177
  PA Wrist Image Analysis
    Practice, 182
Wrist: PA Oblique Projection
  (Lateral Rotation), 182
  PA Oblique Wrist Analysis
    Practice, 186
Wrist: Lateral Projection
  (Lateromedial), 186
  Lateral Wrist Analysis
    Practice, 191
Wrist: Ulnar Deviation,
  PA Axial Projection
  (Scaphoid), 192
  PA Axial (Scaphoid) Analysis
    Practice, 197
Wrist: Carpal Canal (Tunnel)
  (Tangential, Inferosuperior
  Projection), 198
Forearm: AP Projection, 199
  AP Forearm Analysis
    Practice, 203
Forearm: Lateral Projection
  (Lateromedial), 203
  Lateral Forearm Analysis
    Practice, 207

Elbow: AP Projection, 207
  AP Elbow Analysis
    Practice, 212
Elbow: AP Oblique Projections
  (Medial and Lateral
  Rotation), 212
  AP Oblique Elbow Analysis
    Practice, 216
Elbow: Lateral Projection
  (Lateromedial), 217
  Lateral Elbow Analysis
    Practice, 222
Elbow: Axiolateral Elbow Projection
  (Coyle Method), 223
  Axiolateral Elbow (Coyle
  Method) Analysis
    Practice, 226
Humerus: AP Projection, 226
Humerus: Lateral Projection
  (Lateromedial and
  Mediolateral), 229
  Lateral Humeral Analysis
    Practice, 233

OBJECTIVES

After completion of this chapter, you should be able to do the following:

- Identify the required anatomy on upper extremity projections.
- Describe how to properly position the patient, image receptor (IR), and central ray (CR) on upper extremity projections.
- List the image analysis guidelines for upper extremity projections with accurate positioning.
- State how to reposition the patient properly when upper extremity projections with poor positioning are produced.
- Discuss how to determine the amount of patient or CR adjustment required to improve upper extremity projections with poor positioning.
- State the kilovoltage (kV) that is routinely used for upper extremity projections, and describe which anatomic structures will be visible when the correct technical factors are used.

- List the soft tissue structures that are of interest on upper extremity projections. State where they are located and describe why their visualization is important.
- Explain how wrist and elbow rotations affect the position of the radial and ulnar styloids.
- Discuss how a patient with large, muscular, or thick proximal forearms should be positioned for good posteroanterior (PA) and lateral wrist projections to be obtained.
- State the carpal bone changes that occur when the wrist is extended, deviated, or ulnar- and radial-deviated in the PA and lateral projections.
- Describe how the positioning procedure is adjusted if wrist projections are ordered with a request that more than one fourth of the distal forearm be included.
- Explain how and why the CR is adjusted for the PA ulnar-deviated scaphoid projection if a proximal or

distal scaphoid fracture is in question and if a patient cannot adequately ulnar-flex.
- List palpable structures used to identify the location of the elbow and glenohumeral joints.
- Explain how the patient is positioned if only one joint can be placed in its true position for AP and lateral forearm and humeral projections.

- Discuss how hand- and wrist-positioning will affect visualization of the radial tuberosity on lateral elbow projections.
- State why the patient's humerus is never rotated if a humeral fracture is suspected.

KEY TERMS

carpal canal
concave
convex
distal
extension
external rotation
fat pad

flexion
internal rotation
joint effusion
lateral
medial
palmar
pronate

pronator fat stripe
proximal
radial deviation
scaphoid fat stripe
ulnar deviation

IMAGE ANALYSIS GUIDELINES

Technical Data. When the technical data in Table 4-1 are followed, or adjusted as needed for additive and destructive patient conditions (see Table 2-6), along with the best practices discussed in Chapters 1 and 2, all upper extremity projections will demonstrate the image analysis guidelines in Box 4-1 unless otherwise indicated.

FINGER: PA PROJECTION

See Table 4-2, (Figures 4-1 and 4-2).
Phalangeal Soft Tissue Width and Midshaft Concavity. Finger rotation is controlled by how tightly the palm is placed flat against the IR. When the hand is allowed to relax and the palm is lifted slightly away from

the IR, rotation occurs. Because the thumb prevents the hand from rotating laterally, medial rotation is the most common rotation error. Take a few minutes to study the finger projections in Figure 4-3. Note that in the PA projection, concavity of the phalanges is equal on both sides and in the lateral projection the anterior surface is concave, whereas the posterior surface is slightly convex. Also note that as the finger is rotated medially for a PA oblique projection, the amount of concavity increases on the side toward which the anterior (palmar) surface is rotated, whereas the side toward which the posterior surface rotates demonstrates less concavity. The same observations can be made about the soft tissue that surrounds the phalanges. More soft tissue thickness is present on the anterior hand surface than on the posterior surface, so the side demonstrating the greatest soft tissue width on a rotated PA or a PA oblique projection is the side toward which the anterior surface was rotated. This information can be used to determine whether the finger was medially or laterally rotated when a poorly positioned PA finger has been obtained. If the anterior

TABLE 4-1	Upper Extremity Technical Data			
Projection	kV	Grid	mAs	SID
Finger	55-65		1	40-48 inches (100-120 cm)
Thumb	55-65		1	40-48 inches (100-120 cm)
Hand	55-65		1	40-48 inches (100-120 cm)
Wrist	65-70		2	40-48 inches (100-120 cm)
Forearm	70-75		2	40-48 inches (100-120 cm)
Elbow	70-75		2	40-48 inches (100-120 cm)
Humerus	75-85	Grid*	3	40-48 inches (100-120 cm)
Pediatric	60-70		1-2	40-48 inches (100-120 cm)

*Use grid if part thickness measures 4 inches (10 cm) or more and adjust mAs per grid ratio requirement.

BOX 4-1	Upper Extremity Imaging Analysis Guidelines

- The facility's identification requirements are visible.
- A right or left marker identifying the correct side of the patient is present on the projection and is not superimposed over the VOI.
- Good radiation protection practices are evident.
- Bony trabecular patterns and cortical outlines of the anatomical structures are sharply defined.
- Contrast resolution is adequate to demonstrate the surrounding soft tissue, bony trabecular patterns, and cortical outlines.
- No quantum mottle or saturation is present.
- Scatter radiation has been kept to a minimum.
- There is no evidence of removable artifacts.

TABLE 4-2	PA Finger Projection	
Image Analysis Guidelines (Figure 4-1)	**Related Positioning Procedures (Figure 4-2)**	
• Soft tissue width and midshaft concavity are equal on both sides of phalanges.	• Position finger in PA projection with the palmar surface placed flat against and centered to the IR.	
• There is no soft tissue overlap from adjacent digits.	• Separate fingers slightly.	
• IP and MCP joints are demonstrated as open spaces.	• Fully extend finger.	
• Phalanges are seen without foreshortening.		
• PIP joint is at the center of the exposure field.	• Center the CR to the PIP joint.	
• Finger and half of the MC are included within the exposure field.	• Open the longitudinal collimation to include the distal phalanx and the distal half of the metacarpal.	
	• Transversely collimate to within 0.5 inch (1.25 cm) of the finger skin line.	

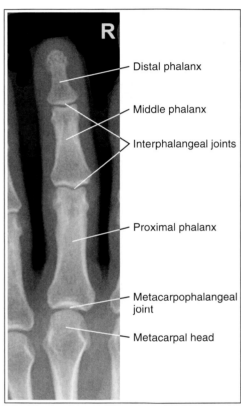

R

Distal phalanx

Middle phalanx

Interphalangeal joints

Proximal phalanx

Metacarpophalangeal joint

Metacarpal head

FIGURE 4-1 PA finger projection with accurate positioning.

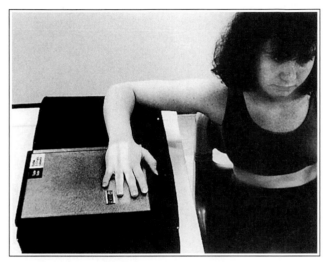

FIGURE 4-2 Proper patient positioning for PA finger projection.

surface is rotated toward the longest second metacarpal (MC) or thumb (Figure 4-4) the finger was externally rotated and if it was rotated toward the shortest fifth MC the finger was internally rotated.

Joint Spaces and Phalanges. The interphalangeal (IP) and metacarpophalangeal (MCP) joint spaces are open and the phalanges are not foreshortened if the finger is fully extended and the CR is perpendicular and centered to the proximal IP (PIP) joint. This finger positioning and CR placement align the joint spaces parallel with the CR and perpendicular to the IR, as shown in Figure 4-5, resulting in open joint spaces. It also prevents foreshortening of the phalanges, because their long axes are aligned parallel with the IR and perpendicular to the CR. The alignment of the CR and IR with the joint spaces and phalanges changes when the finger is flexed (Figure 4-6). This poor alignment causes the phalanges to foreshorten and be superimposed on the joint spaces, closing them (Figure 4-7).

Positioning the Unextendable Finger. If the patient is unable to extend the finger, it may be necessary to use an AP projection to demonstrate open IP and MCP joint spaces and to visualize the phalanges of greatest interest without foreshortening. In this case, investigate the reason the examination is being performed to determine the phalanx and joint space of interest. Then supinate the patient's hand into an AP projection, elevating the proximal metacarpals until the phalanx of interest is parallel with the IR and the joint space of interest is perpendicular to the IR (Figure 4-8). Figures 4-9 and 4-10 demonstrate how patient positioning with respect to the CR determines the anatomy that is visible. For Figure 4-9 the patient was imaged in a PA projection with fingers flexed. For Figure 4-10 the same patient was imaged in an AP projection with the proximal MCs elevated to place the affected proximal phalanges parallel with the IR. Note the difference in demonstration of the joint spaces and proximal phalanx fractures.

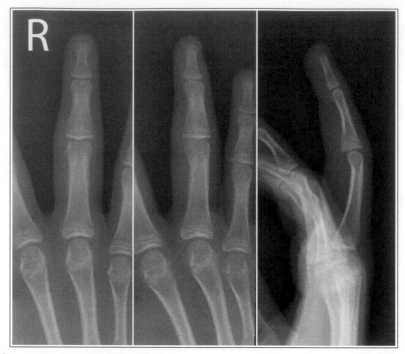

FIGURE 4-3 PA, lateral, PA oblique finger projections for demonstrating soft tissue and phalanx concavity comparison.

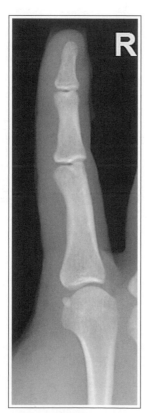

FIGURE 4-4 PA finger projection taken with finger rotated medially.

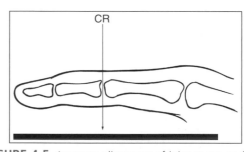

FIGURE 4-5 Accurate alignment of joint space and CR.

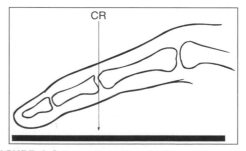

FIGURE 4-6 Poor alignment of joint space and CR.

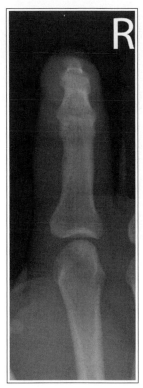

FIGURE 4-7 PA finger projection taken without the CR aligned parallel with the joint spaces and perpendicular to the phalanges.

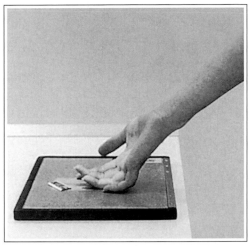

FIGURE 4-8 Patient positioning for AP flexed finger projection.

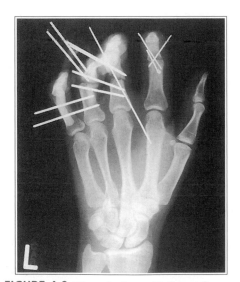

FIGURE 4-9 PA projection with flexed fingers.

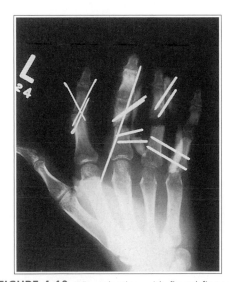

FIGURE 4-10 AP projection with flexed fingers.

PA Finger Analysis Practice

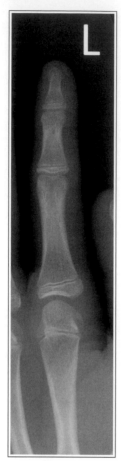

IMAGE 4-1

Analysis. The soft tissue width and the concavity of the phalangeal midshafts on either side of the phalanx are not equal; the finger was rotated for the projection. The side of the phalangeal with the greater concavity and soft tissue width is facing the thumb. The finger was rotated externally.

Correction. Internally rotate the finger, placing it flat against the IR.

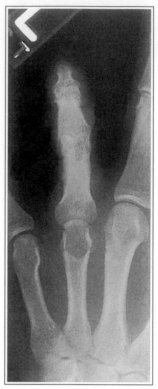

IMAGE 4-2

Analysis. The IP and MP joints are closed, and the distal and middle phalanges are foreshortened. The finger was flexed.

Correction. Extend the finger, and place the palm flat against the IR. If the patient is unable to extend the finger, position it in an AP projection, elevating the proximal MCs until the affected phalanx is parallel with the IR or the affected joint space is perpendicular to the IR.

FINGER: PA OBLIQUE PROJECTION

See Table 4-3, (Figures 4-11 and 4-12).

Phalangeal Soft Tissue Width and Midshaft Concavity. Study the amount of phalangeal midshaft concavity and soft tissue width demonstrated on PA oblique finger projections to verify whether the required 45-degree angle of obliquity is obtained and to determine the proper repositioning movement needed when the projection shows too much or too little obliquity. An accurately positioned 45-degree PA oblique finger demonstrates more phalangeal midshaft concavity and twice as much soft tissue width on the side of the finger that the anterior surface is rotated toward. If the phalangeal midshaft concavity and soft tissue width on both sides of the digit are more nearly equal, the finger was rotated less than the required 45 degrees (Figure 4-13). If the soft tissue width on one side of the digit is more than twice as much as that on the other, and when one aspect of the phalangeal midshaft is concave but the other aspect is slightly convex, the angle of obliquity was more than 45 degrees (Figure 4-14).

TABLE 4-3	PA Oblique Finger Projection	
Image Analysis Guidelines (Figure 4-11)	**Related Positioning Procedures (Figure 4-12)**	
• Twice as much soft tissue width is demonstrated on one side of the phalanges as on the other side. • More concavity is seen on one aspect of the phalangeal midshafts than the others. • There is no soft tissue overlap from adjacent digits. • IP and MCP joints are demonstrated as open spaces. • Phalanges are not foreshortened.	• Begin with finger in PA projection with the palmar surface placed flat against and centered to the IR. • Externally rotate the hand until the affected finger is at a 45-degree angle with IR. • Separate fingers slightly. • Fully extend finger. • Use support on finger as needed to keep finger parallel with IR and prevent motion.	
• PIP joint is at the center of the exposure field. • Finger and half of the MC are included within the exposure field.	• Center a perpendicular CR to the PIP joint. • Open the longitudinal collimation to include the distal phalanx and the distal half of the MC. • Transversely collimate to within 0.5 inch (1.25 cm) of the finger skin line.	

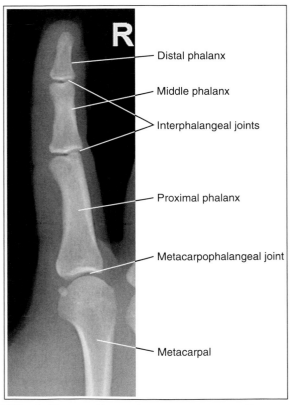

FIGURE 4-11 PA oblique finger projection with accurate positioning.

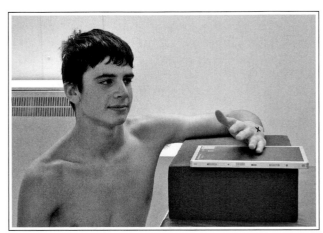

FIGURE 4-12 Proper patient positioning for PA oblique finger projection.

Alternate Second Finger Positioning. When positioning for a second PA oblique finger projection, internally rotating the hand until the finger is at a 45-degree angle with the IR places the second finger at a shorter object–image receptor distance (OID) and will reduce the magnification that will occur with external rotation. This internally rotated finger should meet the same image analysis guidelines as listed herein.

Soft Tissue Overlap. Slight separation of the patient's fingers prevents overlapping of the adjacent finger's soft tissue onto that of the affected finger. Superimposition of these soft tissues makes it difficult to evaluate the soft tissue of the affected finger (Figure 4-15).

Joint Space and Phalanges. When the hand and fingers are rotated to obtain the PA oblique, all but the fifth finger are positioned away from the IR at varying OIDs and naturally tilt toward the IR with their fingertips resting on it. This finger-positioning closes the IP and MCP joint spaces and foreshortens the phalanges (Figure 4-16). It is only if the affected finger remains fully extended and aligned parallel with the IR that the joint spaces will be properly aligned perpendicular and the phalanges properly aligned parallel with the IR. For the shaking finger, an immobilization device placed beneath the distal phalanx to prop finger may be needed. This is especially true when the second and third digits are imaged because they are at the greatest OID.

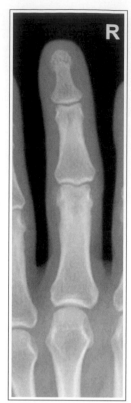

FIGURE 4-13 PA oblique finger projection taken with less than 45 degrees of obliquity.

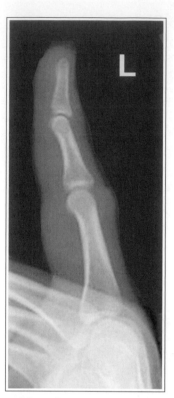

FIGURE 4-14 PA oblique finger projection taken with more than 45 degrees of obliquity.

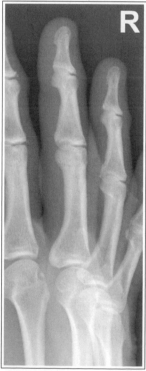

FIGURE 4-15 PA oblique finger projection taken with the soft tissue from adjacent fingers superimposed over the affected finger's soft tissue.

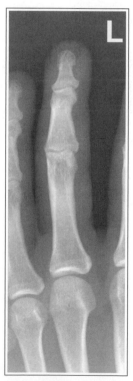

FIGURE 4-16 PA oblique finger projection taken without the finger positioned parallel with the IR.

TABLE 4-4   Lateral Finger Projection

Image Analysis Guidelines (Figure 4-17)	Related Positioning Procedures (Figure 4-18)
• There is no overlap from adjacent fingers.	• Form the hand into a tight fist, with affected finger extended. • Use an immobilization device as needed to help finger extension only if the device does not put stress on the injured area.
• Anterior surface of the middle and proximal phalanges demonstrate midshaft concavity and the posterior surface shows slight convexity. • When visualized, the fingernail is demonstrated in profile.	• Center finger to the IR, with the lateral surface resting on the IR if imaging the second or third finger and medial surface for fourth or fifth finger. • Adjust hand rotation to obtain a lateral projection with fingernail in profile.
• IP joints are demonstrated as open spaces. • Phalanges are not foreshortened. • PIP joint is at the center of the exposure field.	• Align finger parallel with the IR. • Center a perpendicular CR to the PIP joint.
• Entire finger and MC head are included within the exposure field.	• Open the longitudinal collimation to include the distal phalanx and the distal half of the MC. • Transversely collimate to within 0.5 inch (1.25 cm) of the finger skin line.

PA Oblique Finger Analysis Practice

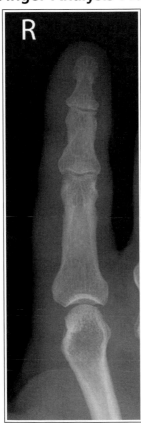

IMAGE 4-3

Analysis. The soft tissue width and midshaft concave are nearly equal on both sides of the phalanx; the finger was positioned at less than 45 degrees of obliquity for the projection.

Correction. Increase the finger obliquity to 45 degrees. Keep finger parallel with the IR.

FINGER: LATERAL PROJECTION

See Table 4-4, Figures 4-17 and 4-18.

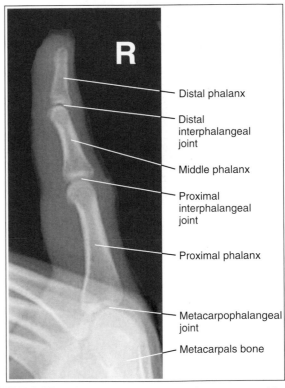

FIGURE 4-17 Lateral finger projection with accurate positioning.

Labels: Distal phalanx; Distal interphalangeal joint; Middle phalanx; Proximal interphalangeal joint; Proximal phalanx; Metacarpophalangeal joint; Metacarpals bone.

Phalangeal Midshaft Concavity. The anterior surface of the middle and proximal phalanges demonstrate midshaft concavity and the posterior surfaces show slight convexity when the lateral finger projection is obtained without rotation. The anterior surface of the finger also demonstrates more than twice as much soft tissue width than the posterior surface. Failing to rotate the finger enough to obtain a lateral projection results in an image that appears more like the PA oblique finger projection, with the concavity demonstrated on both sides of the middle and proximal phalangeal midshafts and the soft tissue width closer to twice as much on the anterior surface when compared with the posterior surface (Figure 4-19).

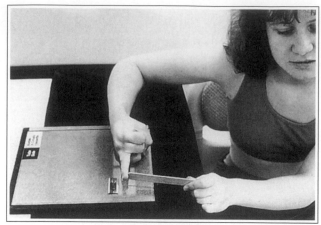

FIGURE 4-18 Proper patient positioning for lateral finger projection.

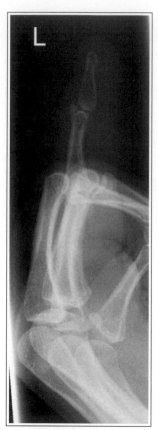

FIGURE 4-20 Lateral finger projection without the unaffected fingers flexed enough to prevent soft tissue or bony superimposition of the affected digit's proximal phalanx.

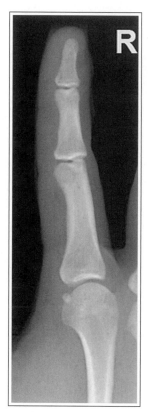

FIGURE 4-19 Lateral finger projection with insufficient finger obliquity.

Adjacent Finger Overlap. To visualize the proximal phalanx on a lateral projection, it may be necessary to extend the affected finger with an immobilization device or to tape the unaffected fingers away from the affected finger. If the unaffected fingers are not drawn away from the proximal phalanx of the affected finger, they will be superimposed on the area, preventing adequate visualization (Figure 4-20).

Finger Fractures. An immobilization device should not be used to extend the finger if a fracture is suspected and the device will cause stress to the fractured area (Figure 4-21) and potentially farther damage. For such

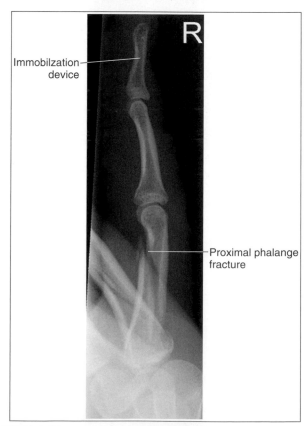

FIGURE 4-21 Lateral finger projection demonstrating a proximal phalanx fracture that is stressed because of the immobilization device that was used to extend the finger.

Immobilzation device

Proximal phalange fracture

TABLE 4-5	AP Thumb Projection	
Image Analysis Guidelines (Figures 4-22 and 4-23)		**Related Positioning Procedures (Figure 4-24)**
• Concavity on both sides of the phalanges and MC midshafts is equal. • There is equal soft tissue width on each side of the phalanges.		• Internally rotate arm until the thumb is centered to the IR in an AP projection, with the nail positioned directly against the IR and not visible on either side.
• IP, MCP, and CM joints are demonstrated as open spaces. • Phalanges are not foreshortened.		• Fully extend the thumb.
• Superimposition of the medial palm soft tissue over the proximal first MC and the CM joint is minimal. • MCP joint is at the center of the exposure field. • Phalanges, MC, and CM joint are included within the exposure field.		• Using the unaffected hand, draw the medial palmar surface away from the thumb without rotating thumb from the AP projection. • Center a perpendicular CR to the MCP joint. • Align the long axis of the thumb and the collimator light line. • Open the longitudinal collimation to include the distal phalanx and CM joint. • Transversely collimate to within 0.5 inch (1.25 cm) of the thumb skin line.

a patient, leave the finger positioned as is. This may result in overlap of other fingers and soft tissue onto the affected area and require the need for additional kV to penetrate through the greater thickness (see Figure 4-20).

Lateral Finger Analysis Practice

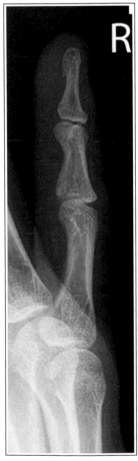

IMAGE 4-4

Analysis. Concavity is demonstrated on both sides of the middle and proximal phalangeal midshafts, indicating that the finger was not adequately rotated for this projection.

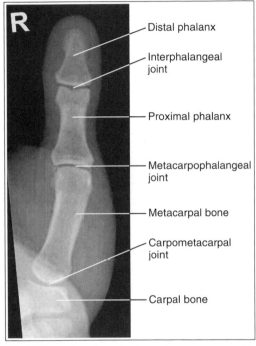

FIGURE 4-22 AP thumb projection with accurate positioning.

Distal phalanx
Interphalangeal joint
Proximal phalanx
Metacarpophalangeal joint
Metacarpal bone
Carpometacarpal joint
Carpal bone

Correction. Increase the degree of finger rotation until the finger is in a lateral projection.

THUMB: AP PROJECTION

See Table 4-5, (Figures 4-22, 4-23 and 4-24).
Phalangeal and Metacarpal Midshaft Concavity and Soft Tissue Width. A nonrotated AP thumb projection demonstrates equal concavity on both sides of the phalangeal and MC midshafts, as well as equal soft tissue widths on both sides of the phalanges. When the thumb is rotated away from an AP projection, the amount of midshaft concavity increases on the side of the thumb toward which the anterior thumb surface rotates and decreases on the side toward which the posterior surface

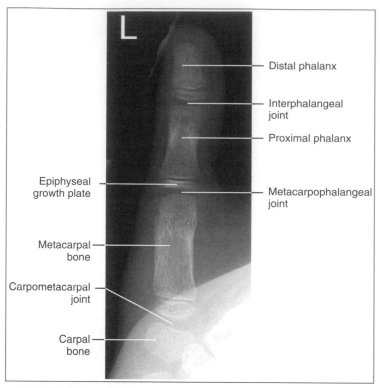

FIGURE 4-23 Accurately positioned pediatric PA thumb projection.

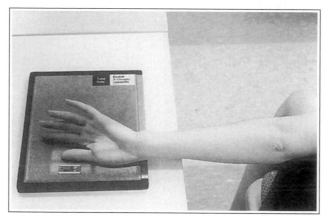

FIGURE 4-24 Proper patient positioning for AP thumb projection.

rotates. The same observation can be made about the soft tissue surrounding the phalanges when the thumb is rotated, with more soft tissue width evident on the side toward which the anterior surface is rotated, and less soft tissue width seen on the side toward which the posterior surface is rotated. If the arm is internally rotated more than needed to bring the thumb in an AP projection, the anterior thumb surface will be demonstrated next to the hand on the projection (Figure 4-25) and when the arm has not been internally rotated enough the posterior thumb surface will be demonstrated toward the hand.

Joint Spaces and Phalanges. The IP, MCP, and CM joint spaces are open, and the phalanges are

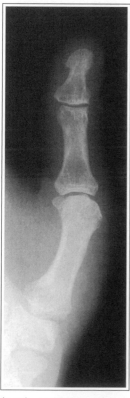

FIGURE 4-25 AP thumb projection taken with hand internally rotated too far.

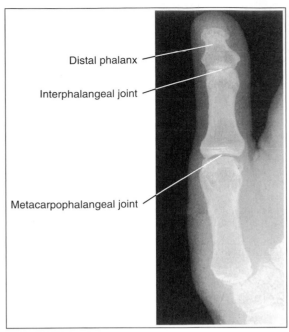

FIGURE 4-26 AP thumb projection taken with the MP joint elevated off the IR and the distal thumb posteriorly extended.

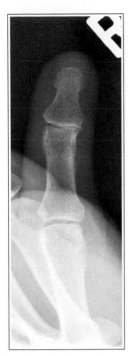

FIGURE 4-27 AP thumb projection taken without the MCs and palmer surface drawn away from the thumb.

demonstrated without foreshortening as long as the thumb is placed flat against and positioned parallel with the IR and the CR is perpendicular and centered to the MCP joint space. This positioning aligns the joint spaces parallel with the CR and perpendicular to the IR and positions the long axes of the phalanges perpendicular to the CR and parallel with the IR. These relationships change when the thumb is flexed or posteriorly extended (hitchhiker's thumb) for the projection. Thumb flexion and extension foreshorten the phalanges and superimpose them over the joint spaces (Figure 4-26).

Palmar Soft Tissue. Minimal palmar soft tissue overlap occurs when the medial palm surface is drawn away from the thumb by using the opposite hand to move it off the proximal thumb region. If the medial surface of the palm is not drawn away from the thumb, the soft tissue and possibly the fourth and fifth MCs obscure the proximal first MC and CM joint (Figure 4-27). One should be careful not to rotate the thumb from the AP projection when drawing soft tissue away.

Thumb and Collimator Alignment. Aligning the long axes of the thumb and collimator light line enables you to collimate tightly without clipping the distal phalanx or proximal metacarpal (Figure 4-28).

Alternate PA Thumb Projection. The image analysis guidelines for the AP thumb projection can be used to evaluate a PA thumb projection (Figure 4-29), with the following modifications. First, the medial palm soft tissue does not overlap the proximal first MC and CM joint. Second, on a PA projection, the CM joint is closed.

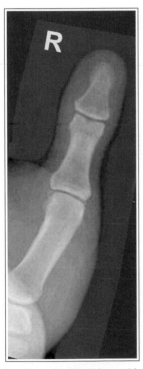

FIGURE 4-28 AP thumb projection taken without the long axis of the thumb aligned with the long axis of the collimated field, causing the proximal MC and the CM joint to be clipped.

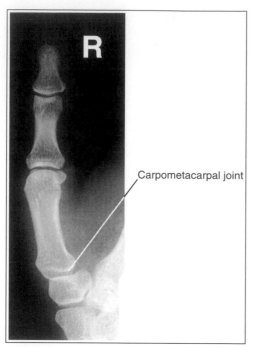

FIGURE 4-29 PA thumb projection with accurate positioning.

Carpometacarpal joint

AP Thumb Analysis Practice

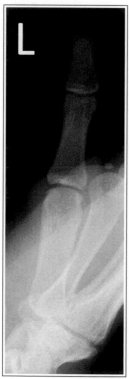

IMAGE 4-5

Analysis. The fifth MC and the medial palm soft tissue are superimposed over the proximal first MC and CM joint. The MCs and palmer surface have not been drawn away from the thumb.

Correction. Using the patient's other hand, draw the medial side of the hand and palmar surface away from the thumb. Make sure that the thumb does not rotate

TABLE 4-6	Lateral Thumb Projection
Image Analysis Guidelines (Figures 4-30 and 4-31)	**Related Positioning Procedures (Figure 4-32)**
• Anterior proximal phalanx and MC demonstrates midshaft concavity, and the posterior proximal phalanx and MC demonstrates slight convexity. • When visualized, the thumbnail is demonstrated in profile.	• Place hand's palmar surface flat against the IR. • Center the thumb on the IR. • Flex the hand and fingers only until the thumb naturally rolls into a lateral projection and thumbnail is in profile.
• IP, MCP, and CM joints are demonstrated as open spaces. • Phalanges are not foreshortened.	• Rotate hand as needed to place in a PA projection. • Extend thumb.
• First proximal MC is only slightly superimposed by the second proximal MC.	• Abduct the thumb, drawing it away from the second finger.
• MCP joint is at the center of the exposure field.	• Center a perpendicular CR to the MCP joint.
• Phalanges, MC, and CM joint are included within the exposure field.	• Align the long axes of the thumb and collimator light field. • Open the longitudinal collimation to include the distal phalanx and CM joint. • Transversely collimate to within 0.5 inch (1.25 cm) of the thumb skin line.

away from an AP projection with this movement and that the patient's opposite hand is not included in the collimation field.

THUMB: LATERAL PROJECTION

See Table 4-6, (Figures 4-30, 4-31, and 4-32).
Phalanx and Metacarpal Midshaft Concavity. When the hand and fingers are accurately flexed and the thumb is in a lateral projection, the midshaft of the proximal phalanx and MC demonstrates concavity on their anterior aspects and slight convexity on their posterior aspects. If the patient's hand is not flexed enough to place the thumb in a lateral projection, the posterior aspects of these midshafts will show some degree of concavity (Figure 4-33). Overflexion of the hand causes superimposition of the second and third proximal MCs onto the proximal first MC, obscuring it (Figure 4-34).
Joint Spaces and Phalangeal. The IP, MCP, and CM joints are visible as open spaces, and the phalanges are not foreshortened as long as the thumb remains in contact and parallel with the IR. Because the fourth and

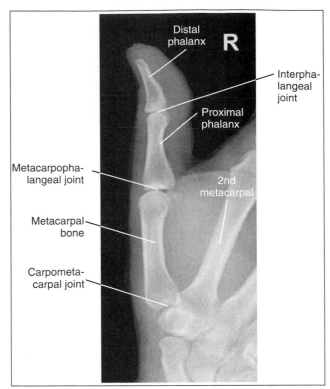

FIGURE 4-30 Lateral thumb projection with accurate positioning.

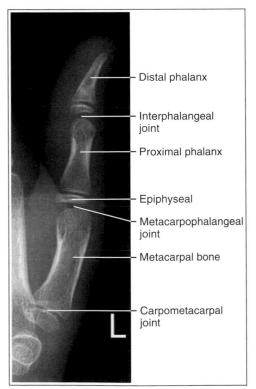

FIGURE 4-31 Accurately positioned pediatric lateral thumb projection.

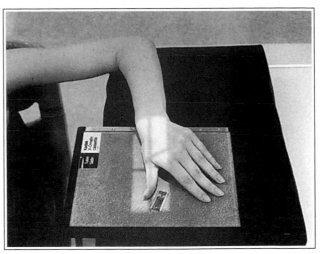

FIGURE 4-32 Proper patient positioning for lateral thumb projection.

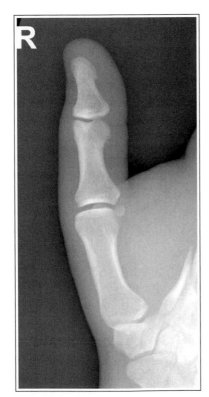

FIGURE 4-33 Lateral thumb projection taken without adequate hand flexion.

fifth fingers are shorter than the second and third, the hand tends to medially rotate slightly when the palm and fingers are flexed, with the finger tips against the IR. This external rotation may cause the proximal thumb to elevate off the IR and result in phalangeal foreshortening and closed joint spaces. Ensure that the hand is in a PA projection and the proximal thumb is positioned adjacent to the IR to prevent this.

Thumb Abduction. Whenever possible, the anatomic part of interest should be demonstrated without superimposition of any structure. For a lateral thumb projection, the proximal MC can be demonstrated with only a very small amount of superimposition if the thumb is abducted away from the palm. Failure to abduct the thumb results in a significant amount of first and second proximal MC overlap and obstruction of the CM joint (Figure 4-35).

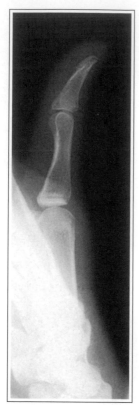

FIGURE 4-34 Lateral thumb projection taken with the hand over-flexed, causing the second and third proximal MCs to superimpose the first proximal MC.

Lateral Thumb Analysis Practice

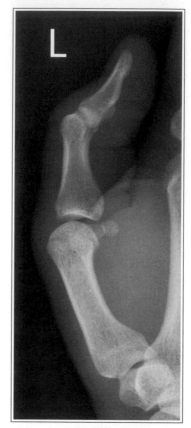

IMAGE 4-6

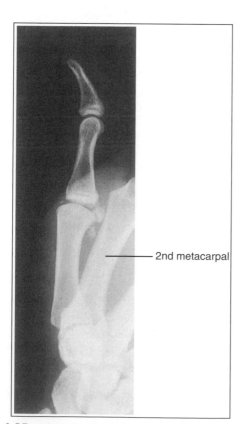

2nd metacarpal

FIGURE 4-35 Lateral thumb projection taken without the thumb abducted.

Analysis. The IP joint is closed and the distal phalanx is foreshortened. The thumb was flexed.

Correction. Extend the thumb and lie flat against the IR.

THUMB: PA OBLIQUE PROJECTION

See Table 4-7, (Figures 4-36, 4-37, and 4-38).

Soft Tissue Width and Phalangeal and Metacarpal Midshaft Concavity. When the thumb is in a 45-degree PA oblique projection, the proximal phalange and metacarpal demonstrate more midshaft concavity and twice as much soft tissue width on the side of the thumb that the anterior thumb surface is rotated toward when compared with the side the posterior surface is rotated toward. If the hand is not placed flat against the IR, but is allowed to flex, the thumb rotates closer to a lateral projection. Such positioning can be identified on a projection by noting the increase in midshaft concavity and soft tissue width seen on the side the anterior thumb surface is rotated toward and the decrease in concavity and soft tissue width seen on the side the posterior thumb surface is rotated toward (Figure 4-39).

TABLE 4-7 | PA Oblique Thumb Projection

Image Analysis Guidelines (Figures 4-36 and 4-37)	Related Positioning Procedures (Figure 4-38)
• Twice as much soft tissue is present on the side of the thumb next to the fingers than the opposite side. • More proximal phalangeal and metacarpal midshaft concavity is present on the side of the thumb next to the fingers than the other side.	• Extend hand and place its palmar surface flat against the IR, placing the thumb at a 45-degree angle with the IR. • Center the thumb on the IR.
• IP, MCP, and CM joints are demonstrated as open spaces. • Phalanges are not foreshortened.	• Keep entire thumb adjacent to the IR.
• MCP joint is at the center of the exposure field. • Phalanges, MC, and CM joint are included within the exposure field.	• Center a perpendicular CR to the MCP joint and IR. • Align the long axes of the thumb and collimator light field. • Open the longitudinal collimation to include the distal phalanx and CM joint. • Transversely collimate to within 0.5 inch (1.25 cm) of the thumb skin line.

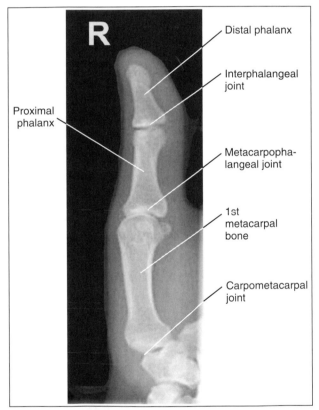

FIGURE 4-36 PA oblique thumb projection with accurate positioning.

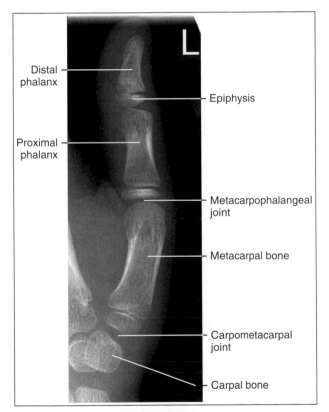

FIGURE 4-37 Accurately positioned pediatric PA oblique thumb projection.

Joint Space, Phalangeal and Metacarpal. The IP, MCP, and CM joint spaces are open and the metacarpal and phalanges are visible without foreshortening when the entire palmar surface remains flat against the IR. Flexion of the hand will result in the hand rotating medially and the thumb tilting downward, causing the IP and MCP joint spaces to close the phalanges to foreshorten (Figure 4-40).

Longitudinal Thumb Alignment. Aligning the long axes of the thumb and collimator light field enables you to collimate tightly without clipping the distal phalanx or proximal metacarpal (Figure 4-41).

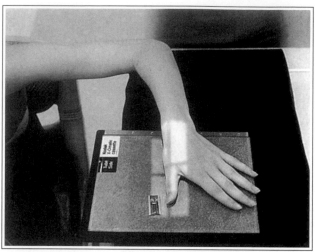

FIGURE 4-38 Proper patient positioning for PA oblique thumb projection.

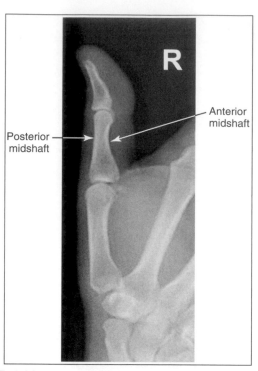

FIGURE 4-39 PA oblique thumb projection taken without the palm placed flat against the IR, causing thumb to be positioned at more than 45 degrees of obliquity.

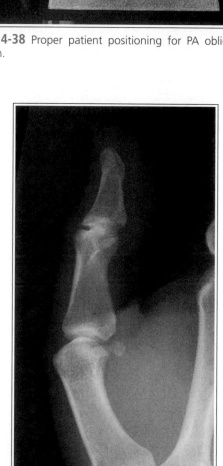

FIGURE 4-40 PA oblique thumb projection taken without the palmer surface and thumb against the IR.

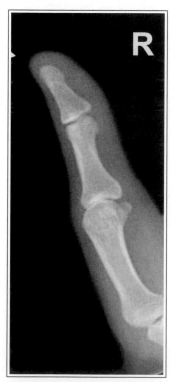

FIGURE 4-41 PA oblique thumb projection taken without the long axis of the thumb aligned with the long axis of the collimated field, causing the proximal MC and the CM joint to be clipped.

PA Oblique Thumb Analysis Practice

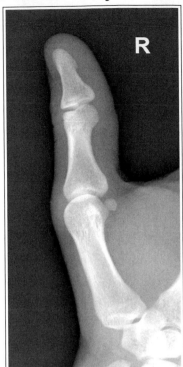

IMAGE 4-7

Analysis. The IP and MCP joints are closed, and the phalanges are foreshortened. The palm surface was not positioned flat against the IR, and the thumb was tilting down toward the IR.

Correction. Place the palmer surface and thumb flat against the IR.

HAND: PA PROJECTION

See Table 4-8, (Figures 4-42 and 4-43).

Soft Tissue Width and Phalangeal and Metacarpal Midshaft Concavity. If the hand is not fully extended and brought flat against the IR but is slightly flexed, it often relaxes and medially rotates. A medially rotated PA hand projection is signified by a narrowing or slight superimposition of the third through fifth MC heads and unequal soft tissue thickness and midshaft concavity on the sides of the phalanges. The MCs also show unequal midshaft concavity and spacing (Figure 4-44). Abducting the patient's arm and placing the forearm and humerus on the same horizontal plane, with the elbow flexed 90 degrees, assists in preventing medial rotation and also demonstrates better wrist positioning. This is especially important if there is a wrist condition that is causing pain to radiate into the hand. When the patient has been positioned in this manner, the ulnar styloid appears in profile on the projection. Lateral rotation of the hand is seldom a problem because the thumb prevents this movement.

Joints Spaces, Phalanges, and Metacarpals. Flexion of the hand causes poor alignment of the IP and CM joint spaces, phalanges, and MCs with the IR and CR, resulting in closed joint spaces and foreshortening of the phalanges and MCs (Figure 4-45). The position of the thumb also changes to closer to or to a lateral projection depending on the degree of hand flexed.

Thumb and Hand Closeness. Keeping the thumb placed close to the hand allows for tighter collimation and better CR placement, as it will put the center of the hand at the third MCP joint. When the thumb is abducted the CR needs to be moved toward the second MCP joint to transversely collimate to within

TABLE 4-8	PA Hand Projection	
Image Analysis Guidelines (Figure 4-42)	**Related Positioning Procedures (Figure 4-43)**
• Soft-tissue outlines of the second through fifth phalanges are uniform. • Distance between the MC heads is equal. • Equal midshaft concavity is seen on both sides of the phalanges and MCs of the second through fifth fingers.	• Pronate and extend the hand and fingers, and place the palmar surface flat against the IR in a PA projection. • Center hand on IR.
• There is no soft tissue overlap from adjacent fingers • IP, MCP, and CM joints are demonstrated as open spaces. • Phalanges are demonstrated without foreshortening. • Thumb demonstrates a 45-degree oblique projection.	• Separate fingers, leaving a slight space between them. • Ensure fingers are fully extended, placing them parallel with the IR.
• Thumb is positioned close to the hand. • Third MCP joint is at the center of the exposure field. • Phalanges, MCs, carpals, and 1 inch (2.5 cm) of the distal radius and ulna are included within the exposure field.	• Position the thumb a small distance from the hand. • Center a perpendicular CR to the third MCP joint. • Open the longitudinal collimation to include the distal phalanges and 1 inch (2.5 cm) of the distal forearm. • Transversely collimate to within 0.5 inch (1.25 cm) of the first and fifth digits' skin line.

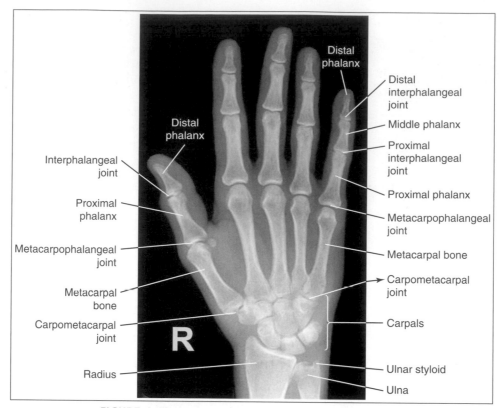

FIGURE 4-42 PA hand projection with accurate positioning.

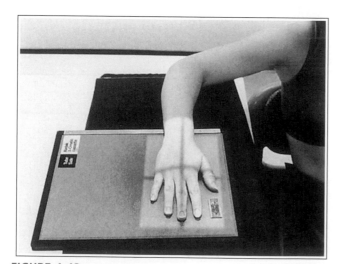

FIGURE 4-43 Proper patient positioning for PA hand projection.

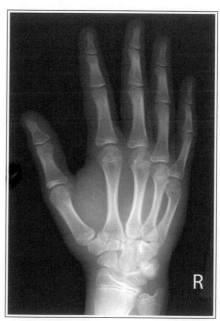

FIGURE 4-44 PA hand projection taken in slight medial rotation.

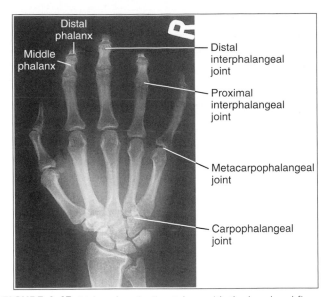

FIGURE 4-45 PA hand projection taken with the hand and fingers flexed.

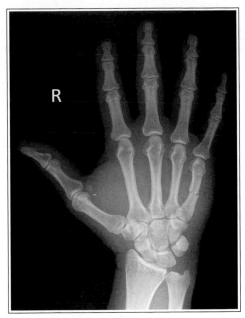

FIGURE 4-46 PA hand projection with thumb positioned too far away from hand.

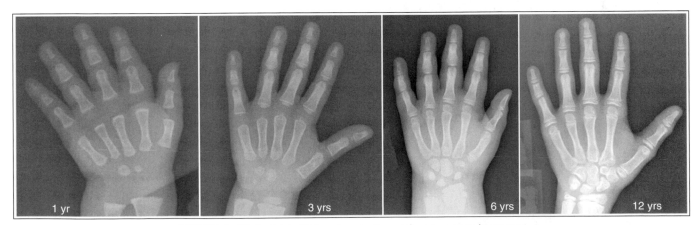

FIGURE 4-47 Pediatric PA hand projections taken to assess bone age.

0.5 inch (1.25 cm) from the first and fifth digits' skin line (Figure 4-46).

Special Condition

Pediatric Bone Age Assessment. A pediatric PA bone age hand is taken to assess the skeletal versus the chronologic age of a child. Because bones develop in an orderly pattern, skeletal age may be assessed from infancy through adolescence. Illness, metabolic or endocrine dysfunction, and taking certain types of medications and therapies are all reasons why a pediatric patient's skeletal and chronologic age may not correspond. A left PA hand and wrist is typically the projection of choice because bony developmental changes are readily visible and easily evaluated. For skeletal age to be evaluated, the phalanges, metacarpals, carpals, and distal radius and ulna must be included in their entirety (Figure 4-47).

PA Hand Analysis Practice

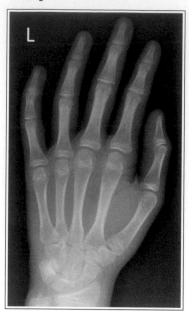

IMAGE 4-8

Analysis. There is unequal midshaft concavity on either side of the phalanges and MCs, and uneven spacing of the MC heads. The hand was in slight external rotation.

Correction. Internally rotate the hand until the palm and fingers are flat against the IR.

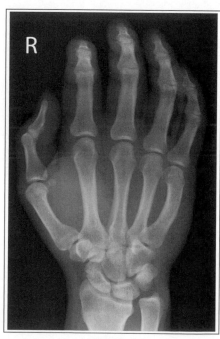

IMAGE 4-9

Analysis. The IP and CM joints are closed, and the phalanges and MCs are foreshortened. The thumb demonstrates a lateral projection. The hand and fingers are flexed for this projection.

Correction. Fully extend the patient's hand and fingers, and then place them flat against the IR. If the patient is

unable to extend the hand and fingers, position them in an AP projection, adjusting the hand position as needed to demonstrate the area of greatest interest without foreshortening.

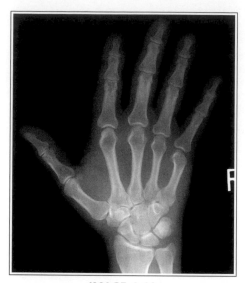

IMAGE 4-10

Analysis. The thumb is in full abduction and the CR was centered to the second MCP joint.

Correction. Position the thumb close to the hand and center the CR to the third MCP joint.

HAND: PA OBLIQUE PROJECTION (LATERAL ROTATION)

See Table 4-9, (Figures 4-48 and 4-49).

Metacarpal Spacing. When positioning for a PA oblique hand projection, it is best to view the hand and not the wrist when confirming the degree of obliquity, as using the wrist can result in a miscalculation of the amount of obliquity. The wrist will demonstrate more than 45 degrees of obliquity when the hand is in the required 45-degree oblique. This is especially true if the humerus and forearm have not been placed on the same horizontal plane as discussed in the PA oblique wrist projection. When the patient has been positioned with the arm on the same horizontal plane, the ulnar styloid is demonstrated in profile medially on the projection.

As the hand is rotated from a PA to lateral projection the amount of MC head and midshaft superimposition goes from no superimposition to total superimposition. If the 45-degree PA oblique hand is obtained with less than 45 degrees of obliquity, the MC relationship is similar to that of a PA projection of the hand with the midshafts of the MCs closer to evenly spaced, and the MC heads seen without superimposition (Figure 4-50). Although an accurate PA oblique hand demonstrates a small space between the fourth and fifth metacarpal midshafts, if the hand is rotated more than 45 degrees, this space is

TABLE 4-9	PA Oblique Hand Projection	
Image Analysis Guidelines (Figure 4-48)		**Related Positioning Procedures (Figure 4-49)**
• Each of the second through fifth MC midshafts demonstrate more concavity on one side than on the other. • First and second MC heads are not superimposed, the third through fifth MC heads are slightly superimposed, and a slight space is present between the fourth and fifth MC midshafts. • There is no soft tissue overlap from the thumb or adjacent fingers. • IP and MCP joints are demonstrated as open spaces. • Phalanges are demonstrated without foreshortening. • Thumb position may vary from a lateral to PA oblique projection. • Thumb is positioned close to the hand. • Third MCP joint is at the center of the exposure field. • Phalanges, MCs, carpals, and one inch (2.5 cm) of the distal radius and ulna are included within the exposure field.		• Begin with the hand's palmar surface positioned against the IR in a PA projection. • Externally rotate the hand until it is at a 45-degree angle with IR. • Center the hand on the IR. • Separate fingers slightly. • Fully extend fingers, aligning them parallel with the IR. • Support finger and hand with sponge as needed to hold extended position • Position thumb within a small distance from the hand. • Center a perpendicular CR to the third MCP joint and IR. • Open the longitudinal collimation to include the distal phalanges and 1 inch (2.5 cm) of the distal forearm. • Transversely collimate to within 0.5 inch (1.25 cm) of the first and fifth digits' skin line.

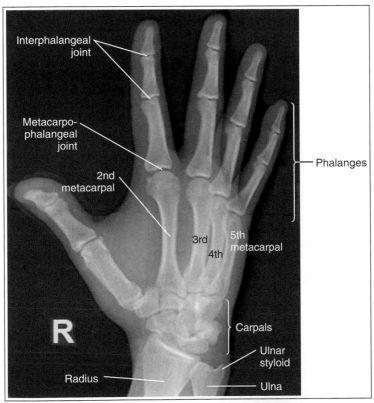

FIGURE 4-48 PA oblique hand projection with accurate positioning.

obscured and the fourth and fifth MC midshafts demonstrate some degree of superimposition (Figure 4-51).

Soft Tissue Overlap. Slightly separating the fingers prevents soft tissue overlapping (Figure 4-52).

Joint Spaces and Phalanges. If the PA oblique hand projection is obtained to only evaluate the metacarpals, it is not uncommon to take the PA oblique projection with the patient's fingers flexed and used to maintain the required obliquity instead of using an immobilization device (Figure 4-53). Before the projection is obtained with flexed fingers, a good patient history should be obtained to confirm that the phalanges will not be evaluated. Such positioning closes the IP joint spaces and foreshortens the phalanges (Figures 4-51 and 4-54).

Thumb Positioning. Keeping the thumb placed close to the hand allows for tighter collimation and better CR placement, as it will put the center of the hand at the third MCP joint (see Figure 4-51).

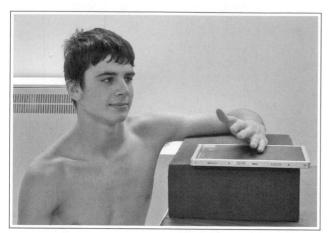

FIGURE 4-49 Proper patient positioning for PA oblique hand projection with extended fingers.

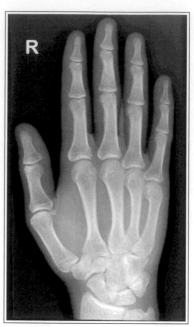

FIGURE 4-50 PA oblique hand projection taken with inadequate hand obliquity.

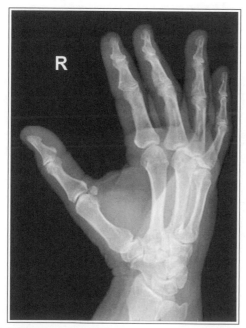

FIGURE 4-51 PA oblique hand projection taken with more than 45 degrees of obliquity and without the fingers positioned parallel with the IR.

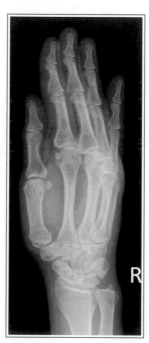

FIGURE 4-52 PA oblique hand projection taken without the fingers spread apart, causing soft tissue and bony structures of adjacent digits to overlap.

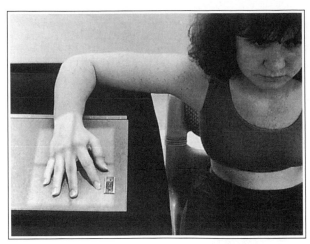

FIGURE 4-53 Proper patient positioning for PA oblique hand projection with flexed fingers.

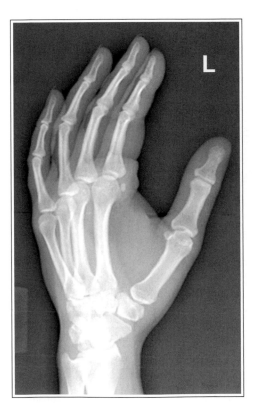

FIGURE 4-54 PA oblique hand projection taken without the fingers positioned parallel with the IR.

PA Oblique Hand Analysis Practice

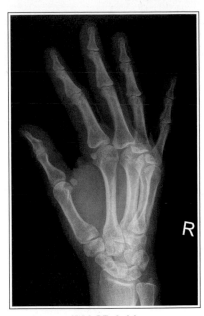

IMAGE 4-11

Analysis. The midshaft of the third through fifth MCs are superimposed. The hand was placed at more than 45 degrees of obliquity. The phalanges are foreshortened, and the IP joint spaces are closed. The fingers are not positioned parallel with the IR, but were instead used to prop the hand.

Correction. Internally rotate the hand until the MCs and IR form a 45-degree angle and extend the fingers, placing them parallel with the IR.

HAND: "FAN" LATERAL PROJECTION (LATEROMEDIAL)

See Table 4-10, (Figures 4-55 and 4-56).

Metacarpal Superimposition. When positioning for a lateral hand projection, it is best to view the superimposition of the patient's knuckles versus the wrist when confirming a true lateral because using the wrist can result in a miscalculation. When the knuckles are superimposed the wrist may demonstrate a slight external rotation. This is especially true if the humerus and forearm have not been placed on the same horizontal plane for the projection, as explained in the lateral wrist projection. The accuracy of a lateral hand projection should then be determined by judging the degree of superimposition of the second through fifth MC heads and midshafts and not the degree of radius and ulna superimposition. If the MC midshafts are not superimposed and the fifth MC is demonstrated anterior to the second through fourth MCs, the hand was slightly externally rotated or supinated (Figure 4-57). The fifth MC can be identified by its length; it is the shorter of the second through fifth MCs. If the MC midshafts are not superimposed and the second MC is demonstrated

TABLE 4-10	Lateral Hand Projection	
Image Analysis Guidelines (Figure 4-55)	**Related Positioning Procedures (Figure 4-56)**
• Second through fifth MCs are superimposed.	• Position the lateral aspect of the hand against the IR. • Adjust hand rotation until the second through fifth knuckles are placed directly on top of one another in a lateral projection. • Center hand on IR.
• Second through fifth digits are separated, demonstrating little superimposition of the proximal bony or soft tissue structures. • Thumb is demonstrated without superimposition of the other digits and is in a PA to slight PA oblique projection.	• Fan the second and third fingers anteriorly and fourth and fifth posteriorly, separating the fingers as far apart as possible without superimposing the thumb.
• IP joints are open. • Phalanges are not foreshortened. • Thumb is positioned close to hand. • MCP joints are at the center of the exposure field. • Phalanges, MCs, carpals, and 1 inch (2.5 cm) of the distal radius and ulna are included within the exposure field.	• Extend and align the fingers and thumb parallel with the IR. • Support fingers and hand as needed to hold position. • Position the thumb within a small distance from the hand. • Center a perpendicular CR to the MCP joint and to IR. • Open the longitudinal collimation to include the distal phalanges and 1 inch (2.5 cm) of the distal forearm. • Transversely collimate to within 0.5 inch (1.25 cm) of the first and fifth digits skin line.

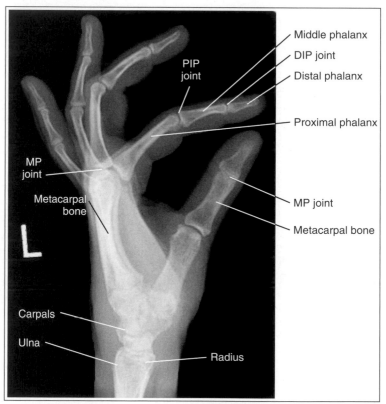

FIGURE 4-55 Lateral hand projection with accurate positioning.

anterior to the third through fifth MCs, the hand was slightly internally rotated or pronated (Figures 4-58 and 4-59). The second MC can also be identified by its length; it is the longest.

Fanned Fingers. To demonstrate the fingers without superimposition on a lateral hand projection, they are fanned by drawing the second and third fingers anteriorly and the fourth and fifth fingers posteriorly. The amount of finger separation obtained depends on the patient's mobility. Immobilization devices are available to help maintain proper positioning. When the fingers are fanned they can be individually studied. If the fingers are not adequately separated they superimpose one another on the projection (see Figure 4-59).

Lateral Hand in Extension. It has been suggested that foreign bodies of the palm can be better localized when the lateral hand projection is taken with the hand and fingers in extension. The image analysis guidelines

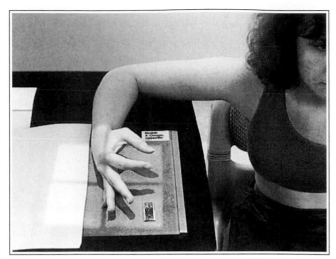

FIGURE 4-56 Proper patient positioning for lateral hand projection.

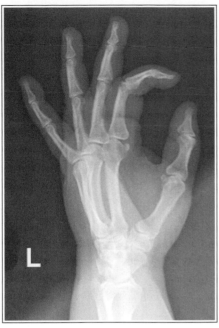

FIGURE 4-58 Lateral hand projection taken with the hand in internal rotation.

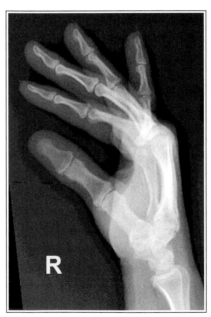

FIGURE 4-57 Lateral hand projection taken with the hand in slight external rotation.

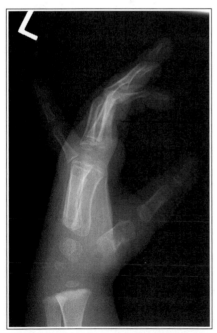

FIGURE 4-59 Pediatric lateral hand projection taken with the hand in slight internal rotation.

for the extended lateral hand projection will be the same as for the fan lateral projection, except that the second through fifth fingers will be superimposed (Figure 4-60).

Lateral Hand in Flexion. It has been suggested that a lateral hand projection obtained with the hand in flexion will better distinguish the degree of anterior or posterior displacement of a fractured metacarpal. The image analysis guidelines for the flexed lateral hand projection will be the same as for the fan lateral projection, except that the hand will be flexed and the second through fifth fingers will be superimposed (Figure 4-61).

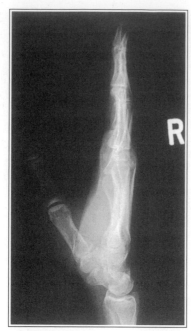

FIGURE 4-60 Lateral hand projection taken with the hand and fingers in full extension.

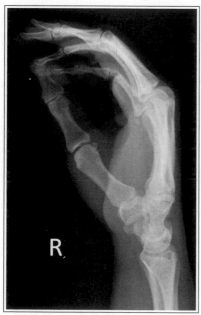

FIGURE 4-61 Lateral hand projection taken with the hand and fingers flexed.

Lateral Hand Analysis Practice

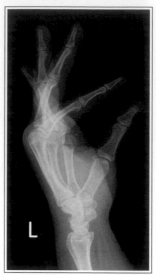

IMAGE 4-12

Analysis. The second through fifth MC midshafts are not superimposed, and the shortest (fifth) MCs anterior to the third through fourth MCs. The hand was externally rotated.

Correction. Internally rotate the hand until the MCs are superimposed.

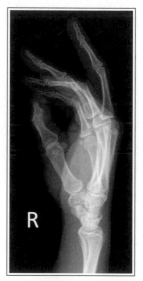

IMAGE 4-13

Analysis. The digits are superimposed and the thumb is foreshortened. Fingers were not fanned and the thumb was not positioned parallel with the IR.

Correction. Fan the second and third fingers anteriorly and the fourth and fifth posteriorly, separating the fingers as far apart as possible without superimposing the thumb, and position the thumb parallel with the IR.

TABLE 4-11	PA Wrist Projection
Image Analysis Guidelines (Figure 4-62)	**Related Positioning Procedures (Figure 4-63)**
• Scaphoid fat stripe is demonstrated. • Ulnar styloid is in profile medially.	• Correctly set the technical data. • Flex the elbow to 90 degrees and abduct the humerus, placing the humerus and forearm on the same horizontal plane.
• Radial styloid is in profile laterally. • Radioulnar articulation is open. • Superimposition of the MC bases is limited. • Radioscaphoid and radiolunate joints are closed. • Anterior and posterior margins of the distal radius are within 0.25 inch (0.6 cm) of each other.	• Rest distal forearm and pronated hand against the IR in PA projection. • Center the wrist on the IR. • Move the proximal forearm off of the IR as needed to position the forearm parallel with the IR.
• Second through fifth CM joint spaces are open. • Scaphoid is only slightly foreshortened. • Lunate is trapezoidal in shape.	• Flex the hand, placing the MCs at a 10- to 15-degree angle with the IR.
• Long axes of the third MC and the midforearm are aligned. • Lunate is positioned distal to the radioulnar articulation.	• Align the long axes of the third MC and the midforearm
• Carpal bones are at the center of the exposure field. • Carpal bones, one fourth of the distal ulna and radius, and half of the proximal MCs are included within the exposure field.	• Center a perpendicular CR to the midwrist. • Open the longitudinal collimation to include half of the MCs and 1 inch (2.5 cm) of distal forearm. • Transversely collimate to within 0.5 inch (1.25 cm) of the skin line.

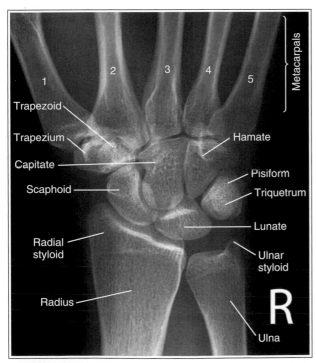

FIGURE 4-62 PA wrist projection with accurate positioning.

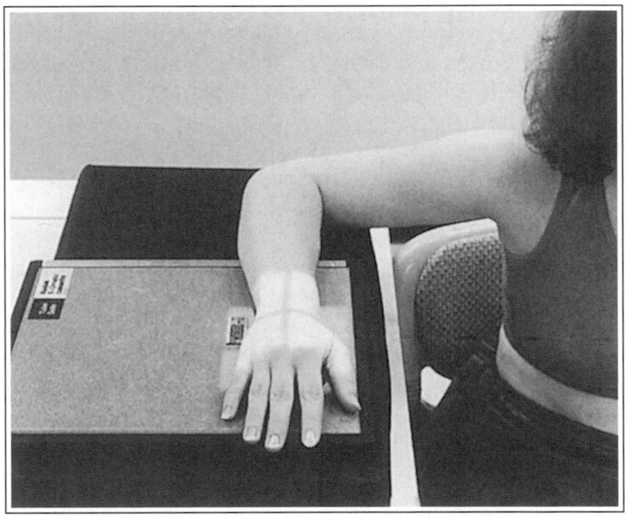

WRIST: PA PROJECTION

See Table 4-11, (Figures 4-62 and 4-63).

Scaphoid Fat Stripe. The scaphoid fat stripe is one of the soft tissue structures that is visible on properly positioned PA wrist projections (Figure 4-64). It is convex and located just lateral to the scaphoid in an uninjured wrist. A change in the convexity of this stripe may indicate to the reviewer the presence of joint effusion or of

FIGURE 4-63 Proper patient positioning for PA wrist projection.

a radial side fracture of the scaphoid, radial styloid process, or proximal first MC. Failing to obtain a true PA projection may result in obscuring this stripe.

Ulnar Styloid. Humerus and elbow positioning determines the placement of the ulnar styloid. Abducting the humerus to position the elbow in a lateral projection with the humeral epicondyles aligned perpendicularly to the IR brings the ulnar styloid in profile and aligns the radius and ulna parallel with each other. The ulna and radius cross each other if the humerus is not abducted but is allowed to remain in a vertical position with the humeral epicondyles aligned closer to parallel with the IR. This inaccurate positioning can be identified on a PA wrist projection by viewing the ulnar styloid, which is no longer demonstrated in profile (Figure 4-65).

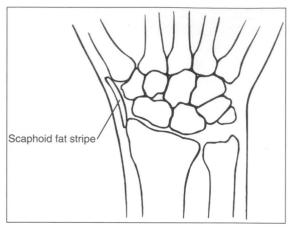

FIGURE 4-64 Location of scaphoid fat stripe. *(From Martensen K II: Radiographic positioning and analysis of the wrist,* In-Service Reviews in Radiologic Technology, *16[5], 1992.)*

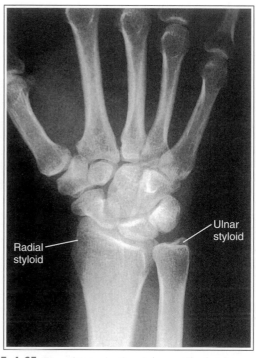

FIGURE 4-65 PA wrist projection taken with the humerus in a vertical position with the humeral epicondyles closer to parallel with the IR and wrist in slight external rotation.

Radial Styloid, Radioulnar Articulation and MC Bases. Wrist rotation determines the position of the radial styloid, openness of the radioulnar articulation, and degree of MC base superimposition.

External hand and wrist rotation (Figures 4-65 and 4-66) causes the:
- Medially located carpal bones and MC bases to demonstrate increased superimposition and decreased intercarpal and MC joint space visualization
- Laterally located carpal bones and MC bases to demonstrate less superimposition, and increased intercarpal and MC joint space visualization
- Radioulnar articulation to close

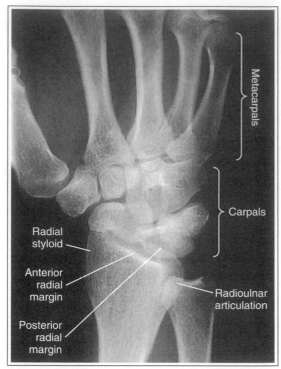

FIGURE 4-66 PA wrist projection taken with the wrist in external rotation and the proximal forearm slightly elevated.

Internal hand and wrist rotation (Figure 4-67) causes the:
- Laterally located carpal bones and MC bases to demonstrate increased superimposition and decreased intercarpal and MC joint space visualization
- Pisiform and hamate hook to demonstrate increased visibility
- Radioulnar articulation to close

Distal Radius and Radioscaphoid and Radiolunate Joints. The distal radial carpal articular surface is concave and slants approximately 11 degrees from posterior to anterior. When the forearm is positioned parallel with the IR for a PA wrist projection, the slant of the distal radius causes the posterior radial margin to project slightly (0.25 inch or 0.6 cm) distal to the anterior radial margin, obscuring the radioscaphoid and radiolunate joints.

If the proximal forearm is elevated higher than the distal forearm (caused when the patient has a large muscular or thick proximal forearm) the PA wrist demonstrates the posterior radial margin at a distance greater than 0.25 inch (0.6 cm) distal to the anterior margin and increased superimposition of the posterior radius on the scaphoid and lunate (Figures 4-66 and 4-68).

Identifying the Posterior and Anterior Distal Radial Margins. To identify the posterior and anterior radial margins from each other on a PA projection, view the distal radioulnar articulation. The posterior edge of this surface is blunt, whereas the anterior edge is rounded. Study the distal end of a radial skeletal bone to

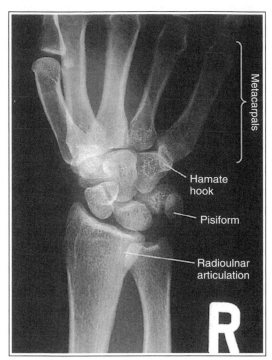

FIGURE 4-67 PA wrist projection taken with the wrist in internal rotation, and the proximal forearm positioned slightly lower than the distal forearm, demonstrating open radiolunate and radioscaphoid joint spaces.

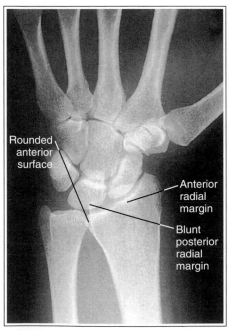

FIGURE 4-68 PA wrist projection taken with the proximal forearm positioned higher than the distal forearm.

familiarize yourself better with this difference. Also notice that with the external wrist rotation the posterior radius superimposes the ulna and with internal rotation the ulna superimposes the anterior radius.

Positioning the Patient with a Thick Proximal Forearm. On a patient with a large muscular or thick proximal forearm, it may be necessary to allow

the proximal forearm to extend off the IR or table to position the forearm parallel with the IR. If the patient is not positioned in this manner, the radius will be foreshortened, demonstrating an excessive amount of radial articular surface, and superimposition of the scaphoid and lunate onto the radius will be greater (see Figure 4-68).

Positioning the Forearm to Demonstrate Open Radioscaphoid and Radiolunate Joints. To superimpose the distal radial margins and to demonstrate radioscaphoid and radiolunate joints as open spaces (see Figure 4-67), the proximal aspect of the forearm should be positioned slightly lower (5 to 6 degrees from horizontal) than the distal forearm.

CM Joint Spaces and Scaphoid Visualization. To understand how the wrist's position changes when the hand is placed against the IR and flexed, view your own wrist in a PA projection with the hand extended flat against a hard surface. Note how in this position the wrist is slightly flexed. Next, begin slowly flexing your hand and notice how the wrist moves from a flexed to an extended position with increased hand flexion. The drawings of the scaphoid, capitate, and lunate bones in Figure 4-69 show how the carpal bone position also varies with this wrist flexion and extension. Study the CM joint space in reference to a perpendicular CR that is centered to the space on the wrist positions illustrated in Figure 4-69. Figures 4-70 and 4-71 demonstrate the changes illustrated in Figure 4-69 on PA wrist radiographic images. For Figure 4-70 the wrist was in flexion (the hand was extended), and for Figure 4-71 the wrist was in extension (the hand was overflexed). Compare these projections with the properly positioned wrist shown in Figure 4-62.

Identifying Causes of Obscured CM Joint Spaces. When the hand is too extended (MCs positioned less than 10 degrees with IR) the PA wrist projection demonstrates obscured third through fifth CM joint spaces and a severely foreshortened scaphoid that has taken a signet ring configuration (a large circle with a smaller circle within it) (see Figure 4-70). When the hand has been overflexed (MCs positioned >15 degrees with IR) the PA wrist projection demonstrates foreshortened MCs, closed second through third CM joint spaces and decreased scaphoid foreshortening (see Figure 4-71). Because the MCs are different lengths and may be positioned at different angles with the IR when the hand is flexed, it is necessary to evaluate each CM joint to determine accurate positioning and position each MC at a 10- to 15-degree angle to the IR to open all the CM joints. Figure 4-72 demonstrates a PA wrist with closed second and third and open fourth and fifth CM joints.

Third MC and Midforearm Alignment. If the long axes of the third MC and the midforearm are aligned, the patient's wrist has been placed in a neutral position, without deviation. Figure 4-73 illustrates how wrist deviation alters the shape of the scaphoid and

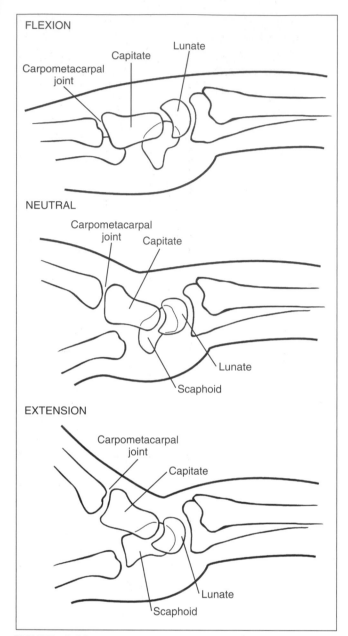

FIGURE 4-69 Lateral wrist in flexion (top), neutral position (middle), and extension (bottom). *(From Martensen K II: Radiographic positioning and analysis of the wrist,* In-Service Reviews in Radiologic Technology, *16[5], 1992.)*

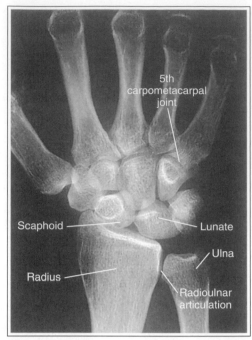

FIGURE 4-70 PA wrist projection taken with the hand and fingers extended, positioning the MCs at less than 10 to 15 degrees with the IR.

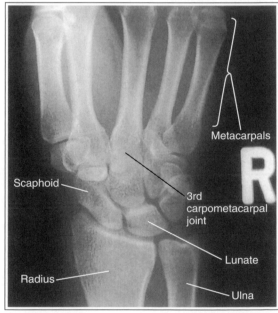

FIGURE 4-71 PA wrist projection taken with the hand and fingers overflexed, positioning the MCs at more than 10 to 15 degrees with the IR.

the position of the lunate in respect to the radioulnar articulation. Radial deviation of the wrist causes the distal scaphoid to tilt anteriorly and demonstrate increased foreshortening as it forms a signet ring configuration on the projection, and the lunate to shift medially, toward the ulna (Figure 4-74). Ulnar deviation of the wrist causes the distal scaphoid to tilt posteriorly and to demonstrate decreased foreshortening, and the lunate to shift laterally, toward the radius (Figure 4-75).

Demonstrating Joint Mobility. Radial and ulnar deviated wrist projections may be specifically requested to demonstrate wrist joint mobility. If this is the case, two PA projections are obtained, one with the wrist in

radial deviation and one with the wrist in ulnar deviation. The radial deviated wrist should demonstrate an excessively foreshortened scaphoid that forms a signet ring configuration and a medially shifted lunate. The ulnar deviated wrist should demonstrate decreased scaphoid foreshortening and a laterally shifted lunate.

CR Centering. Centering the CR to the midwrist is necessary to demonstrate undistorted carpals and open

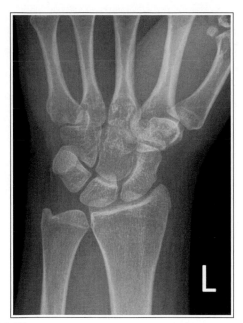

FIGURE 4-72 PA wrist projection with closed second and third and open fourth and fifth CM joint, demonstrating different MC alignments with IR.

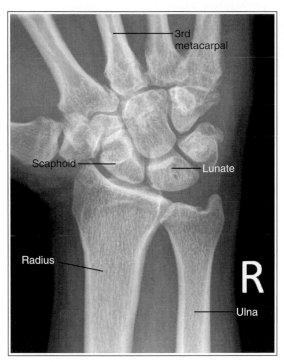

FIGURE 4-74 PA wrist projection taken with the wrist in radial deviation.

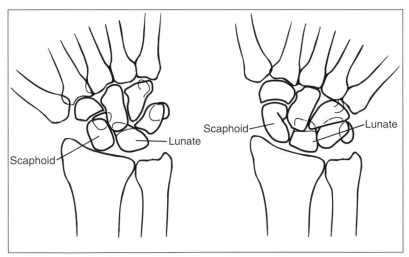

FIGURE 4-73 PA wrist in radial deviation (*left*) and ulnar deviation (*right*). (*From Martensen K II: Radiographic positioning and analysis of the wrist*, In-Service Reviews in Radiologic Technology, *16[5], 1992.*)

intercarpal joint spaces. Centering the CR to the distal forearm in an attempt to include more than one fourth of the distal forearm will result in distorted carpals, closed intercarpal joint spaces, and the posterior radial margin projected more than 0.25 inch (0.6 cm) distal to the anterior margin. If it is necessary to obtain such a projection, the CR should remain on the wrist joint, and

the collimation field should be opened to demonstrate the desired amount of forearm. This method will result in an extended, unnecessary radiation field distal to the metacarpals. A lead strip or apron placed over this extended radiation field protects the patient's phalanges and prevents backscatter from reaching the IR.

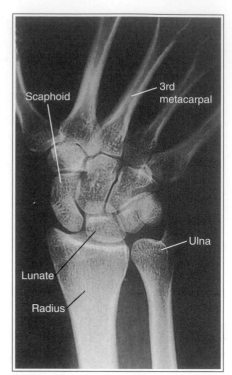

FIGURE 4-75 PA wrist projection taken with the wrist in ulnar deviation.

PA Wrist Image Analysis Practice

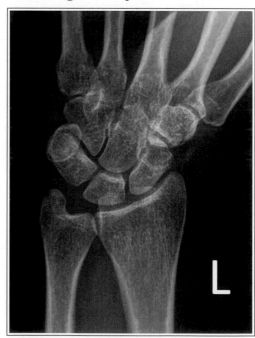

IMAGE 4-14

Analysis. The third MC is not aligned with the long axis of the midforearm, and the second through third CM joints are closed. The wrist was in radial deviation and the MCs were at a greater than 10- to 15-degree angle with the IR.

Correction. Ulnar deviate the wrist until the third MC is aligned with the long axis of the midforearm, and decrease the second through third MC's angle with the IR.

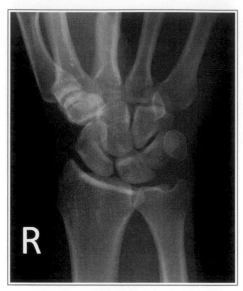

IMAGE 4-15

Analysis. The laterally located carpals and MCs are superimposed, and the radioulnar articulation is close. The wrist was in slight internal rotation for this projection.

Correction. Rotate the wrist externally until it is in a PA projection.

WRIST: PA OBLIQUE PROJECTION (LATERAL ROTATION)

See Table 4-12, (Figures 4-76 and 4-77).

Ulnar Styloid. Humerus and elbow positioning determines the placement of the ulnar styloid. Abducting the humerus to position the elbow in a lateral projection with the humeral epicondyles aligned perpendicularly to the IR brings the ulnar styloid in profile and aligns the radius and ulna parallel with each other. The ulna and radius cross each other if the humerus is not abducted but is allowed to remain in a vertical position with the humeral epicondyles closer to parallel with the IR. This inaccurate positioning can be identified on a PA wrist projection by viewing the ulnar styloid, which is no longer demonstrated in profile.

Alignment of Third MC and Midforearm. If the long axes of the third MC and the midforearm are aligned before the wrist is rotated, the patient's wrist is placed in a neutral position, without deviation. Radial deviation of the wrist causes the distal scaphoid to tilt anteriorly, demonstrates increased foreshortening and positions the scaphoid tuberosity adjacent to the radius, obscuring its visualization (Figure 4-78). Ulnar deviation results in decreased scaphoid foreshortening (Figure 4-82).

TABLE 4-12	PA Oblique Wrist Projection
Image Analysis Guidelines (Figure 4-76)	**Related Positioning Procedures (Figure 4-77)**
• Scaphoid fat stripe is demonstrated. • Ulnar styloid is in profile medially.	• Correctly set the technical data. • Flex the elbow to 90 degrees and abduct the humerus, placing the humerus and forearm on the same horizontal plane. • Rest the distal forearm and pronated hand against the IR in a PA projection. • Center the wrist on IR.
• Scaphoid is demonstrated in partial profile, without a signet ring configuration. • Scaphoid tuberosity is not positioned directly next to the radius.	• Align the long axis of the third MC and the midforearm before the wrist is rotated.
• Anterior and posterior articulating margins of the distal radius are within 0.25 inch (0.6 cm) of each other.	• Move the proximal forearm off of the IR as needed to position the forearm parallel with the IR.
• Second CM and the scaphotrapezial joint spaces are demonstrated as open spaces. • Trapezoid and trapezium are demonstrated without superimposition. • Trapeziotrapezoidal joint space is open. • About one fourth of the trapezoid superimposes the capitate. • Fourth and fifth MC midshafts demonstrate a small separation between them.	• Flex the hand until the second MC is placed at a 10- to 15-degree angle with the anterior plane of the wrist. • Externally rotate the hand and wrist until the wrist forms a 45-degree angle with the IR.
• Carpal bones are at the center of the exposure field. • Carpal bones, one fourth of the distal ulna and radius, and half of the proximal MCs are included within the exposure field.	• Center a perpendicular CR to the midwrist area and IR. • Open the longitudinal collimation to include half of the MCs. • Transversely collimate to within 0.5 inch (1.25 cm) of the skin line.

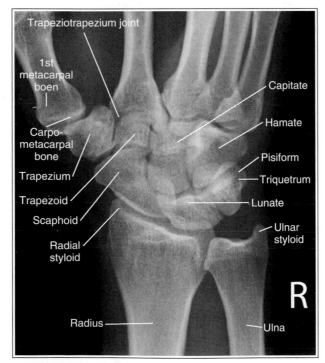

FIGURE 4-76 PA oblique wrist projection with accurate positioning.

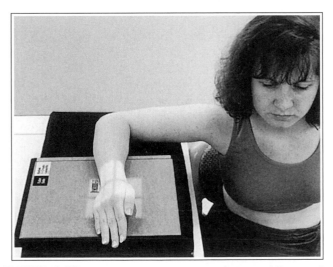

FIGURE 4-77 Proper patient positioning for PA oblique wrist projection.

Distal Radius and Radioscaphoid and Radiolunate Joints.

The articular surface of the distal radius is concave and slants approximately 11 degrees from posterior to anterior. When the forearm is positioned parallel with the IR for the PA oblique wrist projection, the slant of the distal radius causes the posterior radial margin to project slightly (0.25 inch or 0.6 cm) distal to the anterior radial margin, obscuring the radioscaphoid and radiolunate joints. If the proximal forearm is elevated higher than the distal forearm (caused when the patient has a large muscular or thick proximal forearm) the projection will demonstrate the posterior radial margin at a distance greater than 0.25 inch (0.6 cm) distal to the anterior margin and increased superimposition of the posterior radius on the scaphoid and lunate (Figures 4-79 and 4-82).

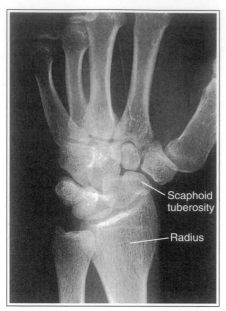

FIGURE 4-78 PA oblique wrist taken with the wrist in radial deviation.

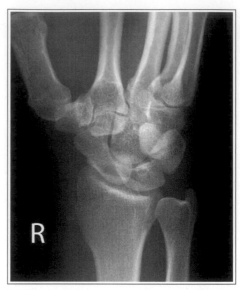

FIGURE 4-80 PA oblique wrist projection with more than 45 degrees of wrist obliquity, the second MC positioned at greater than 10 to 15 degrees with the anterior arm plane, and the proximal forearm elevated.

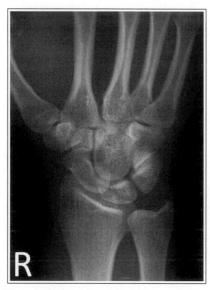

FIGURE 4-79 PA oblique wrist taken with proximal forearm elevated and less than 45 degrees of wrist obliquity.

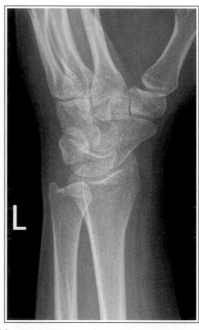

FIGURE 4-81 PA oblique wrist projection taken with more than 45 degrees of wrist obliquity, the proximal forearm elevated, and the second MC positioned at greater than 10 to 15 degrees with the anterior arm plane.

Positioning Patient with Thick Proximal Forearm or to Demonstrate Open Radioscaphoid and Radiolunate Joints. See PA wrist for explanation (Figure 4-83).

Second CM and Scaphotrapezial Joint Spaces. For the PA oblique wrist, the second CM and the scaphotrapezial joint spaces are opened by flexing the hand until the second MC is placed at a 10- to 15-degree angle with the IR (and with the anterior plane of the wrist). This same hand flexion needs to occur on the PA oblique wrist to demonstrate an open second CM joint space, but because the MCs are not positioned adjacent to the IR, the angle needs to be maintained with the anterior plane of the wrist. If the second MC is positioned more than

a 15-degree angle with the anterior wrist plane, a portion of the second MC base superimposes the trapezoid, closing the second CM and scaphotrapezial joints (Figures 4-80 and 4-81). Because the wrist obliquity elevates the distal MC, seldom is a projection obtained that demonstrates the trapezoid superimposing the second MC base that is caused by placing the MC at a degree that is less than 10 degrees.

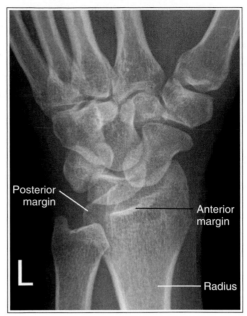

FIGURE 4-82 PA oblique wrist projection taken with the ulnar deviation and the proximal forearm elevated.

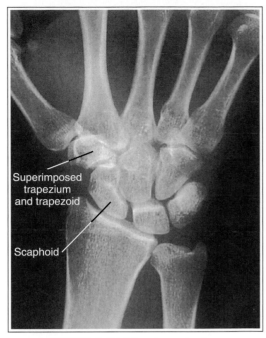

FIGURE 4-84 PA wrist projection.

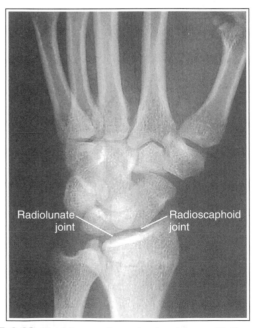

FIGURE 4-83 PA oblique wrist projection taken with the proximal forearm positioned slightly lower than the distal forearm, causing the radiolunate and radioscaphoid joint spaces to be open.

Trapezoid, Trapezium, and Trapeziotrapezoidal Joint Space. When judging the degree of wrist obliquity for a PA oblique projection, it is best to judge the amount of wrist obliquity and not hand obliquity. The obliquity of the hand and wrist are not always equal when they are rotated, especially if the humerus and forearm are not positioned on the same horizontal plane for the projection. On a PA wrist projection (Figure 4-84), the trapezoid superimposes the trapezium, but when the wrist is placed in a 45-degree PA oblique projection the trapezium is drawn from beneath the trapezoid, providing clear visualization of both carpal bones and the joint space (trapeziotrapezoidal) between them (Figure 4-76). The 45-degree PA oblique also rotates the trapezoid on top of the capitate, demonstrating about one fourth of the trapezoid superimposing the capitate on the projection.

Identifying Insufficient or Excessive Wrist Obliquity. If the wrist is rotated less than the required 45 degrees, the trapezoid superimposes a portion of the trapezium, closing the trapeziotrapezoidal joint space, less than one fourth of the trapezoid superimposes the capitate, and the fourth and fifth MC midshafts demonstrate a larger separation (Figure 4-79). If wrist obliquity is more than the required 45 degrees, the trapezium superimposes the trapezoid, closing the trapeziotrapezoidal joint space, more than one fourth of the trapezoid superimposes the capitate, and the fourth and fifth MC midshafts are superimposed (Figures 4-80 and 4-81).

PA Oblique Wrist Analysis Practice

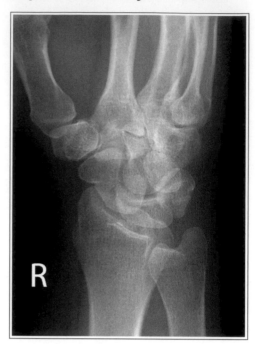

IMAGE 4-16

Analysis. The scaphoid is foreshortened and positioned adjacent to the radius, the trapeziotrapezoidal joint space is closed, more than one fourth of the trapezoid superimposes the capitate, the fourth and fifth MC midshafts are superimposed, the posterior radial margin is at a distance greater than 0.25 inch distal to the anterior margin, and the second MC base superimposes the trapezoid closing the second CM and scaffold trapezoidal joint. The wrist was radial deviated, at greater than 45

degrees oblique with the IR, and taken with the proximal forearm elevated, and the second MC was at a greater angle in 10 to 15 degrees with the anterior wrist plane. **Correction.** Align the long axis of the third MC and the midforearm, decrease the degree of external rotation, depress the proximal forearm, and decrease the angle of the second MC with the anterior arm plane.

WRIST: LATERAL PROJECTION (LATEROMEDIAL)

See Table 4-13, (Figures 4-85 and 4-86).
Pronator Fat Stripe. The pronator fat stripe is one of the soft tissue structures that are demonstrated on lateral wrist projections (Figure 4-87). It is located parallel to the anterior (volar) surface of the distal radius, is normally convex, and lies within 0.25 inch (0.6 cm) of the radial cortex. Bowing or obliteration of this fat stripe may be the only indication of a subtle radial fracture. Failure to obtain a true lateral projection will obscure this stripe.

Ulnar Styloid. The ulnar styloid is demonstrated in profile when the patient's elbow is in a lateral projection, with the humerus abducted and the humeral epicondyles aligned perpendicularly to the IR. If the humerus is not abducted to this degree, the ulnar styloid will not be demonstrated in profile (Figures 4-88 and 4-89).

Elbow and Humerus Positioning. In contrast to positioning the forearm and humerus on the same horizontal plane for a lateral wrist projection, a lateral wrist projection may be taken with zero forearm rotation. For this to be accomplished the humerus is not abducted and the elbow is placed in an AP projection, with the humeral epicondyles aligned parallel with the IR (Figure 4-90).

TABLE 4-13	Lateral Wrist Projection
Image Analysis Guidelines (Figure 4-85)	**Related Positioning Procedures (Figure 4-86)**
• Pronator fat stripe is demonstrated. • Ulnar styloid is demonstrated in profile posteriorly.	• Correctly set the technical data. • Flex the elbow to 90 degrees and abduct the humerus, placing the humerus and forearm on the same horizontal plane.
• Anterior aspects of the distal scaphoid and pisiform are aligned. • Distal radius and ulna are superimposed. • Distal aspects of the distal scaphoid and pisiform are aligned.	• Externally rotate arm and rest the medial forearm and hand against IR midline in lateral projection. • Center the wrist on the IR. • Move the proximal forearm off of the IR as needed to position the forearm parallel with the IR. • Align the long axes of the third MC and midforearm.
• Second through fifth MCs are placed at a 10- to 15-degree angle with the anterior plane of the wrist. • Thumb is parallel with the forearm. • Trapezium is demonstrated without superimposition of the first proximal MC. • First MC is demonstrated without foreshortening.	• Flex the hand until the second through fifth MCs are placed at a 10- to 15-degree angle with the anterior plane of the wrist. • Align the first MC parallel with the forearm. • Depress the thumb, placing the first and second MC at the same horizontal level.
• Carpal bones are at the center of the exposure field. • Carpal bones, one fourth of the distal ulna and radius, and half of the proximal MCs are included within the exposure field.	• Center a perpendicular CR to the midwrist area and IR. • Open the longitudinal collimation to include half of the MCs and 1 inch (2.5 cm) of the distal forearm. • Transversely collimate to within 0.5 inch (1.25 cm) of the skin line.

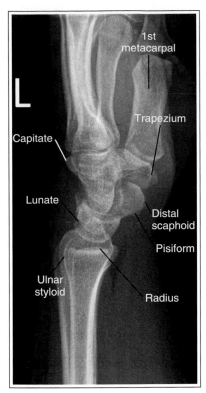

FIGURE 4-85 Lateral wrist projection with accurate positioning.

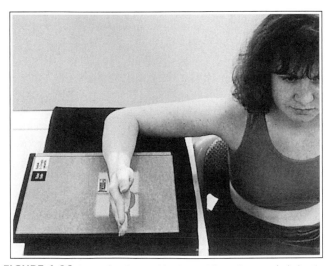

FIGURE 4-86 Lateral wrist positioning without humeral abduction and with humeral epicondyles aligned paralel with IR.

Such positioning rotates the ulnar styloid out of profile, demonstrating it distal to the midline of the ulnar head (see Figures 4-89 and 4-94). Because forearm rotation has been eliminated, the ulnar head also shifts closer to the lunate. This positioning allows for more accurate measuring of the ulnar length. Department policy determines which humerus positioning is performed in your facility.

Anterior Alignment of the Distal Scaphoid and Pisiform. The relationship between the pisiform and distal aspect of the scaphoid can best be used to discern whether a lateral wrist projection has been obtained. On

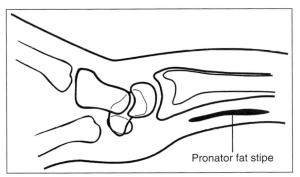

FIGURE 4-87 Location of pronator fat stripe. *(From Martensen K II: Radiographic positioning and analysis of the wrist, In-Service Reviews in Radiologic Technology, 16[5], 1992.)*

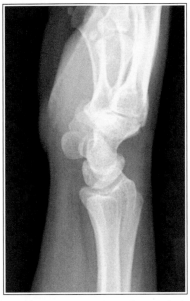

FIGURE 4-88 Lateral wrist projection taken with the humeral epicondyles aligned parallel with the IR, the wrist in external rotation, and without the thumb positioned parallel with the IR.

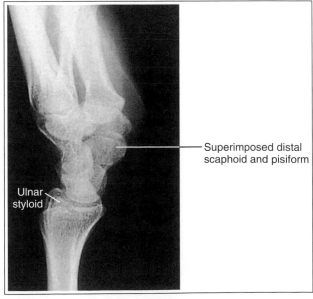

FIGURE 4-89 Lateral wrist projection taken with the humeral epicondyles aligned parallel with the IR.

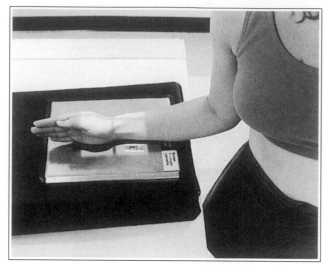

FIGURE 4-90 Lateral wrist positioning without humeral abduction.

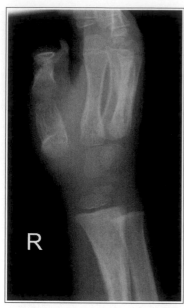

FIGURE 4-92 Pediatric lateral wrist projection taken with the wrist in internal rotation.

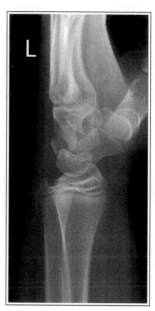

FIGURE 4-91 Pediatric lateral wrist projection taken with the wrist in internal rotation and without the thumb positioned parallel with the IR.

a lateral projection, these two carpals should be superimposed, with their anterior aspects aligned. It is with wrist rotation that this alignment changes. If the anterior aspect of the distal scaphoid is positioned posterior to the anterior aspect of the pisiform, the patient's wrist was externally rotated (see Figure 4-88). If the anterior aspect of the distal scaphoid is positioned anterior to the anterior aspect of the pisiform, the patient's wrist was internally rotated (Figures 4-91 and 4-92).

An alternate method of determining how to reposition a rotated lateral wrist projection uses the radius and ulna. The ulna is positioned anterior to the radius when the wrist was externally rotated and the ulna is positioned posterior to the radius when the wrist was internally rotated. Because the radius is wider than the ulna, this method is not as exact as viewing the pisiform and distal scaphoid relationship, and should not be the preferred method.

Distal Alignment of the Distal Scaphoid and Pisiform. To obtain a neutral lateral wrist projection, align the long axes of the third metacarpal and the midforearm parallel with the IR. This is accomplished by looking at the anterior or posterior surface of the hand and forearm. The wrist is radial deviated or ulnar deviated when the proximal forearm is higher or lower than the distal forearm, respectively. With radial and ulnar deviation, the distal scaphoid moves but the pisiform's position remains relatively unchanged. Radial deviation of the wrist forces the distal scaphoid to move anteriorly and proximally (Figure 4-93), causing the distal aspect of the distal scaphoid to be positioned proximal to the distal aspect of the pisiform (Figure 4-94). Ulnar deviation shifts the distal scaphoid posteriorly and distally (see Figure 4-93), causing the distal aspect of the distal scaphoid to be positioned distal to the distal aspect of the pisiform (Figure 4-95). The degree of pisiform and distal scaphoid separation is usually very small, because the technologist would be unlikely to position a patient in maximum wrist deviation without being aware of the positioning error. To obtain optimal lateral wrist projections, however, you must learn to eliminate even small degrees of deviation.

Positioning Patient with Thick Proximal Forearm. For a patient with a large muscular or thick proximal forearm, it may be necessary to allow the proximal forearm to hang off the IR or table to maintain a neutral wrist position (Figure 4-96). If the patient is not

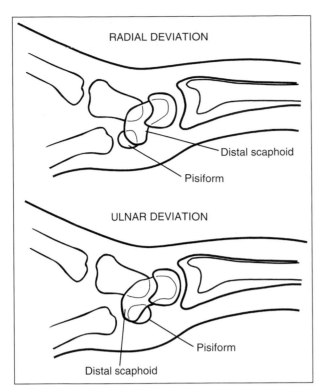

FIGURE 4-93 Lateral wrist in radial deviation (*top*) and ulnar deviation (*bottom*).

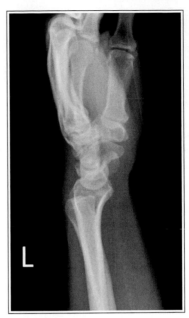

FIGURE 4-95 Lateral wrist projection with the wrist in ulnar deviation and the humeral epicondyles aligned parallel with IR.

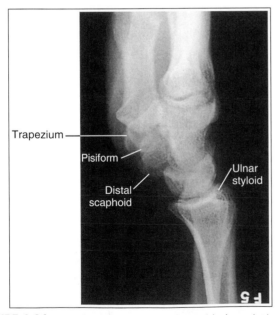

FIGURE 4-94 Lateral wrist projection taken with the wrist in radial deviation and the humeral epicondyles aligned parallel with the IR.

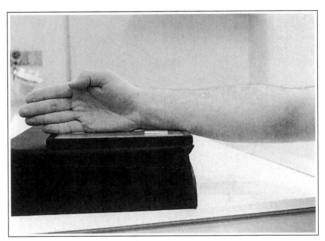

FIGURE 4-96 Positioning of patient with thick proximal forearm.

positioned in this manner, radial deviation of the wrist will result. If the proximal forearm does not remain level but is allowed to depress lower than the distal forearm in this situation, ulnar deviation will result.

Metacarpals and Thumb Alignment with the Forearm. Wrist projections are to be taken in the neutral position, without flexion and extension of the wrist unless special requests are made. To place the wrist

neutral for the lateral projection, the metacarpals are positioned at a 10- to 15-degree angle with the anterior plane of the wrist and the thumb aligned parallel with the forearm. In wrist flexion the lunate and distal scaphoid tilts anteriorly (see Figure 4-94). In wrist extension the lunate and distal scaphoid tilts posteriorly (Figure 4-98).

Lateral Projections Taken for Wrist Joint Mobility. Lateral flexion and extension projections of the wrist may be specifically requested to demonstrate wrist joint mobility. These projections are completed by positioning the patient in maximum allowable flexion and extension as demonstrated in Figures 4-97 and 4-98, respectively.

Thumb Positioning and Trapezium Visualization. To obtain optimal demonstration of the trapezium, depress the thumb until it is at the same horizontal level as the

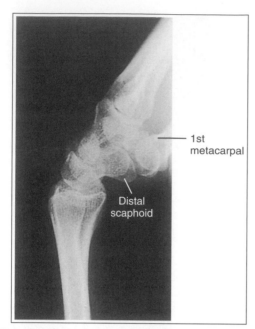

FIGURE 4-97 Lateral wrist projection taken with the wrist flexed.

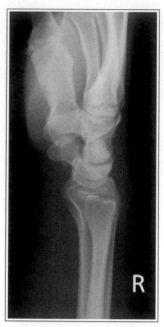

FIGURE 4-99 Lateral wrist projection taken without the thumb being positioned parallel with the IR.

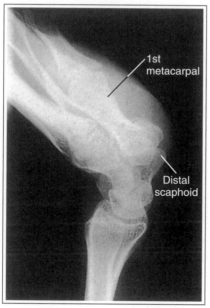

FIGURE 4-98 Lateral wrist projection taken with the wrist extended.

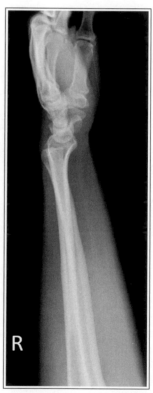

FIGURE 4-100 Lateral wrist projection taken with CR positioned distal to the wrist to include more than one fourth of the distal forearm.

second MC. This positioning places the trapezium and MC parallel with the IR, demonstrating them without superimposition. If the distal first MC is not depressed, it is foreshortened, and its proximal aspect is superimposed over the trapezium (Figures 4-91 and 4-99).

CR Centering. Centering the CR to the midwrist is necessary to demonstrate undistorted carpals and open intercarpal joint spaces. Centering the CR to the distal forearm in an attempt to include more than one fourth of the distal forearm will result in the distal scaphoid being projected distal to the pisiform (Figure 4-100). If it is necessary to obtain a projection that includes more of the forearm, the CR should remain on the wrist joint,

and the collimation field opened to demonstrate the desired amount of forearm. This method results in an extended, unnecessary radiation field distal to the metacarpals. A lead strip or apron placed over this extended radiation field protects the patient's phalanges and prevents backscatter from reaching the IR.

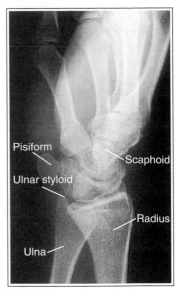

FIGURE 4-101 Mediolateral wrist projection.

Alternate Mediolateral Wrist Projection. Routinely, the lateral wrist projection is taken with the ulnar side of the wrist against the IR (lateromedial projection). If, instead, the radial side of the wrist was placed against the IR (mediolateral projection) to obtain a lateral wrist projection, the ulna and pisiform are visualized anterior to the radius and scaphoid, respectively, and the ulnar styloid is demonstrated in profile anteriorly (Figure 4-101).

Lateral Wrist Analysis Practice

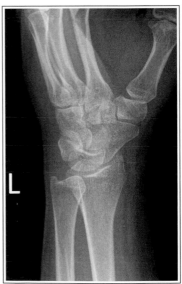

IMAGE 4-17

Analysis. The anterior aspect of the distal scaphoid is anterior to the anterior aspect of the pisiform, and the radius is anterior to the ulna. The wrist was internally rotated

Correction. Externally rotate the wrist until the wrist is in a lateral projection.

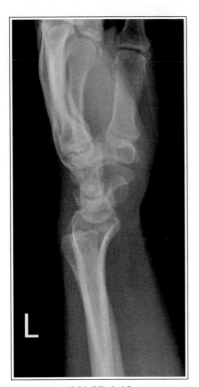

IMAGE 4-18

Analysis. The distal aspect of the distal scaphoid is demonstrated distal to the pisiform. The wrist was in ulnar deviation.

Correction. Place the wrist in a neutral position by aligning the long axis of the third MC and the midforearm parallel with the IR.

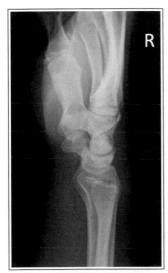

IMAGE 4-19

Analysis. The first proximal MC is superimposed over the trapezium. The thumb was not depressed, placing it and the second MC at the same horizontal level.

Correction. Depress the thumb, placing it and the second MC at the same horizontal level.

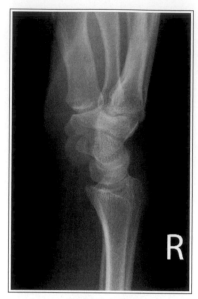

IMAGE 4-20

Analysis. The anterior aspect of the pisiform is shown anterior to the anterior aspect of the distal scaphoid. The wrist was externally rotated.

Correction. Internally rotate the wrist until the wrist is in a lateral projection.

WRIST: ULNAR DEVIATION, PA AXIAL PROJECTION (SCAPHOID)

See Table 4-14, (Figures 4-102 and 4-103).

Scaphotrapezium and Scaphotrapezoidal Joint Spaces. The scaphotrapezium and scaphotrapezoidal joint spaces are aligned at a 15-degree angle to the IR when the patient's hand is pronated and fully extended.

On the PA axial projection, because the required 15-degree proximal (toward the elbow) CR angle aligns the x-ray beam with these joints they are demonstrated as open spaces. If the hand is not extended and the palm placed flat against the IR, but rather is flexed, the second MC is superimposed over the trapezoid and trapezium, closing the scaphotrapezium and scaphotrapezoidal joint spaces (Figures 4-104 and 4-107).

Scaphoid and Scaphocapitate and Scapholunate Joint Spaces. In a neutral PA projection of the wrist, the distal scaphoid tilts anteriorly and the scaphoid's

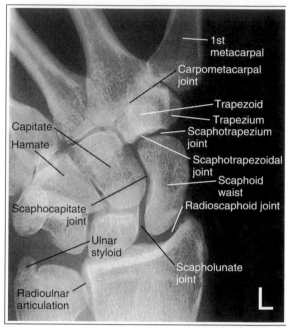

FIGURE 4-102 Ulnar-deviated, PA axial (scaphoid) wrist projection with accurate positioning.

TABLE 4-14	PA Axial (Scaphoid) Wrist Projection
Image Analysis Guidelines (Figure 4-102)	**Related Positioning Procedures (Figure 4-103)**
• Scaphoid fat stripe is demonstrated. • Ulnar styloid is in profile medially.	• Correctly set the technical data. • Flex the elbow to 90 degrees and abduct the humerus, placing the humerus and forearm on the same horizontal plane. • Rest the distal forearm and pronated hand against the IR in a PA projection. • Center the wrist on the IR.
• Scaphotrapezium and scaphotrapezoidal joint spaces are open. • Scaphoid is demonstrated without foreshortening or excessive elongation. • Scaphocapitate and scapholunate joint spaces are open. • Radioscaphoid joint space is open.	• Extend the hand, and place its palmar surface flat against the IR. • Ulnar deviate the wrist until the long axis of the first MC and the radius are aligned and the wrist externally rotates to a 25-degree angle with the IR. • Move the proximal forearm off of the IR as needed to position the proximal forearm slightly higher (2 degrees) than the distal forearm.
• Scaphoid waist is demonstrated. • Scaphoid is at the center of the exposure field.	• Center a 15-degree proximally angled CR to the scaphoid.
• Carpal bones, radiolunar articulation, and proximal first through fourth MCs are included within the exposure field.	• Open the longitudinal collimation to include the first through fourth MC bases and 1 inch (2.5 cm) of the distal radius. • Transversely collimate to within 0.5 inch (1.25 cm) of the skin line.

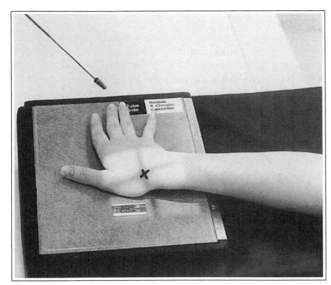

FIGURE 4-103 Proper patient positioning for ulnar-deviated, PA axial (scaphoid) wrist projection. X indicates the location of the scaphoid.

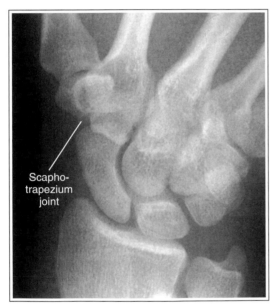

FIGURE 4-104 PA axial wrist projection taken without the hand extended and palm placed flat against the IR.

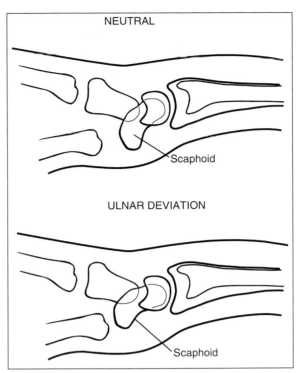

FIGURE 4-105 Lateral wrist in neutral position (*top*) and in ulnar deviation (*bottom*).

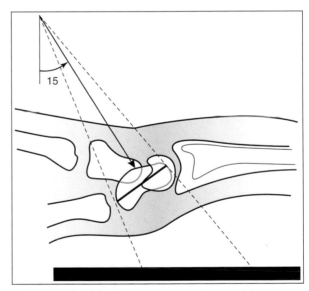

FIGURE 4-106 Proper alignment of CR and fracture.

long axis is at approximately a 20-degree angle with the IR, causing foreshortening distortion of the scaphoid on the projection (Figures 4-62 and 4-105). To offset some of this foreshortening and better demonstrate the scaphoid, the patient's wrist is placed in maximum ulnar deviation and a 15-degree proximal CR angulation is directed to the long axis of the scaphoid for a PA axial scaphoid projection. Maximum ulnar deviation has been accomplished when the first metacarpal is aligned with the radius and it moves the distal scaphoid posteriorly about 5 degrees, bringing the scaphoid's long axis closer to perpendicular to the CR and decreasing scaphoid foreshortening on the projection (Figure 4-106).

When maximum ulnar deviation and the 15-degree proximal CR angle are used the CR is aligned perpendicular to the scaphoid waist, which is where 70% of all scaphoid fractures occur (Figure 4-107).

Compensating for Inadequate Ulnar Deviation. Many patients with suspected scaphoid fractures are unable to achieve maximum ulnar wrist deviation and the 5-degree posterior shift of the distal scaphoid. This places the scaphoid's long axis at a greater angle with the CR and the projection will demonstrate

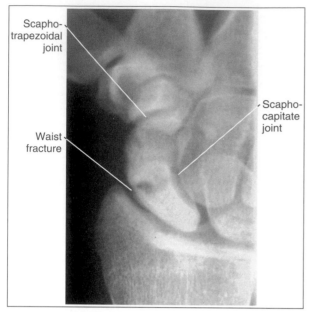

FIGURE 4-107 PA axial wrist projection demonstrating a scaphoid waist fracture, and taken without the hand extended and palm placed flat against the IR and the wrist in maximum ulnar deviation.

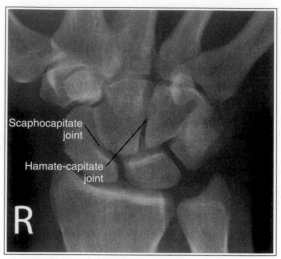

FIGURE 4-108 PA axial wrist projection taken without the wrist in maximum ulnar deviation and without external wrist rotation.

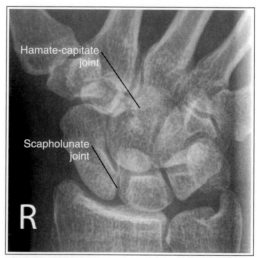

FIGURE 4-109 PA axial wrist projection taken with the wrist externally rotated more than needed.

increased scaphoid foreshortening unless the CR angulation is increased to a 20-degree proximal angle to compensate.

Medial Wrist Rotation upon Ulnar Deviation. When the humerus is abducted and positioned parallel with the IR, and the elbow placed in a flexed lateral position, as the patient's wrist is ulnar deviated it naturally rotates medially about 25 degrees, opening the scaphocapitate and scapholunate joint spaces. One can judge how accurately the humerus, forearm, and elbow have been positioned by evaluating the location of the ulnar styloid. Accurate positioning places the ulnar styloid in profile medially. If the humerus is positioned as described and the scaphocapitate joint space is closed and the capitate and hamate are demonstrated without superimposition, the degree of obliquity was insufficient (Figures 4-107 and 4-108). If the scapholunate joint space is closed and the capitate and hamate demonstrate some degree of superimposition, the wrist was rotated more than needed (Figure 4-109). Excessive medial wrist obliquity often occurs when the humerus and forearm are not positioned on the same horizontal plane and the elbow is placed in an AP projection, demonstrating the ulnar styloid distal to the midline of the ulnar head (Figure 4-110).

Radioscaphoid Joint Space. The distal radial carpal articular surface is concave and slants approximately 11 degrees from posterior to anterior when the forearm is positioned parallel with the IR. That is why the posterior radial margin is seen 0.25 inch (0.6 cm) distal to the anterior margin on a PA wrist projection when a perpendicular CR is used. With the 15-degree proximal CR angulation that is used for the PA axial scaphoid the posterior radial margin is projected proximally and is seen proximal to the anterior radial margin on the projection (Figure 4-111). To demonstrate an open radioscaphoid joint, the anterior and posterior margins of the distal radius need to be superimposed. This superimposition is accomplished by elevating the proximal forearm very slightly (2 degrees) above the distal forearm (Figure 4-112).

Positioning Patient with Thick Proximal Forearm. For a patient with a large muscular or thick proximal forearm, it may be necessary to allow the proximal forearm to hang off the IR or table to align the CR with the distal radial surface. If the patient is not positioned in this manner, the posterior radial margin will superimpose the proximal scaphoid and lunate (see Figure 4-111).

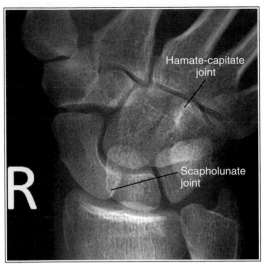

FIGURE 4-110 PA axial wrist projection taken with the humeral epicondyles parallel with the IR and wrist externally rotated more than needed.

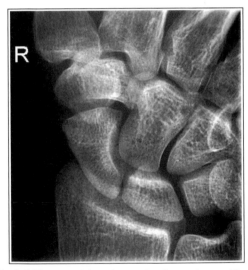

FIGURE 4-111 PA axial wrist projection taken with proximal forearm elevated slightly above the distal forearm.

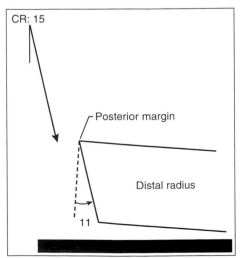

FIGURE 4-112 Alignment of CR and distal radius to obtain open radioscaphoid joint.

CR Angulation. One goal of the PA axial projection is to demonstrate the scaphoid without foreshortening and is accomplished by aligning the CR perpendicular to the long axis of the scaphoid. Scaphoid foreshortening occurs when the CR is not angled enough to align it perpendicular to the scaphoid's long axis. Another goal is to demonstrate the scaphoid with the least amount of elongation. A slight amount of elongation of the scaphoid occurs on all PA axial projections because the IR is not positioned perpendicular to the CR or parallel with the scaphoid's long axis (see Figure 4-106). It is when the CR and IR angles is acute that excessive scaphoid elongation occurs.

Adjusting CR Angulation to Align with Fracture. The scaphoid is the most commonly fractured carpal bone. One reason for this is its location among the other carpal bones. Two rows of carpal bones exist, a distal row and a proximal row, with joint spaces between them that allow the wrist to move. The scaphoid bone, however, is aligned partially with both these rows, with no joint space. When an individual falls on an outstretched hand, the wrist is hyperextended, causing the proximal and distal carpal rows to flex at the joints, and a great deal of stress is placed on the narrow waist of the scaphoid. This stress often results in a fracture at the scaphoid waist.

Three areas of the scaphoid may be fractured: the waist, which sustains approximately 70% of the fractures; the distal end, which sustains 20% of the fractures; and the proximal end, which sustains 10% (Figure 4-113). Because scaphoid fractures can be at different locations on the scaphoid, precise positioning and CR angulation are essential to obtain the optimum demonstration of this bone. When a fracture is suspected

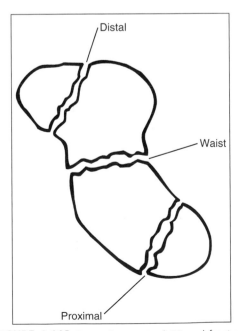

FIGURE 4-113 Poor alignment of CR and fracture.

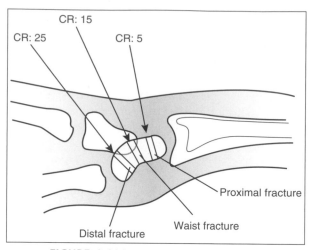

FIGURE 4-114 Sites of scaphoid fracture.

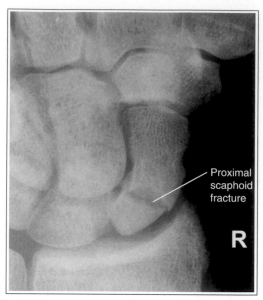

FIGURE 4-116 PA axial wrist projection taken with a 5-degree proximal CR angle demonstrating a proximal scaphoid fracture.

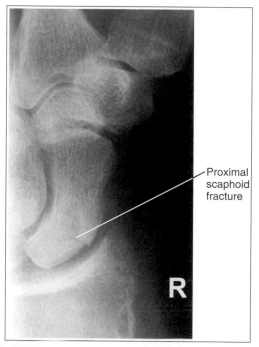

FIGURE 4-115 PA axial wrist projection taken with a 15-degree proximal CR angle demonstrating a proximal scaphoid fracture.

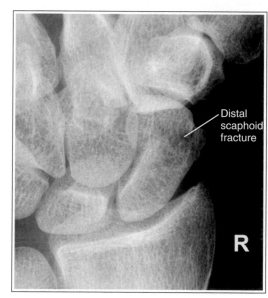

FIGURE 4-117 Distal scaphoid fracture.

because of persistent pain and obliteration of the fat stripe but no fracture has been demonstrated on routine projections, it may be necessary to use different CR angulation to align it perpendicular to the scaphoid location of interest and parallel with a fracture line if present (Figure 4-114). A decrease of 5 to 10 degrees in CR angulation better demonstrates the proximal scaphoid. Compare Figures 4-115 and 4-116. These projections demonstrate a proximal fracture. Figure 4-115 was taken with the typical 15-degree proximal angle, and Figure 4-116 was taken with a 5-degree proximal angle. Note the increase in fracture line visualization in Figure 4-116. Increase the CR angle by 5 to 10 degrees, with a maximum of 25 degrees, to demonstrate a distal

scaphoid fracture best (Figure 4-117). Angulations of more than 25 degrees project the proximal first metacarpal onto the distal scaphoid, obscuring the area of interest (Figure 4-118).

Collimation. Although technologists are taught to collimate as tightly as possible for radiation protection and scatter radiation reduction reasons, one should not collimate too tightly on the PA axial projection. Failing to include the other carpal bones and at least 0.5 inch (1.25 cm) of each of the surrounding anatomic structures on the projection eliminates the opportunity to identify how to improve positioning when a poor projection has been created, as these structures are used in the determination.

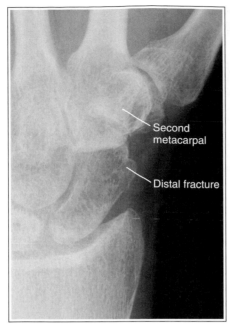

FIGURE 4-118 PA axial wrist projection taken with a 30-degree proximal CR angle and the hand and fingers positioned flat against the IR. A distal scaphoid fracture is present, but not well demonstrated because the CR angulation was too great.

PA Axial (Scaphoid) Analysis Practice

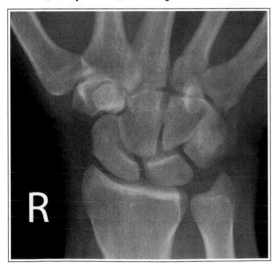

IMAGE 4-21

Analysis. The scaphocapitate joint is closed and the hamate-capitate joint is open. The wrist was not ulnar deviated enough to adequately externally rotate the wrist.

Correction. If patient is unable to increase the degree of ulnar deviation, slightly externally rotate the wrist.

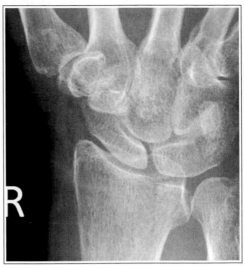

IMAGE 4-22

Analysis. The scaphotrapezium and scaphotrapezoidal joint spaces are closed, the scaphocapitate joint is closed and the hamate-capitate joint is open, and the radioscaphoid joint is closed. The hand was not extended and the palm placed flat against the IR, the wrist was not externally rotated enough, and the proximal forearm was elevated.

Correction. Extend the hand and place the palm flat against the IR and slightly externally rotate the wrist, and move the proximal forearm off of the IR until it is only slightly higher than the distal forearm.

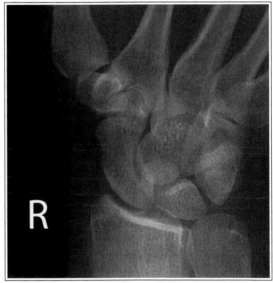

IMAGE 4-23

Analysis. The scaphotrapezium and scaphotrapezoidal joint spaces are closed, the scapholunate joint is closed, and the capitate and hamate demonstrate some degree of superimposition. The hand was not extended and the palm placed flat against the IR, and the wrist was externally rotated more than needed.

Correction. Extend hand and place the palm flat against the IR and slightly decrease the degree of external wrist rotation.

TABLE 4-15	Tangential, Inferosuperior (Carpal Canal) Wrist Projection	
Image Analysis Guidelines (Figure 4-119)	**Related Positioning Procedures (Figure 4-120)**	
• Carpal canal is visualized in its entirety. • Carpal bones are demonstrated with only slight elongation.	• Rest the distal forearm and pronated hand against the IR in a PA projection. • Center the wrist to the IR. • Hyperextend the wrist by having the patient grasp the fingers with the unaffected hand and gently pull them posteriorly until the long axis of the MCs are positioned close to vertical, with the wrist remaining in contact with the IR. • Align the CR at a 25- to 30-degree proximal angle.	
• Pisiform is demonstrated without superimposition of the hamulus of the hamate.	• Rotate the hand 10 degrees internally (toward the radial side) or until the fifth MC is perpendicular to the IR.	
• Carpal canal is at the center of the exposure field.	• Center the CR to the center of the palm of the hand.	
• Trapezium, distal scaphoid, pisiform and hamulus of the hamate are included within the exposure field.	• Open the longitudinal and transverse collimations to within 0.5 inch (1.25 cm) of the skin line.	

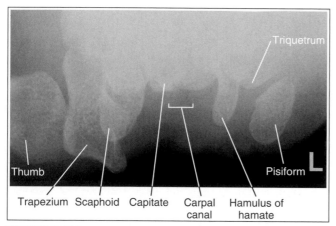

FIGURE 4-119 Carpal canal projection of the wrist with accurate positioning.

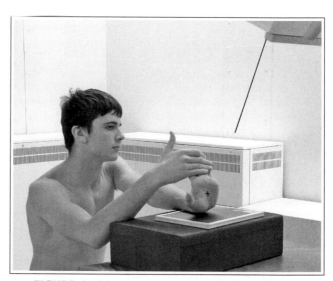

FIGURE 4-120 Proper carpal canal wrist positioning.

WRIST: CARPAL CANAL (TUNNEL) (TANGENTIAL, INFEROSUPERIOR PROJECTION)

See Table 4-15, (Figures 4-119 and 4-120).

The carpal canal position is used to evaluate the carpal canal for the narrowing that results in carpal canal syndrome and demonstrate fractures of the pisiform and hamulus of the hamate. The carpal canal is a passageway formed anteriorly by the flexor retinaculum, posteriorly by the capitate, laterally by the scaphoid and trapezium, and medially by the pisiform and hamate (Figure 4-121).

Carpal Canal Visualization. To show the carpal canal and demonstrate the carpals with only slight elongation, the MCs are positioned as close to vertical as the patient allows, with the wrist staying in contact with the IR, and a proximal angle is placed on the CR. If the MCs can be placed vertical a 25-degree proximal angle is used and a 30-degree angle is used if the patient cannot bring the hand to a completely vertical position but can bring it within 15 degrees of vertical. When imaging a patient who is unable to extend the wrist enough to place the

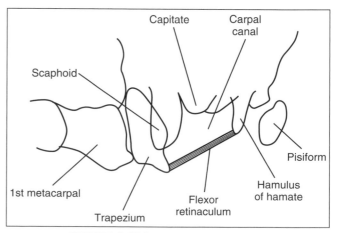

FIGURE 4-121 Carpal canal anatomy.

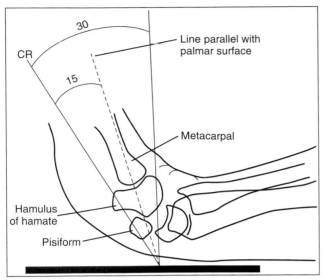

FIGURE 4-122 CR alignment for insufficient wrist extension.

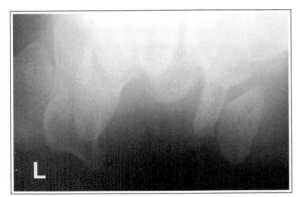

FIGURE 4-123 Carpal canal wrist taken with the CR and IR angle being too acute.

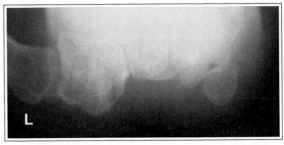

FIGURE 4-124 Carpal canal wrist taken with too great of a CR and palmer surface angle.

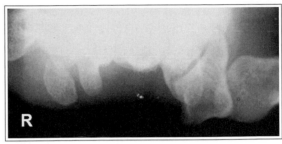

FIGURE 4-125 Carpal canal wrist taken with too small of a CR and palmer surface angle.

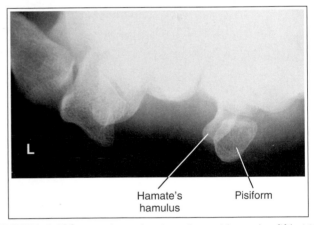

Hamate's hamulus   Pisiform

FIGURE 4-126 Carpal canal wrist taken without the fifth MC aligned perpendicular to the IR.

metacarpals to within 15 degrees of vertical, the CR angle needs to be increased. To determine the degree of angulation to use, first align the CR so that it is parallel with the patient's palmar surface, and then increase the angle an additional 15 degrees proximally (Figure 4-122). The resulting projection demonstrates adequate visualization of the carpal bones and carpal canal, although there will be increased elongation as the angle between the CR and IR becomes more acute (Figure 4-123).

If the angle between the CR and metacarpals is too great, the carpal canal will not be fully demonstrated and the carpal bones will be foreshortened (Figure 4-124). If the angle between the CR and metacarpals is too small, the carpal canal is not fully demonstrated and the bases of the hamulus process, pisiform, and scaphoid are obscured by the MC bases (Figure 4-125).

Pisiform and Hamulus Process. Fractures of the pisiform and hamulus process are best demonstrated when they are seen without superimposition. This is accomplished by rotating the patient's hand 10 degrees internally (toward the radial side) or until the fifth MC is aligned perpendicularly to the IR. If the hand is not internally rotated, the pisiform will be superimposed over the hamulus process on the projection (Figure 4-126).

FOREARM: AP PROJECTION

See Table 4-16, (Figures 4-127 and 4-128).
Wrist and Distal Forearm Positioning. Rotation of the distal forearm results from inaccurate positioning of the hand and wrist. If the wrist and hand are not positioned in an AP projection but are rotated, the radial styloid is no longer in profile and the distal radius and ulna and MC bases demonstrate increased superimposition. To identify which way the wrist is rotated, evaluate the MC and carpal bones. When the wrist and hand are

TABLE 4-16	AP Forearm Projection	
Image Analysis Guidelines (Figure 4-127)	**Related Positioning Procedures (Figure 4-128)**	
• Brightness is uniform across the entire forearm.	• Center the forearm to the IR in an AP projection, with the wrist placed at the anode end of the tube and the elbow at the cathode end.	
• Radial styloid is demonstrated in profile laterally. • Superimposition of the MC bases and of the radius and ulna is minimal. • Radial tuberosity is demonstrated in profile medially. • Radius and ulna run parallel.	• Supinate the hand, positioning the second through fifth knuckles against IR.	
• Ulnar styloid is projected distally to the midline of the ulnar head. • One eighth (0.25 inch) of the radial head superimposes the ulna.	• Position the humeral epicondyles parallel with the IR.	
• Olecranon process is situated within the olecranon fossa. • Coronoid process is visible on end.	• Extend the elbow.	
• Forearm midpoint is at the center of the exposure field.	• Center a perpendicular CR to the forearm midpoint.	
• Wrist and elbow joints and forearm soft tissue are included within the exposure field.	• Open the longitudinal collimation field to include the wrist and elbow. • Transversely collimate to within 0.5 inch (1.25 cm) of the skin line.	

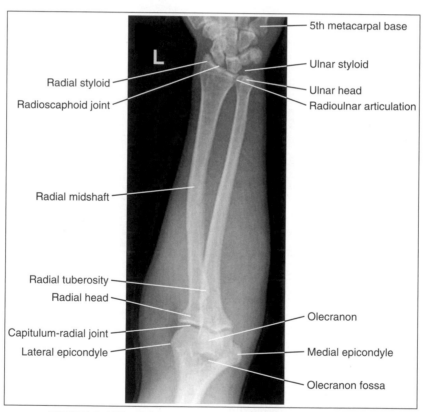

FIGURE 4-127 AP forearm projection with accurate positioning.

internally rotated, the laterally located first and second MC bases and carpal bones are superimposed, and the medially located MCs bases, pisiform, and hamate hook are better demonstrated (Figures 4-129 and 4-130). If the wrist and hand are externally rotated, the medially located fourth and fifth MC bases and carpal bones will be superimposed, whereas the laterally located MCs bases and carpal bones will demonstrate less superimposition.

Radial Tuberosity. When the distal humerus is positioned with the epicondyles parallel with the IR, the relationship of the radius and ulna is controlled by wrist positioning. To place the radius and ulna parallel and the radial tuberosity in profile medially, position the wrist and hand in an AP projection. When the hand and wrist are pronated, the radius crosses over the ulna, and the radial tuberosity is rotated posteriorly, out of profile (Figure 4-131).

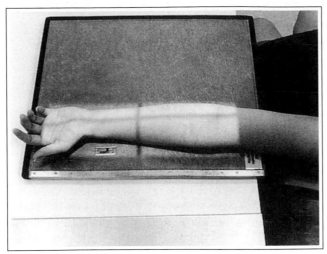

FIGURE 4-128 Proper AP forearm positioning.

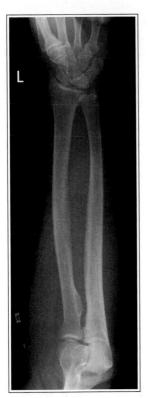

FIGURE 4-130 AP forearm projection taken with the wrist internally rotated and the elbow externally rotated.

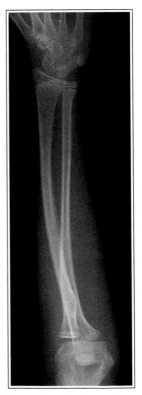

FIGURE 4-129 AP forearm projection taken with accurate elbow positioning and the wrist internally rotated.

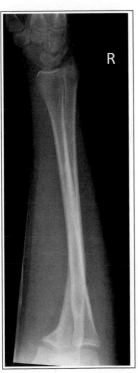

FIGURE 4-131 AP forearm projection taken with the wrist in a PA projection.

Humerus and Elbow Positioning. Proximal forearm rotation results when the humeral epicondyles are poorly positioned. Rotation can be identified on the projection when more or less than one eighth of the radial head superimposes the ulna and when the humeral epicondyles are not visualized in profile. When more than one eighth of the radial head is superimposed over the ulna, the elbow has been internally rotated (Figure 4-146). When less than one eighth of the radial head is superimposed over the ulna, the elbow has been externally rotated (see Figure 4-130).

Ulnar Styloid. The position of the ulnar styloid is determined by the position of the humerus and elbow. When the humerus and elbow positions are adjusted but the wrist position is maintained, it is the ulna that rotates and changes position. Positioning the humeral epicondyles parallel with the IR for the AP projection of the forearm places the ulnar styloid posterior to the head of the ulna. If the elbow is rotated internally and the wrist remains in an AP projection, then the ulnar styloid is demonstrated laterally, next to the radius. If the elbow is rotated externally and the wrist remains in an AP projection, then the ulnar styloid is demonstrated in profile medially.

Elbow Flexion. The positions of the olecranon process and fossa and the coronoid process on an AP forearm projection are determined by the amount of elbow flexion. Accurate forearm positioning requires us to position the elbow in full extension, which places the olecranon process within the olecranon fossa and demonstrates the coronoid process on end. When a forearm projection is taken with the elbow flexed and the proximal humerus elevated (Figure 4-132), the olecranon process moves away from the olecranon fossa and the coronoid process shifts proximally. How far the olecranon process is from the fossa depends on the degree of elbow flexion. The greater the elbow flexion, the farther the olecranon process is positioned away from the fossa and the more foreshortened is the distal humerus.

CR Centering and Openness of Wrist and Elbow Joint Spaces

Distal Forearm. The distal radial carpal articular surface is concave and slants at approximately 11 degrees from posterior to anterior. When the wrist and forearm are placed in an AP projection and the CR is centered to the midforearm, diverged x-rays record the structures much as if the CR were angled toward the wrist joint. If this angle of divergence is parallel with the AP slant of the distal radius, the resulting projection shows superimposed distal radial margins and open radioscaphoid and radiolunate joint spaces. If the angle of divergence is not parallel with the AP slant of the distal radius, as when the patient has a muscular proximal forearm or the patient's forearm is long and more diverged x-rays are used, the projection shows the distal radial carpal articular surface and the radiocarpal joint spaces are closed.

Proximal Forearm. The image analysis guidelines for the elbow on an AP forearm projection are slightly different from those of an AP elbow projection because of the difference in CR centering between the two projections. For the AP forearm projection, diverged x-rays record the elbow joint instead of straight x-rays, much the same as if the CR were angled toward the elbow joint. The AP elbow projection demonstrates an open elbow joint, whereas the AP forearm projection demonstrates the radial head projected into the elbow joint. The longer the patient's forearm is, the more the radial head will be projected proximally.

Positioning for Fracture

Distal Forearm. Patients with known or suspected fractures may be unable to position both the wrist and elbow joints into an AP projection simultaneously. In such cases, position the joint closer to the fracture in a true position. When the fracture is situated closer to the wrist joint, the wrist joint and distal forearm should meet the requirements for an AP projection, but the elbow and proximal forearm may demonstrate an AP oblique or lateral projection. It may be necessary to position the distal forearm in a PA projection when an AP projection is difficult for the patient (Figure 4-133).

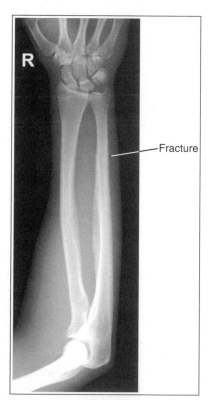

FIGURE 4-133 A forearm taken with the wrist in a PA projection and the elbow in a lateral projection, and demonstrating a distal forearm fracture.

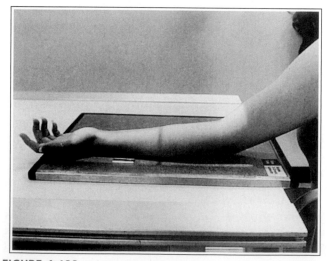

FIGURE 4-132 Patient positioned for AP forearm projection with flexed humerus.

Proximal Forearm. When the fracture is situated closer to the elbow joint, the elbow joint and proximal forearm should meet the requirements for an AP projection, whereas the wrist and distal forearm may demonstrate an AP oblique projection.

Including Wrist and Elbow. Position the forearm on the IR so at least half of the hand and all the elbow soft tissue remains on the IR. After centering the CR, longitudinally collimate until the collimator's light extends just beyond the wrist and elbow. Because the x-rays used to record the wrist and elbow are at an angle, the wrist and elbow will be projected more distally and proximally on the actual image, moving about 1 inch (2.5 cm) beyond where the collimator's light ends.

AP Forearm Analysis Practice

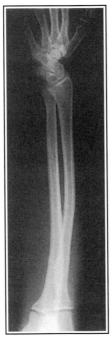

IMAGE 4-24

Analysis. The elbow has been accurately positioned. The first and second MC bases and the laterally located carpal bones are superimposed, and the medially located carpal bones and pisiform are well demonstrated. The wrist was internally rotated.

Correction. While maintaining the AP projection of the elbow, rotate the wrist and hand externally until the hand and wrist are in an AP projection.

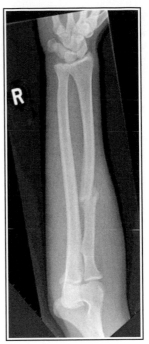

IMAGE 4-25

Analysis. The radial styloid is not demonstrated in profile, the laterally located first and second MC bases and the carpal bones are superimposed, and the medially located carpals are better demonstrated. The wrist was internally rotated. Less than one eighth of the radial head is superimposed over the ulna. The elbow was externally rotated.

Correction. Rotate the wrist and hand externally until they are in an AP projection, and rotate the elbow internally until the humeral epicondyles are parallel with the IR.

FOREARM: LATERAL PROJECTION (LATEROMEDIAL)

See Table 4-17, (Figures 4-134 and 4-135).

Soft Tissue Structures. Soft tissue structures of interest include the anterior and posterior fat pads and the supinator fat stripe at the elbow and pronator fat stripe at the wrist (see Figure 4-136). The elbow's anterior fat pad is situated anterior to the distal humerus, and the elbow's supinator fat stripe is visible parallel to the anterior aspect of the proximal radius. A change in the shape or placement of these fat structures indicates joint effusion and elbow injury. The elbow's posterior fat pad is normally obscured on a negative lateral forearm image because of its location within the olecranon fossa. On elbow injury, joint effusion pushes this pad out of the fossa, allowing it to be visualized proximally and posterior to the olecranon process. The wrist's pronator fat stripe is demonstrated parallel to the anterior surface of the distal radius. Bowing or obliteration of this fat stripe may be the only indication of subtle radial fractures.

TABLE 4-17	Lateral Forearm Projection	
Image Analysis Guidelines (Figure 4-134)	**Related Positioning Procedures (Figure 4-135)**
• Brightness is uniform across the forearm	• Center the forearm to the IR in a lateral projection, with the wrist placed at the anode end of the tube and the elbow at the cathode end.
• Anterior aspect of the distal scaphoid and the pisiform are aligned. • Distal radius and ulna are superimposed. • Radial tuberosity is not demonstrated in profile.	• Abduct the humerus and flex the elbow to 90 degrees, and then rest the ulnar side of the forearm against the IR, with the wrist placed at the anode end of the tube. • Center the forearm on the IR. • Externally rotate distal forearm until wrist is in a lateral projection.
• Ulnar styloid is demonstrated in profile posteriorly. • Elbow joint space is open. • Anterior aspects of the radial head and coronoid process are aligned.	• Position the humerus parallel with the IR.
• Forearm midpoint is at the center of the exposure field. • Wrist and elbow joints and forearm soft tissue are included within the exposure field.	• Center a perpendicular CR to the forearm midpoint. • Open the longitudinal collimation field to include the wrist and elbow. • Transversely collimate to within 0.5 inch (1.25 cm) of the skin line.

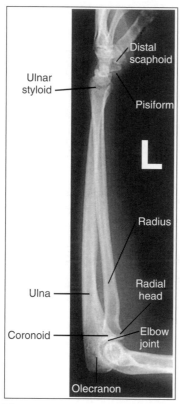

FIGURE 4-134 Lateral forearm projection with accurate positioning.

When the elbow is flexed 90 degrees, displacement of the anterior or posterior fat pads can be used as a sign to determine diagnosis. Poor elbow positioning, however, also displaces these fat pads and consequently simulates joint pathology. When the elbow is extended, nonpathologic displacement of the anterior and posterior fat pads may result from intraarticular pressure and the olecranon's position within the olecranon fossa.

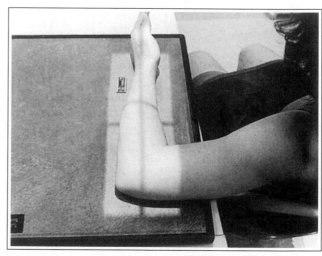

FIGURE 4-135 Proper patient positioning for lateral forearm projection.

Wrist and Distal Forearm Positioning

Radius and Ulna Alignment. On a lateral forearm projection with accurate wrist and distal forearm positioning, the distal radius and ulna are superimposed. If the wrist and distal forearm are internally rotated, the radius is visible anterior to the ulna (see Figure 4-137). If the wrist and distal forearm are externally rotated, the radius is visible posterior to the ulna.

Radial Tuberosity. Visibility of the radial tuberosity on a lateral forearm projection is determined by the position of the wrist, when the elbow is accurately positioned with the humeral epicondyles aligned perpendicular to the IR. When the wrist is placed in a lateral projection, the radial tuberosity is situated on the medial aspect of the radius and is superimposed by the radius, and is not demonstrated in profile (see Figure 4-134). If the wrist is externally rotated, the radial tuberosity is

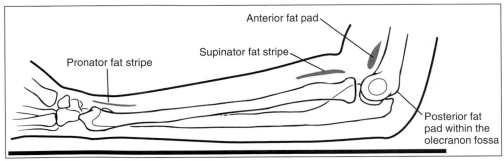

FIGURE 4-136 Placement of wrist and elbow soft tissue.

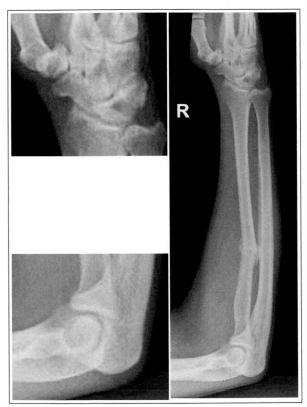

FIGURE 4-137 Lateral forearm projection taken with the wrist internally rotated.

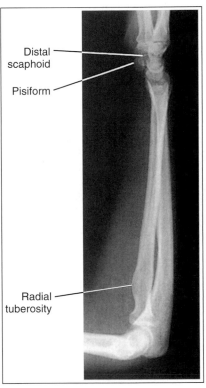

FIGURE 4-138 Lateral forearm projection taken with the wrist externally rotated.

demonstrated anteriorly (Figure 4-138), and if the wrist is internally rotated 40 degrees or more the radial tuberosity is seen posteriorly.

Humerus and Elbow Positioning. Accurate humeral positioning aligns the anterior aspects of the radial head and coronoid process. If the proximal humerus is elevated, the anterior aspect of the radial head is positioned posterior to the coronoid process and the proximal radius and ulna demonstrate increased superimposition (Figures 4-139 and 4-140). If the proximal humerus is depressed, the anterior aspect of the radial head is positioned anterior to the coronoid process.

CR Centering and Openness of Elbow Joint Space. To obtain an open elbow joint on a lateral elbow projection, the distal forearm is elevated as needed to align the humeral epicondyles perpendicular to the IR. This same alignment is not performed for the lateral forearm projection and yet in most cases the elbow joint will be demonstrated as an open space. This occurs because the CR is centered to the midforearm and the diverged x-rays used to image the elbow align parallel with the slant

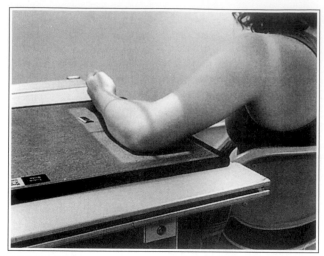

FIGURE 4-139 Lateral forearm projection taken with the proximal humerus elevated.

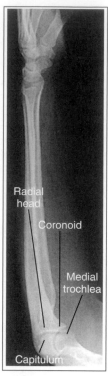

FIGURE 4-140 Lateral forearm projection taken with the proximal humerus elevated.

of the humeral epicondyles and the elbow joint space (Figure 4-141).

Effect of Muscular or Thick Forearm. Because the patient's forearm rests on its medial (ulnar) surface, the size of the proximal and distal forearm affects the appearance of the elbow joint space. For a patient with a muscular or thick proximal forearm, which is therefore elevated higher than the distal forearm, the radial head will be projected into the elbow joint spaces and the resulting projection demonstrates a closed elbow joint space (Figure 4-142).

Positioning for Fracture. Patients with known or suspected fractures may be unable to position both the wrist and elbow joint into a lateral projection simultaneously. In such cases, position the joint closer to the fracture in the true position (Figure 4-143).

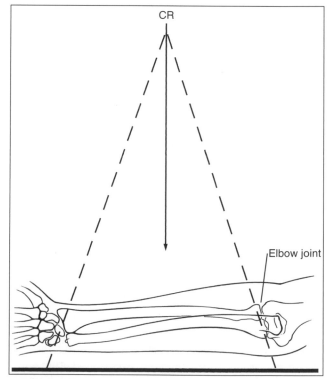

FIGURE 4-141 Alignment of x-ray divergence on distal forearm. *CR,* Central ray.

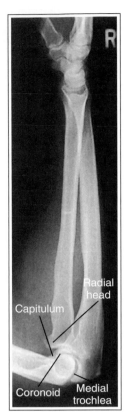

FIGURE 4-142 Lateral forearm projection taken on a patient with a muscular or thick proximal forearm.

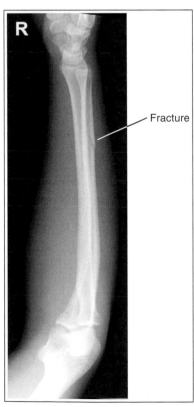

FIGURE 4-143 Lateral forearm projection taken with the wrist in a lateral projection and the elbow in an AP oblique projection, and demonstrating a distal forearm fracture.

Lateral Forearm Analysis Practice

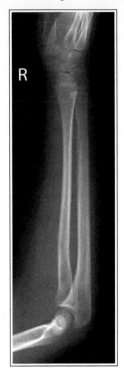

IMAGE 4-26

Analysis. The elbow is accurately positioned. The distal scaphoid is anterior to the pisiform and the radius is anterior to the ulna. The wrist and hand are internally rotated.

Correction. Externally rotate the wrist and hand until the wrist is in a lateral projection.

ELBOW: AP PROJECTION

See Table 4-18, (Figures 4-144 and 4-145).

Humeral Epicondyles and Radial Head and Ulna Relationship. Rotation of the elbow is a result of poor humeral epicondyle positioning and can be identified on an AP elbow projection when the epicondyles are not visualized in profile, and more or less than one eighth (0.25 inch [0.6 cm]) of the radial head superimposes the ulna. If the epicondyles are not demonstrated in profile, evaluate the degree of radial head superimposition of the ulna to determine how to reposition for an AP projection. If more than one eighth of radial head is superimposed over the ulna, the elbow has been medially (internally) rotated (Figure 4-146). If less than one eighth of the radial head is superimposed over the ulna, the elbow has been laterally (externally) rotated (Figures 4-147 and 4-148).

Radial Tuberosity. The alignment of the radius and ulna is determined by the position of the humerus and the wrist and hand. When the humerus is accurately positioned for an AP elbow projection, with the humeral epicondyles parallel with the IR, the radial tuberosity is

TABLE 4-18	AP Elbow Projection	
Image Analysis Guidelines (Figure 4-144)		**Positioning Procedures (Figure 4-145)**
• Medial and lateral humeral epicondyles are demonstrated in profile. • One eighth (0.25 inch) of the radial head superimposes the ulna.		• Center the elbow to the IR in an AP projection. • Align the humeral epicondyles parallel with the IR.
• Radial tuberosity is in profile medially. • Radius and ulna are parallel.		• Externally rotate the wrist to an AP projection.
• Elbow joint space is open. • Radial head articulating surface is not demonstrated. • Olecranon process is situated within the olecranon fossa.		• Fully extend the elbow.
• Elbow joint is at the center of the exposure field.		• Center a perpendicular CR to the midelbow joint located at a level 0.75 inch (2 cm) distal to the medial epicondyle.
• Elbow joint, one fourth of the proximal forearm and distal humerus, and the lateral soft tissue are included within the exposure field.		• Open the longitudinal collimation field to include one fourth of the proximal forearm and distal humerus. • Transversely collimate to within 0.5 inch (1.25 cm) of the skin line.

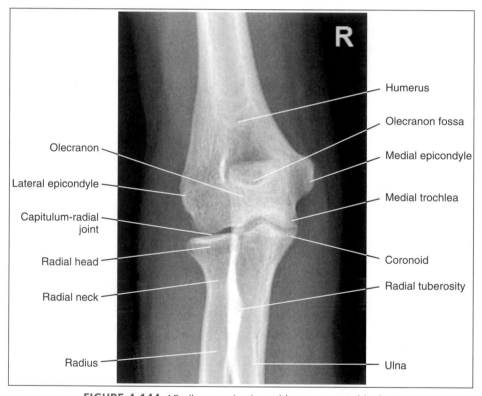

FIGURE 4-144 AP elbow projection with accurate positioning.

demonstrated in profile medially and the radius and ulna are aligned parallel with each other as long as the wrist is in an AP projection. If the wrist cannot be brought into an AP projection, the AP elbow projection will demonstrate varying radial and ulnar relationships and radial tuberosity visualizations. When the wrist has been internally rotated to a PA projection, the radius crosses over the ulna and the radial tuberosity is rotated posteriorly, out of profile (Figures 4-131 and 4-149).

Elbow Flexion. Flexion of the elbow joint distorts the elbow structures and draws the olecranon from the olecranon process on an AP projection (see Figure 4-148).

How a flexed elbow is positioned with respect to the IR determines which elbow structures are distorted. If the flexed elbow is obtained with the humerus placed parallel with the IR and the forearm elevated as demonstrated in Figure 4-150, the resulting projection demonstrates an undistorted distal humerus, whereas the proximal forearm is distorted, visualizing a closed elbow joint space and the radial head articulating surface imaged partially on end (Figure 4-151). If the flexed elbow is obtained with the forearm placed parallel with the IR and the humerus elevated as demonstrated in Figure 4-152, the resulting projection demonstrates an

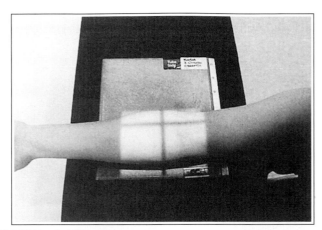

FIGURE 4-145 Proper patient positioning for AP elbow projection.

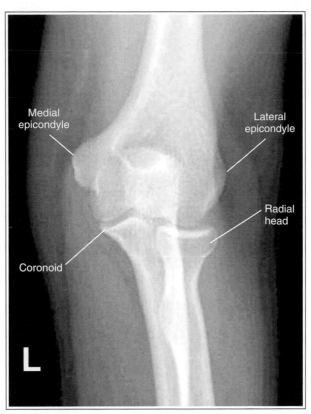

Medial epicondyle

Lateral epicondyle

Radial head

Coronoid

L

FIGURE 4-146 AP elbow projection taken with the elbow in slight internal rotation.

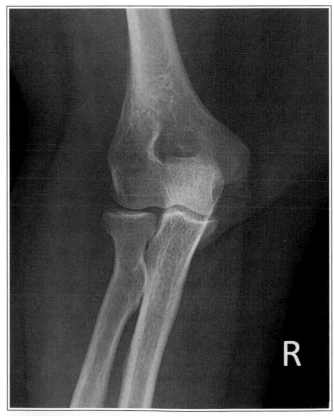

R

FIGURE 4-147 AP elbow projection taken with the elbow in external rotation.

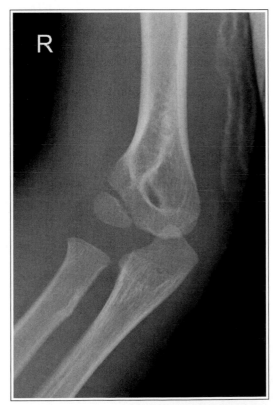

R

FIGURE 4-148 Pediatric AP elbow projection taken with the elbow in external rotation and slight flexion.

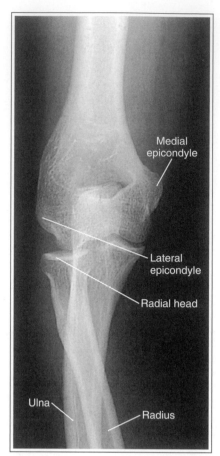

FIGURE 4-149 AP elbow projection taken with the hand and wrist pronated.

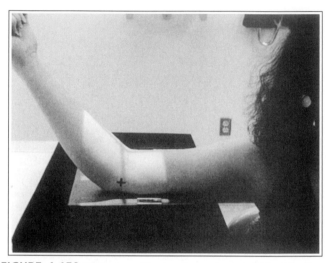

FIGURE 4-150 Patient positioning for nonextendable AP elbow projection—humerus parallel with IR.

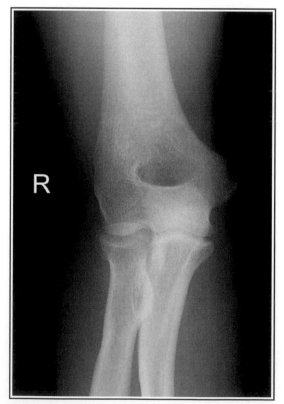

FIGURE 4-151 AP elbow projection taken with the humerus positioned parallel with the IR and the distal forearm elevated.

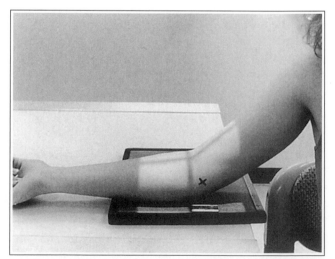

FIGURE 4-152 Patient positioning for nonextendable AP elbow projection—forearm parallel with IR.

undistorted proximal forearm and an open elbow joint space, and a foreshortened distal humerus (Figure 4-153). If a flexed elbow is resting on the posterior point of the olecranon, with the proximal humerus and the distal forearm elevated as shown in Figure 4-154, both the humerus and the forearm are foreshortened as described. The severity of the distortion increases with increased elbow flexion.

Positioning for the Flexed Elbow. An AP elbow projection that cannot be fully extended should be obtained using two separate exposures as demonstrated in Figures 4-152 and 4-154. When evaluating the projections for accuracy use only the image analysis guidelines that pertain to the part that was positioned parallel with the IR. The elbow joint space will be demonstrated as an open space only when the forearm is positioned parallel with the IR (see Figure 4-153).

CR Centering. To obtain the desired open elbow joint space along with the forearm being placed parallel with the IR as described, the CR also needs to be centered to the elbow joint. When the CR is centered proximal to the elbow joint space, the capitulum is projected into the joint and when the CR is centered distal to the elbow joint, the radial head is projected into the joint space (Figure 4-155). Poor CR placement also distorts the radial head, causing its articulating surface to be demonstrated. The degree of joint closure depends on how far the CR is positioned from the elbow joint, which determines how diverged the x-rays will be that record the elbow joint. The farther away from the joint the CR is centered, the more the elbow joint space is obscured and the more of the radial head articulating surface is demonstrated.

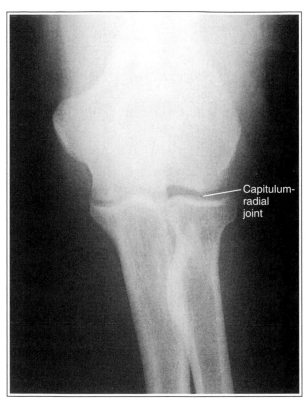

Capitulum-radial joint

FIGURE 4-153 AP elbow projection taken with the proximal humerus elevated and the forearm positioned parallel with the IR.

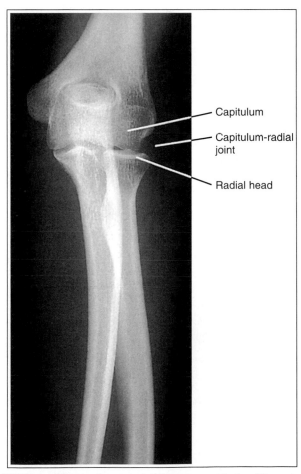

Capitulum

Capitulum-radial joint

Radial head

FIGURE 4-155 AP elbow projection taken with the CR centered distal to the joint space and demonstrating a closed elbow joint space.

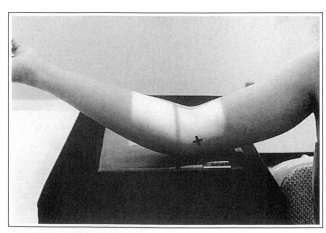

FIGURE 4-154 Proper nonextendable AP elbow positioning.

AP Elbow Analysis Practice

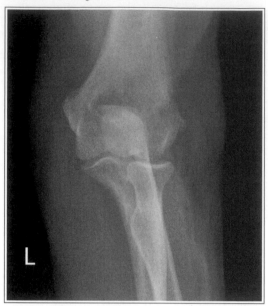

IMAGE 4-27

Analysis. The humeral epicondyles are not in profile and more than one eighth of the radial head is superimposed over the ulna. The elbow was medially rotated.
Correction. Rotate the elbow externally until the humeral epicondyles are parallel with the IR.

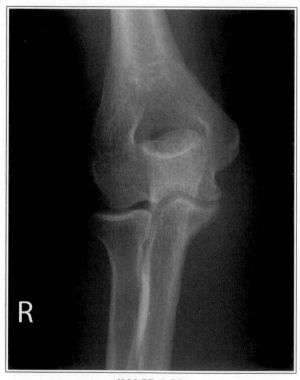

IMAGE 4-28

Analysis. The humeral epicondyles are not in profile and less than one eighth of the radial head is superimposing the ulna. The elbow was laterally rotated.
Correction. Rotate the elbow internally until the humeral epicondyles are parallel with the IR.

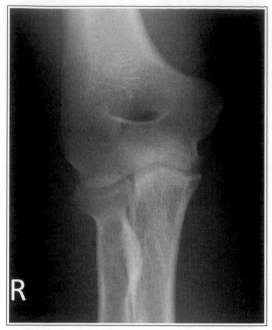

IMAGE 4-29

Analysis. The distal humerus is demonstrated without foreshortening, but the proximal forearm is severely distorted. If the humerus was positioned parallel with the IR, the distal forearm was elevated.
Correction. If possible, fully extend the elbow. If the patient is unable to extend the elbow, this is an acceptable projection of the distal humerus. A second AP projection of the elbow should be taken with the forearm positioned parallel with the IR.

ELBOW: AP OBLIQUE PROJECTIONS (MEDIAL AND LATERAL ROTATION)

See Table 4-19, (Figures 4-156, 4-157, 4-158, and 4-159).
Humeral Epicondyles

Medial Oblique (Internal Rotation). An accurately rotated AP medial oblique elbow projection demonstrates the coronoid process in profile and three fourths of the radial head superimposes over the ulna and is accomplished when the humeral epicondyles are placed at a 45-degree oblique with the IR. If the humeral epicondyles are at less than 45 degrees of obliquity, less than three fourths of the radial head superimposes the ulna (Figure 4-160). If the humeral epicondyles are at more than 45 degrees of obliquity, more than three fourths of the radial head superimposes the ulna (Figure 4-161).

Lateral Oblique (External Rotation). Accurate positioning for an AP lateral oblique elbow projection rotates the radius away from the ulna, demonstrating the ulna without radial superimposition and is accomplished when the humeral epicondyles are placed at a 45-degree oblique with the IR. If the humeral epicondyles are at less than 45 degrees of obliquity, the radial head and/or the radial tuberosity still partially superimpose the ulna

TABLE 4-19	AP Oblique Elbow Projection
Image Analysis Guidelines (Figures 4-156 and 4-157)	**Related Positioning Procedures (Figures 4-158 and 4-159)**

• Medial oblique:
  • Coronoid process, trochlear notch, and medial aspect of the trochlea are seen in profile.
  • Three fourths of the radial head superimposes the ulna.
• Lateral oblique:
  • Capitulum and radial head are seen in profile.
  • Ulna is demonstrated without radial head, neck, and tuberosity superimposition.
  • Radioulnar joint is open.
	• Center the elbow on the IR in an AP projection.
	• Medial oblique: Internally rotate the arm until the humeral epicondyles form a 45-degree angle with the IR.
	• Lateral oblique: Externally rotate the arm until the humeral epicondyles form a 45-degree angle with the IR.

• Medial oblique:
  • Trochlea-coronoid process joint is open.
  • Coronoid process articulating surface is not demonstrated.
• Lateral oblique:
  • Capitulum-radial head joint space is open.
  • Radial head articulating surface is not demonstrated.
	• Fully extend the elbow.

• Elbow joint is at the center of the exposure field. • Elbow joint, one fourth of the proximal forearm and distal humerus, and the lateral soft tissue are included within the exposure field.	• Center a perpendicular CR to the midelbow. • Open the longitudinal collimation field to include one fourth of the proximal forearm and distal humerus. • Transversely collimate to within 0.5 inch (1.25 cm) of the skin line.

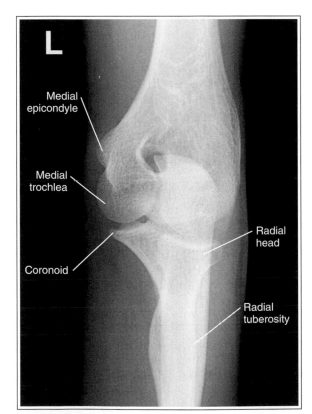

FIGURE 4-156 Internally rotated AP oblique elbow projection with accurate positioning.

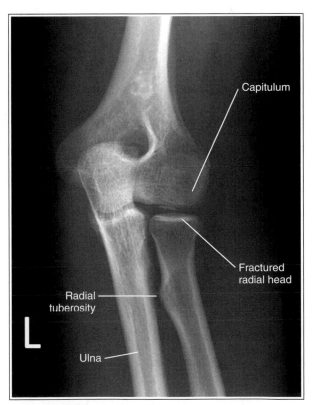

FIGURE 4-157 Externally rotated AP oblique elbow projection with accurate positioning.

(Figure 4-162). If the humeral epicondyles are at more than 45 degrees of obliquity, the coronoid process partially superimposes the radial head, the radial tuberosity and ulna demonstrate no superimposition, and the radial tuberosity is no longer in profile (Figure 4-163).

Elbow Flexion. Flexion of the elbow also distorts the AP oblique elbow projections. With elbow flexion, the olecranon process moves away from the olecranon fossa and the coronoid process shifts proximally. How the flexed elbow is positioned with respect to the IR

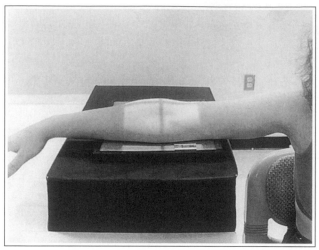

FIGURE 4-158 Proper patient positioning for internal AP oblique elbow projection.

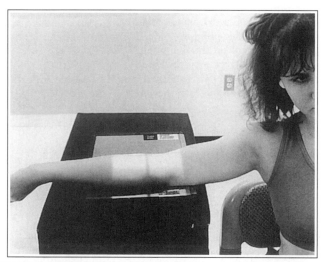

FIGURE 4-159 Proper patient positioning for external AP oblique elbow projection.

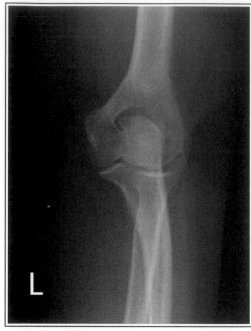

FIGURE 4-160 Internal AP oblique elbow projection taken with less than 45 degrees of elbow obliquity.

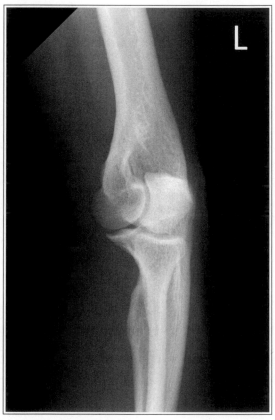

FIGURE 4-161 Internal AP oblique elbow projection taken with more than 45 degrees of elbow obliquity.

determines which elbow structures are distorted on the projection. If the flexed elbow is obtained with the humerus placed parallel with the IR and the distal forearm elevated, the projection shows an undistorted distal humerus, whereas the proximal forearm is foreshortened, visualizing closed capitulum-radial head (medial oblique) or trochlear-coronoid process (lateral oblique) joint spaces with the articulating surfaces of the radial head or trochlea visualized, respectively (Figure 4-164). If the forearm is positioned parallel with the IR and the proximal humerus is elevated, the projection shows an undistorted proximal forearm, an open capitulum-radial head (medial oblique) or trochlear-coronoid process (lateral oblique) joint space and a foreshortened distal humerus. If a flexed elbow is resting on the posterior point of the olecranon, with the proximal humerus and the distal forearm elevated, both the humerus and the forearm are foreshortened as described.

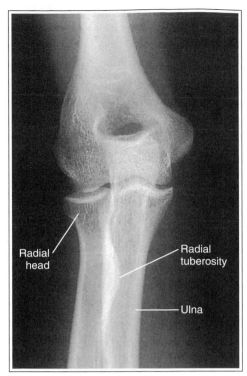

FIGURE 4-162 External AP oblique elbow projection taken with less than 45 degrees of elbow obliquity and the distal forearm slightly elevated.

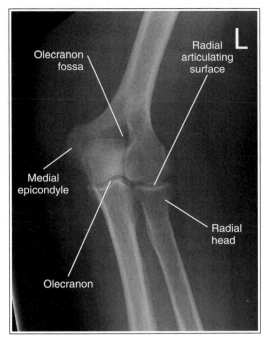

FIGURE 4-164 External AP oblique elbow projection taken with the distal forearm elevated.

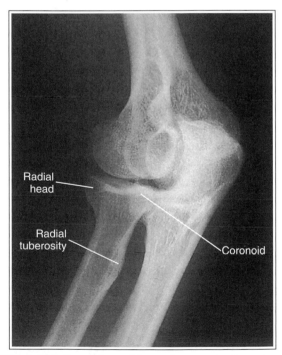

FIGURE 4-163 External AP oblique elbow projection taken with more than 45 degrees of elbow obliquity.

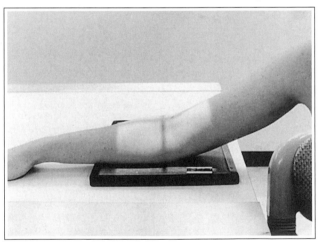

FIGURE 4-165 Proper patient positioning for AP oblique elbow projection with a flexed elbow.

The severity of the distortion increases with increased elbow flexion.

Positioning for the Flexed Elbow. For AP oblique elbow projections, if the patient's condition prevents full elbow extension, the anatomic structure (forearm or humerus) of greatest interest should be positioned parallel with the IR. This is discerned by obtaining a good patient history and looking at images obtained in the past of the same structure. If the radial head or coronoid process is of interest, position the forearm parallel with the IR (Figure 4-165). If the capitulum or medial trochlea is of interest, position the humerus parallel with the IR. When evaluating the projections, follow the image analysis guidelines that relate to the structure (forearm or humerus) that was positioned parallel with the IR to determine projection acceptability. The elevated forearm or humerus, respectively, will demonstrate distortion and will be of less value for diagnosis.

Elbow Joint Spaces

CR Centering. To obtain open capitulum-radial and trochlear-coronoid process joint spaces, the CR must also be centered to the joint spaces as well as the forearm positioned parallel with the IR. When the CR is centered proximal to the joint spaces, the structures of the distal humerus are projected into the joints, and when the CR is centered distal to the joint spaces, the structures of the proximal forearm are projected into the joint spaces. Poor CR positioning also distorts the radial head and coronoid process, causing their articulating surface to be visualized. The degree of joint closure and radial head and coronoid process distortion depends on how far the CR is positioned from the elbow joint. The farther away from the joint the CR is centered, the more the joint spaces will be obscured, and the more the articulating surfaces of the radial head and coronoid process will be demonstrated.

AP Oblique Elbow Analysis Practice

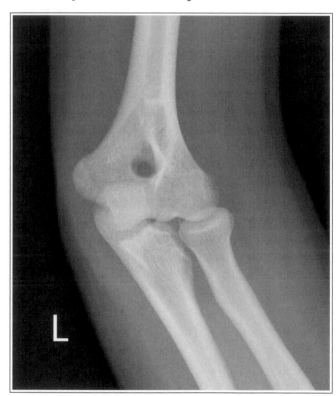

IMAGE 4-30 External rotation.

Analysis. The olecranon process is drawn slightly away from the olecranon fossa, the capitulum-radial joint space is closed, and the radial articulating surface is demonstrated. The forearm was not positioned parallel with the IR.

Correction. If possible, fully extend the elbow. If the patient is unable to fully extend the elbow and the radial head is of interest, position the forearm parallel with the IR and allow the proximal humerus to be elevated.

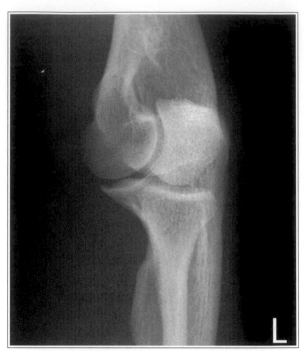

IMAGE 4-31 Internal rotation.

Analysis. The radial head is entirely superimposed on the ulna. Elbow obliquity was more than 45 degrees.

Correction. Decrease the degree of internal obliquity until the humeral epicondyles are angled at 45 degrees with the IR.

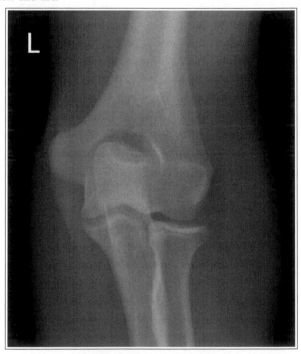

IMAGE 4-32 External rotation.

Analysis. The radial head and tuberosity are partially superimposed over the ulna. The degree of elbow obliquity was less than 45 degrees.

Correction. Increase the degree of external obliquity until the humeral epicondyles are angled at 45 degrees with IR.

TABLE 4-20	Lateral Elbow Projection	
Image Analysis Guidelines (Figure 4-166)	**Related Positioning Procedures (Figure 4-167)**	
• Anterior, posterior and supinator fat pads are demonstrated • Elbow is flexed 90 degrees.	• Correctly set the technical data. • Abduct the humerus and flex the elbow to 90 degrees. • Rest the ulnar side of the elbow against the IR. • Center the elbow to the IR.	

• Humerus demonstrates three concentric arcs, which are formed by the trochlear sulcus, capitulum, and medial trochlea.
 	
Humerus Positioning
• Distal surfaces of the capitulum and medial trochlea are nearly aligned.
• Anterior surfaces of the radial head and the coronoid process are aligned.
 	
Forearm Positioning
• Elbow joint is open.
• Anterior surfaces of the capitulum and medial trochlea are near aligned.
• Proximal surfaces of the radial head and the coronoid process are aligned.
	• Align the humeral epicondyles perpendicular to the IR.
	  • Humeral adjustments align the proximal and distal aspects of the humeral epicondyles.
	  • Distal forearm adjustments align the anterior and posterior aspects of the humeral epicondyles.	

• Radial tuberosity is not demonstrated in profile. • Elbow joint is at the center of the exposure field. • Elbow joint, one fourth of the proximal forearm and distal humerus, and the lateral soft tissue are included within the exposure field.	• Externally rotate the wrist and hand to a lateral projection. • Center a perpendicular CR to the midelbow. • Open the longitudinal collimation field to include one fourth of the proximal forearm and distal humerus. • Transversely collimate to within 0.5 inch (1.25 cm) of the skin line.	

ELBOW: LATERAL PROJECTION (LATEROMEDIAL)

See Table 4-20, (Figures 4-166 and 4-167).

Elbow Soft Tissue Structures. To evaluate a lateral elbow projection, the reviewer not only analyzes the bony structure, but also studies the placement of the soft tissue fat pads. Three fat pads of interest are present on a lateral elbow projection, the anterior and posterior fat pads and the supinator fat stripe. The anterior fat pad should routinely be seen on all lateral elbow projections when adequate exposure factors are used. This pad is formed by the superimposed coronoid process and radial pads and is situated immediately anterior to the distal humerus (Figure 4-168). A change in the shape or placement of the anterior fat pad may indicate joint effusion and elbow injury. The posterior fat pad is normally obscured on a negative lateral elbow projection because of its location within the olecranon fossa. When an injury occurs, joint effusion pushes this pad out of the fossa, allowing it to be visualized proximal and posterior to the olecranon fossa. The supinator fat stripe is visible parallel to the anterior aspect of the proximal radius (see Figure 4-168). Displacement of this fat stripe is useful for diagnosing fractures of the radial head and neck.

Elbow Flexion and Fat Pad Visualization. When the elbow is flexed 90 degrees, the forearm can be elevated to align the anatomic structures of the distal humerus properly, and displacement of the anterior and posterior fat pads can be used as signs to determine diagnosis.

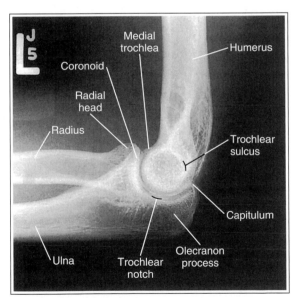

FIGURE 4-166 Lateral elbow projection with accurate positioning.

If the elbow is not adequately flexed, these fat pads can be displaced by poor positioning instead of joint pathology, interfering with their diagnostic usefulness. When the arm is extended, nonpathologic displacement of the anterior fat pad results from intraarticular pressure placed on the joint. Nonpathologic displacement of the posterior fat pad is a result of positioning of

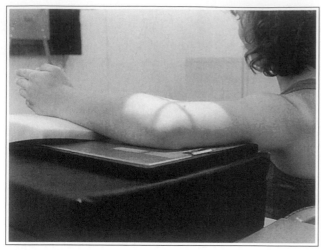

FIGURE 4-167 Proper patient positioning for lateral elbow projection.

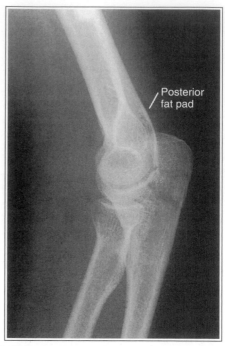

FIGURE 4-169 Lateral elbow projection taken with the elbow extended and the hand and wrist pronated.

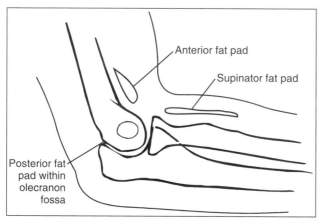

FIGURE 4-168 Locations of fat pads on lateral elbow projection. *(From Martensen K III: The elbow,* In-Service Reviews in Radiologic Technology, *14[11], 1992.)*

the olecranon within the olecranon fossa, which causes proximal and posterior displacement of the pad (Figure 4-169).

Humeral Epicondyles. A lateral elbow projection is obtained when the proximal humerus and distal forearm are positioned so the humeral epicondyles are situated directly on top of each other, placing an imaginary line drawn between them perpendicular to the IR. This positioning aligns the trochlear sulcus, capitulum, and medial trochlea into three concentric (having the same center) arcs (Figure 4-170). The trochlear sulcus is the small center arc. It moves very little when a positional change is made and works like a pivoting point between the capitulum and medial aspect of the trochlea. The largest of the arcs is the medial aspect of the trochlea. It is demonstrated very close to and slightly superimposed on the curve of the trochlear notch. The intermediate-sized arc is the capitulum. When these three arcs are in accurate alignment, the elbow joint is visualized as an open

space and the anterior and proximal surfaces of the radial head and coronoid process are aligned.

Proximal humerus positioning (elevation and depression) determines the alignment of the distal surfaces of the capitulum and medial trochlea, and the anterior alignment of the radial head and coronoid process, whereas distal forearm positioning (depression and elevation) determines the anterior alignment of the capitulum and medial trochlea and the proximal alignment of the radial head and coronoid process. Carefully evaluate projections that show poor positioning, as both forearm and humeral corrections may be needed to obtain accurate positioning.

Proximal Humerus Mispositioning. If the proximal humerus is elevated (Figure 4-171), the distal capitulum surface is demonstrated too far distal to the distal surface of the medial trochlea and the radial head is placed too far posteriorly to the coronoid process (Figure 4-172). If the proximal humerus is depressed (positioned lower than the distal humerus) (Figure 4-173), the distal capitulum surface is demonstrated too far proximal to the distal medial trochlear surface and the radial head is positioned too far anteriorly to the coronoid process (Figures 4-174 and 4-175).

Distal Forearm Mispositioniong. When the distal forearm is positioned too close to the IR (depressed) (Figure 4-176), the projection shows the capitulum too far anteriorly to the medial trochlea and the radial head distally to the coronoid process (Figures 4-177 and 4-178). When the distal forearm is positioned too far

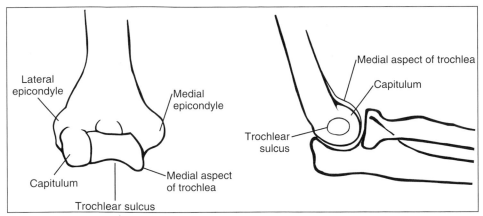

FIGURE 4-170 AP (*left*) and lateral (*right*) projections showing anatomy of the distal humerus. *(From Martensen K III: The elbow, In-Service Reviews in Radiologic Technology, 14[11], 1992.)*

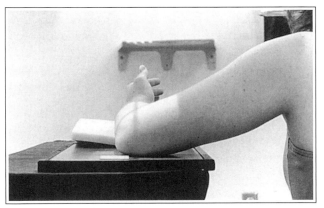

FIGURE 4-171 Patient positioned for lateral elbow projection with elevated proximal humerus.

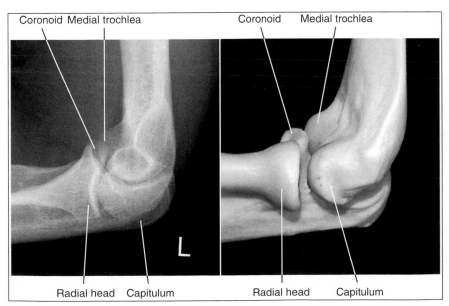

FIGURE 4-172 Lateral elbow projection taken with the proximal humerus elevated.

from the IR (elevated) (Figure 4-179), the projection shows the capitulum too far posteriorly to the medial trochlea and the radial head proximally to the coronoid process (Figure 4-180).

Radial Tuberosity. Visibility of the radial tuberosity on the lateral projection is determined by the position of the wrist. When the wrist is placed in a lateral projection, the radial tuberosity is not demonstrated on the projection as it is situated on the medial aspect of the radius and is superimposed by the radius. When the wrist is externally rotated, the radial tuberosity is rotated to the anterior arm surface and is demonstrated in profile anteriorly (Figure 4-181). Internal wrist rotation rotates the radial tuberosity to the posterior arm surface and demonstrates it posteriorly (Figure 4-182).

Positioning for Radial Head Fractures. Lateral elbow projections taken with the wrist in different projections

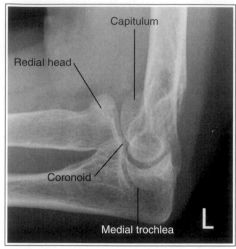

FIGURE 4-175 Lateral elbow projection taken with the proximal humerus and distal forearm depressed.

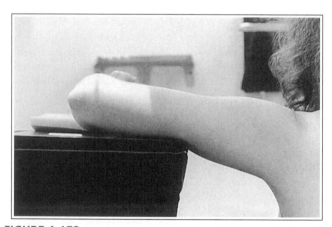

FIGURE 4-173 Patient positioned for lateral elbow projection with depressed proximal humerus.

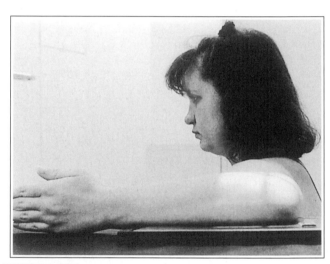

FIGURE 4-176 Patient positioned for lateral elbow projection with depressed distal forearm.

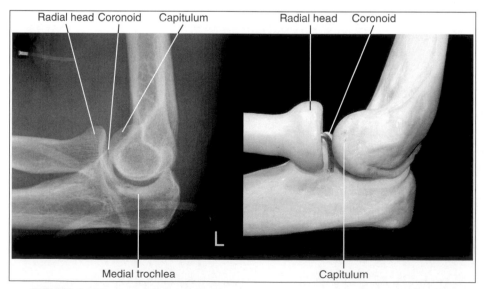

FIGURE 4-174 Lateral elbow projection taken with the proximal humerus depressed.

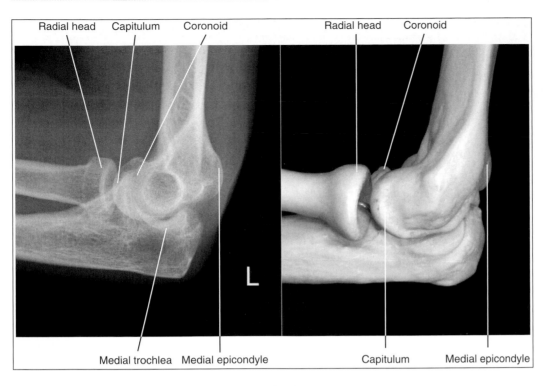

Radial head   Capitulum   Coronoid

Radial head   Coronoid

L

Medial trochlea   Medial epicondyle

Capitulum   Medial epicondyle

FIGURE 4-177 Lateral elbow projection taken with the distal forearm depressed.

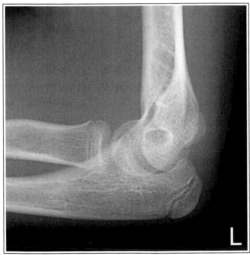

L

FIGURE 4-178 Pediatric lateral elbow projection taken with the distal forearm depressed.

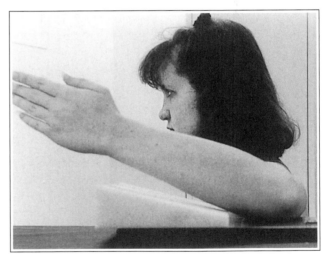

FIGURE 4-179 Patient positioned for lateral elbow projection with elevated distal forearm.

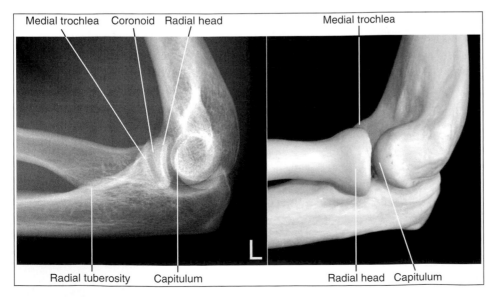

Medial trochlea   Coronoid   Radial head

Medial trochlea

L

Radial tuberosity   Capitulum

Radial head   Capitulum

FIGURE 4-180 Lateral elbow projection taken with the distal forearm positioned too far away from the IR and the wrist internally rotated.

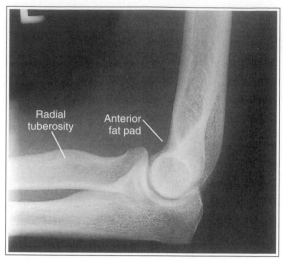

FIGURE 4-181 Lateral elbow projection taken with the wrist externally rotated.

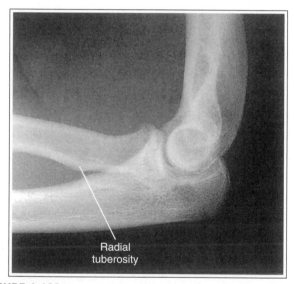

FIGURE 4-182 Lateral elbow projection taken with the wrist internally rotated.

(AP oblique, lateral, PA oblique, and PA) are often obtained to study the circumference of the radial head and neck for fractures; they are referred to as *radial head projections*. These projections are evaluated using the same lateral elbow guidelines listed in the preceding with the exception of the placement of the radial tuberosity, which will change with wrist rotation as indicated.

Lateral Elbow Analysis Practice

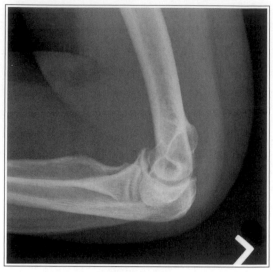

IMAGE 4-33

Analysis. The radial head is positioned too far posteriorly on the coronoid process and the distal surface of the capitulum is demonstrated too far distally to the distal surface of the medial trochlea. The proximal humerus was elevated.

Correction. Lower the proximal humerus until the humeral epicondyles are superimposed and the humerus is positioned parallel with the IR.

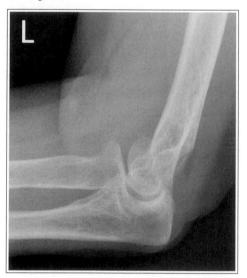

IMAGE 4-34

Analysis. The radial head is positioned anterior to the coronoid process, and the capitulum is too far proximal to the medial trochlea. The proximal humerus was depressed.

Correction. Elevate the proximal humerus until the humeral epicondyles are superimposed and the humerus is positioned parallel with the IR.

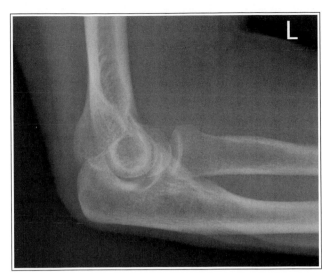

IMAGE 4-35

Analysis. The radial head is distal to the coronoid process, and the capitulum is too far anteriorly to the medial trochlea. The patient was placed with the distal forearm positioned too close to the IR.

Correction. Elevate the distal forearm until the humeral epicondyles are superimposed.

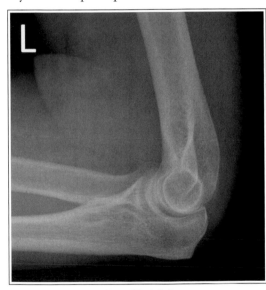

IMAGE 4-36

Analysis. The radial head is proximal to the coronoid process and the capitulum is too far posteriorly to the medial trochlea. The patient was positioned with the distal forearm placed too far away from the IR.

Correction. Lower the distal forearm until the humeral epicondyles are superimposed.

ELBOW: AXIOLATERAL ELBOW PROJECTION (COYLE METHOD)

See Table 4-21, (Figures 4-183 and 4-184).

The radial axiolateral elbow projection is a special projection taken when a fracture of the radial head or capitulum is suspected.

TABLE 4-21	Axiolateral Elbow Projection
Image Analysis Guidelines (Figure 4-183)	**Related Positioning Procedures (Figure 4-184)**
• Elbow is flexed 90 degrees	• Abduct the humerus and flex the elbow to 90 degrees. • Rest the ulnar side of the elbow against the IR. • Center the elbow to the IR.

Humerus Position
• Capitulum is proximal to the medial trochlea, demonstrating no superimposition.
• Radial head superimposes only the anterior tip of the coronoid process.
Forearm Position
• Elbow joint is open.
• Anterior surfaces of the capitulum and medial trochlea are nearly aligned.
• Proximal surfaces of the radial head and coronoid process are aligned.
	• Align the humeral epicondyles perpendicular to the IR.
	  • Humeral adjustments align the proximal and distal aspects of the humeral epicondyles.
	  • Distal forearm adjustments align the anterior and posterior aspects of the humeral epicondyles.
	• Angle the CR 45 degrees proximally.

Lateral Wrist • The anterior and posterior surfaces of the radial head are seen in profile. **PA Wrist** • The medial and lateral surfaces of the radial head are seen in profile.	• Position the wrist and hand in a lateral or PA projection to demonstrate the radial head surfaces of interest.
• The radial head is at the center of the exposure field.	• Center the CR to the midelbow.
• One fourth of the proximal forearm and distal humerus and the lateral soft tissue are included within the exposure field.	• Open the longitudinal collimation field to include one fourth of the proximal forearm and distal humerus. • Transversely collimate to within 0.5 inch (1.25 cm) of the skin line.

Humerus and CR Angulation. To project the capitulum proximal to the medial trochlea and the radial head anterior to the coronoid process on an axiolateral elbow projection, the elbow is placed in a lateral projection and a 45-degree proximal (toward the shoulder) angle is placed on the CR (see Figure 4-184). This combination of positioning and angulation projects the anatomic structures (radial head and capitulum) situated farther from the IR proximal to those structures (coronoid process and medial trochlea) situated closer to the IR.

If the CR is angled accurately but the proximal humerus is depressed lower than the distal humerus,

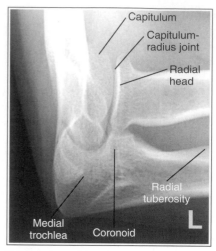

FIGURE 4-183 Axiolateral (Coyle method) elbow projection with accurate positioning.

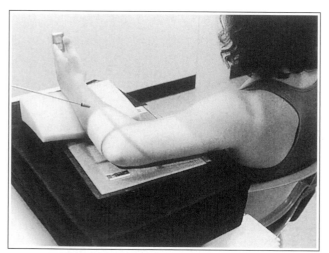

FIGURE 4-184 Proper patient positioning for axiolateral (Coyle method) elbow projection.

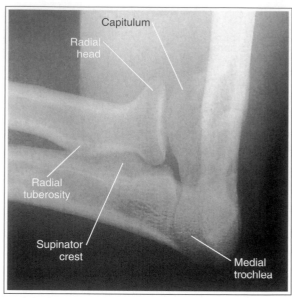

FIGURE 4-185 Axiolateral elbow projection taken with the proximal humerus depressed and the radial tuberosity demonstrated in partial profile, indicating that the wrist was in a PA oblique projection.

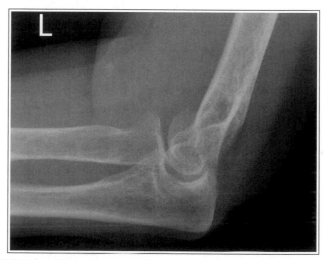

FIGURE 4-186 Axiolateral elbow projection taken with the proximal humerus elevated.

the cortices of the medial trochlea and capitulum are not clearly defined, the coronoid process is free of radial head superimposition, and the proximal radius superimposes the ulnar supinator crest (a sharp, prominent ridge running along the lateral margin of the ulna that divides the ulna's anterior and posterior surfaces; Figure 4-185). The same projection can also result if the patient is accurately positioned but the CR is angled more than 45 degrees. If the CR is accurately angled but the proximal humerus is elevated, the medial trochlea demonstrates some capitular superimposition and the radial head superimposes over more than the tip of the coronoid process (Figure 4-186). The same projection can result if the patient is accurately positioned but the CR is angled less than 45 degrees.

Elbow Flexion and CR Alignment. With 90 degrees of elbow flexion, the 45-degree CR angle and proper CR alignment with the elbow accurately causes the capitulum to move proximally and the radial head to move anteriorly. If more or less than 90 degrees of elbow flexion is used, the CR traverses the distal humerus, proximal forearm, or both at an alignment that will not move the capitulum and/or radiation head in the desired direction. A projection obtained with more than 90 degrees of elbow flexion and the CR aligned accurately with the proximal forearm, but poorly with the distal humerus, will accurately project the radial head anterior to the coronoid process, but it will also project it into the distal humerus, obscuring its visualization (Figure 4-187).

Forearm. The openness of the elbow joint space, the anterior alignment of the capitulum and medial trochlea, and the proximal alignment of the radial head and coronoid process are affected when the distal forearm is

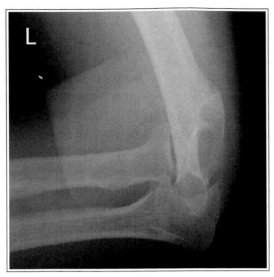

FIGURE 4-187 Axiolateral elbow projection taken with the elbow flexed more than 90 degrees.

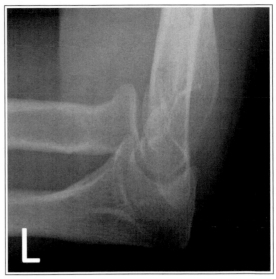

FIGURE 4-189 Axiolateral elbow projection taken with the distal forearm positioned too far away from the IR and the wrist in a lateral projection.

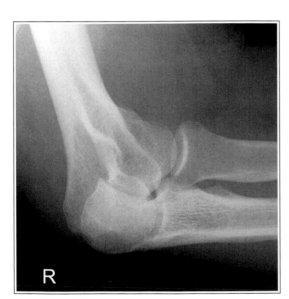

FIGURE 4-188 Axiolateral elbow projection taken with the distal forearm depressed and the wrist placed in a lateral projection.

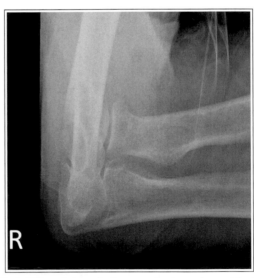

FIGURE 4-190 Axiolateral elbow projection taken with the wrist in a PA projection and demonstrating the radial tuberosity and medial aspect of the radial head in profile.

positioned. If the distal forearm is positioned too close to the IR (depressed), the projection shows a closed elbow joint space and shows the capitulum too far anterior to the medial trochlea and the radial head distal to the coronoid process (Figure 4-188). If the distal forearm is positioned too far away from the IR (elevated), the projection shows the capitulum too far posterior to the medial trochlea and the radial head proximal to the coronoid process (Figure 4-189).

Wrist and Hand. As with the lateral projection, the position of the wrist determines which surfaces of the radial head are placed in profile, but it is different than discussed for the lateral projection because of the

45-degree CR angle that is used for the axiolateral projection. If the patient's wrist is in an AP projection, the radial tuberosity and medial aspect of the radial head are demonstrated in profile on the posterior arm surface and the lateral aspect of the radial head appears in profile on the anterior arm surface (Figure 4-190). If the wrist is in a lateral projection, the radial tuberosity is not demonstrated in profile but is superimposed by the radius. In this position, the anterior aspect of the radial head is demonstrated in profile on the anterior arm surface and the posterior aspect of the radial head is demonstrated in profile on the posterior arm surface (Figures 4-188 and 4-189).

Axiolateral Elbow (Coyle Method) Analysis Practice

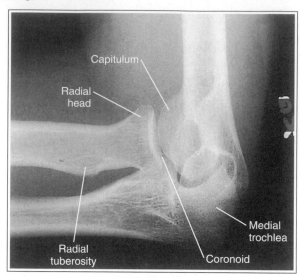

IMAGE 4-37

Analysis. The capitulum-radius joint space is closed, the radial head is demonstrated distal to the coronoid process, and the capitulum is demonstrated too far anterior to the medial trochlea. The distal forearm was depressed. The radial head is superimposed over more than just the tip of the coronoid process, and the medial trochlea and capitulum demonstrate slight superimposition. The proximal humerus was elevated. The lateral and medial surfaces of the radial head are in profile. The wrist was placed in a PA projection.

Correction. Elevate the distal forearm and depress the proximal humerus until the humeral epicondyles are aligned perpendicular to the IR.

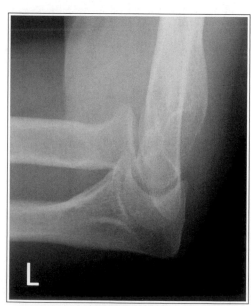

IMAGE 4-38

Analysis. The radial head is superimposed over more than just the tip of the coronoid process, and the medial

trochlea and capitulum demonstrate slight superimposition. The proximal humerus was elevated. The radial head is demonstrated proximal to the coronoid process and the capitulum is demonstrated too far posterior to the medial trochlea. The distal forearm was elevated. The anterior and posterior surfaces of the radial head are demonstrated. The wrist was placed in a lateral projection.

Correction. Depress the proximal humerus and the distal forearm until the humeral epicondyles are aligned perpendicular to the IR.

HUMERUS: AP PROJECTION

See Table 4-22, (Figures 4-191, 4-192, and 4-193).
Humeral Epicondyles. Rotation of the humerus is a result of poor humeral epicondyle positioning. When the humeral epicondyles and the greater tuberosity are not

TABLE 4-22	AP Humerus Projection	
Image Analysis Guidelines (Figures 4-191 and 4-192)	**Related Positioning Procedures (Figure 4-193)**
• There is uniform brightness across the humerus.	• Position the elbow at the anode end of tube and the wrist at the cathode end.
Distal Humerus • Medial and lateral humeral epicondyles are demonstrated in profile. • One eighth of the radial head superimposes the ulna (about 0.25 inch [0.6 cm]). **Proximal Humerus** • Greater tubercle is demonstrated in profile laterally. • Humeral head is demonstrated in profile medially. • Vertical cortical margin of the lesser tubercle is visible about halfway between the greater tubercle and the humeral head.	• Position patient in a supine or upright AP projection with the affected arm extended and centered to IR. • Supinate the hand and wrist, and externally rotate the arm until the humeral epicondyles are aligned parallel with the IR.
• Humeral midpoint is at the center of the exposure field.	• Center a perpendicular CR to the humeral midpoint, IR, and grid.
• Shoulder and elbow joints and the lateral humeral soft tissue are included within the exposure field.	• Open the longitudinal collimation field until it extends 1 inch (2.5 cm) beyond the elbow and shoulder joints. • Transversely collimate to within 0.5 inch (1.25 cm) of the skin line laterally and the coracoid medially.

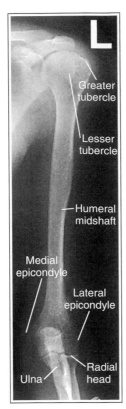

FIGURE 4-191 AP humerus projection with accurate positioning.

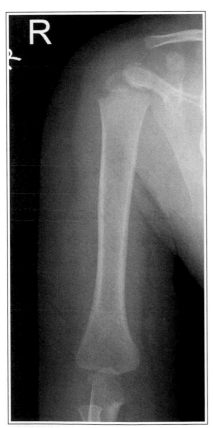

FIGURE 4-192 Pediatric AP humerus projection with accurate positioning.

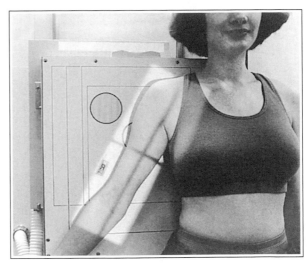

FIGURE 4-193 Proper patient positioning for AP humerus projection—collimator head rotated.

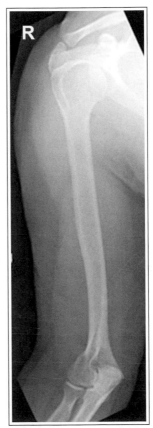

FIGURE 4-194 AP humerus projection taken with the arm externally rotated.

demonstrated in profile, measure the amount of radial head superimposition on the ulna to determine how the patient should be repositioned. If less than one eighth of the radial head superimposes the ulna, the humerus has been externally rotated more than needed to obtain an AP projection (Figure 4-194). If more than one eighth of the radial head superimposes the ulna, the humerus has not been externally rotated enough to bring the humeral epicondyles parallel with the IR (Figure 4-195).

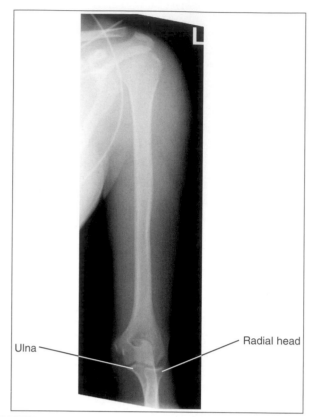

FIGURE 4-195 AP humerus projection taken with the arm internally rotated.

Ulna — Radial head

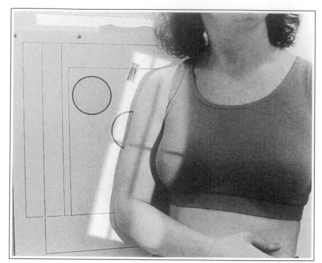

FIGURE 4-196 Patient positioning for AP humerus projection when fracture is located close to shoulder.

Positioning for Humeral Fracture. When a fracture of the humerus is suspected or a follow-up projection is being taken to assess healing of a humeral fracture, the patient's arm should not be externally rotated to obtain the AP projection because external rotation of the arm increases the risk of radial nerve damage. For such an examination, the joint closer to the fracture should be aligned in the true AP projection. If the fracture site is situated closer to the shoulder joint and the arm cannot be externally rotated, the greater tuberosity is placed in profile by rotating the patient's body toward the affected humerus 35 to 40 degrees (Figure 4-196). Depending on the amount of humeral rotation at the fracture site, the proximal and the distal humerus may or may not be an AP projection at the same time (Figure 4-197). If the fracture is situated closer to the elbow joint, extend the arm and rotate the patient's body toward the affected humerus until the humeral epicondyles are aligned parallel with the IR. Depending on the amount of humeral rotation at the fracture site, the greater tubercle may or may not be in profile.

Field Size and Collimation. The collimated field should extend at least 1 inch (2.5 cm) beyond each joint space to ensure that the joints are included in the exposure field. The elbow is located approximately 0.75 inch (2 cm) proximal to the medial epicondyle. The shoulder joint is located at the same level as the palpable coracoid.

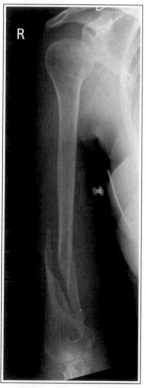

FIGURE 4-197 AP humerus projection demonstrating a fractured humerus.

For a patient with a long humerus, it may be necessary to position the humerus somewhat diagonally on the IR to obtain the needed IR length. For the computed radiography system, it is not advisable to position the part diagonally unless the system is set to handle this alignment. If using the DR system for this positioning, the collimator head can be turned or rotated to align the long axis of the collimated light field with the long axis of the humerus to allow for tight collimation.

HUMERUS: LATERAL PROJECTION (LATEROMEDIAL AND MEDIOLATERAL)

See Table 4-23, (Figures 4-198, 4-199, 4-200, and 4-201). **Mediolateral versus Lateromedial Projections.** The alignment of the distal surfaces of the capitulum and medial trochlea varies depending on the method used to obtain the projection. Two methods can be used to position the patient for a lateral humerus projection,

mediolateral and lateromedial. The first method positions the patient's body in an upright PA projection, with the arm internally rotated until the humeral epicondyles are perpendicular to the IR; this is termed a *mediolateral projection* (see Figure 4-200). In this position it is important that the body maintains a PA projection. Do not allow the patient to rotate the body toward the affected humerus instead. Such body obliquity causes an increase in tissue thickness at the proximal humerus compared

TABLE 4-23	Lateral Humerus Projection	
Image Analysis Guidelines (Figures 4-198 and 4-199)	**Related Positioning Procedures (Figures 4-200 and 4-201)**
• Gray shades are uniform across the humerus.	• Position the elbow at the anode end of tube.
Proximal Humerus	• Position patient in a supine or upright AP or PA projection with the affected humerus centered to the IR.
• Lesser tubercle is demonstrated in profile medially.	• Flex the elbow and supinate the hand.
• Humeral head and greater tubercle are superimposed.	• Internally rotate the arm until humeral epicondyles are aligned perpendicular to IR.
Distal Humerus	
• Anterior surfaces of the capitulum and medial trochlea are nearly aligned.	
• Humeral midpoint is at the center of the exposure field.	• Center a perpendicular CR to the humeral midpoint, IR and grid.
• Shoulder and elbow joints and the lateral humeral soft tissue are included within the exposure field.	• Open the longitudinal collimation field until it extends 1 inch (2.5 cm) beyond the elbow and shoulder joints.
	• Transversely collimate to within 0.5 inch (1.25 cm) of the skin line laterally and the coracoid medially.

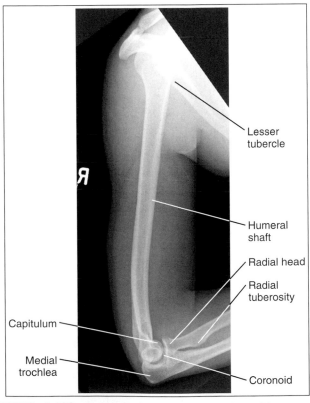

FIGURE 4-198 Mediolateral humerus projection with accurate positioning.

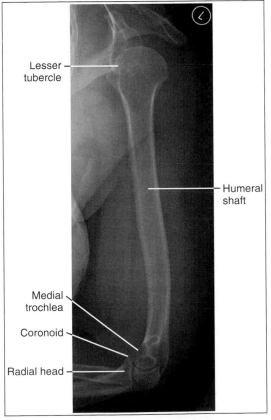

FIGURE 4-199 Lateromedial humerus projection with accurate positioning.

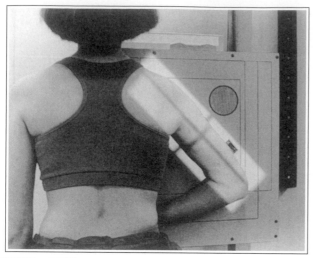

FIGURE 4-200 Proper patient positioning for mediolateral humerus projection.

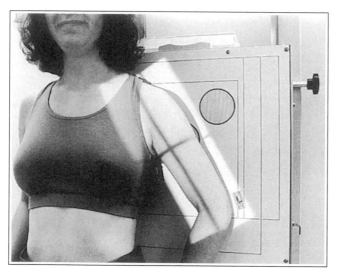

FIGURE 4-201 Proper patient positioning for lateromedial humerus projection.

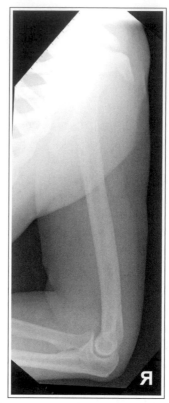

FIGURE 4-202 Mediolateral humerus projection taken with the torso rotated toward the humerus, increasing the tissue thickness at the proximal humerus.

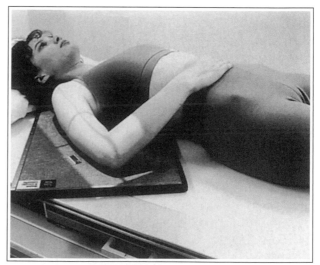

FIGURE 4-203 Patient positioned for lateromedial humerus projection with poor distal humerus alignment.

with the distal humerus, because the shoulder tissue is superimposed over the proximal humerus (Figure 4-202), resulting in lower contrast resolution in this area.

The second method positions the patient's body in an AP projection, with the arm internally rotated until the humeral epicondyles are perpendicular to the IR; this is termed a *lateromedial projection* (see Figure 4-201). If the patient's forearm is positioned across the body in an attempt to flex the elbow 90 degrees and the distal humerus is not brought away from the IR enough to position the humeral epicondyles perpendicular to the IR (Figure 4-203), the projection demonstrates the capitulum posterior to the medial trochlea, a distorted proximal forearm, and the lesser tubercle in partial profile (Figure 4-204).

The difference in the anatomic relationships of the distal humerus between the mediolateral and lateromedial projections is a result of x-ray beam divergence. For

a lateral humerus projection, the CR is centered to the midhumeral shaft, which is located approximately 5 inches (13 cm) from the elbow joint. Because the elbow joint is placed so far away from the CR, diverged x-ray beams are used to image the elbow joint. This causes the anatomic structures positioned farthest from the IR to be diverged more distally than the anatomic structures positioned closest to the IR. In the mediolateral

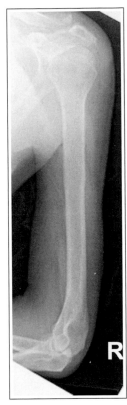

FIGURE 4-204 Lateromedial humerus projection taken with insufficient internal rotation to position the humeral epicondyles perpendicular to the IR.

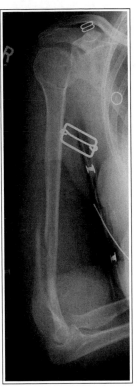

FIGURE 4-205 Lateral humerus projection demonstrating a fractured humerus.

projection, the medial trochlea is placed farther from the IR than the capitulum. Consequently x-ray beam divergence will project the medial trochlea distal to the capitulum. In the lateromedial projection the capitulum is situated farther from the IR; therefore the x-ray beam divergence will project it distally to the medial trochlea.

Positioning for Humeral Fracture. When a fracture of the humerus is suspected or a follow-up projection is being taken to assess healing of a fracture, the patient's forearm or humerus should not be rotated to obtain a lateral projection. Rotation of the forearm and humerus would increase the risk of radial nerve damage and displacement of the fracture fragments space (Figure 4-205). Because the forearm should not be rotated for a trauma examination, a lateral projection of the proximal and distal humerus must be obtained by positioning the patient differently.

Distal Humeral Fracture. Obtain a lateral distal humerus projection by gently sliding an IR between the patient and the distal humerus. Adjust the IR until the epicondyles are positioned perpendicularly to the IR. Place a flat contact protecting shield between the patient and the IR to absorb any radiation that would penetrate the IR and expose the patient. Finally center the CR perpendicularly to the IR and distal humerus (Figure 4-206). This positioning should demonstrate a true

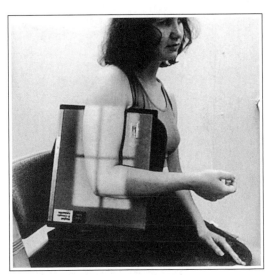

FIGURE 4-206 Proper patient positioning for distal humerus fracture.

lateral projection of the distal humerus with superimposition of the epicondyles and of the radial head and coronoid process (Figure 4-207).

Proximal Humeral Fracture. A lateral projection can be achieved by positioning the patient in one of two ways when a proximal humeral fracture is suspected. The first method is best done with the patient in the scapular Y, PA axial projection. For this projection, begin by placing the patient in a PA upright projection

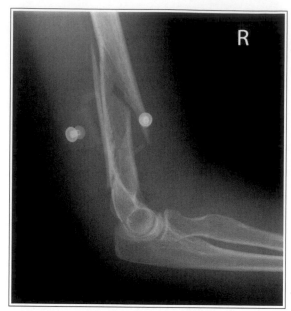

FIGURE 4-207 Lateral distal humerus projection demonstrating a fractured distal humerus.

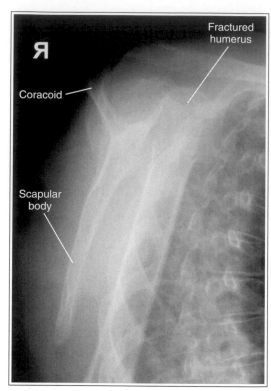

FIGURE 4-209 Accurately positioned AP oblique (scapular Y) shoulder projection demonstrating a fractured proximal humerus.

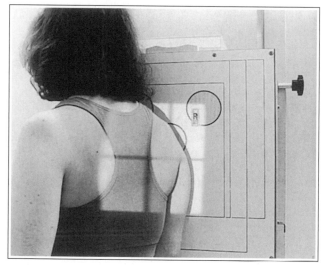

FIGURE 4-208 Proper scapular Y, PA oblique projection positioning of patient for proximal humerus fracture.

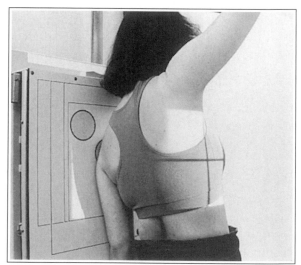

FIGURE 4-210 Proper transthoracic lateral positioning of patient for proximal humerus fracture.

with the humerus positioned as is, and then rotate the patient toward the affected humerus (≈45 degrees) until the scapular body is in a lateral projection (Figures 4-208 and 4-209). Precise positioning and evaluating points for this projection can be studied by referring to the discussion of the scapular Y, PA axial projection in Chapter 5.

Alternate Transthoracic Lateral Humerus Projection. The second method of obtaining a lateral projection of the fractured proximal humerus can be accomplished with the transthoracic lateral projection (Figure 4-210). The patient's body is placed in a lateral position with the affected humerus resting against the grid IR, and the unaffected arm is raised above the patient's head. To prevent superimposition of the shoulders on the projection, either (1) elevate the unaffected shoulder by tilting the upper midsagittal plane toward the IR and using a horizontal CR, or (2) position the shoulders on the same transverse plane and angle the CR 10 to 15 degrees cephalically. Then, direct the CR to the midthorax at the level of the affected shoulder. Use

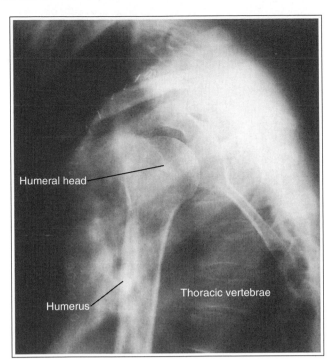

FIGURE 4-211 Transthoracic lateral projection of the proximal humerus with accurate positioning.

Lateral Humeral Analysis Practice

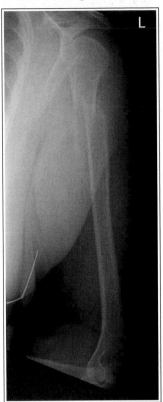

IMAGE 4-39

breathing technique to blur the vascular lung markings and axillary ribs. With this technique, a long exposure time (3 seconds) is used while the patient breathes shallowly (costal breathing) during the exposure. A transthoracic lateral projection with accurate positioning should sharply demonstrate the affected proximal humerus halfway between the sternum and the thoracic vertebrae, without superimposition of the unaffected shoulder (Figure 4-211).

Analysis. There is poor contrast resolution between the proximal and distal humerus, because the torso was rotated toward the humerus instead of staying in a PA projection. A proximal humerus fracture is present.

Correction. When a fracture is suspected the arm should not be rotated to obtain a lateral humerus projection—instead the alternate PA oblique (scapular Y) projection should be obtained.

OUTLINE

Shoulder: AP Projection, 235
  AP Shoulder Analysis
    Practice, 241
Shoulder: Inferosuperior Axial
  Projection (Lawrence
  Method), 242
  Inferosuperior Axial Shoulder
    Analysis Practice, 247
Glenoid Cavity: AP Oblique
  Projection (Grashey Method), 248
  AP Oblique Shoulder Analysis
    Practice, 252
Scapular Y: PA Oblique
  Projection, 252
  PA Oblique (Scapular Y) Shoulder
    Analysis Practice, 257

Proximal Humerus: AP Axial
  Projection (Stryker "Notch"
  Method), 258
  AP Axial (Stryker Notch)
    Shoulder Analysis
    Practice, 260
Supraspinatus "Outlet":
  Tangential Projection (Neer
  Method), 261
  Tangential (Outlet) Shoulder
    Analysis Practice, 263
Clavicle: AP Projection, 264
  AP Clavicle Analysis
    Practice, 266
Clavicle: AP Axial Projection
  (Lordotic Position), 266

Acromioclavicular (AC) Joint:
  AP Projection, 267
Scapula: AP Projection, 270
  AP Scapular Analysis
    Practice, 273
Scapula: Lateral Projection
  (Lateromedial or
  Mediolateral), 273
  Lateral Scapular Analysis
    Practice, 277

OBJECTIVES

After completion of this chapter, you should be able to do the following:

- Identify the required anatomy on shoulder, clavicular, acromioclavicular (AC) joint, and scapular projections.
- Describe how to properly position the patient, image receptor (IR), and central ray (CR) for projections of the shoulder, clavicle, AC joint, and scapula.
- List the image analysis guidelines and the related positioning procedure for projections of the shoulder, clavicle, AC joint, and scapula.
- State how to properly reposition the patient when shoulder, clavicular, AC joint, and scapular projections show poor positioning.
- State the technical factors routinely used for shoulder, clavicular, AC joint, and scapular projections and describe which anatomic structures are visible when the correct technique factors are used.
- State where the humerus is positioned if a shoulder dislocation is demonstrated on the AP and PA oblique (scapular Y) shoulder projections.

- Discuss how the visualization of the proximal humerus changes as the humeral epicondyles are placed at different angles to the IR.
- Explain how the scapula moves when the humerus is abducted.
- List the anatomic structures that form the Y on a PA oblique (scapular Y) shoulder projection.
- State how the lateral and medial borders of the scapula can be identified.
- Discuss why non–weight-bearing and weight-bearing projections are required when AC joints are imaged.
- Describe how the shoulder is retracted to obtain an AP projection of the scapula.
- Discuss which anatomic structures must move to allow the humerus to abduct.
- Describe the effect of humeral abduction on the degree of patient obliquity needed to position the scapula in a lateral projection.

KEY TERMS

abduct
anterior shoulder dislocation
bilateral
Hill-Sachs defect

longitudinal foreshortening
protract
recumbent
retract

supraspinatus outlet
transverse foreshortening
unilateral
weight-bearing

IMAGE ANALYSIS GUIDELINES

Technical Data. When the technical data in Table 5-1 are followed, or adjusted as needed for additive and destructive patient conditions (see Table 2-6), along with the best practices discussed in Chapters 1 and 2, all shoulder projections will demonstrate the image analysis guidelines listed in Box 5-1 unless otherwise indicated.

SHOULDER: AP PROJECTION

See Table 5-2, (Figures 5-1, 5-2, and 5-3).

Shoulder Movements

Supine versus Upright. The AP projection of the shoulder positions the scapular body at 35 to 45 degrees of obliquity, with the lateral scapula situated more anteriorly than the medial scapula. This positioning causes

TABLE 5-1	Shoulder Technical Data					
Projection	kV	Grid	AEC	mAs	SID	
AP, shoulder	75-85	Grid	Center		40-48 inches (100-120 cm)	
Inferosuperior axial, shoulder	75-85			5	40-48 inches (100-120 cm)	
AP oblique (Grashey method), glenoid cavity	75-85	Grid	Center		40-48 inches (100-120 cm)	
PA oblique (scapular Y), shoulder	75-85	Grid		5	40-48 inches (100-120 cm)	
AP axial (Stryker notch method), proximal humerus	75-85	Grid		5	40-48 inches (100-120 cm)	
Tangential (Neer Method), supraspinatus outlet	75-85	Grid		5	40-48 inches (100-120 cm)	
AP and AP axial, clavicle	75-85	Grid		3	40-48 inches (100-120 cm)	
AP, AC joint	70-80	Grid		3	40-48 inches (100-120 cm) Unilateral or 72 inches (183 cm) Bilateral	
AP, scapula	75-85	Grid	Center		40-48 inches (100-120 cm)	
Lateral, scapula	75-85	Grid		5	40-48 inches (100-120 cm)	
Pediatric	60-70			1-2.5	40-48 inches (100-120 cm)	

TABLE 5-2	AP Shoulder Projection
Image Analysis Guidelines (Figure 5-1)	**Related Positioning Procedures (Figures 5-2 and 5-3)**
• Scapular body demonstrates minimal transverse foreshortening and ½ of the scapular body is visualized without thorax superimposition. • Clavicle is demonstrated with minimal longitudinal foreshortening and with the medial clavicular end positioned next to the lateral edge of the vertebral column. • *Nondislocated shoulder:* Glenoid cavity is partially demonstrated with the humeral head superimposing it. • *Dislocated shoulder:* Glenoid cavity is partially demonstrated with the humeral head positioned inferior to the glenoid cavity.	• Center shoulder to the table or upright IR in an AP projection. • Position the shoulders at equal distances from the IR, aligning the midcoronal plane parallel with the IR.
• Scapular body is demonstrated without longitudinal foreshortening. • Midclavicle superimposes the superior scapular angle. • Humerus is demonstrated without abduction. • *Neutral Humerus:* Greater tubercle is partially seen in profile laterally and the humeral head is partially seen in profile medially. • *Alternate externally rotated humerus:* Greater tubercle is seen in profile laterally and the humeral head in profile medially. An arrow or word marker is present that indicates external rotation. • *Alternate internally rotated humerus:* Lesser tubercle is seen in profile medially and the humeral head is superimposed by the greater tubercle. An arrow or word marker is present that indicates internal rotation. • An arrow marker or word marker is present that indicates the direction the humerus was rotated if alternate humerus rotation was used.	• Straighten the upper midcoronal plane, aligning it parallel with the IR. • Position the humerus next to the body. • Place the patient's palm against the thigh, aligning the humeral epicondyles at a 45-degree angle with the IR. • *Alternate externally rotated humerus:* Externally rotate the arm until the humeral epicondyles are aligned parallel with the IR. Place an arrow or word marker on the IR indicating external rotation. • *Alternate internally rotated humerus:* Internally rotate the arm until the humeral epicondyles are aligned perpendicular to the IR. Place an arrow or word marker on the IR indicating internal rotation.
• Superior scapular body is at the center of the exposure field.	• Center a perpendicular (horizontal if upright) CR 1inch (2.5 cm) inferior to the coracoid process.
• Glenohumeral joint, clavicle, proximal third of the humerus, and superior scapula are included within the exposure field.	• Center the IR and grid to the CR. • Longitudinally collimate to include the top of the shoulder. • Transversely collimate to the medial clavicular end and within 0.5 inch (1.25 cm) of the lateral humeral skin line.

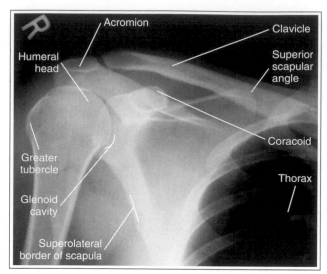

FIGURE 5-1 Upright AP shoulder projection with accurate positioning.

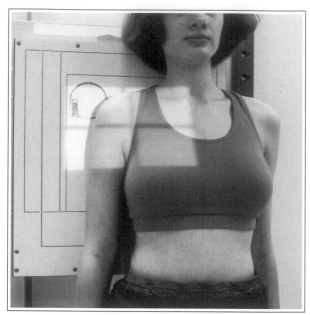

FIGURE 5-3 Accurately positioned AP shoulder projection obtained with humeral epicondyles positioned at a 45-degree angle with IR.

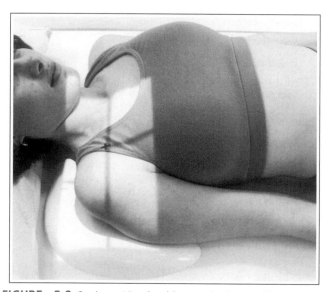

FIGURE 5-2 Supine AP shoulder projection with accurate positioning.

BOX 5-1 | Shoulder Imaging Analysis Guidelines

- The facility's identification requirements are visible.
- A right or left marker identifying the correct side of the patient is present on the projection and is not superimposed over the VOI.
- Good radiation protection practices are evident.
- Bony trabecular patterns and cortical outlines of the anatomical structures are sharply defined.
- Contrast resolution is adequate to demonstrate the surrounding soft tissue, bony trabecular patterns, and cortical outlines.
- No quantum mottle or saturation is present.
- Scatter radiation has been kept to a minimum.
- There is no evidence of removable artifacts.

---

the scapular body to demonstrate transverse foreshortening and the glenoid cavity to be visible on an AP projection. The exact amount of scapular foreshortening and glenoid cavity that is demonstrated is affected by the degree of shoulder retraction. When the projection is obtained in a supine position there is greater shoulder retraction in comparison to when the shoulder is obtained in an upright position because of the gravitation pull placed on the shoulder and the degree of forced thoracic spinal straightening that occurs as the patient lies on the firm imaging table. The supine method is the preferred method because it causes shoulder retraction and the scapular body to be positioned more nearly parallel with the IR, demonstrating decreased transverse foreshortening of the scapular body and glenoid cavity visualization.

Midcoronal Plane Positioning and Shoulder Rotation. Rotation on an AP shoulder projection affects the degree of thorax superimposition over the scapular body, the degree of clavicular foreshortening, and the relationship of the medial clavicular end to the lateral edge of the vertebral column. When the patient is rotated toward the affected shoulder, placing it closer to IR, the resulting projection demonstrates increased thoracic superimposition over the scapular body, increased clavicular foreshortening, and the medial clavicular end rotates away from the lateral edge of the vertebral column (Figure 5-4). When the patient is rotated away from the affected shoulder, placing it farther from the IR, the resulting projection demonstrates decreased thoracic superimposition over the scapular body, decreased clavicular foreshortening, and the medial clavicular end superimposing the vertebral column (Figure 5-5).

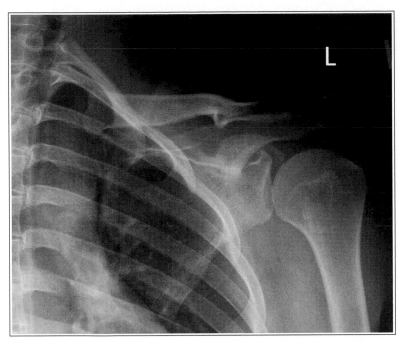

FIGURE 5-4 AP shoulder projection taken with patient rotated toward the affected shoulder.

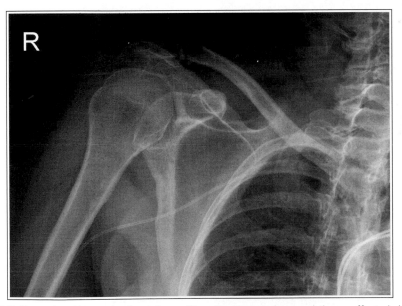

FIGURE 5-5 AP shoulder projection taken with patient rotated toward the unaffected shoulder.

Midcoronal Plane Tilting. When the midcoronal plane is straightened and aligned parallel with the IR, the scapula body is demonstrated without longitudinal foreshortening and the midclavicle superimposes the superior scapular angle. It is tilting of this plane with the IR that causes the scapula to longitudinally foreshorten and changes the relationship of the midclavicle and superior scapular angle. If the upper midcoronal plane is tilted anteriorly (forward), the superior scapular angle will be demonstrated superior to the midclavicle on the projection (Figures 5-6 and 5-7). If the upper midcoronal plane is tilted posteriorly (backward), the superior scapular angle will be shown inferior to the midclavicle (Figure 5-8). Anterior and posterior upper midcoronal plane tilting will also result in increased longitudinal foreshortening of the scapular body.

Kyphotic Patients. The kyphotic patient's increase in spinal convexity prevents the upper midcoronal plane from being straightened and positioned parallel with the IR and situates the scapula more anteriorly as in maximum shoulder protraction. As a result, AP shoulder projections obtained with the patient positioned as close

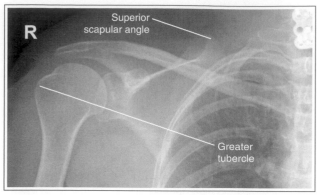

FIGURE 5-6 AP shoulder projection taken with the midcoronal plane tilted anteriorly.

to the routine for the projection as the patient can accommodate will demonstrate the superior scapular angle superior to the midclavicle and longitudinal scapular foreshortening, and increased transverse scapular foreshortening and glenoid cavity visualization. Figure 5-9 demonstrates an AP shoulder obtained on a nonkyphotic and kyphotic patient for comparison.

There are alternative positioning methods to better demonstrate the scapular body with minimal foreshortening. One method keeps the midcoronal plane parallel

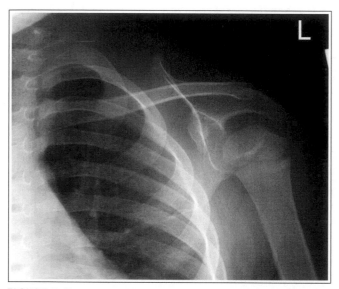

FIGURE 5-7 Pediatric AP shoulder projection taken with the mid-coronal plane tilted anteriorly.

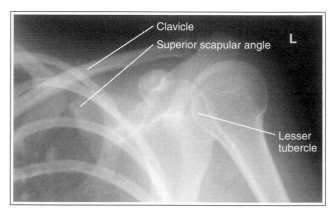

FIGURE 5-8 AP shoulder projection taken with the mid-coronal plane tilted posteriorly.

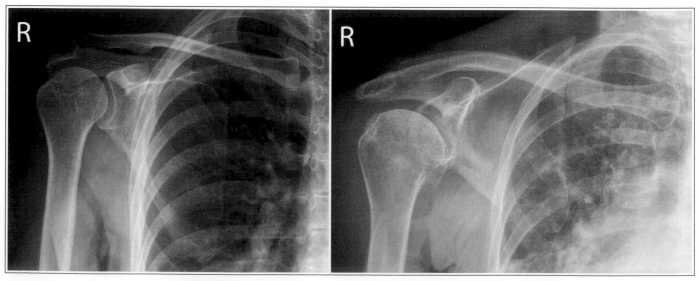

FIGURE 5-9 Nonkyphotic and kyphotic AP shoulder projections.

with the IR and uses a cephalic CR angulation to offset the longitudinal foreshortening. With this method, the CR is angled until it is perpendicular with the scapular body. Because the IR is not perpendicular to the CR for this method, there will be elongation that will increase as the CR to IR angle becomes more acute. The second method is to lean the patient's shoulders and upper thoracic vertebrae posteriorly to place the upper midcoronal plane at an angle with the IR that brings the scapular body parallel with the IR and use a horizontal CR. The kyphotic patient will also be unable to retract the shoulder to decrease the transverse scapular foreshortening that is caused by the condition, though they can be rotated toward the affected shoulder to decrease it.

Humerus Positioning

Humeral Epicondyles. The position of the humeral epicondyles with respect to the IR determines whether the greater tubercle and humeral head or the lesser tubercle will be in partial or full profile on an AP shoulder projection. The technologist can ensure they have the tubercle and humeral head positioned accurately before they expose the projection by understanding the relationship between the humeral epicondyles and these structures. The palpable lateral epicondyle is aligned with the greater tubercle, and the palpable medial epicondyle is aligned with the humeral head. This means that when the humeral epicondyles are palpated and positioned so they are aligned parallel with the IR, the AP shoulder projection demonstrates the greater tubercle in profile laterally and humeral head in profile medially (Figures 5-10 and 5-11). The lesser tubercle is anteriorly located at right angles to the greater tubercle and humeral head. To position the lesser tubercle in

profile, the anterior aspect of the proximal humerus must be in profile and is accomplished by aligning the humeral epicondyles perpendicular to the IR (Figures 5-12 and 5-13).

For a routine AP shoulder projection, the humerus is placed in neutral rotation and is accomplished by positioning the humeral epicondyles at a 45-degree angle with the IR (see Figure 5-3). The resulting projection demonstrates the greater tubercle partially in profile laterally and the humeral head partially in profile medially (see Figure 5-1). If the projection is obtained demonstrating the greater tubercle in profile laterally and the humeral head in profile medially, the arm was externally

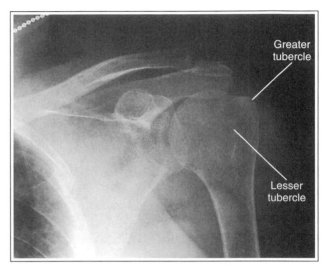

FIGURE 5-11 Accurately positioned AP shoulder projection obtained with humeral epicondyles positioned parallel with IR.

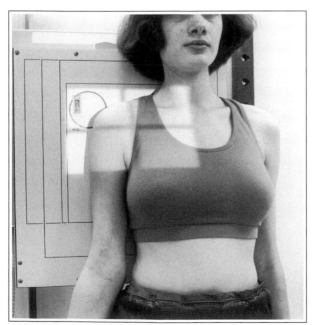

FIGURE 5-10 Proper positioning for an externally rotated AP shoulder projection.

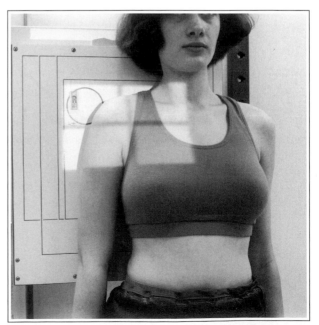

FIGURE 5-12 Proper positioning for an internally rotated AP shoulder projection.

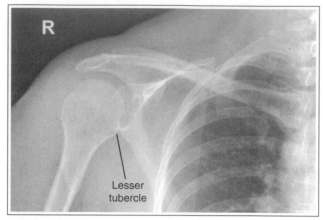

FIGURE 5-13 Accurately positioned AP shoulder projection obtained with the humeral epicondyles positioned perpendicular to IR.

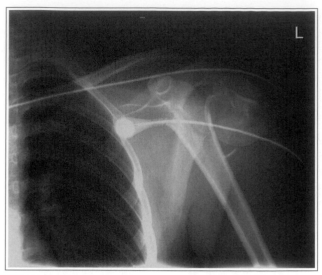

FIGURE 5-14 AP shoulder projection demonstrating a proximal humeral head fracture.

rotated more than needed to obtain a neutral rotation (see Figure 5-11). If the projection is obtained demonstrating the lesser tubercle in profile medially and the humeral head and greater tubercle superimposed, the arm was internally rotated (see Figure 5-13). Internal humeral rotation also causes shoulder protraction, which moves the scapula anteriorly, transversely foreshortening the scapular body and increasing the amount of the glenoid cavity demonstration.

AP Shoulder Projections Taken for Mobility. AP shoulder projections obtained in external and internal rotation may be specifically requested to demonstrate shoulder mobility. These projections are completed as described in Table 5-2 (see Figures 5-10 and 5-12) and should demonstrate the greater or lesser tubercle, respectively, if accurately positioned.

Humeral Fractures. AP shoulder projections on patients with suspected humerus fractures should be obtained with the humerus positioned as it is, without attempting to rotate it into position, avoiding further displacement and nerve damage. In this case, the acceptable projection will have varying tubercle demonstration and relationships between the glenoid cavity and humeral head. For example, a proximal humeral head fracture may demonstrate the humeral head shifted away from the glenoid cavity, often not seeming to be associated with the humerus at all, and does not demonstrate the tubercles (Figures 5-14 and 5-15).

Shoulder Dislocations. AP shoulder projections on patients with suspected shoulder dislocations should be obtained with the humerus positioned as is, without attempting to rotate it into position. Shoulder dislocations result in positioning of the humeral head anteriorly or posteriorly and inferiorly to the glenoid cavity. Anterior dislocation, which is more common (95%), results in the humeral head being demonstrated anteriorly, beneath the coracoid process (Figures 5-16 and 5-17). Posterior dislocations, which are uncommon (2%-4%),

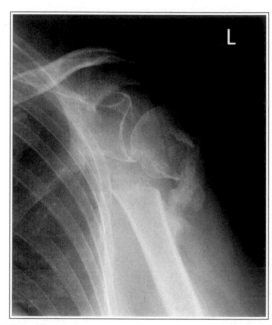

FIGURE 5-15 AP shoulder projection demonstrating a proximal humeral head fracture.

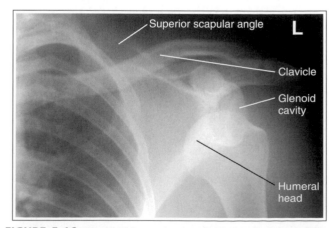

FIGURE 5-16 AP shoulder projection demonstrating an anterior shoulder dislocation.

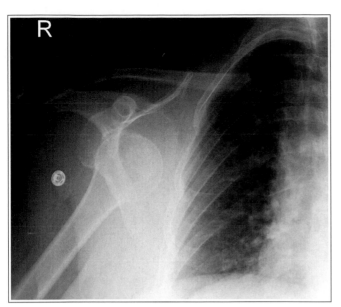

FIGURE 5-17 AP shoulder projection demonstrating an anterior dislocation.

result in the humeral head being demonstrated posteriorly, beneath the acromion process or spine of the scapula. On AP shoulder projections the dislocation is identified by the humeral head being demonstrated inferior to the glenoid cavity. A PA oblique (transscapular Y) projection must be obtained to confirm its anterior or posterior location.

AP Shoulder Analysis Practice

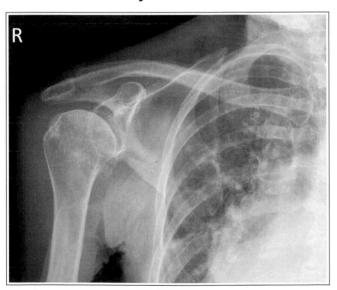

IMAGE 5-1

Analysis. The superior scapular angle is demonstrated superior to the midclavicle. The upper midcoronal plane was tilted anteriorly.
Correction. Straighten the midcoronal plane, aligning it parallel with the IR.

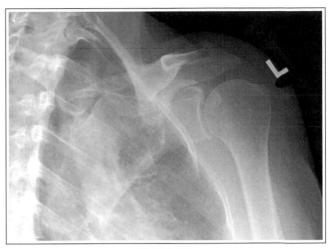

IMAGE 5-2

Analysis. The glenoid cavity is almost in profile, with only a small amount of the articulating surface demonstrated, the superolateral border of the scapula is superimposed by the thorax, and the clavicle is longitudinally foreshortened. The patient was rotated toward the affected shoulder. The greater tubercle is in profile.
Correction. Rotate the patient away from the affected shoulder into an AP projection, until the shoulders are positioned at equal distances from the table, aligning the midcoronal plane parallel with the IR.

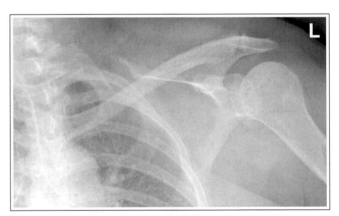

IMAGE 5-3

Analysis. The scapular body is drawn from beneath the thorax and is foreshortened, the glenoid cavity is demonstrated on end, and the medial clavicular end is superimposed over the vertebral column. The patient was rotated toward the unaffected shoulder. The superior scapular angle is demonstrated superior to the midclavicle. The upper midcoronal plane was tilted anteriorly. The lesser tubercle is in profile.
Correction. Rotate the patient toward the affected shoulder into an AP projection, with the shoulders positioned at equal distances from the table, and straighten the midcoronal plane.

SHOULDER: INFEROSUPERIOR AXIAL PROJECTION (LAWRENCE METHOD)

See Table 5-3, (Figures 5-18, 5-19, 5-20, and 5-21).
Humeral Abduction and CR Alignment. To obtain an open glenohumeral joint space the CR must be aligned parallel with the joint space and glenoid cavity. Because no palpable structures are present to help align the CR with the glenohumeral joint, the technologists must rely on our knowledge of scapular movement on humeral abduction to align it. Abduction of the arm is accomplished by combined movements of the glenohumeral joint and the scapula as it glides around the thoracic cavity. The ratio of movement in these two articulations

TABLE 5-3	Inferosuperior Axial Shoulder Projection
Image Analysis Guidelines (Figures 5-18, 5-19 and 5-20)	**Related Positioning Procedures (Figure 5-21)**
• Inferior and superior margins of the glenoid cavity are superimposed, demonstrating an open glenohumeral joint space. • Lateral edge of the coracoid process base is aligned with the inferior margin of the glenoid cavity. • Long axis of the humeral shaft is seen with minimal foreshortening	• Position patient in a supine position with the affected shoulder placed next to the lateral edge of the imaging table. • Abduct the affected arm to 90 degrees with the body. • Align a horizontal CR 30-35 degrees with the lateral body surface, bringing it parallel with the glenohumeral joint space. • Position the IR vertically at the top of the affected shoulder and align it perpendicular to the CR.
• Humeral head is at the center of the exposure field.	• Center the horizontal CR to the midaxillary region at the level of the coracoid process.
Per facility requirement: • *Parallel epicondyles:* Lesser tubercle is seen in profile anteriorly. • *45-degree epicondyles:* Lesser tubercle is seen in partial profile anteriorly and the posterolateral aspect of the humeral head is seen in profile posteriorly.	• Extend the arm and rest the elbow on a support. *Per facility requirement:* • Externally rotate the arm until the humeral epicondyles are positioned parallel with the floor. • Externally rotate the arm until the humeral epicondyles are positioned at a 45-degree angle with the floor.
• Coracoid process is demonstrated in profile. • Coracoid base is fully visualized anterior to the scapular neck. • Posterior shoulder and humeral structures are included.	• Confirm that the upper back has not arched, but remains in contact with the table, as the arm is externally rotated. • Elevate the shoulder 2-3 inches (5-7.6 cm) from the table with a sponge or folded washcloth.
• Medial aspect of the coracoid is included.	• Laterally flex the neck and turn the face toward the unaffected shoulder. • Place the top edge of the IR snugly against the neck.
• Glenoid cavity, coracoid process, scapular spine, acromion process, and one third of the proximal humerus are included within the exposure field.	• Open the longitudinal collimation slightly beyond the coracoid process. • Transversely collimate to within 0.5 inch (1.25 cm) of the proximal humeral skin line.

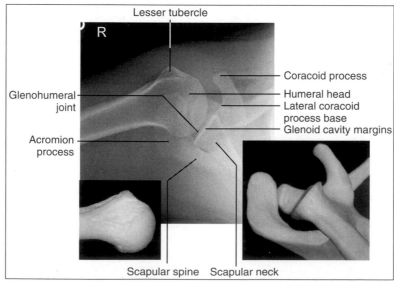

FIGURE 5-18 Inferosuperior axial shoulder projection with accurate positioning obtained with humeral epicondyles positioned parallel with floor.

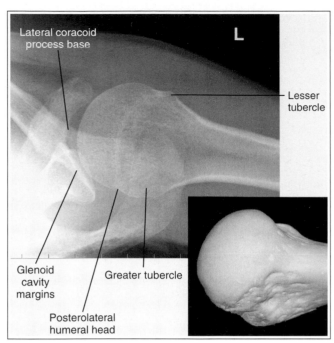

FIGURE 5-19 Inferosuperior axial shoulder projection with accurate positioning obtained with humeral epicondyles positioned at 45 degrees with floor.

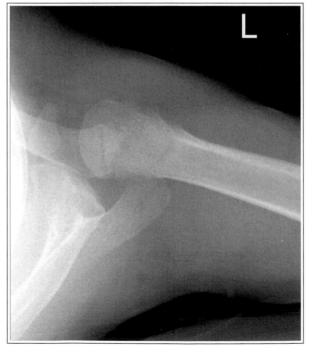

FIGURE 5-20 Pediatric inferosuperior axial shoulder projection with accurate positioning.

is two parts glenohumeral joint to one part scapulothoracic, with the initial movement (60 degrees of abduction) being primarily glenohumeral joint.

In a patient who is not experiencing severe pain with the 90-degree humeral abduction, the scapular

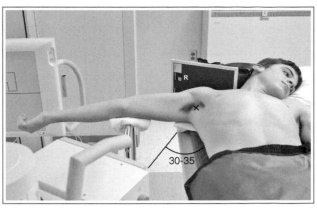

FIGURE 5-21 Proper inferosuperior axial shoulder positioning.

movement angles the glenoid cavity to approximately 30 to 35 degrees with the lateral body surface (Figure 5-22). Consequently, to align the CR parallel with the glenohumeral joint on such a patient, the angle between the lateral body surface and CR is 30 to 35 degrees. This angle is best accomplished by first determining the 23- and 45-degree angles and then aligning the CR between these two angles. Thirty-four degrees is halfway between the 23- and 45-degree angles (see Figure 5-21).

If a patient is unable to abduct the arm to the full 90 degrees, the angle between the lateral body surface and CR needs to be decreased to align it parallel with the glenohumeral joint (Figure 5-23). Because the first 60 degrees of humeral abduction involves primarily movement of the glenohumeral joint without accompanying scapulothoracic movement, the angle between the CR and lateral body surface is approximately 20 degrees when the humerus is abducted up to 60 degrees. As the degree of abduction increases from 60 to 90 degrees, the CR to lateral body surface angle is incrementally increased from 20 to 35 degrees.

Inaccurate alignment of the CR with the glenohumeral joint space can be identified on a projection by the increased demonstration of the articulating surface of the glenoid cavity and misalignment of the inferior margin of the glenoid cavity with the lateral edge of the coracoid process base. Whether the angle between the CR and the lateral body surface should be increased or decreased when a poor projection is obtained can be determined by viewing the relationship of the coracoid process base to the inferior margin of the glenoid cavity. Because the inferior margin of the glenoid cavity is situated farther from the IR than the coracoid base, it will be projected to one side of the lateral edge of the coracoid process base instead of being aligned with it if the CR is aligned inaccurately. If the CR to lateral body surface angle is too small, the inferior glenoid cavity margin will be projected laterally to the lateral edge of the coracoid process base. (Closely compare the coracoid process base and glenoid cavity relationships in Figures 5-18 and 5-24.) If the angle is too large, the inferior margin will

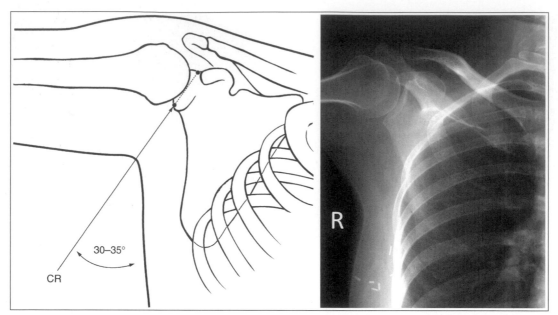

FIGURE 5-22 Placement of glenoid cavity with arm abducted 90 degrees. *CR,* Central ray.

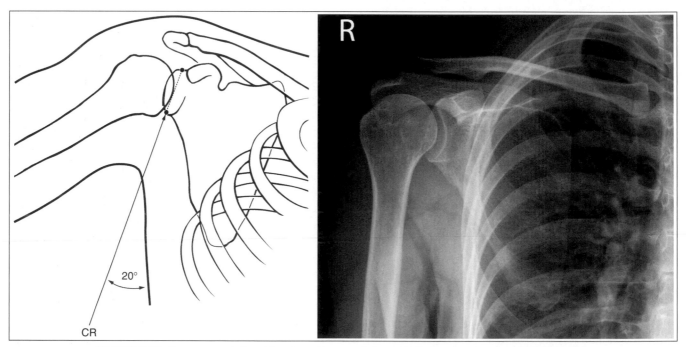

FIGURE 5-23 Placement of glenoid cavity with arm abducted less than 90 degrees. *CR,* Central ray.

be projected medially to the lateral edge of the coracoid process base (Figure 5-25).

Humerus Positioning

Humeral Fracture or Shoulder Dislocation. On a patient with suspected humeral fracture or shoulder dislocation, the humerus should not be abducted or rotated to avoid farther displacement and nerve damage (Figures 5-26 and 5-27). To obtain a lateral projection of the shoulder and humerus when a fracture or dislocation is

suspected, perform the PA oblique (scapular Y) projection as described later in the chapter.

Humerus Foreshortening. Humeral shaft foreshortening is unavoidable on an inferosuperior axial shoulder projection because the CR cannot be aligned parallel with the glenohumeral joint and perpendicular to the humerus at the same time. As a result, the humeral shaft will always demonstrate some degree of foreshortening, although it can be kept to a minimum as long as the

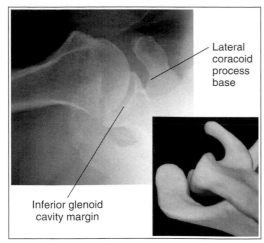

FIGURE 5-24 Inferosuperior axial shoulder projection taken with too small of a CR to lateral body surface angle.

Lateral coracoid process base

Inferior glenoid cavity margin

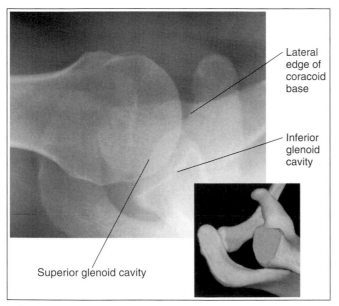

Lateral edge of coracoid base

Inferior glenoid cavity

Superior glenoid cavity

FIGURE 5-25 Inferosuperior axial shoulder projection taken with too large of a CR to lateral body surface angle

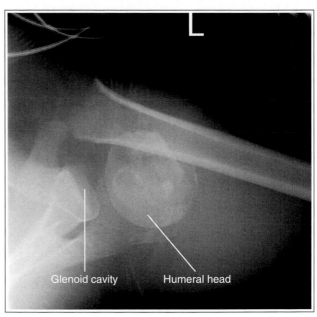

Glenoid cavity   Humeral head

FIGURE 5-26 Inferosuperior axial shoulder projection demonstrating a humeral head fracture.

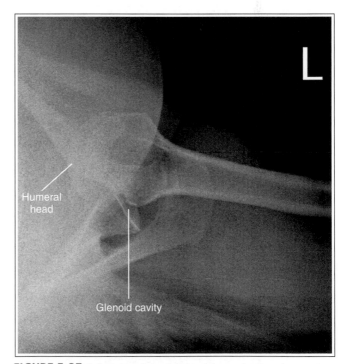

Humeral head

Glenoid cavity

FIGURE 5-27 Inferosuperior axial shoulder projection demonstrating an anterior dislocation and a Hill-Sachs defect.

patient is able to abduct the arm to 90 degrees. On the patient who is unable to abduct the arm to 90 degrees, the humeral shaft demonstrates excessive foreshortening, as identified by the on-end appearance that it will take (Figure 5-28).

Humerus Rotation. The position of the humeral epicondyles with respect to the IR determines which of the humeral head's anatomical structures will be seen in profile on the inferosuperior axial shoulder. Your facility analysis guidelines define whether having the lesser tubercle or the posterolateral aspect of the humeral head in profile is the optimal visualization.

Lesser Tubercle in Profile. To demonstrate the lesser tubercle in profile anteriorly, externally rotated the arm

until the humeral epicondyles are positioned parallel with the floor (see Figure 5-18).

Posterolateral Humeral Head in Profile. To demonstrate the posterolateral humeral head in profile posteriorly and the lesser tubercle in partial profile anteriorly the arm is externally rotated until the humeral epicondyles are placed at a 45-degree angle with the floor (see Figure 5-21). The lateral epicondyle is positioned closer to the floor. This humerus positioning is especially helpful in identifying the Hill-Sachs defect. The Hill-Sachs defect is a notch defect (compression fracture) in the postero-lateral aspect of the humeral head created by impinge-ment of the articular surface of the humeral head against the anteroinferior rim of the glenoid cavity that results from anterior shoulder dislocations (see Figure 5-27). If the humerus is externally rotated more than needed to position the humeral epicondyles at a greater than

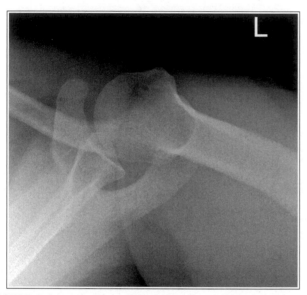

FIGURE 5-28 Inferosuperior axial shoulder projection taken with the arm abducted less than 90 degrees.

45-degree angle with the floor, the lesser tubercle and posterior lateral humeral head will not be demonstrated; instead, the greater tubercle will be demonstrated to some degree posteriorly with it being in profile if the epicondyles are positioned perpendicular to the floor (Figures 5-29 and 5-30). For some patients, this degree of external rotation can only be accomplished by involving the vertebral column as described in the next section.

Coracoid Process and Base. The coracoid process is demonstrated in profile and the coracoid base is seen without scapular neck superimposition when the scapu-lar body remains parallel with the table. With excessive external arm rotation or if the patient's elbow is flexed and the hand of the affected arm is used to hold the IR in place, the upper thoracic vertebrae arches upward, causing the inferior scapular body to tilt anteriorly, the coracoid to move behind the scapular neck and be less visible and demonstrate a widening of the space between the scapular neck and acromion (Figure 5-31).

Including the Posterior Surface. To ensure that the scapular spine and other posterior shoulder structures are included, elevate the patient's shoulder 2 to 3 inches (5-7.6 cm) from the table with a sponge or folded wash-cloth. If the shoulder is not elevated, all aspects of the posterior shoulder and humeral structures may not be included on the projection (Figure 5-32).

Including the Medial Coracoid. To include the medial coracoid, laterally flex the neck and turn the face away from the affected shoulder. This position will allow the IR to be placed more medially in respect to the patient and includes more of the coracoid. If this medial IR placement is not accomplished, the coracoid and other medial structures will not be included (Figure 5-33).

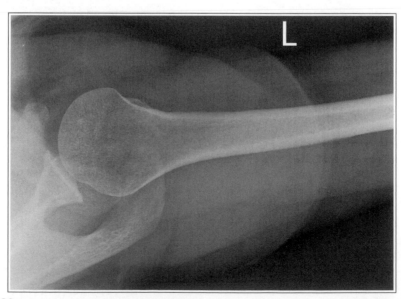

FIGURE 5-29 Inferosuperior axial shoulder projection taken with the arm externally rotated more than 45 degrees with the floor.

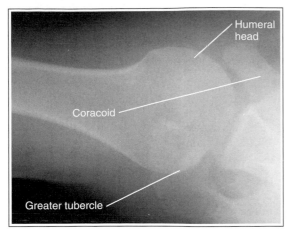

FIGURE 5-30 Inferosuperior axial shoulder projection taken with the arm externally rotated more than 45 degrees with the floor.

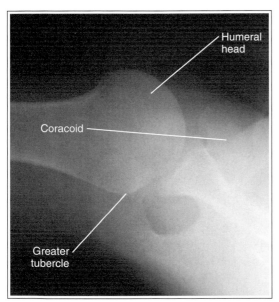

FIGURE 5-31 Inferosuperior axial shoulder projection taken with the upper thoracic vertebrae arching upwardly.

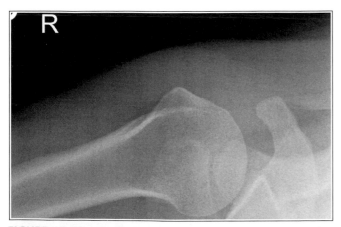

FIGURE 5-32 Inferosuperior axial shoulder projection taken without the shoulder elevated 2 to 3 inches from the table.

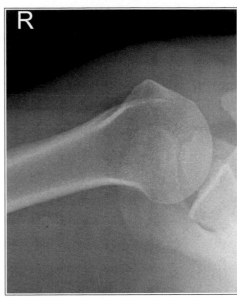

FIGURE 5-33 Inferosuperior axial shoulder projection taken without adequate lateral neck flexion and the IR positioned enough medially.

Inferosuperior Axial Shoulder Analysis Practice

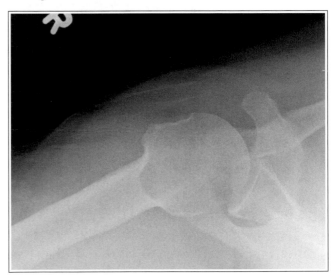

IMAGE 5-4

Analysis. The glenohumeral joint is closed, and the inferior glenoid cavity margin is demonstrated medially to the lateral edge of the coracoid process base and superior glenoid cavity margin, indicating that the angle between the lateral body surface and the CR was too large. The humerus is foreshortened and the humeral head is distorted. The arm is not abducted 90 degrees with the body.

Correction. Decrease the angle between the lateral body surface and CR. If possible, have the patient abduct the humerus to 90 degrees from the body. If the patient cannot abduct the humerus, no humeral corrective movement is necessary.

TABLE 5-4	AP Oblique Projection (Grashey Method)
Image Analysis Guidelines (Figures 5-34 and 5-35)	**Related Positioning Procedures (Figure 5-36)**
• Glenoid cavity is demonstrated in profile and the glenohumeral joint space is open. • Tip of the coracoid process is superimposing the humeral head by about 0.25 inch (0.6 cm). • Glenoid cavity is shown without thorax superimposition. • Clavicle is longitudinally foreshortened and is horizontally situated.	• Center the shoulder to the upright IR in an AP projection with the arm dangling freely by side. • Rotate the body toward the affected shoulder until the midcoronal plane is at a 35- to 45-degree angle with the IR or until coracoid process and acromion angle are superimposed. • Distribute the weight evenly between the feet. • Position shoulders on the same horizontal plane, preventing the patient from leaning against the IR.
• Superior margin of the coracoid process is aligned with the superior margin of the glenoid cavity.	• Straighten the upper midcoronal plane, aligning vertically.
• Glenohumeral joint is at the center of the exposure field. • Glenoid cavity, humeral head, coracoid and acromion processes, and lateral clavicle are included within the exposure field.	• Center a horizontal CR to the coracoid process. • Center the IR and grid to the CR. • Open the longitudinal collimated field enough to include the top of shoulder. • Transversely collimate to within 0.5 inches (1.25 cm) of the lateral humeral skin line.

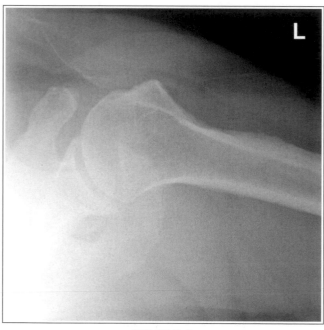

IMAGE 5-5

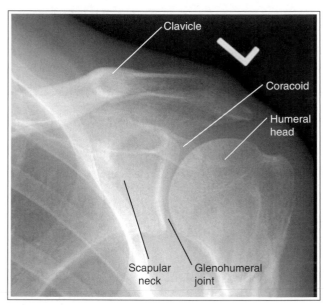

FIGURE 5-34 AP oblique (Grashey) shoulder projection with accurate positioning.

Analysis. The glenohumeral joint is closed, and the inferior glenoid cavity margin is demonstrated lateral to the coracoid process base. The angle between the lateral body surface and the CR was less than required to align the CR parallel with the glenohumeral joint.

Correction. Increase the angle between the lateral body surface and the CR to 30 to 35 degrees.

GLENOID CAVITY: AP OBLIQUE PROJECTION (GRASHEY METHOD)

See Table 5-4, (Figures 5-34, 5-35, and 5-36).

Midcoronal Plane Positioning and Shoulder Rotation. To place the glenoid cavity in profile and obtain an open glenohumeral joint space, the patient's scapular body is positioned parallel with the IR by rotating the patient 35 to 45 degrees. The amount of patient obliquity that is needed varies between patients because of differences in posture, shoulder roundedness, kyphosis, and degree of shoulder protraction. One method of determining the amount of patient obliquity necessary for all types of variations is to palpate the coracoid process and acromion angle and then rotate the patient toward the affected shoulder until the coracoid process is superimposed over the acromion angle, aligning an imaginary line connecting them perpendicular to the IR (Figures 5-37 and 5-38).

Poor body obliquity will be identified on an AP oblique projection as a closed glenohumeral joint space. Whether the body has been rotated too much or too little

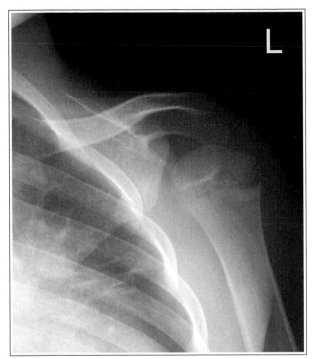

FIGURE 5-35 Pediatric AP oblique (Grashey) shoulder projection with accurate positioning.

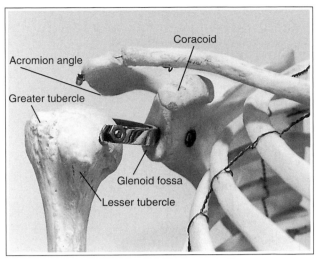

FIGURE 5-37 Location of coracoid process.

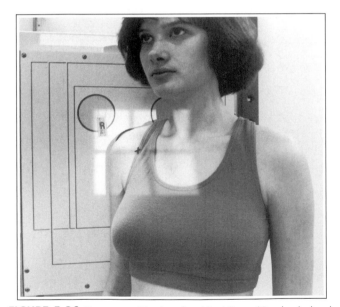

FIGURE 5-36 Proper positioning for AP oblique (Grashey) shoulder projection.

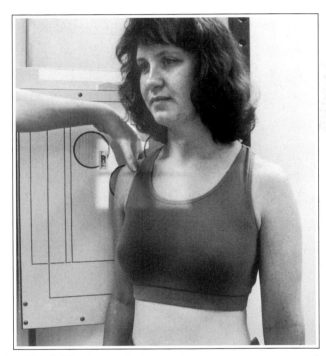

FIGURE 5-38 Alignment of coracoid and acromion processes for AP oblique (Grashey) shoulder projection.

to accomplish this closed joint can be determined by evaluating the relationship of the coracoid process with the humeral head, the degree of thorax superimposition on the glenoid cavity and scapular neck, and the degree of longitudinal clavicle foreshortening. When repositioning for excessive or insufficient obliquity, remember that the glenohumeral joint space is narrow and that the necessary repositioning movement is only half the distance demonstrated between the anterior and posterior

margins of the glenoid cavity. In most cases, you need to move the patient only a few degrees to obtain an open joint space, so it is important to carefully evaluate and make mental notes on how the patient was positioned for the initial examination. If a repeat is necessary, start with the patient position used for the initial examination and then adjust the position from this starting point. If obliquity was excessive, the glenohumeral joint space is closed, more than 0.25 inch (0.6 cm) of the lateral tip of the coracoid process is superimposed over the humeral head, the thorax demonstrates increased glenoid cavity and scapular neck superimposition, and the clavicle

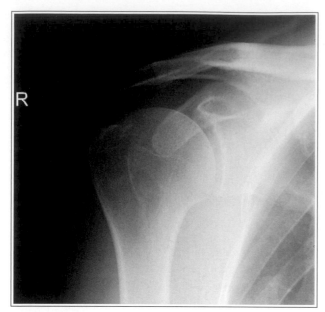

FIGURE 5-39 AP oblique (Grashey) shoulder projection taken with excessive obliquity.

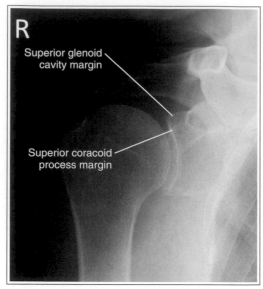

FIGURE 5-41 AP oblique (Grashey) shoulder projection taken with the upper midcoronal plane tilted anteriorly.

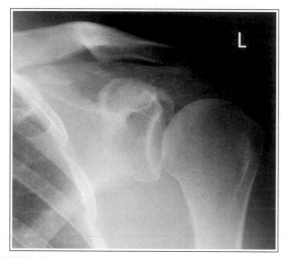

FIGURE 5-40 AP oblique (Grashey) shoulder projection taken with insufficient obliquity.

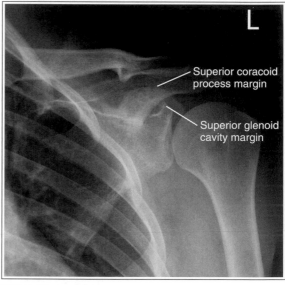

FIGURE 5-42 AP oblique (Grashey) shoulder projection taken with the upper midcoronal plane tilted posteriorly.

demonstrates excessive longitudinal foreshortening (Figure 5-39). If obliquity was insufficient, the glenohumeral joint space is closed, the lateral tip of the coracoid process demonstrates less than 0.25 inch (0.6 cm) of humeral head superimposition, the thorax is not superimposed over the scapular neck, and the clavicle demonstrates little longitudinal foreshortening (Figure 5-40).
Midcoronal Plane Tilting. When the midcoronal plane is straightened and aligned vertically, the superior margin of the coracoid is aligned with the superior margin of the glenoid cavity. If the upper midcoronal plane is tilted anteriorly, the superior margin of the coracoid process will be demonstrated inferior to the superior margin of the glenoid cavity (Figure 5-41). If the upper midcoronal

plane is tilted posteriorly, the superior margin of the coracoid process will be demonstrated superior to the superior margin of the glenoid cavity (Figure 5-42).
Kyphotic Patient. The kyphotic patient's increase in spinal convexity prevents the upper midcoronal plane from being straightened and situates the scapula more anteriorly as in maximum shoulder protraction. As a result, AP shoulder projections obtained with the patient positioned as close to the routine for the projection as the patient can accommodate will demonstrate the superior margin of the coracoid demonstrated inferior to the superior margin of the glenoid cavity. The alternate

positioning methods used in the AP shoulder projection can be used here to offset this appearance.

The kyphotic patient will also require increased obliquity to position the glenoid cavity in profile and the resulting projection will demonstrate the thorax closer to or superimposed over the glenohumeral joint space.

Shoulder Protraction. Protraction of the shoulder occurs as a result of pressure that is placed on the affected shoulder when the patient leans against IR. The sternoclavicular and AC joints function cooperatively to allow the shoulder to be drawn anteriorly. When the shoulder is protracted, the scapula glides around the thorax, moving it anteriorly. This increase in anterior shoulder positioning places the scapular body at a larger starting angle with the IR, therefore requiring an increase in patient obliquity to bring the scapular body parallel with the IR for the AP oblique projection. A projection obtained with the patient leaning against the IR and adequately rotated will demonstrate an open glenohumeral joint, but more of the thorax will be superimposed over the glenoid cavity (Figure 5-43).

Recumbent Position. Shoulder protraction also occurs and requires an increase in patient obliquity when the projection is performed on a recumbent patient. In the recumbent position, the pressure of the body on the affected shoulder when the patient is rotated forces the shoulder to protract and shift superiorly. Projections taken with the patient in this position demonstrate the glenoid cavity situated slightly superiorly and the clavicle aligned more vertically, and superimposing the scapular neck (Figure 5-44). When evaluating an AP oblique shoulder projection on a recumbent patient, the relationship between the lateral tip of the coracoid process and the humeral head described above is also used to reposition the patient for excessive or insufficient obliquity. If obliquity was excessive, the glenohumeral joint is closed, the lateral tip of the coracoid process is superimposed over more than 0.25 inch (0.6 cm) of the humeral head, and the clavicle is superimposed over the scapular neck (Figure 5-45). If the obliquity was insufficient, then the glenohumeral joint is closed, the lateral tip of the coracoid process is superimposed over less than 0.25 inch (0.6 cm) of the humeral head, and the clavicle is not superimposed over the scapular neck (Figure 5-46).

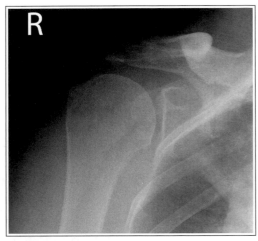

FIGURE 5-43 AP oblique (Grashey) shoulder projection taken with the patient leaning against the IR.

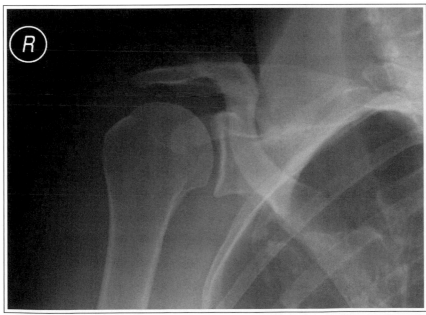

FIGURE 5-44 Supine AP oblique (Grashey) shoulder projection demonstrating the glenoid cavity situated superiorly and the clavicle aligned vertically.

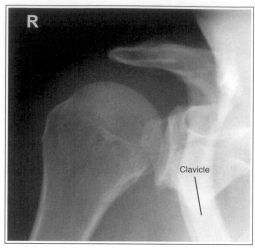

FIGURE 5-45 Supine AP oblique (Grashey) shoulder projection taken with excessive obliquity.

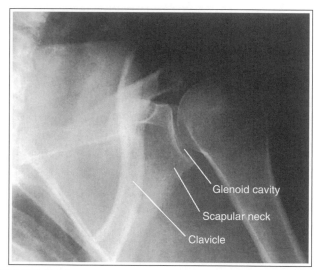

FIGURE 5-46 Supine AP oblique (Grashey) shoulder projection taken with insufficient obliquity.

AP Oblique Shoulder Analysis Practice

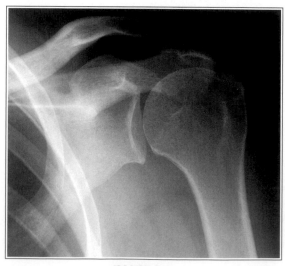

IMAGE 5-6

Analysis. The glenohumeral joint space is closed, the lateral tip of the coracoid process superimposed is less than 0.25 inch (0.6 cm) of the humeral head, and the clavicle demonstrates little foreshortening. Patient obliquity was insufficient. The superior margin of the coracoid process is superior to the superior margin of the glenoid cavity. The upper midcoronal plane was tilted posteriorly.

Correction. Increase the degree of patient obliquity and straighten the midcoronal plane, aligning it parallel with the IR.

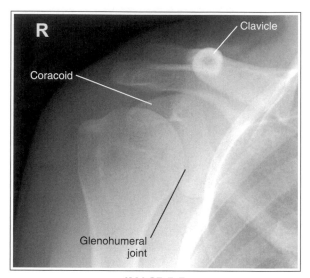

IMAGE 5-7

Analysis. The glenohumeral joint space is closed, more than 0.25 inch (0.6 cm) of the lateral tip of the coracoid process is superimposed over the humeral head, and the clavicle demonstrates excessive longitudinal foreshortening. Patient obliquity was excessive.

Correction. Decrease the degree of patient obliquity.

SCAPULAR Y: PA OBLIQUE PROJECTION

See Table 5-5, (Figures 5-47 and 5-48).

Midcoronal Plane Positioning and Shoulder Rotation. If the patient's arm is allowed to hang freely, the scapular body is placed in a lateral projection when the midcoronal plane is positioned at a 45-degree angle with the IR. The exact degree of obliquity varies with differences in shoulder roundness, which requires decreased obliquity, or humeral abduction and shoulder retraction, which requires increased obliquity. One method of determining the amount of patient obliquity necessary for all types of variations is to palpate the coracoid process and the acromion angle, and rotate the patient until an imaginary line drawn between them is aligned parallel with the IR, positioning the vertebral border of the scapula between them. This positioning sets up the Y formation,

TABLE 5-5	PA Oblique (Scapular Y) Shoulder Projection

Image Analysis Guidelines (Figure 5-47)	Related Positioning Procedures (Figure 5-48)
• Scapular body is in a lateral projection, with superimposed lateral and vertebral scapular borders. • Scapular structures form a Y, with the scapular body as the leg and the acromion and coracoid processes as the arms. • Glenoid cavity is demonstrated on end at the converging point of the arms and leg of the Y. • *No Injury:* Glenoid cavity and humeral head, and the scapular body and the humeral shaft are superimposed. • *Shoulder dislocation:* Glenoid cavity does not superimpose the humeral head. • *Proximal humerus fracture:* Glenoid cavity superimposes the humeral head, but the scapular body does not superimpose the humeral shaft.	• Center the shoulder to the upright IR in a PA projection. • Rotate the patient's body toward the affected shoulder until the midcoronal plane is at a 45-degree angle with the IR or until an imaginary line drawn between the coracoid process and acromion is aligned parallel with the IR, positioning the vertebral border of the scapula between them. • Affected arm is allowed to hang freely.
• Scapula is demonstrated without longitudinal foreshortening. • Clavicle and superior scapular angle are visualized at the same transverse level.	• Straighten the upper midcoronal plane.
• Midscapular body is at the center of the exposure field.	• Center a horizontal CR to the vertebral (medial) border of the scapula, halfway between the inferior scapular and acromial angles.
• Scapula, including the inferior and superior angles, the coracoid and acromion processes, and the proximal humerus, are included within the exposure field.	• Center the IR and grid to the CR. • Open the longitudinal collimation enough to include the acromion process and inferior scapular angles. • Transversely collimate to within 0.5 inches (1.25 cm) of the lateral humeral skin line.

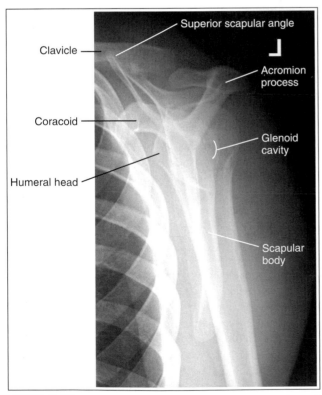

FIGURE 5-47 PA oblique (scapular Y) shoulder projection with accurate positioning.

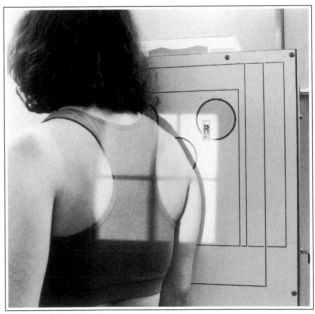

FIGURE 5-48 Proper PA oblique (scapular Y) positioning.

with the scapular body positioned between the acromion and coracoid processes.

If the patient obliquity is not accurate for the scapular Y position, the Y formation of the scapula is not formed, the vertebral and lateral borders of the scapular body are not superimposed but are visualized next to each other, and the glenoid cavity is not demonstrated on end. To determine whether patient obliquity needs to be increased or decreased to superimpose the vertebral and lateral borders of scapular body and position the glenoid cavity

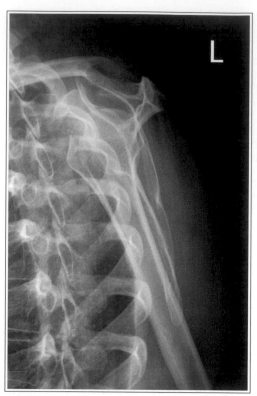

FIGURE 5-49 PA oblique (scapular Y) shoulder projection taken with excessive obliquity.

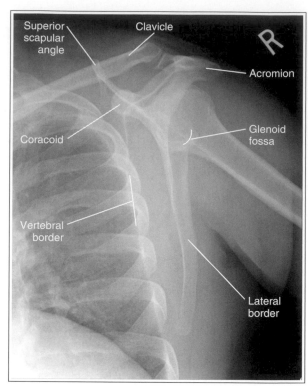

FIGURE 5-50 PA oblique (scapular Y) shoulder projection taken with insufficient obliquity.

on end, identify the borders of the scapula. The lateral border is thick, with two cortical outlines that are separated by approximately 0.25 inch (0.6 cm), whereas the cortical outline of the vertebral border demonstrates a single thin line. If the lateral border is superimposed by the thorax or is positioned closer to the thorax than the vertebral border, the obliquity was excessive (Figure 5-49). If the vertebral border superimposes the thorax or is demonstrated closer to the thorax than the lateral border, patient obliquity was insufficient (Figure 5-50). The glenoid cavity will rotate in the same direction as the lateral border.

Midcoronal Plane. When the upper thoracic spine is straightened and the midcoronal plane is aligned vertically, the scapula body is demonstrated without longitudinal foreshortening and the superior scapular angle and clavicle are demonstrated on the same transverse plane. Longitudinal foreshortening on a PA oblique projection is a result of leaning the patient's upper midcoronal plane and shoulder toward or away from the IR. When the patient is leaning toward the IR, the clavicle is demonstrated inferior to the superior scapular angle (Figure 5-51) When the patient it leaning away from the IR, the clavicle is seen superior to the superior scapular angle (Figure 5-52).

Kyphotic Patient. On a patient with spinal kyphosis the scapula is situated such that longitudinal foreshortening of the body will occur even on an accurately positioned PA oblique projection. To offset this curvature

and obtain a scapula with reduced foreshortening, the CR may be angled until it is aligned perpendicular to the vertebral scapular border. For the PA oblique projection, the angulation would be caudal and, for AP oblique projection, the angulation would be cephalad.

Dislocated Shoulder and Proximal Humeral Fracture. Two indications for the PA oblique projection are to diagnose shoulder dislocations and proximal humeral fractures. When present, these indications will align the glenoid cavity and scapular body with the humeral head and shaft differently as indicated in Table 5-5. This relational change should not be a positioning concern to the imaging technologist. As long as the scapula is positioned in a Y formation, proper positioning has been obtained.

Detecting Shoulder Dislocation. The cortical outline of the glenoid cavity is visible as a circular density at the junction of the coracoid and acromion processes and the scapular body. Normally, the humeral head is superimposed over this junction. When the humeral head is not positioned over the glenoid cavity, a shoulder dislocation exists and will result in positioning of the humeral head anterior or posterior and inferior to the glenoid cavity. An anterior dislocation results in the humeral head being demonstrated anteriorly, beneath the coracoid process (Figure 5-53). A posterior dislocation results in the humeral head being demonstrated posteriorly, beneath the acromion process (Figure 5-54).

Detecting Proximal Humeral Fracture. A PA oblique projection taken of a patient with a proximal

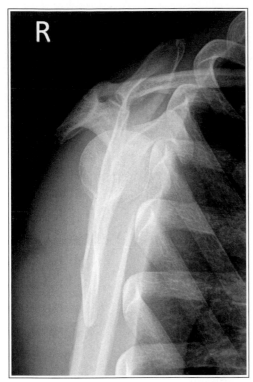

FIGURE 5-51 PA oblique (scapular Y) shoulder projection taken with the upper mid-coronal plane tilted anteriorly.

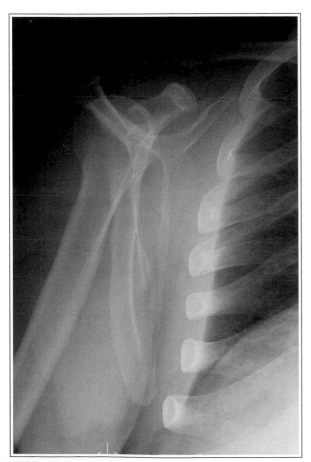

FIGURE 5-52 PA oblique (scapular Y) shoulder projection taken with the upper midcoronal plane tilted posteriorly.

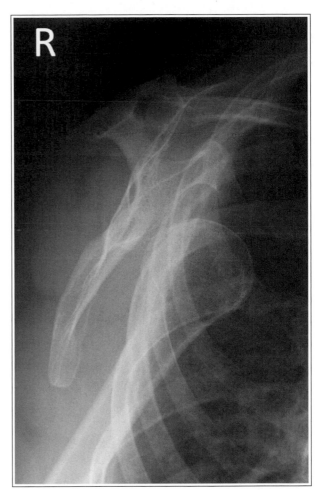

FIGURE 5-53 PA oblique (scapular Y) shoulder projection demonstrating an anterior dislocation.

humeral fracture will typically demonstrate superimposition of the humeral head and glenoid cavity, but the humeral shaft will be positioned anteriorly or posteriorly to the scapular body (Figure 5-55). It is important that correct Y formation of the scapula be accomplished when a fracture is suspected, because poor formation may result in misdiagnosis. Figures 5-55 and 5-56 are projections from the same patient. Compare the accuracy of the scapular Y formation and the alignment of the humeral head and shaft on these projections.

AP Oblique Projection

AP Oblique Projection for the Recumbent Patient.
For a patient who is recumbent and unable to stand, the scapular Y formation can be obtained by means of an AP oblique projection. To position the patient, palpate the acromion and coracoid processes and vertebral scapular borders in the same way as described for the standing PA oblique projection, except rotate the patient toward the unaffected shoulder. The anatomic relationship of the bony structures of the scapula and clavicle should be aligned identically on PA and AP oblique projections. The AP oblique projection, however, demonstrates increased magnification of the scapula and humerus (Figure 5-57).

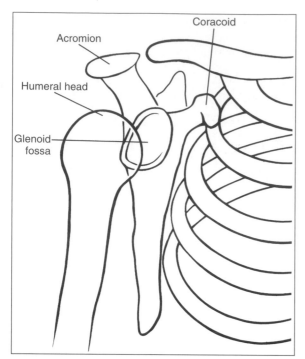

FIGURE 5-54 PA oblique (scapular Y) shoulder projection demonstrating a posterior.

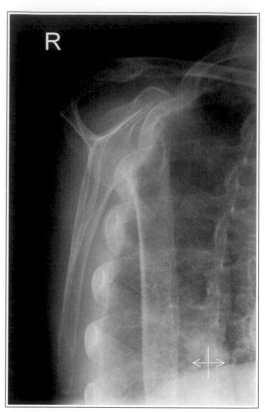

FIGURE 5-55 PA oblique (scapular Y) shoulder projection demonstrating a proximal humeral fracture.

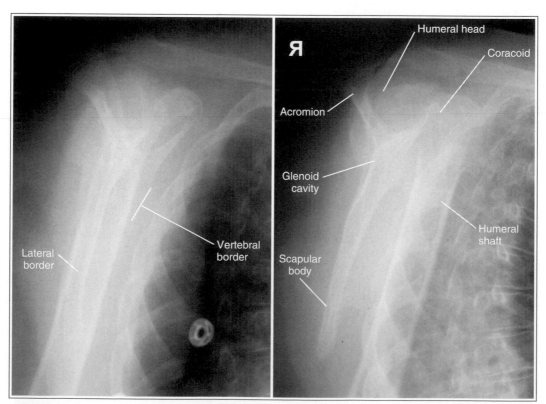

FIGURE 5-56 PA oblique (scapular Y) shoulder projections demonstrating a proximal humeral fracture on the same patient as in Fig. 5-55, with insufficient obliquity and accurate positioning.

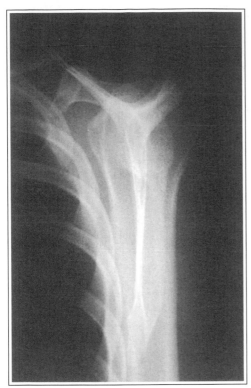

FIGURE 5-57 Properly positioned AP oblique (scapular Y) shoulder projection.

PA Oblique (Scapular Y) Shoulder Analysis Practice

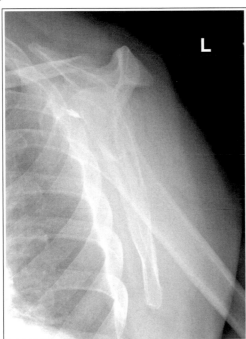

IMAGE 5-8

Analysis. The lateral and vertebral borders of the scapula are demonstrated without superimposition, and the glenoid cavity is not demonstrated on end but is seen laterally. The vertebral scapular borders are

demonstrated next to the ribs. The patient was insufficiently rotated.

Correction. Increase the patient obliquity.

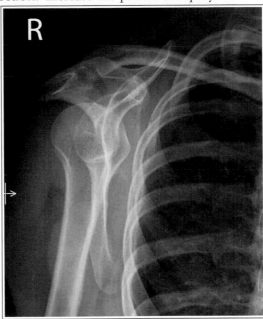

IMAGE 5-9

Analysis. The scapular body, acromion, and coracoid processes are accurately aligned, but the superior scapular angle is demonstrated superior to the clavicle. The scapula is foreshortened. The patient's upper midcoronal plane was leaning toward the IR.

Correction. Straighten the upper midcoronal plane, aligning it parallel with the IR.

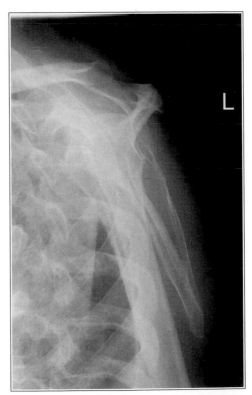

IMAGE 5-10

Analysis. The lateral and vertebral borders of the scapula are demonstrated without superimposition, and the glenoid cavity is not demonstrated on end but is shown medially. The lateral scapular borders are demonstrated next to the ribs. The patient was rotated more than needed to superimpose the borders of the scapular body.

Correction. Decrease the patient obliquity.

PROXIMAL HUMERUS: AP AXIAL PROJECTION (STRYKER "NOTCH" METHOD)

See Table 5-6, (Figures 5-58 and 5-59).

Midcoronal Plane Positioning and Shoulder Rotation. Shoulder rotation on an AP axial projection is detected by evaluating the relationship of the coracoid process with the conoid tubercle (an eminence on the inferior surface of the clavicle to which the conoid ligament is attached). The coracoid process is situated just lateral to the conoid tubercle on a nonrotated projection. If the patient is rotated away from the affected shoulder, the coracoid process is situated medial to this position and more of the glenoid cavity will be demonstrated, and if the patient is rotated toward the affected shoulder, the coracoid process is situated lateral to this position and less of the glenoid cavity will be demonstrated.

Humerus and Humeral Head Positioning. The AP axial projection is taken to diagnose the Hill-Sachs defect of the shoulder. To demonstrate the posterolateral aspect of the humeral head in profile and visualize a Hill-Sachs defect when present, the degree of CR angulation and humeral abduction and the alignment of the humerus with the midsagittal plane must be accurate. To

TABLE 5-6	AP Axial Shoulder Projection (Stryker "Notch" Method)
Image Analysis Guidelines (Figure 5-58)	**Related Positioning Procedures (Figure 5-59)**
• The coracoid process is situated just lateral to the conoid tubercle of the clavicle. • Only a small amount of the glenoid cavity is visualized.	• Position the patient supine in an AP projection with the shoulders at equal distances from the table.
• Posterolateral aspect of the humeral head is in profile laterally. • Greater and lesser tubercles are seen in partial profile, laterally and medially respectively. • Coracoid process superimposes the lateral clavicle.	• Abduct the affected arm until the humerus is vertical (90 degrees with torso and parallel with the midsagittal plane). • Flex the elbow and place the palm of the hand on the top of the patient's head. • Angle the CR 10 degrees cephalically.
• Coracoid process is at the center of the exposure field.	• Center the CR to the coracoid process. The coracoid process must be palpated to determine its location prior to abducting the humerus.
• Humeral head, coracoid process, lateral clavicle, glenoid cavity, and upper third of the scapular body are included within the exposure field.	• Center the IR and grid to the CR. • Open the longitudinal collimated field enough to include the top of the shoulder. • Transversely collimate to within 0.5 inch (1.25 cm) of the lateral humeral skin line.

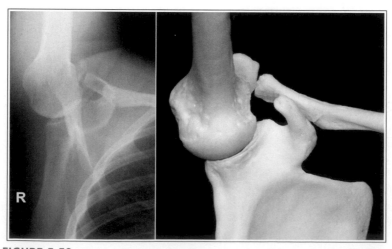

FIGURE 5-58 AP axial (Stryker) shoulder projection with accurate positioning.

distinguish if the poor visualization is caused by poor CR alignment or poor humeral abduction, evaluate the coracoid process and lateral clavicular relationship. When the CR is angled at the correct 10-degree cephalic angulation, the tip of the coracoid process is superimposed over the lateral clavicle. If this relationship is demonstrated, the technologist knows that the correct CR angulation was used and poor visualization of the posterolateral humeral head was caused by poor humeral abduction; and if this relationship is not demonstrated, the technologist knows that the CR was inaccurately set.

Poor Midcoronal Plane Positioning or CR Angulation. If the upper thoracic vertebrae arches upward, causing the upper midcoronal plane to tilt posteriorly, or if less than a 10-degree cephalad CR angle is used,

the coracoid process is demonstrated inferior to the clavicle and the CR will not be properly aligned with the humeral head, obscuring the posterolateral humeral head. The humeral shaft will also demonstrate increased foreshortening (Figure 5-60). If the midcoronal plane is tilted anteriorly or if more than a 10-degree cephalad angle is used, the coracoid process will be demonstrated superior to the clavicle and the humeral shaft will demonstrate decreased foreshortening.

Humeral Abduction. The posterolateral aspect of the humeral head will be obscured when the CR is accurately angled, but the humerus is poorly abducted. If the humerus is abducted beyond vertical, the proximal humerus will be demonstrated with decreased foreshortening (Figure 5-61). If the humerus is abducted to a

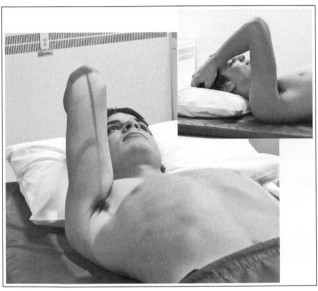

FIGURE 5-59 Proper AP axial (Stryker) shoulder projection positioning.

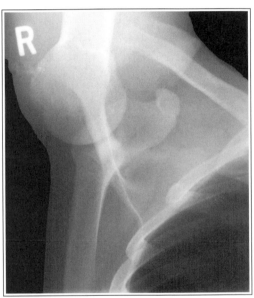

FIGURE 5-60 AP axial (Stryker) shoulder projection taken with inadequate cephalic CR angulation.

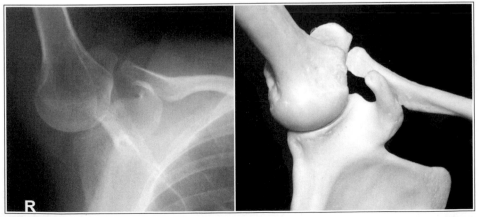

FIGURE 5-61 AP axial (Stryker) shoulder projection taken with the humerus abducted beyond vertical and the distal humerus tilted laterally.

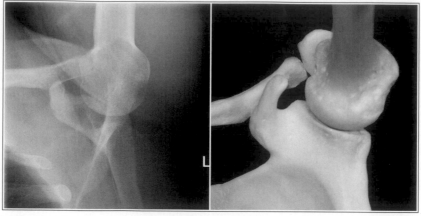

FIGURE 5-62 AP axial (Stryker) shoulder projection taken with the humerus abducted less than vertical.

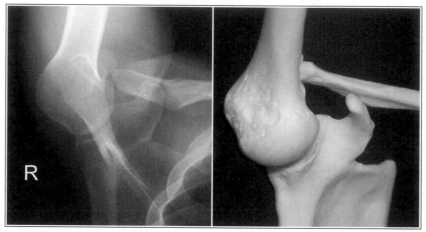

FIGURE 5-63 AP axial (Stryker) shoulder projection with the distal humerus tilted medially.

position that is less than vertical, the humeral shaft will demonstrate increased foreshortening (Figure 5-62).

Distal Humeral Tilting. When the CR is accurately angled and the humerus is accurately abducted, visibility of the posterolateral aspect of the humeral head is also dependent on the degree of medial and lateral tilt of the distal humerus. When the humerus is positioned vertically and parallel with the midsagittal plane, the posterolateral humeral head is demonstrated. If the distal humerus was allowed to tilt laterally the humerus is rotated, the lesser tubercle appears in profile medially, and the greater tubercle and posterolateral humeral head are obscured (see Figure 5-61). If the distal humerus was allowed to tilt medially the lesser tubercle is obscured, and the greater tubercle is demonstrated in profile laterally (Figure 5-63).

AP Axial (Stryker Notch) Shoulder Analysis Practice

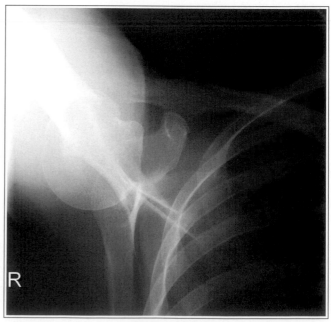

IMAGE 5-11

Analysis. The coracoid process is inferior to the clavicle. The upper thoracic vertebrae were arched upward, causing the upper midcoronal plane to tilt posteriorly or less than a 10-degree cephalic CR angle was used. The humeral shaft demonstrates excessive foreshortening. The humerus was elevated less than vertically. The lesser tubercle is demonstrated in profile and the posterior lateral humeral head is obscured. The humerus was tilted laterally.

Correction. Have patient flatten the upper thoracic vertebrae against the table and assure that a 10-degree cephalic CR angle was used; abduct the humerus to 90 degrees with the torso and align it vertically.

SUPRASPINATUS "OUTLET": TANGENTIAL PROJECTION (NEER METHOD)

See Table 5-7, (Figures 5-64, 5-65, and 5-66).

Arm Position and Shoulder Obliquity. The degree of body obliquity required to obtain a lateral scapula varies with the degree of arm abduction. When the tangential outlet projection is obtained with the patient's arm abducted and hand resting on the hip (Figure 5-66), the shoulder is retracted as the patient is rotated because the IR prevents the humerus from rotating with the body. This shoulder retraction causes the scapula to glide

TABLE 5-7	Tangential Supraspinatus Outlet Projection (Neer Method)
Image Analysis Guidelines (Figure 5-64)	**Related Positioning Procedures (Figures 5-65 and 5-66)**
• Lateral and vertebral scapular borders are superimposed, demonstrating a lateral scapula. • Scapular structures form a Y, with the scapular body as the leg and the acromion and coracoid processes as the arms. • Glenoid cavity is demonstrated on end at the converging point of the arms and leg of the Y.	• Center the shoulder to the upright IR in a PA projection. • Allow the affected arm to freely hang or abduct and rest hand on hip. • Rotate the patient's body toward the affected shoulder until the midcoronal plane is at a 45-degree angle with the IR if the arm is hanging freely or a 60-degree angle with the IR if the arm is abducted.
• Supraspinatus outlet is open and the inferior aspect of the lateral clavicle and acromion are demonstrated in profile. • Lateral clavicle and acromion process form a smooth continuous arch. • Superior scapular angle is at the level of the coracoid process tip and is positioned about 0.5 inch (1.25 cm) inferior to the clavicle.	• Straighten the upper midcoronal plane, aligning it vertically. • Angle the CR 10 to 15 degrees caudally.
• AC joint is at the center of the exposure field. • Acromion process, lateral clavicle, superior scapular spine, coracoid process, and half of the scapular body are included within the exposure field.	• Center the CR to the superior aspect of the humeral head. • Center the IR and grid to the CR. • Open the longitudinal collimation enough to include the acromion process and lateral clavicle. • Transversely collimate to within 0.5 inch (1.25 cm) of the lateral humeral skin line.

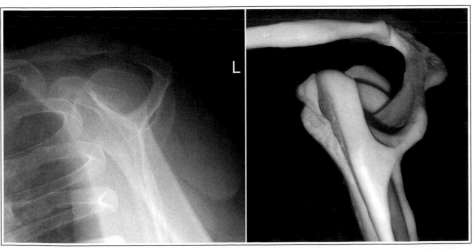

FIGURE 5-64 Tangential (outlet) shoulder projection with accurate positioning.

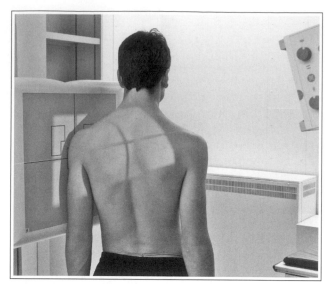

FIGURE 5-65 Proper tangential (outlet) shoulder projection with arm dangling (nonabducted).

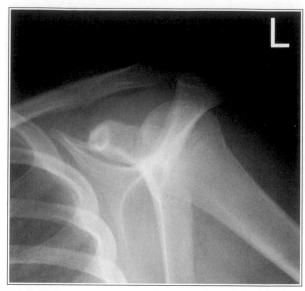

FIGURE 5-67 Tangential (outlet) shoulder projection taken with insufficient obliquity.

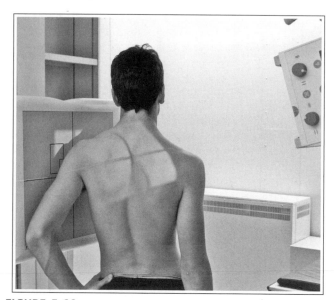

FIGURE 5-66 Proper tangential (outlet) shoulder projection with arm abducted.

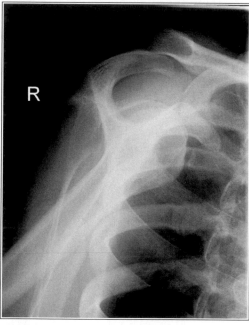

FIGURE 5-68 Tangential (outlet) shoulder projection taken with excessive obliquity.

around the thoracic cavity, moving it toward the spinal column. When the scapula is in this posterior position, the patient's body needs to be rotated more to bring the scapular body to a lateral projection. When the patient's arm is allowed to hang freely for the projection, the shoulder is not retracted, resulting in the scapular body being positioned more anteriorly and therefore requiring less obliquity to bring it into a lateral projection (see Figure 5-65).

If the patient obliquity is not accurate for the tangential projection, the Y formation of the scapula is not attained, the vertebral and lateral borders of the scapular body are not superimposed but are demonstrated next to each other, and the glenoid cavity is not demonstrated

on end. To determine whether patient obliquity needs to be increased or decreased to superimpose the vertebral and lateral borders of the scapular body and position the glenoid cavity on end, identify the borders of the scapula. If the vertebral border superimposes the thorax or is demonstrated closer to the thorax than the lateral border, patient obliquity was insufficient (Figure 5-67). If the lateral border is superimposed by the thorax or is positioned closer to the thorax than the vertebral border, the obliquity was excessive (Figure 5-68). The glenoid cavity will move in the same direction as the lateral scapular border.

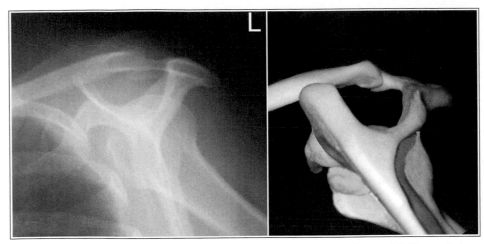

FIGURE 5-69 Tangential (outlet) shoulder projection taken without the caudal CR angulation.

Using Palpable Structures to Determine Accurate Obliquity. The exact degree of obliquity varies with differences in shoulder roundness, which requires decreased obliquity, or humeral abduction and shoulder retraction, which requires increased obliquity. One method of determining the amount of patient obliquity necessary for all types of variations when the arm is allowed to hang freely is to palpate the coracoid process and the acromion angle, and align an imaginary line drawn between them parallel with the IR, positioning the vertebral scapular border between them. This positioning sets up the Y formation, with the scapular body positioned between the acromion and coracoid processes. This method is not reliable when the abducted arm position is used because the increased soft tissue thickness will prevent reliable palpation of the scapular borders.

Midcoronal Plane and CR Alignment. The supraspinatus muscle runs along the supraspinatus fossa, beneath the acromion, and attaches to the greater tubercle. Narrowing of the supraspinatus outlet is caused by a variation in the shape or slope of the acromion or acromioclavicular joint because of spur or osteophyte formations. This narrowing is the primary cause of shoulder impingement and rotator cuff tears. The tangential projection is taken to identify the formation of spurs or osteophytes on the inferior surfaces of the lateral clavicle and acromion process angle. To bring these surfaces in profile so the presences of spur and osteophyte formations can be identified, the midcoronal plane is positioned vertically and the CR angled 10 to 15 degrees caudally and centered to the AC joint. Accurate positioning can be identified by the superior scapular angle being at the level of the coracoid process tip and visible about 0.5 inch (1.25 cm) inferior to the clavicle.

If the tangential outlet projection is taken without the 10- to 15-degree caudal CR angle, with the patient's upper midcoronal plane tilted anteriorly toward the IR, or with the CR centered too inferiorly, the supraspinatus outlet narrows and the superior scapular angle is visualized closer than 0.5 inch (1.25 cm) inferior to the clavicle (Figure 5-69). The supraspinatus outlet will be closed and the superior scapular angle seen superior to the clavicle if the CR is angled in the wrong direction or if the CR is kept horizontal and the upper midcoronal plane is allowed to tilt anteriorly (Figure 5-70).

Tangential (Outlet) Shoulder Analysis Practice

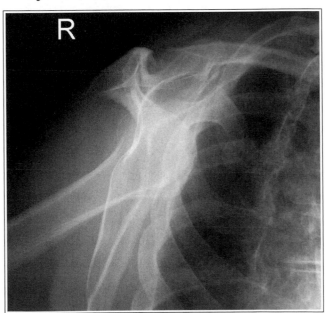

IMAGE 5-12

Analysis. The lateral and vertebral borders of the scapula are demonstrated without superimposition. The lateral border is demonstrated next to the ribs. The patient was rotated more than necessary to superimpose the borders of the scapular body. The supraspinatus outlet is closed and the superior scapular angle is seen superior to the lateral clavicle. The projection was taken without the 10- to 15-degree caudal CR angle or with the patient's upper midcoronal plane tilted anteriorly toward the IR.

Correction. Decrease the degree of patient rotation, ensure that the 10- to 15-degree caudal CR angle was used, and straighten the upper midcoronal plane, aligning it parallel with the IR.

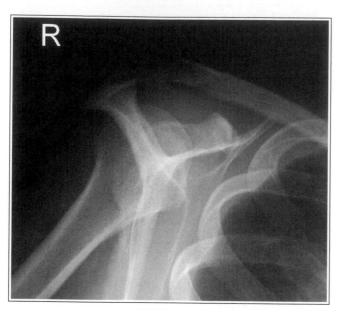

IMAGE 5-13

Analysis. The lateral and vertebral borders of the scapular are demonstrated without superimposition, and the glenoid cavity is not demonstrated on end but is demonstrated laterally. The patient was not rotated enough to superimpose the scapular body.

Correction. Increase the patient obliquity.

CLAVICLE: AP PROJECTION

See Table 5-8, (Figures 5-71 and 5-72).

Midcoronal Plane Positioning and Clavicle Rotation. Rotation and therefore longitudinal foreshortening on an AP clavicle projection is detected by evaluating the relationships of the medial clavicular end with the vertebral column. The medial clavicular end lies next to

TABLE 5-8	AP Clavicle Projection	
Image Analysis Guidelines (Figure 5-71)	**Related Positioning Procedures (Figure 5-72)**
• Medial clavicular end lies next to the lateral edge of the vertebral column.	• Center the midclavicle to the table or upright IR in an AP projection. • Position the shoulders at equal distances from the IR.
• Clavicle and superior scapular angle are visualized at the same transverse level.	• Straighten the upper midcoronal plane, aligning it parallel with the IR.
• Midclavicle is at the center of the exposure field.	• Center a perpendicular CR to the midclavicle.
• Clavicle and the acromion process are included within the exposure field.	• Center the IR and grid to the CR. • Open the longitudinal and transverse collimation enough to include the clavicle.

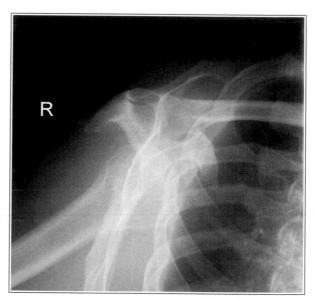

FIGURE 5-70 Tangential (outlet) shoulder projection taken with CR angled cephalically.

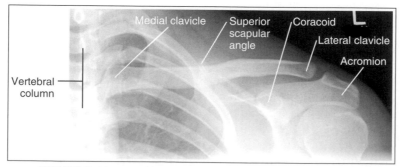

FIGURE 5-71 AP clavicular projection with accurate positioning.

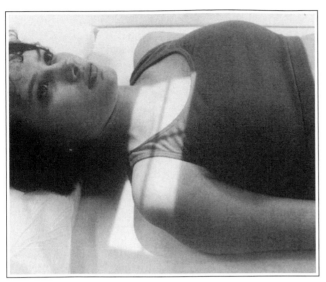

FIGURE 5-72 Proper AP clavicular positioning.

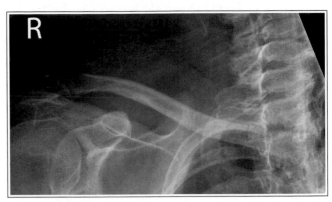

FIGURE 5-73 AP clavicular projection taken with the patient rotated toward the unaffected shoulder.

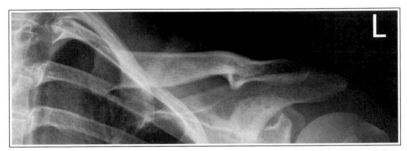

FIGURE 5-74 AP clavicular projection taken with the patient rotated toward the affected shoulder.

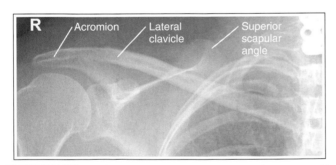

FIGURE 5-75 AP clavicular projection taken with the upper midcoronal plane tilted anteriorly.

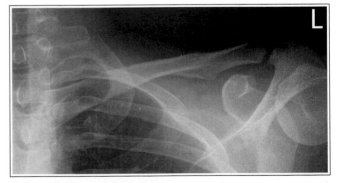

FIGURE 5-76 AP clavicular projection taken with the upper midcoronal plane tilted posteriorly.

the lateral edge of the vertebral column when rotation is not demonstrated on the projection. If the patient is rotated away from the affected clavicle, the medial end of the clavicle is superimposed over the vertebral column (Figure 5-73). If the patient is rotated toward the affected clavicle, the medial end of the clavicle draws away from the vertebral column and the clavicle is longitudinally foreshortened (Figure 5-74).

Midcoronal Plane Tilting. Inferosuperior foreshortening of the clavicle results when the upper midcoronal plane is not positioned parallel with the IR, but instead is allowed to tilt anteriorly or posteriorly. Accurate positioning places the superior scapular angle and clavicle at the same transverse level. If the upper midcoronal plane is tilted anteriorly, the superior scapular angle will be demonstrated superior to the clavicle (Figure 5-75). If the upper midcoronal plane is tilted posteriorly, the superior scapular angle is shown inferior to the clavicle (Figure 5-76).

AP Clavicle Analysis Practice

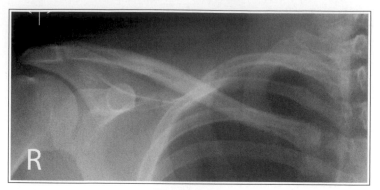

IMAGE 5-14

Analysis. The medial end of the clavicle is drawn away from the lateral edge of the vertebral column. The patient was rotated toward the affected shoulder.

Correction. Rotate the patient away from the affected shoulder until the shoulders are positioned at equal distances from the IR.

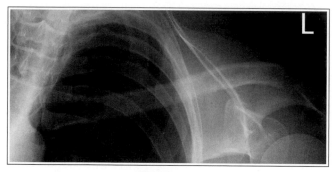

IMAGE 5-15

Analysis. The superior scapular angle is projected superiorly to the midclavicle. The upper midcoronal plane was tilted anteriorly

Correction. Straighten the upper thoracic vertebrae until the mid-coronal plane is aligned parallel with the IR.

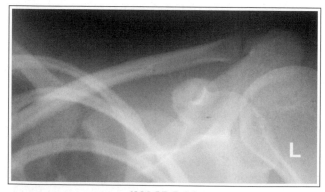

IMAGE 5-16

Analysis. The superior scapular angle is projected inferiorly to the midclavicle. The upper midcoronal plane was tilted posteriorly. The medial clavicular is not

included on the projection. The CR was positioned too laterally.

Correction. Straighten the upper thoracic vertebrae until the midcoronal plane is aligned parallel with the IR, center the CR approximately 1 inch (2.5 cm) medially, and open collimation enough to include the medial end of the clavicle.

CLAVICLE: AP AXIAL PROJECTION (LORDOTIC POSITION)

See Table 5-9, (Figures 5-77 and 5-78).

Midcoronal Plane Positioning and Clavicle Rotation. Rotation on an AP axial clavicle projection is detected by evaluating the relationships of the medial clavicular end with the vertebral column. If the patient is rotated away from the affected clavicle, the medial end of the clavicle is superimposed over the vertebral column. If the patient is rotated toward the affected clavicle, the medial end of the clavicle is drawn away from the vertebral column and the clavicle is longitudinally foreshortened (see Figures 5-73 and 5-74) Rotation on the AP and AP axial clavicle projections are similar, but the clavicle on the AP axial projection would be situated more superiorly on the thorax.

CR Angulation. A 15- to 30-degree cephalic CR angle is used on the axial projection of the clavicle to project

TABLE 5-9	AP Axial Clavicle Projection	
Image Analysis Guidelines (Figure 5-77)	**Related Positioning Procedures (Figure 5-78)**
• Medial clavicular end lies next to the lateral edge of the vertebral column.	• Center the midclavicle to the table or upright IR in an AP projection. • Position the shoulders at equal distances from the IR.
• Superior scapular angle is visualized 0.5 inch (1.25 cm) inferior to the clavicle.	• Straighten the upper midcoronal plane, aligning it parallel with the IR.
• Medial end of clavicle is superimposed over the first, second, or third rib. • Middle and lateral thirds of clavicle are seen superior to the acromion process and the clavicle bows upwardly.	• Angle the CR 15-30 degrees cephalically.
• Midclavicle is at the center of the exposure field. • Clavicle and the acromion process are included within the exposure field.	• Center the CR to the midclavicle. • Center the IR and grid to the CR. • Open the longitudinal and transverse collimation enough to include the clavicle

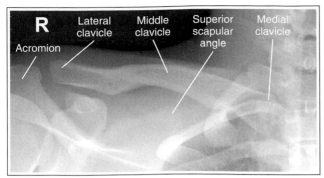

FIGURE 5-77 AP axial clavicular projection with accurate positioning.

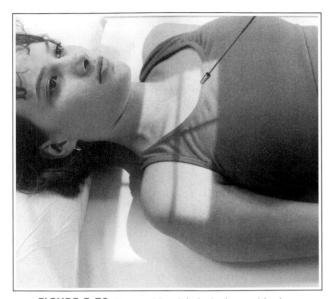

FIGURE 5-78 Proper AP axial clavicular positioning.

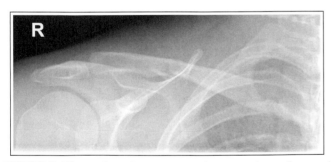

FIGURE 5-79 AP clavicular projection demonstrating a fractured clavicle.

more of the clavicle superior to the thorax region and to demonstrate the degree of fracture displacement, when present. Even though the amount of angulation used may vary among radiology departments, all projections result in superior movement of the clavicle. The larger the angle, the more superiorly the clavicle is projected. Ideally, because 80% of clavicle fractures occur at the middle third and 15% at the lateral third, the CR should be angled enough to project the lateral and middle thirds of the clavicle superior to the thorax and scapula. Compare the projections in Figures 5-79 and 5-80, and

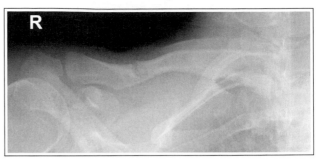

FIGURE 5-80 AP axial clavicular projection demonstrating a fractured clavicle.

note how an increase in cephalic angulation has projected the lateral and middle thirds of the clavicle above the scapula. The clavicle fracture demonstrated on these projections is obvious, but a subtle nondisplaced fracture could be obscured by the scapular structures if an AP axial projection were not included in the examination.

ACROMIOCLAVICULAR (AC) JOINT: AP PROJECTION

See Table 5-10, (Figures 5-81, 5-82, 5-83, and 5-84).

Exam Indication. To evaluate the AC joint for possible injury to the AC ligament, which extends between the lateral clavicular end and the acromion process, the AP projection is taken first without weights. Then a second AP projection is taken with the patient holding 5- to 8-lb weights (Figure 5-84). If injury to the AC ligament has occurred, the AC joint space is wider on the weight-bearing projection than on the projection taken without weights. For the weight-bearing projection, equal weights should be attached to the arms, regardless of whether the examination is unilateral (one side) or bilateral (both sides), keeping the shoulders on the same transverse plane. Attach the weights to the patient's wrists or slide them onto the patient's forearms after the elbows are flexed to 90 degrees, and instruct the patient to allow the weights to depress the shoulders.

Midcoronal Plane Positioning and Clavicle Rotation. Rotation on an AP AC joint projection is detected by evaluating the relationships of the lateral clavicle with the acromion apex and of the scapular body with the thoracic cavity. If the patient was rotated toward the affected AC joint, the lateral end of the clavicle and the acromion apex are rotated out of profile, resulting in a narrowed or closed AC joint. The thoracic cavity also moves toward the scapular body, increasing the amount of scapular body superimposition (Figure 5-85, right shoulder). If the patient is rotated away from the affected AC joint, the lateral end of the clavicle and the acromion apex demonstrate a slightly greater AC joint space with only a small amount of rotation and may be closed with a greater degree of rotation. The scapular body demonstrates decreased thoracic cavity superimposition (see Figure 5-85, left shoulder).

TABLE 5-10 | **AP Acromioclavicular Joint Projection**

Image Analysis Guidelines (Figures 5-81 and 5-82)	Related Positioning Procedures (Figures 5-83 and 5-84)
• Lateral clavicle is horizontal. • About 0.125 inch (0.3 cm) of space is present between the lateral clavicle and acromial apex. • Lateral clavicle demonstrates minimal acromion process superimposition. • Clavicle and the superior scapular angle are demonstrated at the same transverse level.	• Center the AC joint to the upright IR in an AP projection. • Position the shoulders at equal distances from the IR. • Places shoulders on the same transverse plane. • Position the midcoronal plane vertically, aligning it parallel with the IR.
• AC joint is at the center of the exposure field for both the non–weight-bearing and weight-bearing exposures.	• Center a perpendicular CR to the AC joint of interest.
• Lateral clavicle, acromion process and superior scapular angle are included within the exposure field.	• Center the IR to the CR. • Open the longitudinally and transversely collimated field to include one half of the clavicle and the coracoid process.
• A word or arrow marker, point downward, is present on projection that was obtained with the patient holding weights.	• Obtain an AP projection without weights and one with the patient holding 5-8 lb weights. • Place a word or arrow marker on the IR to indicate the projection that was obtained with the patient holding weights.

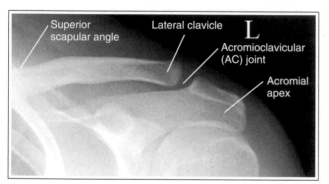

FIGURE 5-81 AP acromioclavicular joint projection (without weights) with accurate positioning.

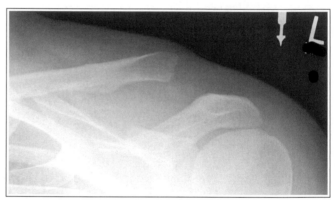

FIGURE 5-82 AP acromioclavicular joint projection (with weights) with accurate positioning.

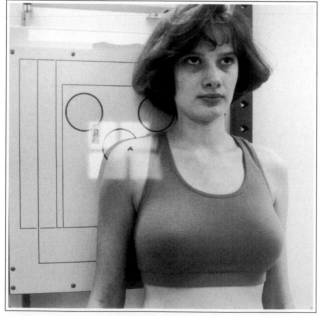

FIGURE 5-83 Proper AP acromioclavicular joint positioning (without weights).

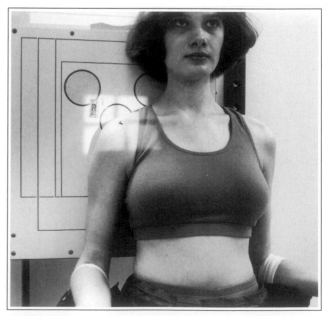

FIGURE 5-84 Proper AP acromioclavicular joint positioning (with weights).

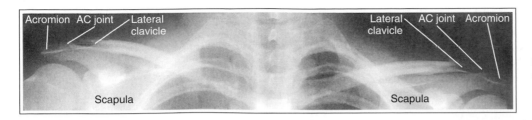

FIGURE 5-85 Bilateral AP acromioclavicular joint projection demonstrating rotation.

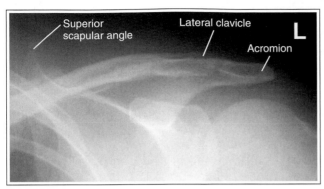

FIGURE 5-86 AP acromioclavicular joint projection taken with the upper midcoronal plane tilted anteriorly.

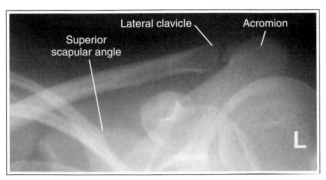

FIGURE 5-87 AP acromioclavicular joint projection taken with the upper midcoronal plane tilted posteriorly.

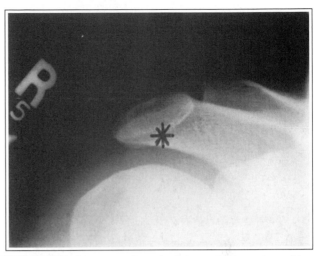

FIGURE 5-88 AP acromioclavicular joint projection taken without weights and showing good centering. Star indicates location of central ray.

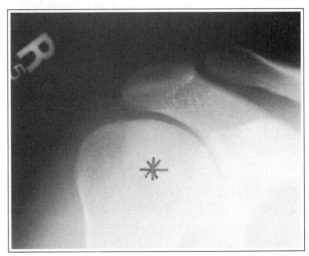

FIGURE 5-89 AP acromioclavicular joint projection taken with weights and showing poor centering. Star indicates location of central ray.

Midcoronal Plane Tilting. Inferosuperior foreshortening of the clavicle and acromion process results when the upper midcoronal plane is allowed to tilt anteriorly or posteriorly. When the projection is obtained with the midcoronal plane tilted, the clavicle and the acromion process are imaged at an angle instead of the desired AP projection, changing the relationships between clavicle and superior scapular angle and the lateral clavicle and acromion process and potentially obscuring an AC ligament injury. This mispositioning is best identified when the superior scapular angle is included on the projection. If the upper midcoronal plane is tilted anteriorly, the lateral clavicle will demonstrate increased acromion process superimposition and the superior scapular angle will be demonstrated superior to the clavicle (Figure 5-86). If the upper midcoronal plane is tilted posteriorly, the lateral clavicle will demonstrate decreased acromion process superimposition and the superior scapular angle will be visible inferior to the clavicle (Figure 5-87).

Kyphotic Patient. For the kyphotic patient a cephalic CR angulation can be used to offset the forward angle

of the scapula. The CR should be angled enough to align it perpendicular to the scapular body.

CR Centering. Because the shoulders are depressed when weights are used, the AC joint moves inferiorly when the patient is given weights for the second exposure. Repalpate for the AC joint on this projection to ensure that the CR is centered at the same location for both without and with weight projections. Failure to center in the same location for both projections may result in a false separation reading as the x-ray beam divergence transverses the AC joint differently. Compare Figures 5-88 and 5-89, which are projections of the same patient, taken without weights and with weights, respectively. Because the CR was not centered in the same location, it is uncertain whether the separation demonstrated on the weight-bearing projection is a result of ligament injury or poor CR centering. The AC joint is located by palpating along the clavicle until the most lateral tip is reached, and then moving about 0.5 inch (1 cm) inferiorly.

Exam Variations

AP Axial Projection (Alexander Method). An AP axial projection (Alexander Method) of the AC joint is taken with a 15-degree cephalic CR angle centered at the level of the AC joint. This projection demonstrates the AC joint superior to the acromion process.

Bilateral AC Joint Projection. See Figure 5-90.

Some facilities obtain bilateral projections of the AC joint as a routine. For this, place the patient in an upright AP projection with shoulders at equal distance to the upright IR and the midcoronal plane vertical. Center the midsagittal plane to the center of the IR and then center a perpendicular CR to the midsagittal plane at a level

1-inch (2.5 cm) superior to the jugular notch. Open the longitudinally collimated field to approximately a 5-inch (10-cm) field size and transversely collimate the full IR length. Make an exposure without weights and an exposure with weights. The unilateral AC joint method is recommended over this bilateral because it reduces exposure to the thyroid and uses less diverged x-rays to record the AC joints. If the bilateral method is used, a long 72-inch (183 cm) SID is used to reduce magnification and allow both joints to fit on one IR.

SCAPULA: AP PROJECTION

See Table 5-11, (Figures 5-91 and 5-92).

Humeral Abduction. Abduction of the humerus is accomplished by combined movements of the shoulder joint and rotation of the scapula around the thoracic cage. The ratio of movement in these two articulations is two parts glenohumeral to one part scapulothoracic. When the arm is abducted, the lateral scapula is drawn from beneath the thoracic cavity and the glenoid cavity

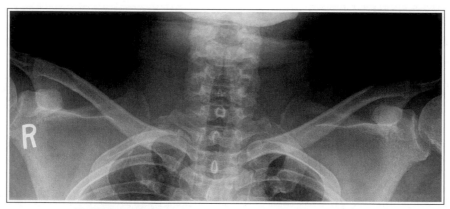

FIGURE 5-90 Bilateral AP acromioclavicular joint projection.

TABLE 5-11	AP Scapula Projection
Image Analysis Guidelines (Figure 5-91)	**Related Positioning Procedures (Figure 5-92)**
• Anterior and posterior margins of the glenoid cavity are nearly superimposed.	• Place the patient in a supine AP projection, with the scapula centered to the IR.
• Lateral scapular border is seen without thoracic cavity superimposition, while the thoracic cavity is superimposing the vertebral border.	• Abduct the affected arm to 90 degrees with the torso.
• Superior scapular angle is seen without clavicular superimposition.	• Flex the elbow and rotate the arm externally, resting the forearm against the table.
• Humeral shaft demonstrates 90 degrees of abduction.	
• Scapula is demonstrated without longitudinal foreshortening.	• Align the upper midcoronal plane parallel with the IR.
• Superior scapular angle is slightly (0.25 inch [0.6 cm]) inferior to the clavicle.	
• Midscapular body is at the center of the exposure field.	• Center a perpendicular CR 2 inches (5 cm) inferior to the coracoid process.
• Scapula is included within the exposure field.	• Center the IR and grid to the CR.
	• Open the longitudinal collimation to the top of the shoulder.
	• Transversely collimate to within 0.5 inch (1.25 cm) of the lateral body skin line.
• Scapular structures situated in the thorax demonstrate adequate contrast resolution.	• Take the exposure after suspended expiration.

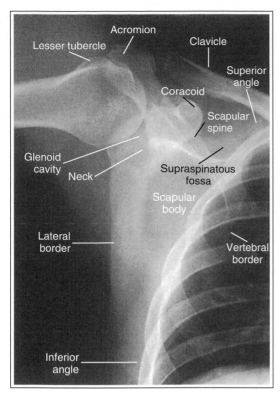

FIGURE 5-91 AP scapular projection with accurate positioning.

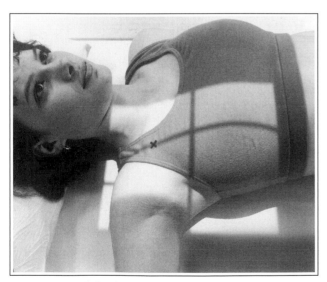

FIGURE 5-92 Proper AP scapular positioning.

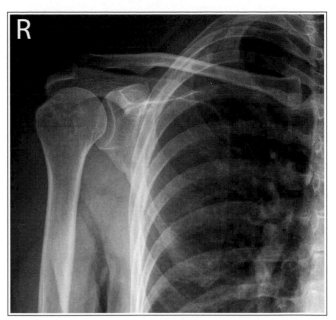

FIGURE 5-93 AP scapular projection taken without abduction.

moves superiorly. Because the first 60 degrees of humeral abduction involves primarily movement of the glenohumeral joint without accompanying scapular movement, it takes at least 90 degrees of humeral abduction to demonstrate the lateral border of the scapula without thoracic cavity superimposition, and the supraspinatus fossa and superior angle without clavicle superimposition. The farther the arm is abducted, the more of the lateral scapular body that is demonstrated without thoracic cavity superimposition. With less than 60 degrees of humeral abduction, the inferolateral border of the

scapula is superimposed by the thoracic cavity and the clavicle is superimposed over the superior scapular angle (Figure 5-93).

Shoulder Retraction. In an AP projection with the patient's arm placed against the side, the scapular body is placed at a 35- to 45-degree angle with the IR. This positioning results in the projection demonstrating transverse foreshortening of the scapular body. To reduce this transverse foreshortening and better visualize the scapular body the humerus is abducted, the elbow is flexed, and the hand is supinated by rotating the arm externally (see Figure 5-92). The humeral abduction causes the scapula to glide around the thoracic surface, moving the inferior scapular angle and lateral scapular body from beneath the thorax. The elbow flexion and hand supination cause the shoulder to retract by placing pressure on the lateral aspect of the scapular body that will result in it moving posteriorly and the scapular body foreshortening to decrease. To take advantage of gravity and obtain maximum shoulder retraction, the projection is taken with the patient in a supine position. Poor retraction of the shoulder is identified by evaluating the foreshortening of the scapular body and glenoid cavity. If the patient's arm is not sufficiently abducted and the shoulder retracted, the scapular body demonstrates excessive foreshortening and the glenoid cavity is demonstrated somewhat on end (Figure 5-94).

Midcoronal Plane Tilting. Longitudinal foreshortening of the scapular body is caused by poor midcoronal plane positioning and may result when the AP scapular projection is taken with the patient in the upright position or when the patient is kyphotic. Foreshortening is prevented by straightening the upper thoracic vertebrae and positioning the midcoronal plane parallel with the IR. A longitudinally foreshortened scapula can be identified on

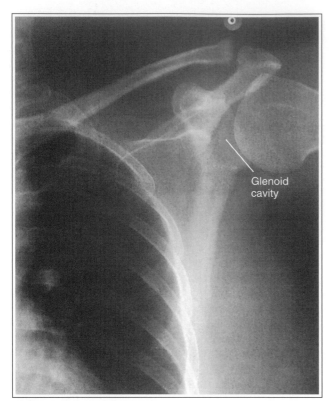

FIGURE 5-94 AP scapular projection taken without adequate shoulder retraction.

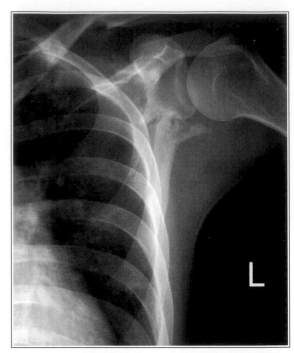

FIGURE 5-95 AP scapular projection demonstrating a scapular fracture.

an AP scapular projection that has the arm adequately abducted when the superior scapular angle is more or less than 0.25 inch (0.6 cm) inferior to the clavicle. When the superior scapular angle is demonstrated less than 0.25 inch (0.6 cm) from the clavicle, the upper midcoronal plane was tilted anteriorly. When the superior scapular angle appears more than 0.25 inch (0.6 cm) inferior to the clavicle, the upper midcoronal plane was tilted posteriorly.

Kyphotic Patient. Longitudinal foreshortening of the scapular body on the kyphotic patient can be improved by angling the CR cephalically until it is perpendicular to the scapular body.

Respiration. Although the AP thickness is approximately the same across the entire scapula, the overall brightness is not uniform. On AP scapular projections, the medial portion of the scapula, which is superimposed by the thoracic cavity, demonstrates less brightness than the lateral scapula, which is superimposed by the soft tissue of the shoulder girdle. This brightness difference is a result of the difference in atomic density that exists between the air-filled thoracic cavity and the bony shoulder structures. The thoracic cavity is largely composed of air, which contains very few atoms in a given area, whereas the shoulder structures contain a higher concentration of atoms. As the radiation goes through the patient's body, fewer photons are absorbed in the thoracic cavity than in the shoulder girdle, because there are fewer atoms with which the photons can interact.

Consequently, more photons penetrate the thoracic cavity to expose the IR than penetrate the shoulder girdle. Taking the exposure on expiration can help increase the contrast resolution in the portion of the scapula that is superimposed by the thoracic cavity by reducing the air and slightly compressing the tissue in this area.

Exam Variations

Breathing Technique. Patient respiration also determines how well the scapular details are demonstrated. Some positioning textbooks suggest that a breathing technique be used to better visualize the vertebral border and medial scapular body through the air-filled lungs. Although visualization of this anatomy would be improved with such a technique, it is difficult to obtain a long enough exposure time (3 seconds) to blur the ribs and vascular lung markings adequately when the overall exposure necessary for an AP scapula projection is so small. If an adequate exposure time cannot be set to use the breathing technique, the exposure should be taken on expiration.

Positioning for Trauma. Trauma patients often experience great pain with arm abduction. Because of this pain, the abduction movement may take place almost entirely at the glenohumeral articulation, instead of involving the combined movements of the glenohumeral and scapulothoracic articulations. When the scapulothoracic articulation is not involved with the movement of humeral abduction, the inferolateral border and inferior angle of the scapula may remain superimposed by the thoracic cavity, and the supraspinatus fossa and superior border may remain superimposed by the clavicle (Figure 5-95). In this situation, little can be done to draw the scapula away from the thoracic cavity, although the exposure can be taken on expiration and a decrease in exposure used that will better demonstrate the parts of the scapula superimposed by the thorax. An AP scapular body projection can be obtained in a trauma situation by using the AP oblique (Grashey) shoulder projection, as discussed earlier in this chapter. In this projection the patient is rotated toward the affected shoulder, bringing the scapula body AP. If the arm is not adequately abducted and the scapula does not move from beneath the thorax, the CR should be centered 0.5 inch (1 cm) more medial.

AP Scapular Analysis Practice

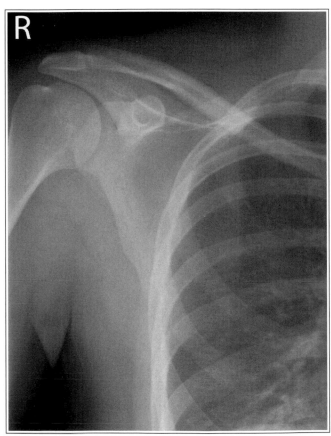

IMAGE 5-17

Analysis. The inferolateral border of the scapula is superimposed by the thoracic cavity, and the superior angle is superimposed by the clavicle. The humerus was not adequately abducted.
Correction. Abduct the humerus to a 90-degree angle with the torso.

SCAPULA: LATERAL PROJECTION (LATEROMEDIAL OR MEDIOLATERAL)

See Table 5-12, (Figures 5-96, 5-97, and 5-98).
Humerus Positioning. Eighty percent of scapular fractures involve the body or neck of the scapula. The neck

TABLE 5-12 | Lateral Scapula Projection

Image Analysis Guidelines (Figure 5-96)	Related Positioning Procedures (Figures 5-97 and 5-98)
• Superior scapular angle and clavicle are at the same transverse level.	• *Upright PA Projection:* Center the shoulder to the upright IR in a PA projection. • *Supine AP Projection:* Position the patient in a supine AP projection, with the shoulder centered to the IR. • Straighten the upper midcoronal plane, aligning it parallel with the IR.
• Scapular body is in a lateral projection, with superimposed lateral and vertebral scapular borders. • Scapular body and thoracic cavity are not superimposing.	• Draw the affected arm across the chest so that the hand can grasp the unaffected shoulder. • Abduct the humerus to 90 degrees or allow the humerus to rest against the chest per facility requirements. • *PA Projection:* Rotate patient toward affected shoulder until the midcoronal plane is at a 45- to 60-degree angle with IR. • *AP Projection:* Rotate patient away from the affected shoulder until the midcoronal plane is at a 45- to 60-degree angle with IR.
• Midscapular body is at the center of the exposure field.	• Center a perpendicular CR to the midscapular body.
• Entire scapula is included within the exposure field.	• Center the IR and grid to the CR. • Open the longitudinal collimation enough to include both the acromion and inferior scapular angles. • Transversely collimate to within 0.5 inch (1.25 cm) of the lateral skin line.

of the scapula is best visualized on the AP projection, because it is demonstrated on end in the lateral projection. If a fracture of the scapular body is present or suspected, the lateral projection is taken to demonstrate the anterior and the posterior alignment of the fracture. To demonstrate the scapular body best, position its long axis parallel with the long axis of the IR by abducting the humerus to a 90-degree angle with the patient's body (Figures 5-98 and 5-99). This positioning causes the scapula to glide anteriorly around the thoracic cavity and tilts the glenoid fossa slightly upward, placing the long axis of the scapular body parallel with the IR (see Figure 5-96). The humerus is also drawn away from the superior scapular body, allowing it to be visualized without humeral superimposition.

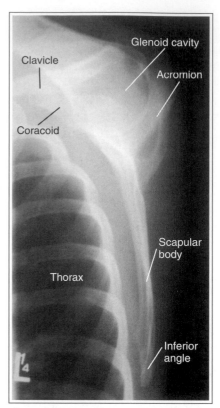

FIGURE 5-96 Lateral scapular projection taken with the arm abducted to 90 degrees and the long axis of the scapular body aligned parallel with the IR.

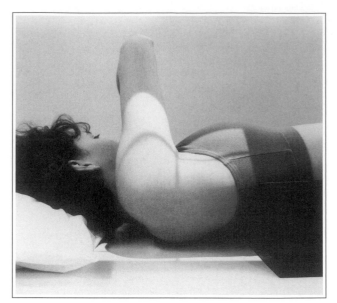

FIGURE 5-98 Lateral scapular positioning with the arm abducted to 90 degrees.

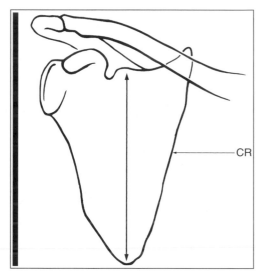

FIGURE 5-99 Long axis of scapular body parallel with image receptor. *CR,* Central ray.

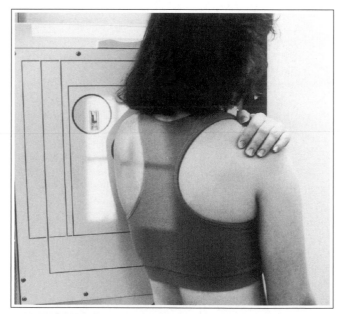

FIGURE 5-97 Proper standing lateral scapular positioning.

If the humerus is not abducted but rests on the patient's chest, with the patient still grasping the opposite shoulder, the vertebral border of the scapula is positioned parallel with the IR (Figures 5-100 and 5-101). This arm positioning produces a projection similar to that obtained for the PA oblique (scapular Y) projection, where the superior scapular body is superimposed over the glenoid cavity and the proximal humerus, the coracoid and acromion processes are visible in profile, and the glenoid cavity is demonstrated on-end (Figure 5-102). If humeral abduction is increased above 90 degrees, with the patient still grasping the opposite shoulder, the lateral border of the scapula is placed parallel with the IR (Figures 5-103 and 5-104). This positioning distorts the superior scapular body and demonstrates the superior scapular angle and scapular spine below the coracoid and acromion processes, respectively (Figure 5-105).

Midcoronal Plane Positioning and Scapular Obliquity. The degree of body obliquity required to superimpose the scapular borders depends on the degree of humeral abduction. As the humerus is abducted, the

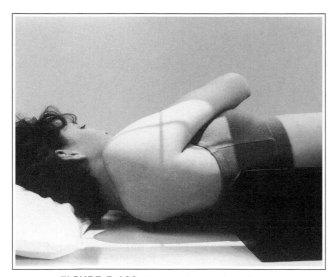

FIGURE 5-100 Arm resting against thorax.

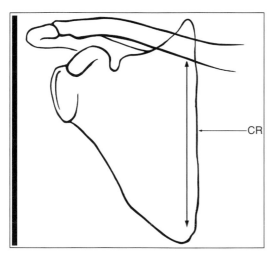

FIGURE 5-101 Vertebral border of scapula parallel with image receptor. *CR,* Central ray.

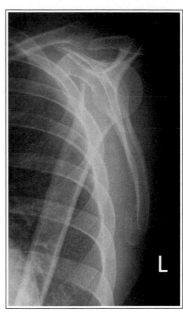

FIGURE 5-102 Lateral scapular projection taken with the arm resting on the patient's chest and the vertebral border of the scapular positioned parallel with the IR.

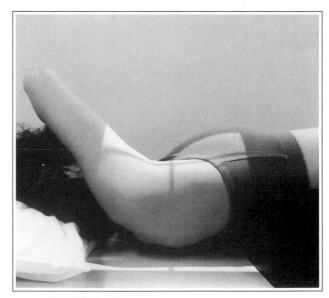

FIGURE 5-103 Arm elevated above 90 degrees.

inferior angle of the scapula glides around the thoracic cage, moving the scapula more anteriorly. The more the humerus is abducted, the more the scapula glides around the thorax and the less body obliquity that is needed to superimpose the vertebral and lateral scapular borders. One method of determining the degree of body rotation needed for all arm positions is to use the palpable lateral and vertebral scapular borders. Because the superior portions of the lateral and vertebral borders are heavily covered with muscles, it is best to palpate them just superior to the inferior scapular angle. Adjusting the degree of arm abduction while palpating will move the location of the inferior angle and help in locating the inferior angle and scapular borders. Once the scapular borders are located, position the arm in the desired degree of abduction and rotate the body until the vertebral border of the scapula is superimposed over the lateral border and the inferior scapular angle is positioned in profile.

Detecting Inaccurate Obliquity. If the body was not accurately rotated for a lateral scapular projection, the borders of the scapula are not superimposed. When such a projection has been produced, one can determine whether patient obliquity was excessive or insufficient by identifying the scapular borders. If the lateral border is superimposed by the thorax or is positioned closer to the thorax than the vertebral border, the obliquity was insufficient (Figure 5-106). If the vertebral border superimposes the thorax or is demonstrated closer to the thorax than the lateral border, patient obliquity was excessive (Figure 5-107).

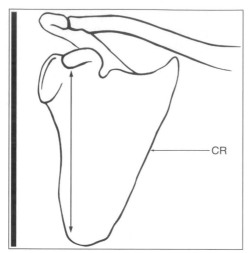

FIGURE 5-104 Lateral border of scapula parallel with image receptor. *CR,* Central ray.

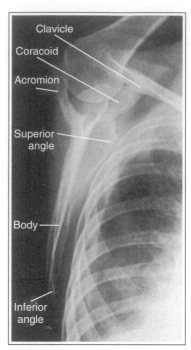

FIGURE 5-105 Lateral scapular projection taken with the arm elevated above 90 degrees and the lateral borders of scapula positioned parallel with the IR.

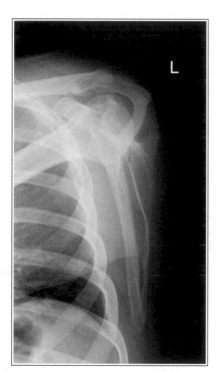

FIGURE 5-106 Lateral scapular projection taken with insufficient obliquity.

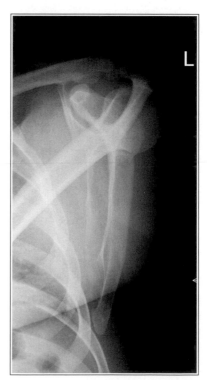

FIGURE 5-107 Lateral scapular projection taken with excessive obliquity.

Lateral Scapular Analysis Practice

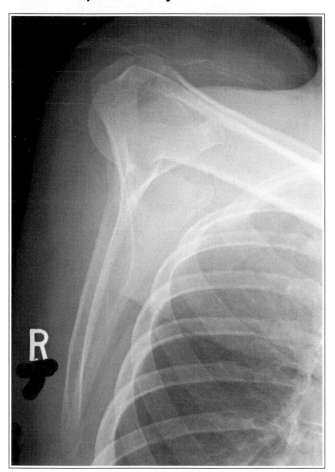

IMAGE 5-18

Analysis. The lateral and vertebral borders of the scapular demonstrate without superimposition. The vertebral border is demonstrated next to the ribs. The patient was insufficiently rotated.

Correction. Increase the degree of patient obliquity.

Lower Extremity

OUTLINE

Toe: AP Axial Projection, 279
  AP Axial Toe Analysis
    Practice, 283
Toe: AP Oblique Projection, 284
  AP Oblique Toe Analysis
    Practice, 286
Toe: Lateral Projection (Mediolateral
  and Lateromedial), 286
  Lateral Toe Analysis
    Practice, 289
Foot: AP Axial Projection
  (Dorsoplantar), 290
  AP Axial Foot Analysis
    Practice, 294
Foot: AP Oblique Projection
  (Medial Rotation), 294
  AP Oblique Foot Analysis
    Practice, 297
Foot: Lateral Projection
  (Mediolateral and
  Lateromedial), 298
  Lateral Foot Analysis
    Practice, 304
Calcaneus: Axial Projection
  (Plantodorsal), 305
  Axial Calcaneal Analysis
    Practice, 307

Calcaneus: Lateral Projection
  (Mediolateral), 308
  Lateral Calcaneal Analysis
    Practice, 311
Ankle: AP Projection, 311
  AP Ankle Analysis Practice, 313
Ankle: AP Oblique Projection
  (Medial Rotation), 314
  AP Oblique Ankle Analysis
    Practice, 317
Ankle: Lateral Projection
  (Mediolateral), 318
  Lateral Ankle Analysis
    Practice, 322
Lower Leg: AP Projection, 322
  AP Lower Leg Analysis
    Practice, 324
Lower Leg: Lateral Projection
  (Mediolateral), 325
  Lateral Lower Leg Analysis
    Practice, 328
Knee: AP Projection, 328
  AP Knee Analysis Practice, 333
Knee: AP Oblique Projection
  (Medial and Lateral Rotation), 333
  AP Oblique Knee Analysis
    Practice, 337

Knee: Lateral Projection
  (Mediolateral), 337
  Lateral Knee Analysis
    Practice, 344
Intercondylar Fossa: PA Axial
  Projection (Holmblad
  Method), 345
  PA Axial Knee Analysis
    Practice, 348
Intercondylar Fossa: AP Axial
  Projection (Béclère Method), 348
Patella and Patellofemoral Joint:
  Tangential Projection (Merchant
  Method), 351
  Tangential (Merchant) Patella
    Analysis Practice, 355
Femur: AP Projection, 355
  Distal Femur, 355
  Proximal Femur, 357
  AP Femur Analysis
    Practice, 359
Femur: Lateral Projection
  (Mediolateral), 360
  Proximal Femur, 362
  Lateral Femur Image Analysis
    Practice, 365

OBJECTIVES

After completion of this chapter, you should be able to do the following:

- Identify the required anatomy on lower extremity projections.
- Describe how to position the patient, image receptor (IR), and central ray (CR) for proper lower extremity projections.
- List the image analysis requirements for accurate positioning for lower extremity projections.
- State how to reposition the patient properly when lower extremity projections with poor positioning are produced.
- Discuss how to determine the amount of patient or CR adjustment required to improve lower extremity projections with poor positioning.
- State the kilovoltage routinely used for lower extremity projections, and describe which anatomic structures are visible when the correct technique factors are used.
- Describe which aspects of a toe's phalanges are concave and which are convex.

- State how the CR angulation is adjusted for an AP axial toe projection when the patient is unable to extend the toe fully.
- Discuss how the degree of CR angulation is adjusted for an AP axial foot projection and how the degree of obliquity is adjusted for an AP oblique foot projection in patients with high and low longitudinal arches.
- State how one can determine from two different patients' AP oblique foot projections which patient's foot has the higher longitudinal arch.
- State how the height of a patient's longitudinal arch can be evaluated on a lateral foot projection.
- State which anatomic structures are referred to as the *talar domes* on a lateral foot, calcaneal, or ankle projection.
- Describe how the CR angulation is adjusted when a patient is unable to dorsiflex the foot for an axial calcaneal projection.

- State how the medial and lateral talar domes can be identified on a lateral foot, calcaneal, or ankle projection with poor positioning.
- Explain why the IR must extend beyond the knee and ankle joints when the lower leg is imaged.
- Explain how the patient is positioned if only one of the joints can be in the true position for AP or lateral lower leg projections.
- Explain how the CR angulation used for AP and oblique knee projections is determined by the thickness of the patient's upper thigh and buttocks, and discuss why this adjustment is required.
- Describe a valgus and a varus knee deformity.
- State how to determine what CR angulation to use for an AP knee projection in a patient who cannot fully extend the knee.
- Describe a patella subluxation, and state how it is demonstrated on an AP knee projection.
- State which anatomic structures are placed in profile on medial and lateral oblique knee projections with accurate positioning.
- List the soft tissue structures of interest found on lower leg projections. State where they are located and why their visualization is important.
- State how the patient's knee is positioned for a lateral knee projection if a patella fracture is suspected.
- State the relationship of the medial and lateral femoral condyles, and describe the degree of femoral inclination demonstrated in a patient in an erect and lateral recumbent position.

- State the femoral length and pelvic width that demonstrate the least amount of femoral inclination.
- Describe two methods that can be used to distinguish the medial and lateral femoral condyles from each other on a lateral knee projection with poor positioning.
- State two ways that the patient and CR angle can be aligned to accomplish superimposed femoral condyles for a lateral knee projection.
- Describe how patellar subluxation is demonstrated on a tangential (axial) projection knee projection.
- State the importance of securing the legs and instructing the patient to relax the quadriceps femoris muscles for a tangential (axial) projection knee projection.
- Explain how the positioning setup for a tangential (axial) projection is adjusted for a patient with large posterior calves.
- State why a 72-inch (183-cm) source–image receptor distance (SID) is required for a tangential (axial) projection knee projection.
- Discuss the importance of including the femoral soft tissue on all femoral projections.
- Explain how a distal and proximal AP and lateral femoral projection is obtained in a patient with a suspected fracture.
- State why the patient's leg is never rotated when a femoral fracture is suspected.

KEY TERMS

abductor tubercle
dorsal
dorsiflexion
dorsoplantar
intermalleolar line

lateral mortise
plantar
plantar-flexion
subluxation
talar domes

tarsi sinus
valgus deformity
varus deformity

IMAGE ANALYSIS GUIDELINES

Technical Data. When the technical data in Table 6-1 are followed, or adjusted as needed for additive and destructive patient conditions (see Table 2-6), along with the best practices discussed in Chapters 1 and 2, all upper extremity projections will demonstrate the image analysis guidelines in Box 6-1 unless otherwise indicated.

TOE: AP AXIAL PROJECTION

See Table 6-2, (Figures 6-1, 6-2, 6-3, and 6-4).
Phalangeal Midshaft Concavity and Soft Tissue Width. Take a few minutes to compare the toe projections in Figure 6-5. Note that in an AP projection, concavity of the midshaft of the proximal phalanx is equal on both sides and in the lateral projection the posterior

(plantar) surface of the proximal phalanx demonstrates more concavity than the anterior (dorsal) surface. Also note that as the toe is rotated for an AP oblique projection, the amount of concavity increases on the side toward which the posterior surface is rotated, whereas the side toward which the anterior surface is rotated demonstrates less concavity. The same observations can be made about the soft tissue that surrounds the phalanges. Equal soft tissue width is demonstrated on each side of the AP toe, there is more soft tissue thickness on the posterior surface than the anterior surface on a lateral toe, and the side demonstrating the greatest soft tissue width on an AP oblique toe is the side toward which the posterior surface is rotated.

Look for this midshaft concavity and soft tissue width variation to indicate rotation on a toe projection. When the toe is rotated laterally, the phalangeal soft tissue

TABLE 6-1	Lower Extremity Technical Data				
Projection	**kV**	**Grid**		**mAs**	**SID**
Toe	55-60			2	40-48 inches (100-120 cm)
Foot	60-70			2	40-48 inches (100-120 cm)
Axial (dorsoplantar), calcaneus	70-75			3	40-48 inches (100-120 cm)
Lateral, calcaneus, and ankle	60-70			2	40-48 inches (100-120 cm)
Ankle, AP and AP oblique	60-75			3	40-48 inches (100-120 cm)
Lower Leg	70-80			3	40-48 inches (100-120 cm)
Knee	65-75 70-85	Grid*		4	40-48 inches (100-120 cm)
Femur	80-85	Grid		5	40-48 inches (100-120 cm)
Pediatric	60-70			1-2	40-48 inches (100-120 cm)

*Use grid if part thickness measures 4 inches (10 cm) or more and adjust mAs per grid ratio requirement.

TABLE 6-2	AP Axial Toe(s) Projection

Image Analysis Guidelines (Figures 6-1, 6-2, and 6-3)	**Related Positioning Procedures (Figure 6-4)**
• Midshaft concavity and soft tissue width are equal on both sides of phalanges.	• Place the patient in a supine or seated position, flex the knee, and place the plantar foot surface on the IR in an AP projection. • Center the toe to the IR.
• IP and MTP joints are open. • Phalanges are seen without foreshortening. • No soft tissue or bony overlap from adjacent digits is present. • Toe: MTP joint is at the center of the exposure field. • Toes: Third MTP joint is at the center of the exposure field. • Phalanges and half of the metatarsal(s) are included within the exposure field.	• Extend the toe(s) and place a 10- to 15-degree proximal (toward the calcaneus) angle on the CR. • Separate the toes enough to see small spaces between them. • Toe: Center the CR to the MTP joint. • Toes: Center the CR to the third MTP. • Longitudinally collimate to include the toe(s) and the distal half of the metatarsal(s) (collimation field extends 2 inches [5 cm] proximal to the between-toe interconnecting tissue). • Transversely collimate to within 0.5 inch (1.25 cm) of the toe or foot skin line.

BOX 6-1	Lower Extremity Technical Data Imaging Analysis Guidelines

- The facility's identification requirements are visible.
- A right or left marker identifying the correct side of the patient is present on the projection and is not superimposed over the VOI.
- Good radiation protection practices are evident.
- Bony trabecular patterns and cortical outlines of the anatomic structures are sharply defined.
- Contrast resolution is adequate to demonstrate the surrounding soft tissue, bony trabecular patterns, and cortical outlines.
- No quantum mottle or saturation is present.
- Scattered radiation has been kept to a minimum.
- There is no evidence of removable artifacts.

width and midshaft concavity are greater on the side positioned away from the lateral foot surface (Figure 6-6). When the toe is rotated medially, the phalangeal soft tissue width and midshaft concavity are greater on the side positioned away from the medial foot surface

(Figure 6-7). If the patient's toenail is visualized, which is often the case with the first toe, it can also be used to determine the direction of toe rotation. The nail rotates in the same direction as the foot.

Joint Spaces and Phalanges. The interphalangeal (IP) and metatarsophalangeal (MTP) joint spaces are open and the phalanges are demonstrated without foreshortening when the toe(s) was fully extended and a 10- to 15-degree proximal (toward the calcaneus) CR was centered to the MTP joint(s). The CR angulation is required to align the CR closer to parallel with the joint spaces and perpendicular to the phalanges, preventing closed joint spaces and foreshortened phalanges (Figure 6-8).

CR Angulation for Nonextendable Toes. For patients who have flexed toes that will not extend and would require greater than a 15-degree CR angulation for the CR to be aligned accurately with the joint space or phalange, the toes and forefoot may be elevated on a radiolucent sponge to bring the phalanges more parallel with the IR. If this is not done the angle between the CR and IR will be too acute, causing excessive elongation distortion. Unfortunately, this elevation will cause magnification distortion and needs to be kept to a minimum.

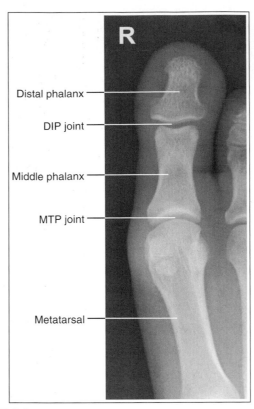

FIGURE 6-1 First AP axial toe projection with accurate positioning. DIP, Distal interphalangeal; MTP, metatarsophalangeal.

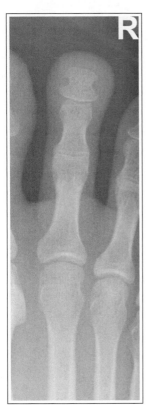

FIGURE 6-2 Second AP axial toe projection with accurate positioning.

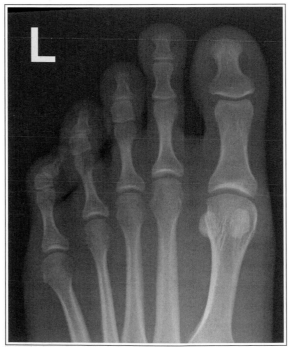

FIGURE 6-3 AP axial projection of the toes with accurate positioning.

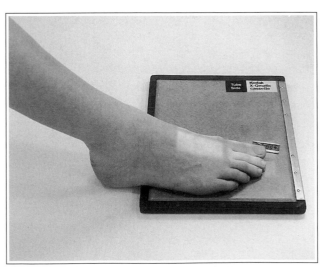

FIGURE 6-4 Proper patient positioning for AP axial toe projection.

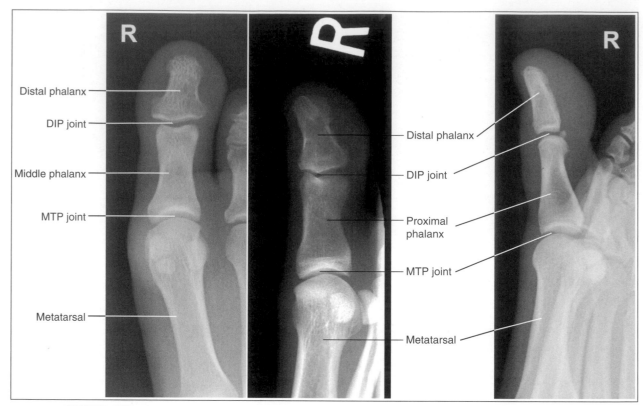

FIGURE 6-5 AP, lateral, AP like toe projections for demonstrating soft tissue and phalanx concavity comparison.

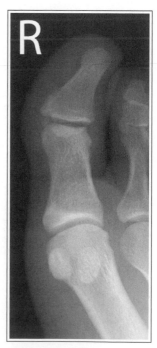

FIGURE 6-6 AP axial toe projection taken with the toe rotated laterally.

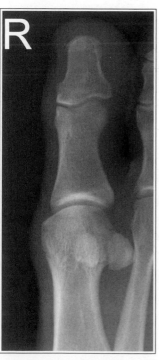

FIGURE 6-7 AP axial toe projection taken with the toe rotated medially.

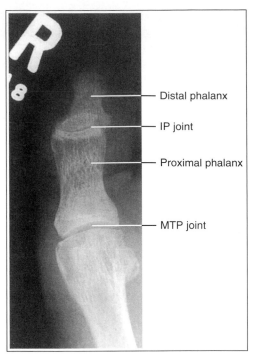

FIGURE 6-8 AP axial toe projection taken without the CR aligned parallel with the IP and MTP joint spaces.

- Distal phalanx
- IP joint
- Proximal phalanx
- MTP joint

AP Axial Toe Analysis Practice

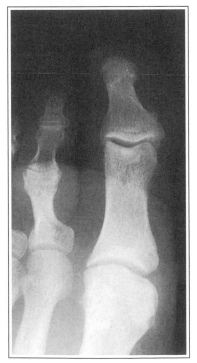

IMAGE 6-1

Analysis. The phalanges demonstrate greater soft tissue width and midshaft concavity on the medial surface. The toe was laterally rotated.

Correction. Medially rotate the foot and toe until they are flat against the IR.

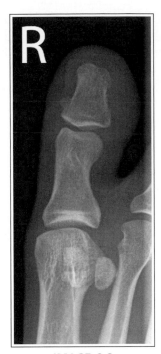

IMAGE 6-2

Analysis. The phalanges demonstrate greater soft tissue width and midshaft concavity on the lateral surface. The toe and foot were medially rotated.

Correction. Laterally rotate the foot until the toe of interest is flat against the IR.

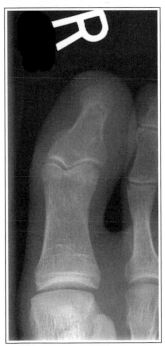

IMAGE 6-3

Analysis. The IP joint spaces are closed, and the distal phalanx is foreshortened. The toe was flexed, and the CR was not aligned parallel with the joint spaces or perpendicular to the distal phalanx.

Correction. If the patient's condition allows, extend the toe, placing it flat against the IR. If the patient is unable

TABLE 6-3 | AP Oblique Toe(s) Projection

Image Analysis Guidelines (Figures 6-9 and 6-10)	Related Positioning Procedures (Figure 6-11)
• Twice as much soft tissue width and more phalangeal concavity are present on the side of the digit rotated away from the IR.	• Place the patient in a supine or seated position, flex the knee, and place the foot on the IR in an AP projection. • Center the toe to the IR. • First through third toe(s): Medially rotate the foot until the toe(s) is at a 45-degree oblique with the IR. • Fourth and fifth toe(s): Laterally rotate the foot until the toe(s) is at a 45-degree oblique with the IR.
• IP and MTP joint spaces are open. • Phalanges are demonstrated without foreshortening.	• Extend the toe(s).
• No soft tissue or bony overlap from adjacent digits. • Toe: MTP joint is at the center of the exposure field. • Toes: The third MTP joint is at the center of the exposure field.	• Separate the toes enough to see small spaces between them. • Toe: Center a perpendicular CR to the MTP joint. • Toes: Center a perpendicular CR to the third MTP joint.
• Phalanges and half of the metatarsal(s) are included within the exposure field.	• Longitudinally collimate to include the toe(s) and the distal half of the metatarsal(s) (collimation field extends 2 inches [5 cm] proximal to the between-toe interconnecting tissue). • Transversely collimate to within 0.5 inch (1.25 cm) of the toe or foot skin line.

to extend the toe, elevate on a radiolucent sponge or until the CR is aligned parallel with the joint space or perpendicular to the phalanx of interest.

TOE: AP OBLIQUE PROJECTION

See Table 6-3, (Figures 6-9, 6-10, and 6-11).

Phalangeal Midshaft Concavity and Soft Tissue Width. When the first through third toes are of interest, the foot is to be rotated medially and when the fourth and fifth toes are of interest, the foot is rotated laterally. The variation in rotation for the different toes is to obtain an AP oblique projection with the least amount of magnification caused by longer object–IR distances (OID).

Rotation Accuracy. To verify the accuracy of rotation on an AP oblique toe and to determine the proper way to reposition the patient when digit obliquity was insufficient or excessive, study the midshaft concavity of the proximal phalanx and compare the soft tissue width on both sides of the digit. A toe projection taken at 45 degrees of obliquity demonstrates more phalangeal midshaft concavity and twice as much soft tissue width on the side positioned farther from the IR. When the midshaft concavity of the proximal phalanx and soft tissue width are closer to equal on both sides of the digit, the toe was not adequately rotated (Figure 6-12). When more than twice the width of soft tissue is present on one side of the digit than on the other and when the posterior aspect of the proximal phalanx's midshaft demonstrates more concavity than the anterior aspect, the toe was rotated more than 45 degrees for the projection (Figure 6-13).

Joint Spaces and Phalanges. The IP and MTP joint spaces are open and the phalanges are demonstrated

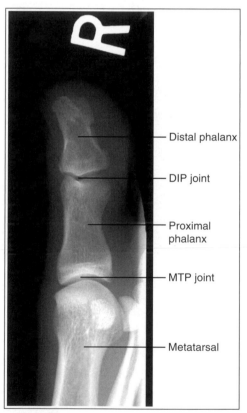

FIGURE 6-9 AP oblique toe projection with accurate positioning. DIP, Distal interphalangeal; MTP, metatarsophalangeal.

without foreshortening when the toe(s) was fully extended and a perpendicular CR was centered to the MTP joint. This toe positioning and CR placement align the joint spaces perpendicular to the IR and parallel with the CR. They also prevent foreshortening of the phalanges, because the long axes of the phalanges are aligned

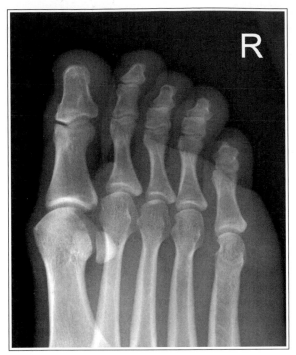

FIGURE 6-10 AP oblique projections of the toes with accurate positioning.

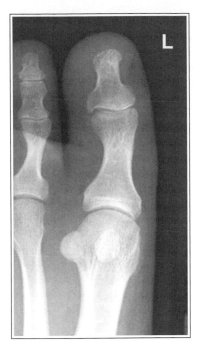

FIGURE 6-12 AP oblique toe projection taken without adequate toe obliquity.

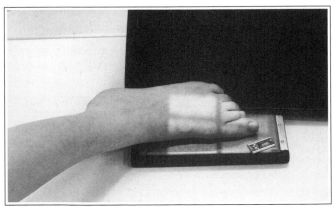

FIGURE 6-11 Proper patient positioning for AP oblique toe projection.

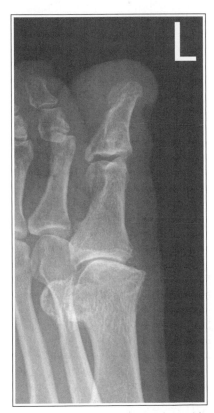

FIGURE 6-13 AP oblique toe projection taken with excessive toe obliquity.

parallel with the IR and perpendicular to the CR. If the toe is not extended, the resulting projection demonstrates closed joint spaces and foreshortened phalanges (Figure 6-14).

CR Angulation for Nonextendable Toes. In patients who are unable to extend their toes, the CR is angled proximally (toward the calcaneus) until it is perpendicular to the toe's phalanx of interest or parallel with the joint space of interest. If this CR angulation results in too acute of a CR to IR angulation, the forefoot may be elevated on a sponge to bring phalanges closer to parallel with the IR and a perpendicular CR used. Unfortunately, this elevation will cause magnification distortion and needs to be kept to a minimum.

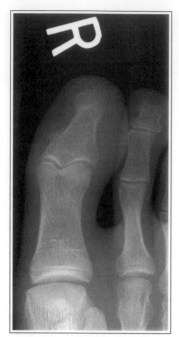

FIGURE 6-14 AP oblique toe projection taken without the CR aligned parallel with the IP and MTP joint spaces.

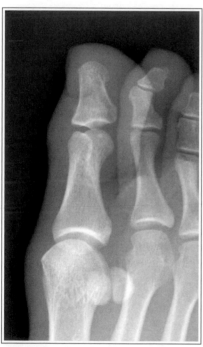

FIGURE 6-15 AP oblique toe projection taken without a small separation between the toes.

Bony and Soft Tissue Overlap. To prevent overlapping of the soft tissue and bony structures, the toes are drawn away from each other enough to provide a small separation between them. It may be necessary to use tape or an immobilization device to maintain this position. If the toes are allowed to overlap, they may superimpose over the affected area (Figure 6-15).

AP Oblique Toe Analysis Practice

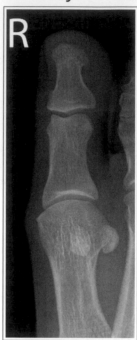

IMAGE 6-4

Analysis. The soft tissue width and midshaft concavity on both sides of the phalanges are almost equal. The toe was rotated less than the required 45 degrees.
Correction. Increase the toe and foot obliquity until the affected toe was at a 45-degree angle with the IR.

TOE: LATERAL PROJECTION (MEDIOLATERAL AND LATEROMEDIAL)

See Table 6-4, (Figures 6-16, 6-17, 6-18 and 6-19).
Phalanx Concavity and Condyle Superimposition. In a lateral projection, the posterior surface of the proximal phalanx demonstrates more concavity than the anterior surface and the condyles of the proximal phalanx are superimposed. Evaluate the degree of metatarsal head superimposition to determine whether the foot and toe was rotated too much or too little when a poor lateral toe is produced. In Figures 6-20 and 6-21 the condyles of the proximal phalanx are not superimposed; the difference between these projections is that the MT heads are shown posterior to the first toe in Figure 6-20 and anterior to the first toe in Figure 6-21. The foot and toe were not rotated enough for the toe to be placed in a lateral projection for Figure 6-20 and was rotated more than needed for Figure 6-21.
Bony and Soft Tissue Overlap. The adjacent toes should be drawn away from the affected toe to prevent overlapping. It may be necessary to use tape or an immobilization device to maintain the unaffected toe's position. Figures 6-18 and 6-19 show how this can be accomplished using tape. If the unaffected toes are not drawn away, they may be superimposed over the affected toe (Figure 6-22).

TABLE 6-4	Lateral Toe Projection
Image Analysis Guidelines (Figures 6-16 and 6-17)	**Related Positioning Procedures (Figures 6-18 and 6-19)**
• Condyles of the proximal phalanx are superimposed.	• Place the patient in a recumbent position, with the knee flexed and the lateral side of the foot against the IR for the first, second, and third toes, and the medial side of the foot against the IR for the fourth and fifth toes. • Center toe to the IR. • Adjust the knee's elevation from the table until the toe is in a lateral projection with the plane of the forefoot aligned perpendicular to the IR.
• There is no soft tissue or bony overlap from adjacent toes.	• Draw the unaffected toes posteriorly away from the affected toe, preventing overlap.
• PIP joint is at the center of the exposure field.	• Center a perpendicular CR to the PIP joint.
• Phalanges and MTP joint space are included within the exposure field.	• Longitudinally collimate to include the toe and the distal half of the metatarsal(s) (collimation field extends 2 inches [5 cm] proximal to the between-toe interconnecting tissue). • Transversely collimate to within 0.5 inch (1.25 cm) of the toe skin line.

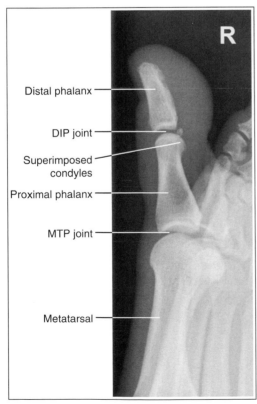

FIGURE 6-16 First lateral toe projection with accurate positioning. DIP, Distal interphalangeal; MTP, metatarsophalangeal.

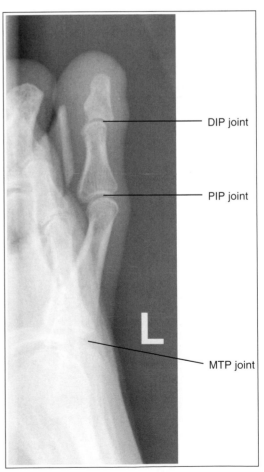

FIGURE 6-17 Second lateral toe projection with accurate positioning. DIP, Distal interphalangeal; MTP, metatarsophalangeal; PIP, proximal interphalangeal.

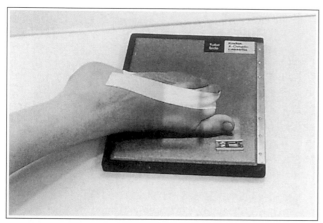

FIGURE 6-18 Proper patient positioning for lateral projection of the first toe.

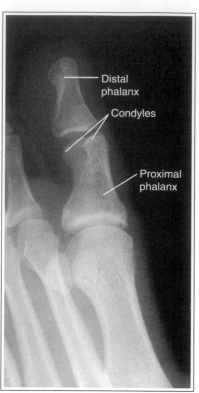

FIGURE 6-20 Lateral toe projection taken without adequate toe obliquity to place the toe in a lateral projection

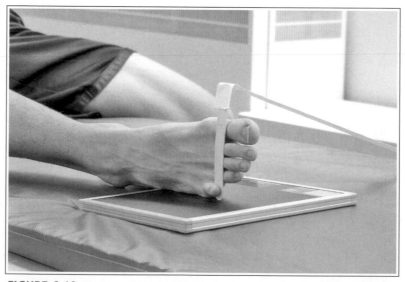

FIGURE 6-19 Proper patient positioning for lateral projection of the fifth toe.

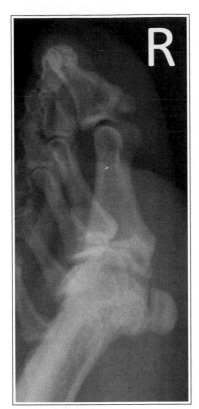

FIGURE 6-21 Lateral toe projection taken with excessive toe obliquity.

Lateral Toe Analysis Practice

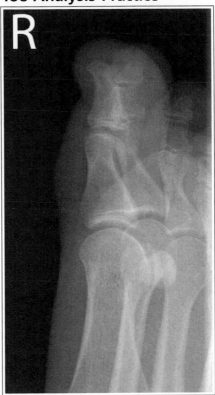

IMAGE 6-5

Analysis. Soft tissue and bony overlap of digits are present. The adjacent unaffected digits were not drawn away from the affected digit.

Correction. The unaffected toes should be drawn away from the affected toe. It may be necessary to use tape or another immobilization device to help the patient maintain this position.

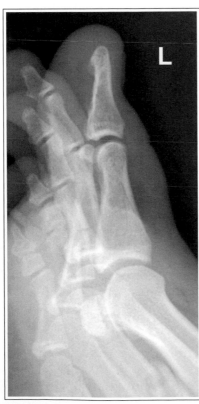

FIGURE 6-22 Lateral toe projection taken without the unaffected toes being drawn away from the affected toe.

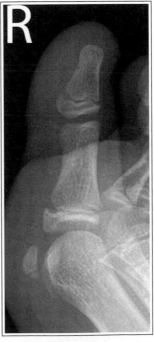

IMAGE 6-6

Analysis. The condyles of the proximal phalanx are not superimposed and the MT heads are shown anterior to the first toe. The foot was rotated more than needed to bring the toe into a lateral projection.

Correction. Decrease the degree of foot rotation until the toe is in a lateral projection.

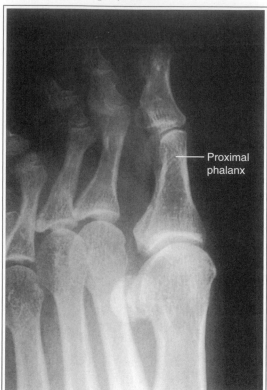

Proximal phalanx

IMAGE 6-7

Analysis. The condyles of the proximal phalanx are not superimposed and the MT heads are shown posterior to the first toe. The foot was under-rotated.

Correction. Increase the degree of foot rotation.

FOOT: AP AXIAL PROJECTION (DORSOPLANTAR)

See Table 6-5, (Figures 6-23 and 6-24).

Metatarsal, Cuneiform, and Talar and Calcaneal Spacing

Medial Arch and Rotation. The medial side of the foot arches up between the heel and the medial three MTP joints to form a visible longitudinal arch. It is because of this medial arch that the medial plantar surface does not always make contact with the IR for an AP foot projection and why it is important to keep the lower leg, ankle, and foot aligned to prevent rotation. If the lower leg, ankle, and foot are not aligned, more pressure can be placed on the medial or lateral plantar surface, causing foot rotation. Study the projections in Figure 6-25 to compare the changes in the relationship among the metatarsals, the cuneiforms, and the amount of talar and calcaneal superimposition that occurs when the foot is rotated. When the foot is laterally rotated, the metatarsal (MT) bases demonstrate increased superimposition, the medial and intermediate cuneiform joint is closed, and the talus moves over the calcaneus, resulting in more than one third of the talus superimposing the calcaneus (<0.75 inch [2 cm] of calcaneal demonstration without talar superimposition). When the foot is medially rotated, the MT bases demonstrate decreased superimposition, the medial and intermediate cuneiform joint is closed, and the talus moves away from the calcaneus, resulting in less than one third of the talus superimposing the calcaneus (>0.75 inch [2 cm] calcaneal visualization without talar superimposition).

Weight-Bearing AP. When positioning the patient for the standing AP foot, keep the feet close together and elevated on the same platform thickness to prevent medial rotation.

TABLE 6-5	AP Axial Foot Projection
Image Analysis Guidelines (Figure 6-23)	**Related Positioning Procedures (Figure 6-24)**
• Equal spacing between the second through fifth MTs • The joint space between the medial (first) and intermediate (second) cuneiforms is demonstrated • About one-third of the talus is superimposing the calcaneus (0.75 inch [2 cm] of the calcaneus is seen without talar superimposition).	• Place the patient in a supine, seated, or standing position, with the plantar foot surface centered on the IR in an AP projection. • Supine only: Align the lower leg, ankle, and foot, keeping equal pressure applied across the plantar surface.
• TMT and navicular-cuneiform joint spaces are open.	• Flex the knee until the foot is as close to a 90-degree angle with the lower leg as possible. • Align the CR perpendicular to the dorsal foot surface, placing a 10- to 15-degree proximal (toward the calcaneus) angle on the CR
• Third MT base is at the center of the exposure field.	• Center the CR to the base of the third metatarsal.
• Proximal calcaneus, talar neck, tarsals, MTs, phalanges, and foot soft tissue are included within the exposure field.	• Longitudinal collimation to include the phalanges. • Transversely collimate to 0.5 inch (1.25 cm) of foot skin line.

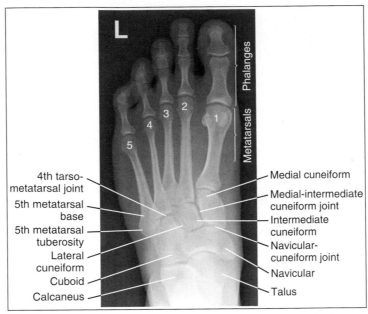

FIGURE 6-23 AP axial foot projection with accurate positioning.

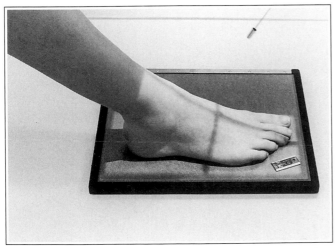

FIGURE 6-24 Proper patient positioning for AP axial foot projection.

Tarsometatarsal and Navicular-Cuneiform Joint Spaces

Determining CR Angulation. The height of the medial longitudinal arch varies between patients and depends on the health of the supporting ligamentous and muscular structures. If these structures fail, the highest point of the arch descends and the TMT and navicular-cuneiform joint spaces are placed at different angles with the IR. To open these joints on an AP foot the CR angulation must be varied per the degree of medial arch height to align it parallel with them. This is typically accomplished by using a 10- to 15-degree proximal (toward the calcaneus) angle. A lower angle is needed when the patient's medial arch is low, and a higher angle is needed for a patient with a high arch. The simplest method of determining the correct angulation to use regardless of the arch height is to align the CR perpendicular to the dorsal surface, as shown in Figure 6-26. This alignment will align the CR parallel with the tarsometatarsal (TMT) joints.

Omitting or employing an inaccurate CR angulation results in obstructed TMT and navicular-cuneiform joint spaces (Figure 6-27).

Ankle Flexion. Having the ankle flexed to a 90-degree angle with the lower leg provides a truer medial arch (Figure 6-28) and will produce less elongation distortion. When the ankle is extended (toes pointed) the longitudinal arch is more elevated, as shown in Figure 6-29, and the CR angle will need to be increased to parallel the TMT joints. This increase in angulation will result in a more acute CR to IR angle, which will result in greater elongation distortion.

Weight-Bearing AP. The CR angulation needed for the non–weight-bearing AP foot in many cases will be less than that needed in the standing position (Figure 6-30). The added body weight will flatten the medial arch, causing the TMT joints to be at a lower angle with the IR and require a decrease in CR angulation to parallel them.

Locating the Base of the Third Metatarsal. To place the third MT base in the center of the projection, center the CR to the midline of the foot at a level 0.5 inch (1.25 cm) distal to the fifth MT tuberosity. The fifth MT tuberosity can be palpated along the lateral foot surface, about halfway between the ball of the foot and the calcaneus.

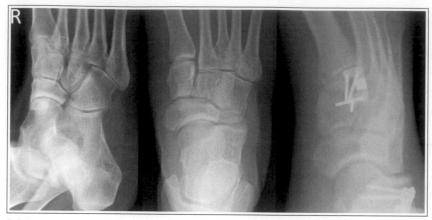

FIGURE 6-25 AP medial oblique, AP, and AP lateral oblique foot projections to compare the changes in the relationship between the MTs and cuneiforms, and the amount of talar and calcaneal superimposition.

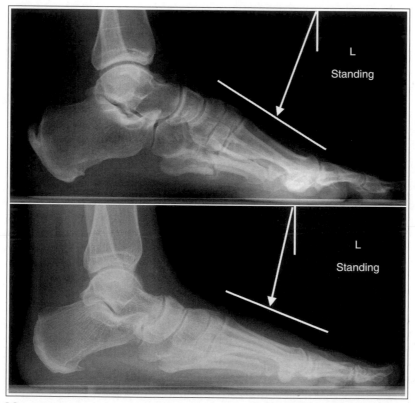

FIGURE 6-26 Lateral foot projections on a patient with a high and low longitudinal arch to demonstrate proper CR alignment to obtain open TMT and navicular-cuneiform joint spaces.

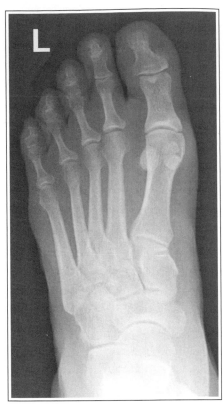

FIGURE 6-27 Lateral foot projection taken with poor CR alignment with the TMT and navicular-cuneiform joint spaces.

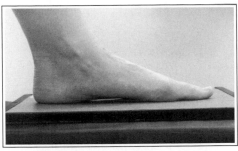

FIGURE 6-28 Lateral foot obtained with the ankle flexed to a 90-degree angle with the lower leg and demonstrating a low medial foot arch (same patient as Figure 6-29).

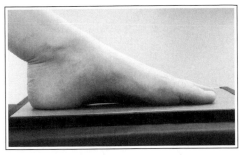

FIGURE 6-29 Lateral foot obtained without the ankle flexed to a 90-degree angle with the lower leg and demonstrating an average medial foot arch (same patient as Figure 6-28).

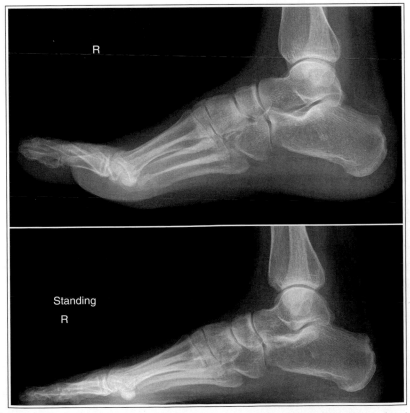

FIGURE 6-30 Lateral foot projections on the same patient demonstrating the effects of weight-bearing versus non–weight-bearing positions on the medial foot arch visualization.

AP Axial Foot Analysis Practice

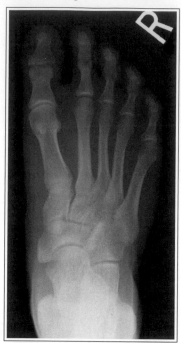

IMAGE 6-8

Analysis. The TMT joint spaces are closed. The CR was not aligned parallel with these joints spaces.
Correction. Direct the CR 10 to 15 degrees proximally or angle the CR until it is perpendicular with the dorsal surface.

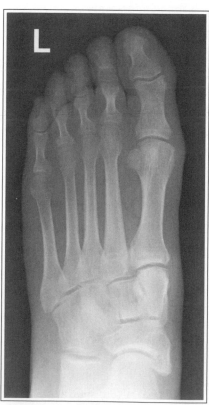

IMAGE 6-9

Analysis. The joint space between the medial and intermediate cuneiforms is closed, the calcaneus demonstrates no talar superimposition, and the MT bases demonstrate decreased superimposition. More pressure was placed on the medial plantar surface than on the lateral surface, resulting in medial foot rotation.
Correction. Rotate the foot laterally until the pressure over the entire plantar surface is equal. The lower leg, ankle, and foot should be aligned.

FOOT: AP OBLIQUE PROJECTION (MEDIAL ROTATION)

See Table 6-6, (Figures 6-31, 6-32, and 6-33).
Cuboid-Cuneiform and Intermetatarsal Joints
Determining Degree of Obliquity. When the cuboid-cuneiform and second through fifth intermetatarsal joints spaces are open, the tarsal sinus and fifth MT base are well demonstrated on an AP oblique foot projection. The amount of rotation required to accomplish these open spaces is dependent on the height of the medial longitudinal arch, with the higher arches requiring more obliquity. If the CR was aligned perpendicular to the dorsal surface for the AP foot as described for the AP foot projection, the degree of angulation determined from this method can be used to indicate the degree of obliquity that is required for the AP oblique foot. If the AP foot CR angulation used was around 5 degrees, indicating a low arch, the patient's foot should be placed at

TABLE 6-6	AP Oblique Foot Projection
Image Analysis Guidelines (Figures 6-31 and 6-32)	**Related Positioning Procedures (Figure 6-33)**
• Cuboid-cuneiform joint space and second through fifth intermetatarsal joint spaces are open. • Tarsi sinus and fifth MT tuberosity are visualized.	• Place the patient in a recumbent or seated position, flex the knee and center the plantar foot surface on the IR. • Flex the knee until the foot is as close to a 90-degree angle with the lower leg as possible. • Medially rotate the leg and foot, keeping them aligned, and placing the plantar surface at a 30- to 60-degree angle with the IR.
• Third MT base is at the center of the exposure field.	• Center a perpendicular CR to the third MT base.
• Phalanges, MTs, tarsals, calcaneus, and foot soft tissue are included within the exposure field.	• Longitudinally collimate to include the phalanges and calcaneus. • Transversely collimate to 0.5 inch (1.25 cm) of foot skin line.

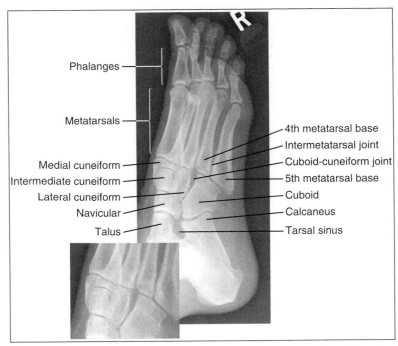

FIGURE 6-31 AP oblique foot projection with accurate positioning in a patient with a high medial arch.

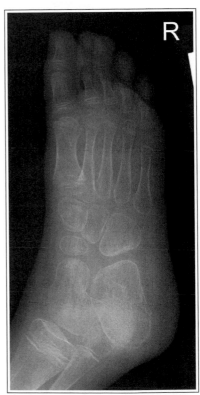

FIGURE 6-32 Pediatric AP oblique foot projection with accurate positioning.

30 degrees of obliquity for the AP oblique foot. If the CR angulation was around 10 degrees, indicating an average arch, the foot should be placed at 45 degrees of obliquity and if the CR angulation was around 15 degrees, indicating a high arch, the foot should be placed

at 60 degrees of obliquity. Figure 6-34 demonstrates an AP oblique foot on a patient with a low, average, and high medial arch. Each demonstrates the required open cuboid-cuneiform and second through fifth intermetatarsal joint, but each was obtained using a different degree of obliquity as noted by the amount of first and second MT base superimposition and the amount of space demonstrated between the MT heads. When the foot is rotated medially, the first MT base rotates beneath the second MT base, with the other MTs following suit, increasing the amount of superimposition and indicating increased obliquity.

Inadequate Obliquity. If the degree of foot obliquity is inadequate for an AP oblique foot, the longitudinally running foot joints (cuneiform-cuboid, navicular-cuboid, and second through fifth intermetatarsal joint spaces) are closed. To determine whether the patient's foot has been underrotated or overrotated, evaluate the intermetatarsal joint space between the fourth and fifth metatarsals. The fourth MT tubercle is a rounded, protruding surface located just distal to the fourth MT base and placed in profile in overrotation. If this joint space is closed and the fourth MT base is superimposed over the fifth MT base, the foot was underrotated (Figure 6-35). If the fourth–fifth intermetatarsal joint space is closed and the fifth proximal MT is superimposed over the fourth MT tubercle, the foot was overrotated (Figure 6-36).

Ankle Flexion. Because the medial arch is pulled higher when the ankle is extended, one must keep the foot and lower leg relationship consistent for the AP and AP oblique foot projections or the degree of obliquity required will not correlate with the CR angulation used for the AP foot.

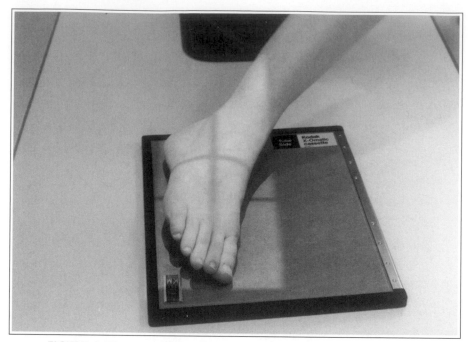

FIGURE 6-33 Proper patient positioning for an AP oblique foot projection.

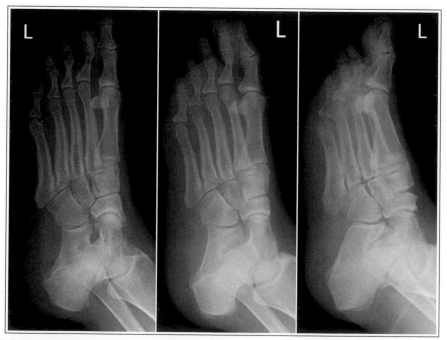

FIGURE 6-34 Accurately positioned AP oblique foot projections taken on patients with a low, average, and high medial foot arch.

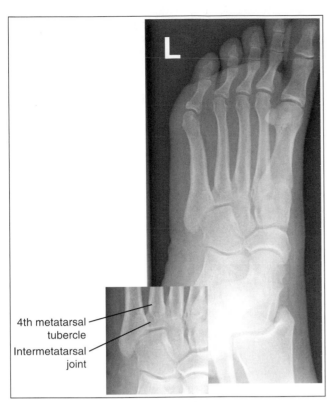

4th metatarsal —
tubercle

Intermetatarsal —
joint

FIGURE 6-35 AP oblique foot projection taken with insufficient foot obliquity.

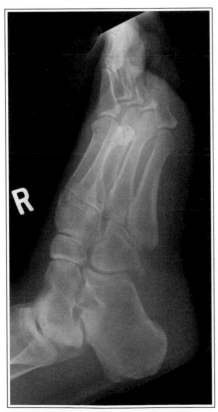

FIGURE 6-36 AP oblique foot projection taken with excessive foot obliquity.

AP Oblique Foot Analysis Practice

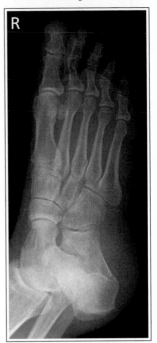

IMAGE 6-10

Analysis. The lateral cuneiforms—cuboid, navicular, cuboid—and third through fifth intermetatarsal joint spaces are closed. The fourth MT tubercle is demonstrated without superimposition of the fifth MT. The foot was not medially rotated enough.

Correction. Increase the degree of medial foot rotation.

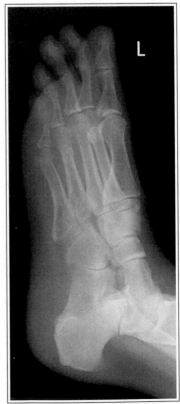

IMAGE 6-11

Analysis. The lateral cuneiforms—cuboid, navicular, cuboid—and intermetatarsal joints spaces are closed, and the fifth proximal MT is superimposed over the fourth MT tubercle. The foot was overrotated.

Correction. Decrease the amount of medial foot rotation.

FOOT: LATERAL PROJECTION (MEDIOLATERAL AND LATEROMEDIAL)

See Table 6-7, (Figures 6-37, 6-38, and 6-39).

Anterior Pretalar and Posterior Pericapsular Fat Pads. Two soft tissue structures located around the foot and ankle may indicate joint effusion and injury: the anterior pretalar fat pad and posterior pericapsular fat pad. The anterior pretalar fat pad is visible anterior to the ankle joint and rests next to the neck of the talus (Figure 6-40). Surrounding the ankle joint is a fibrous, synovium-lined capsule attached to the borders of the tibia, fibula, and talus. On injury or disease invasion the synovial membrane secretes synovial fluid, resulting in distention of the fibrous capsule. Anterior fibrous capsule

TABLE 6-7	Lateral Foot Projection	
Image Analysis Guidelines (Figures 6-37 and 6-38)		**Related Positioning Procedures (Figure 6-39)**
• Contrast and density are adequate to demonstrate the anterior pretalar and posterior pericapsular fat pads.		• Appropriate technical factors are set.
• Long axis of the foot is positioned at a 90-degree angle with the lower leg.		• Start with the patient in a supine or standing position.
• MT heads are superimposed.		• Dorsiflex the foot, placing its long axis at a 90-degree angle with the lower leg.
• Proximal aspects of the talar domes are aligned.		
• Tibiotalar joint is open.		• Extend the knee and align the lower leg parallel with the IR.
• Anterior and posterior aspects of the talar domes are aligned.		
• Distal fibula is superimposed by the posterior half of the distal tibia.		• Externally rotate the affected leg, and oblique the torso as needed to align the lateral foot surface parallel with the IR.
• Distal tarsals are at the center of the exposure field.		• Center the foot to the IR.
		• Center a perpendicular CR to the midline of the foot at the level of the fifth MT base.
• Phalanges, MTs, tarsals, talus, calcaneus, 1 inch (2.5 cm) of the distal lower leg, and foot soft tissue are included within the exposure field.		• Longitudinally collimate to include the toes and calcaneus.
		• Transversely collimate to include 1 inch (2.5 cm) above the medial malleolus.

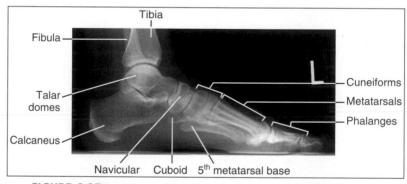

FIGURE 6-37 Mediolateral foot projection with accurate positioning.

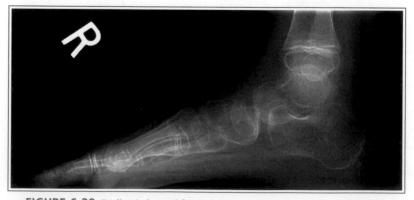

FIGURE 6-38 Pediatric lateral foot projection with accurate positioning.

distention results in displacement of the anterior pretalar fat pad. Because neither the fibrous capsule nor the ankle ligaments can be detected on radiography, displacement of this fat pad indicates joint effusion and the possibility of underlying injuries.

The posterior fat pad is positioned within the indentation formed by the articulation of the posterior tibia and talar bones (see Figure 6-40). This fat pad is displaced

in the same manner as the anterior pretalar fat pad, although it is less sensitive and requires more fluid evasion to be displaced.

Foot Dorsiflexion. In most cases, when a patient is supine and relaxed, the leg rests in external rotation with the foot in plantar flexion. Plantar flexion results in a forced flattening of the anterior pretalar fat pad, reducing its usefulness in the detection of joint effusion.

Foot Dorsiflexion. Appropriate dorsiflexion places the tibiotalar joint in a neutral position and tightens the ligament and muscle structures that will help to keep the foot from resting too heavily on the forefoot and lightly on the heel, more clearly define the medial arch, superimpose the MT heads, and prevent foot rotation. Figure 6-41 demonstrates a lateral foot obtained in dorsiflexion and one obtained in plantar flexion of the

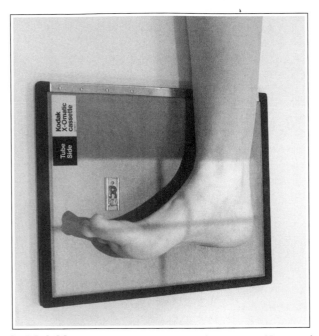

FIGURE 6-39 Lateral foot projection with accurate CR centering and collimation.

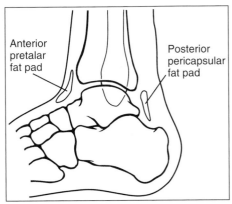

FIGURE 6-40 Location of fat pads.

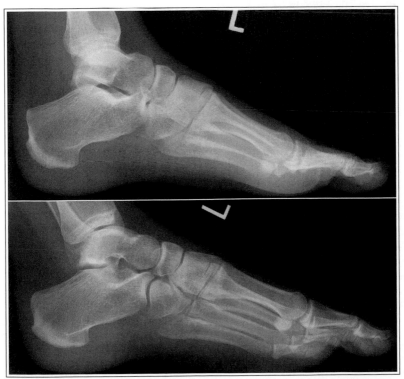

FIGURE 6-41 Lateral foot projections obtained in dorsiflexion and plantar flexion of the same patient.

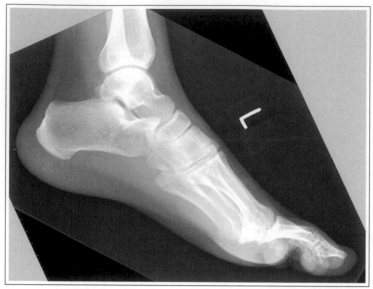

FIGURE 6-42 Accurately positioned lateral foot projection obtained with the patient in plantar flexion.

same patient. Note that the lateral plantar-flexed projection in comparison with the dorsiflexed projection is slightly rotated, does not demonstrate superimposed MT heads, and demonstrates a higher-appearing medial arch. To obtain an accurate lateral foot on a patient who is unable to dorsiflex (Figure 6-42), the knee needs to be slightly flexed and an immobilization support placed beneath it to elevate it the needed amount to place the plantar surfaces of the heel and forefoot perpendicular with the IR.

Proximal Alignment of Talar Domes

Talar Domes. The domes of the talus are formed by the most medial and lateral aspects of the talar's trochlear surface and appear as domed structures that articulate with the tibia on a lateral foot projection. When properly positioned, the talar domes are aligned proximally, anteriorly, and posteriorly, appearing as one, and resulting in an open tibiotalar joint.

Lower Leg Positioning. To obtain correct lower leg and knee positioning for a lateral foot, begin with the patient in a supine position with the leg extended and the foot dorsiflexed (Figure 6-43), and while rotating the patient to bring the lateral foot surface parallel with the IR, keep the leg extended. For most patients, this positioning places the lower leg parallel with the table. If this is not the case, as for a patient with a large upper thigh, the foot and IR is elevated with an immobilization device until the lower leg is brought parallel with the table. Positioning the lower leg parallel aligns the proximal aspects of the talar domes. If the projection is obtained with the proximal or distal lower leg elevated, the resulting projection demonstrates one talar dome visualized proximal to the other.

Repositioning for Poor Lower Leg Positioning. When viewing a lateral foot projection that demonstrates one of the talar domes proximal to the other,

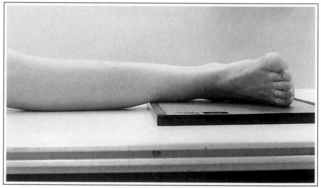

FIGURE 6-43 Accurate positioning of lower leg for a lateral foot projection.

evaluate the height of the medial arch and the degree of narrowing or widening of the talocalcaneal joint to determine which dome is the proximal dome and how to adjust the lower leg to reposition. The height of the arch can be determined by measuring the amount of cuboid demonstrated posterior to the navicular bone. The average lateral foot projection demonstrates approximately 0.5 inch (1.25 cm) of the cuboid, as shown in Figure 6-44. Because the bones that form the foot arch are held in position by ligaments and tendons, weakening of these tissues may result in a decreased or low arch. On a lateral foot projection this decrease in arch height is demonstrated as a decrease in the amount of cuboid demonstrated posterior to the navicular bone. Figure 6-45 shows a lateral foot of a patient with a low longitudinal arch and about 0.25 inch (0.6 cm) of cuboid posterior to the navicular bone, whereas Figure 6-46 shows a patient with a high arch and about 0.75 inch (2 cm) of cuboid posterior to the navicular bones. If the navicular bone is superimposed over more of the cuboid than expected and the talocalcaneal joint is narrowed,

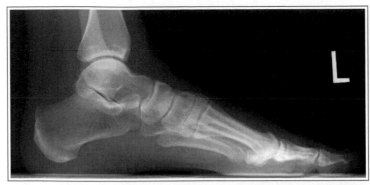

FIGURE 6-44 Lateral foot projection of a patient with an average medial foot arch.

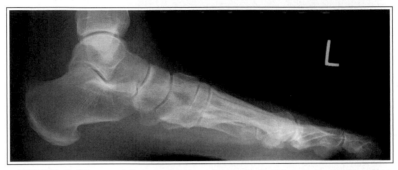

FIGURE 6-45 Lateral foot projection of a patient with a low medial arch.

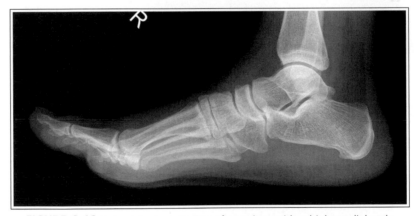

FIGURE 6-46 Lateral foot projection of a patient with a high medial arch.

the lateral dome is the proximal dome and the distal lower leg needs to be elevated or the proximal lower leg depressed by extending the knee to reposition (Figure 6-47). If the navicular bone is superimposed over less of the cuboid than expected and the talocalcaneal joint is wider, the medial dome is the proximal dome and the distal lower leg needs to be depressed or proximal lower leg elevated to reposition (Figures 6-48). The expected arch height can be estimated from the CR angulation used when the AP foot projection was obtained.

Weight-Bearing Lateromedial Foot. When positioning the patient for the standing lateromedial foot, elevate both feet on the same platform thickness and keep the feet positioned close together to prevent the ankles from inverting and causing medial foot rotation, which may reduce the medial arch height and cause the lateral talar dome to be demonstrated proximal to the medial (see Figure 6-47).

Weight-Bearing Mediolateral Foot. When positioning the patient for a standing mediolateral foot, where the patient is standing on one foot only, provide something for the patient to balance the body with so the center of gravity remains in the center of the pelvis. If the center of gravity shifts closer to the affected side when the unaffected foot is raised, the chance of the affected foot rotating laterally increases. Lateral foot rotation will cause the medial arch height to increase and the medial talar dome to be demonstrated proximal to the lateral dome (see Figure 6-48).

Anterior and Posterior Alignment of Talar Domes

Foot Positioning. The anterior and the posterior aspects of the talar domes are aligned on a lateral foot

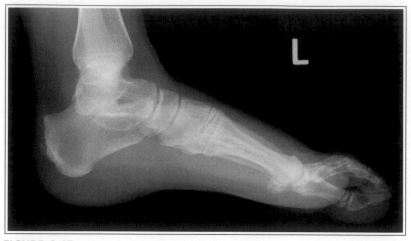

FIGURE 6-47 Lateral foot projection taken with the proximal lower leg elevated.

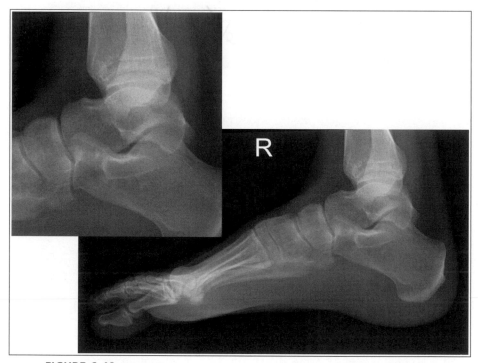

FIGURE 6-48 Lateral foot projection taken with the distal lower leg elevated.

projection when the lateral foot surface is aligned parallel with the IR (Figure 6-49) and even pressure is placed across the entire surface. When the leg is rotated more than needed to place the lateral foot surface parallel with the IR, placing more surface pressure at the forefoot (Figure 6-50), the medial talar dome is demonstrated anterior to the lateral talar dome (Figure 6-51). If the leg is not rotated enough to place the lateral foot surface parallel with the IR, placing more surface pressure at the heel (Figure 6-52), the medial talar dome is demonstrated posterior to the lateral talar dome (Figure 6-53).

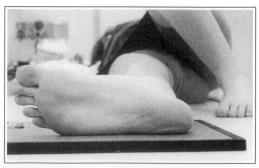

FIGURE 6-49 Accurate positioning of the lateral foot surface.

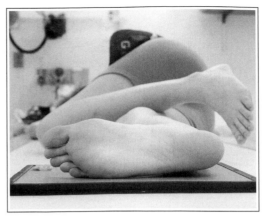

FIGURE 6-50 Poor lateral foot positioning with the calcaneus elevated (leg externally rotated).

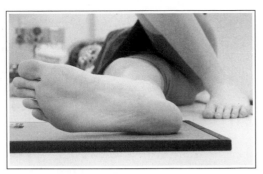

FIGURE 6-52 Poor lateral foot positioning with the calcaneus depressed (leg internally rotated).

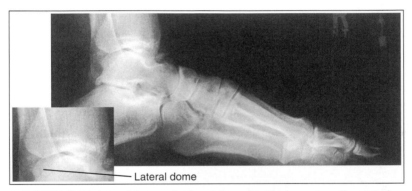

FIGURE 6-51 Lateral foot projection taken with the leg externally rotated.

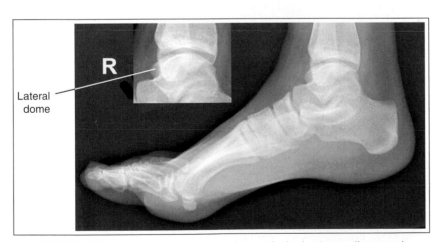

FIGURE 6-53 Lateral foot projection taken with the leg internally rotated.

Using the Tibia and Fibula Relationship to Reposition. When viewing a lateral foot projection that demonstrates one of the talar domes anterior to the other, evaluate the position of the fibula in relation to the tibia to determine how to reposition the patient. The fibula is positioned in the posterior half of the tibia on accurately positioned lateral foot projections. If the fibula is demonstrated more posteriorly than this relationship on a projection, the medial talar dome is anterior and the patient was positioned with the forefoot depressed and the heel elevated (leg too externally rotated), as shown in Figures 6-50 and 6-51. If the fibula is demonstrated more anteriorly than this relationship, the medial talar dome is posterior and the patient was positioned with the forefoot elevated and the heel depressed (leg internal rotation), as shown in Figures 6-52 and 6-53.

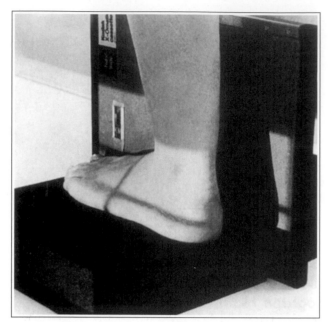

FIGURE 6-54 Lateromedial foot projection with accurate positioning.

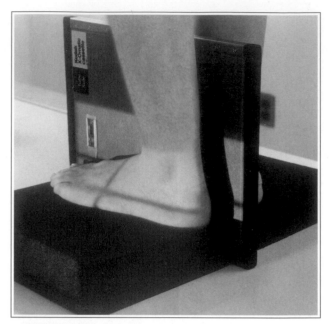

FIGURE 6-56 Poor lateral (lateromedial) foot positioning.

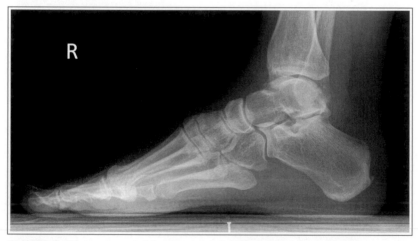

FIGURE 6-55 Lateromedial foot projection taken with the leg internally rotated.

Weight-Bearing Lateromedial Projection. A standing lateromedial foot projection is accomplished by placing the IR against the medial aspect of the foot and aligning the lateral foot surface parallel with the IR, as shown in Figure 6-54. The resulting projection should meet all the analysis requirements listed for the mediolateral projection. The most common misposition for the standing lateromedial projection of the foot shows the medial talar dome positioned anterior to the lateral dome and the distal fibula positioned too posteriorly on the tibia (Figure 6-55). This misposition is a result of aligning the medial foot surface parallel with the IR, as shown in Figure 6-56, rather than the lateral surface. When such a projection is obtained, move the patient's heel away from the IR (leg internally rotated) until the lateral foot surface is parallel with the IR.

Lateral Foot Analysis Practice

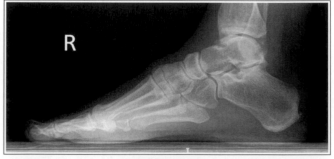

IMAGE 6-12

Analysis. The medial talar dome is positioned anterior to the lateral dome, as indicated by the posterior position of the fibula on the tibia. The lateral foot surface was not positioned parallel with the IR. If this is a mediolateral projection, the forefoot was depressed and the heel was elevated (external rotation). If this is a standing lateral medial projection, the leg was externally rotated to position the medial surface of the foot parallel with the IR.

Correction. Internally rotate the leg until the lateral surface of the foot is parallel with the IR.

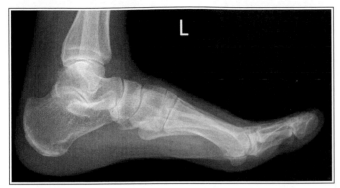

IMAGE 6-13

Analysis. The medial talar dome is positioned posterior to the lateral dome, as indicated by the anterior position of the distal fibula on the tibia. The leg was internally rotated.

Correction. Externally rotate the leg until the foot is parallel with the IR.

CALCANEUS: AXIAL PROJECTION (PLANTODORSAL)

See Table 6-8, (Figures 6-57 and 6-58).

Talocalcaneal Joint Space and Calcaneal Tuberosity

   Foot Positioning. The talocalcaneal joint space is demonstrated as an open space as long as the CR is aligned parallel with it. When the plantar foot surface is positioned vertically, the talocalcaneal joint space is placed at a 40-degree angle with the plane of the IR and is aligned with the 40-degree proximal CR angle. This angulation also aligns the CR nearly perpendicular to the long axis of the calcaneal tuberosity, but because the tuberosity is tilted in relation to the IR, elongation distortion will be present (Figures 6-58 and 6-59).

   Compensating for Dorsiflexion. If the patient's foot is dorsiflexed beyond the vertical position and a 40-degree angulation is used, the talocalcaneal joint space is obscured, and because the CR would be aligned closer to perpendicular with the long axis of the tuberosity, the tuberosity will demonstrate slightly less foreshortening (Figures 6-60 and 6-61). If the patient is unable to reduce the degree of dorsiflexion to open the talocalcaneal joint, the CR needs to be adjusted to parallel it and because the talocalcaneal joint runs closer to perpendicular with the IR in this position, the CR angulation will need to be decreased. To determine the degree of decrease needed, adjust the CR angle until it aligns with the fifth metatarsal base and the point of the distal fibula.

   Compensating for Planter Flexion. Most patients that have trauma to the calcaneal tuberosity will not be able to dorsiflex their foot to 90 degrees with the lower leg. On such a patient, if the projection is obtained with the foot in plantar-flexion, with a 40-degree CR angulation, the talocalcaneal joint space is obscured, and because the CR is aligned closer to parallel with the long axis of the tuberosity, the tuberosity demonstrates foreshortening distortion (Figures 6-62 and 6-63). To open the talocalcaneal joint, the CR angulation needs to be increased until it aligns with the fifth metatarsal base and the point of the distal fibula. This adjusted angulation will demonstrate an open talocalcaneal joint space, and the tuberosity will demonstrate misalignment because of the fracture and elongation if the angle created between the CR and IR is very acute (Figure 6-64). An alternate method to demonstrate the tuberosity when the

TABLE 6-8	Axial Calcaneus Projection
Image Analysis Guidelines (Figure 6-57)	**Related Positioning Procedures (Figure 6-58)**
• Talocalcaneal joint is open. • Calcaneal tuberosity is demonstrated with minimal shape distortion.	• Place the patient in a supine or seated position, with the leg fully extended. • Center the heel to the IR. • Dorsiflex the foot until the plantar surface is perpendicular to the IR. • Place a 40-degree proximal angle on the CR.
• Distal MTs are not demonstrated on the medial or lateral aspect of the foot. • Sustentaculum tali is in profile.	• Position the ankle in an AP projection. • Align the foot straight without inversion or eversion.
• Proximal calcaneal tuberosity is at the center of the exposure field.	• Center the CR to the midline of the foot at the level of the fifth MT base.
• Calcaneal tuberosity and talocalcaneal joint space are included within the exposure field.	• Longitudinally collimate to the heel. • Transversely collimate to within 0.5 inch (1.25 cm) of the heel skin line.

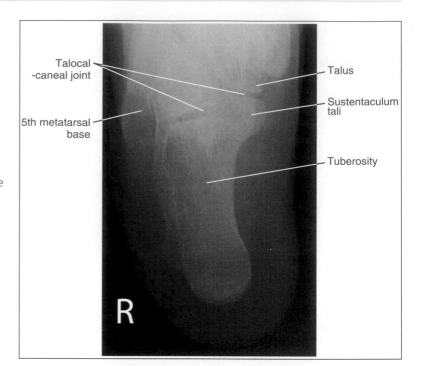

FIGURE 6-57 Axial calcaneal projection with accurate positioning.

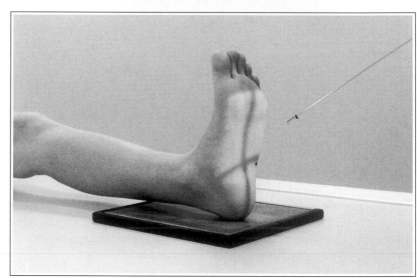

FIGURE 6-58 Proper axial calcaneal projection positioning.

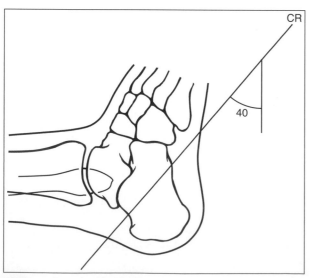

FIGURE 6-59 CR angled 40 degrees with foot in 90-degree position.

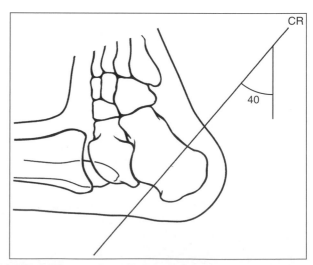

FIGURE 6-60 CR angled 40 degrees with foot in dorsiflexion.

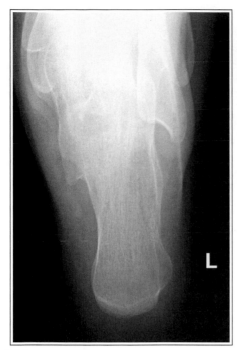

FIGURE 6-61 Axial calcaneal projection taken with poor CR and talocalcaneal joint alignment.

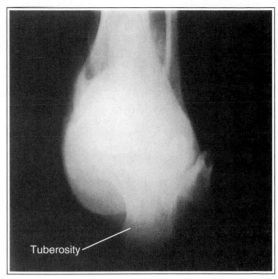

FIGURE 6-63 Axial calcaneal projection taken with poor CR and talocalcaneal joint alignment.

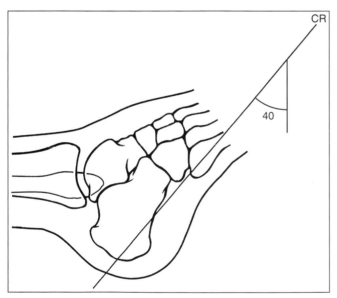

FIGURE 6-62 CR angled 40 degrees with foot in plantar flexion.

foot is plantar-flexed is to elevate the leg, bringing the plantar surface close to perpendicular with the IR, and angle the CR until it is close to perpendicular with the tuberosity; however, unfortunately this will cause increased magnification distortion the farther the heel is positioned away from the IR.

Rotation and Tilting. To prevent calcaneal rotation and tilting, place the ankle in a PA projection and align the foot straight without inversion or eversion. If the ankle is internally rotated or the foot inverted, the first and second metatarsals are demonstrated medially. If the

ankle is externally rotated or the foot everted, the fourth and fifth metatarsals are demonstrated laterally (Figure 6-65).

Axial Calcaneal Analysis Practice

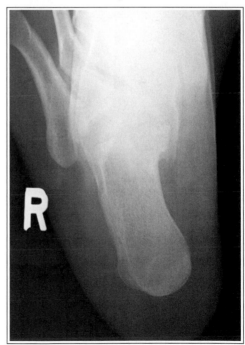

IMAGE 6-14

Analysis. The fourth and fifth MTs are demonstrated on the lateral aspect of the foot. The ankle was externally rotated, or the foot was everted.

Correction. Internally rotate the leg until the ankle is in an AP projection, or bring the foot to a neutral position without eversion.

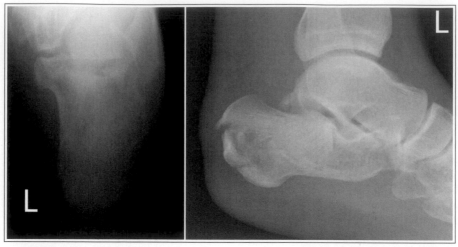

FIGURE 6-64 Axial and lateral calcaneal projections on patient with calcaneal fracture.

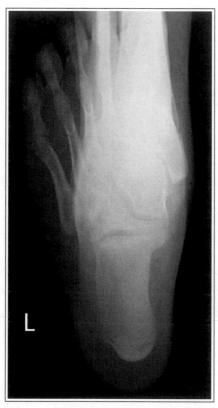

FIGURE 6-65 Axial calcaneal projection taken with external ankle rotation.

TABLE 6-9	**Lateral Calcaneus Projection**
Image Analysis Guidelines (Figure 6-66)	**Related Positioning Procedures (Figure 6-67)**
• Long axis of the foot is positioned at a 90-degree angle with the lower leg.	• Start with the patient in a supine position. • Dorsiflex the foot, placing its long axis at a 90-degree angle with the lower leg.
• Proximal aspects of the talar domes are aligned. • Tibiotalar joint is open.	• Extend the knee and align the lower leg parallel with the table.
• Anterior and posterior aspects of the talar domes are aligned. • Distal fibula is superimposed by the posterior half of the distal tibia.	• Externally rotate the leg, and oblique the torso as needed to align the lateral foot surface parallel with the IR. • Center the ankle to the IR.
• Midcalcaneus is at the center of the exposure field.	• Center a perpendicular CR 1 inch distal to the medial malleolus.
• Tibiotalar joint, talus, calcaneus, and calcaneus-articulating tarsal bones are included within the exposure field.	• Longitudinally collimate to the heel. • Transversely collimate to include 1 inch (2.5 cm) above the medial malleolus.

CALCANEUS: LATERAL PROJECTION (MEDIOLATERAL)

See Table 6-9, (Figures 6-66 and 6-67).

Foot Dorsiflexion. Appropriate dorsiflexion places the tibiotalar joint in a neutral position and tightens the ligament and muscle structures that will help to keep the foot from resting too heavily on the forefoot and lightly on the heel, which may cause the calcaneus to rotate. Trauma to the calcaneal tuberosity prevents most patients from being able to dorsiflex their foot. To obtain an accurate lateral calcaneus on a patient that is unable to dorsiflex, the knee needs to be slightly flexed and an immobilization support placed beneath it to elevate it the needed amount to place the plantar surfaces of the heel and forefoot perpendicular with the IR. Figure 6-68 demonstrates lateral calcaneal projections obtained on a patient with a fractured tuberosity. Note how the fracture is demonstrated differently on these two projections, with only a very small difference in positioning.

Talar Dome Alignment

Lower Leg Positioning. To obtain correct lower leg and knee positioning for a lateral calcaneus, begin with the patient in a supine position with the leg extended and the foot dorsiflexed (see Figure 6-43), and while rotating the patient to bring the lateral foot surface parallel with the IR, keep the leg extended. For most patients, this positioning places the lower leg parallel with the

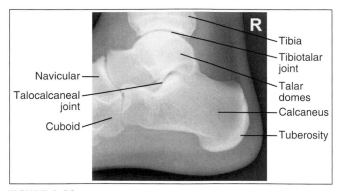

FIGURE 6-66 Lateral calcaneal projection with accurate positioning.

table. If this is not the case, as for a patient with a large upper thigh, the foot and IR should be elevated with an immobilization device until the lower leg is brought parallel with the table. Positioning the lower leg parallel aligns the proximal aspects of the talar domes. If the projection is obtained with the proximal or distal lower leg elevated, the resulting projection demonstrates one talar dome visualized proximal to the other.

Repositioning for Poor Lower Leg Positioning. When viewing a lateral calcaneal projection that demonstrates one of the talar domes proximal to the other, evaluate the height of the medial arch and the degree of narrowing or widening of the talocalcaneal joint to determine which dome is the proximal dome and how to adjust the lower leg to reposition. If the navicular bone is superimposed over more of the cuboid than expected and the talocalcaneal joint is narrowed, the lateral dome is the proximal dome and the distal lower leg needs to be elevated or the proximal lower leg depressed by extending the knee to reposition (Figure 6-69). If the navicular bone is superimposed over less of

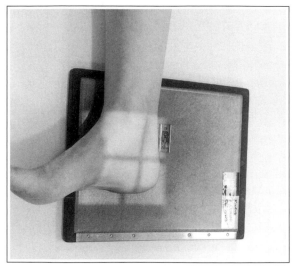

FIGURE 6-67 Accurate lateral calcaneal projection with CR centering and collimation.

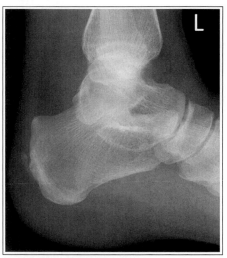

FIGURE 6-69 Lateral calcaneal projection taken with the proximal lower leg elevated.

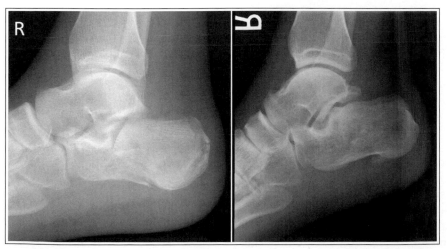

FIGURE 6-68 Lateral calcaneal projection demonstrating a calcaneal fracture.

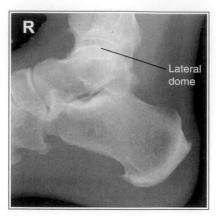

FIGURE 6-70 Lateral calcaneal projection taken with the distal lower leg elevated.

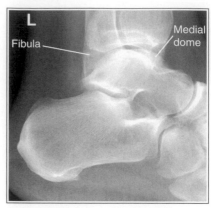

FIGURE 6-73 Lateral calcaneal projection taken with the leg externally rotated.

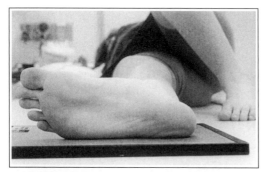

FIGURE 6-71 Proper lateral foot surface positioning for lateral calcaneal projection.

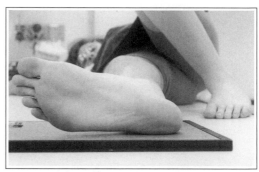

FIGURE 6-74 Poor lateral foot positioning with the calcaneus depressed (leg internally rotated).

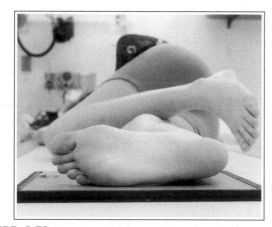

FIGURE 6-72 Poor lateral foot positioning with the calcaneus elevated (leg externally rotated).

placed across the entire surface. When the leg is rotated more than needed to place the lateral foot surface parallel with the IR, placing more surface pressure at the forefoot (Figure 6-72), the medial talar dome is demonstrated anterior to the lateral talar dome (Figure 6-73). If the leg is not rotated enough to place the lateral foot surface parallel with the IR, placing more surface pressure at the heel (Figure 6-74), the medial talar dome is demonstrated posterior to the lateral talar dome (Figure 6-75).

Using the Tibia and Fibula Relationship to Reposition. When viewing a lateral calcaneus projection that demonstrates one of the talar domes anterior to the other, evaluate the position of the fibula in relation to the tibia to determine how to reposition the patient. The fibula is positioned in the posterior half of the tibia on accurately positioned lateral foot projections. If the fibula is demonstrated more posteriorly than this relationship on a projection, the medial talar dome is anterior and the patient was positioned with the forefoot depressed and the heel elevated (leg too externally rotated), as shown in Figures 6-72 and 6-73. If the fibula is demonstrated more anteriorly than this relationship, the medial talar dome is posterior and the patient was positioned with the forefoot elevated and the heel depressed (leg internal rotation), as shown in Figures 6-74 and 6-75.

the cuboid than expected and the talocalcaneal joint is wider, the medial dome is the proximal dome and the distal lower leg needs to be depressed or proximal lower leg elevated to reposition (Figure 6-70).

Foot Positioning. The anterior and the posterior aspects of the talar domes are aligned on a lateral calcaneus projection when the lateral foot surface is aligned parallel with the IR (Figure 6-71) and even pressure is

TABLE 6-10	AP Ankle Projection	
Image Analysis Guidelines (Figure 6-76)		**Related Positioning Procedures (Figure 6-77)**
• Medial mortise is open. • Tibia superimposes one-half of the distal fibula. • Anterior and posterior tibial margins, adjacent to the medial malleolus, are aligned		• Place the patient in a supine or seated position, with the knee fully extended. • Center the ankle joint to the IR. • Dorsiflex the foot to a 90-degree angle with the lower leg. • Rotate leg as needed to place foot in a vertical position.
• Tibiotalar joint space is open. • Tibiotalar joint is at the center of the exposure field. • Tibia is demonstrated without foreshortening. • Distal fourth of the tibia and fibula, the talus, and surrounding ankle soft tissue are included within the exposure field.		• Position the lower leg parallel with the table. • Center a perpendicular CR to the mid-ankle joint, at the level of the medial malleolus. • Longitudinally collimate to include the heel and one fourth of the lower leg. • Transversely collimate to within 0.5 inch (1.25 cm) of the ankle skin line.

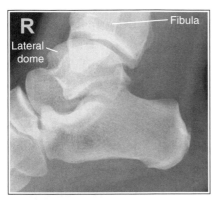

FIGURE 6-75 Lateral calcaneal projection taken with the leg internally rotated.

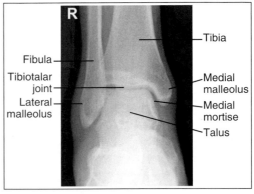

FIGURE 6-76 AP ankle projection with accurate positioning.

Lateral Calcaneal Analysis Practice

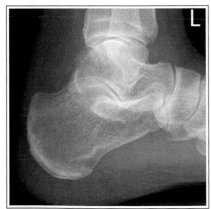

IMAGE 6-15

Analysis. The medial talar dome is positioned posterior to the lateral dome, as indicated by the anterior position of the distal fibula on the tibia. The leg was internally rotated.

Correction. Externally rotate the leg until the lateral foot surface is positioned parallel with the IR.

ANKLE: AP PROJECTION

See Table 6-10, (Figures 6-76 and 6-77).
Medial Mortise. An AP projection of the ankle is obtained by positioning the patient supine on the table,

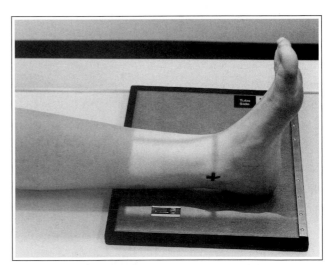

FIGURE 6-77 Proper patient positioning for AP ankle projection.

with the leg fully extended and the foot dorsiflexed until its long axis is placed in a vertical position (see Figure 6-77). In this position, the intermalleolar line (imaginary line drawn between the medial and lateral malleoli) is at a 15- to 20-degree angle with the IR. The medial malleolus is positioned farther from the IR than the lateral malleolus. This malleoli alignment results in the medial mortise (tibiotalar joint) being demonstrated as an open space, alignment of the anterior and posterior tibial margins that are adjacent to the medial mortise, a closed

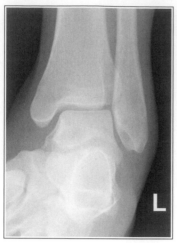

FIGURE 6-78 AP ankle projection of a patient with a ruptured ligament.

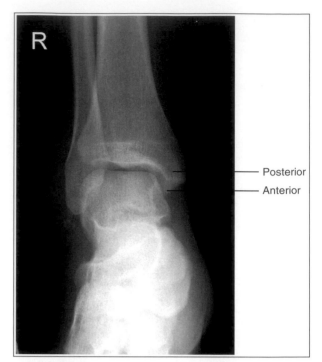

FIGURE 6-80 AP ankle projection taken with the ankle externally rotated.

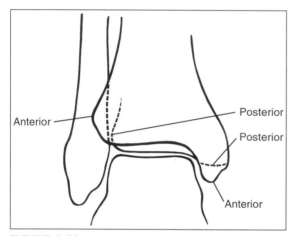

FIGURE 6-79 Anatomy of anterior and posterior ankle.

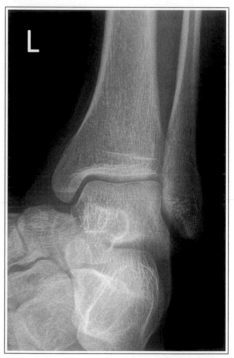

FIGURE 6-81 AP ankle projection taken with the ankle internally rotated.

lateral mortise (fibulotalar joint), and the tibia superimposing about one half of the fibula.

Ruptured Ligament Variation. Contrary to the above description, if the patient has a ruptured ligament the lateral mortise may also be demonstrated as an open space (see Figure 6-78). Such a projection is only acceptable when the medial mortise is also open because it indicates that the projection was obtained without rotation.

Rotation. If the ankle was not positioned in an AP projection but is rotated laterally or medially, the medial mortise is obscured. When an AP ankle demonstrates a closed medial mortise, one can determine which way the patient's leg was rotated by evaluating the amount of tibia superimposition of the fibula and the alignment of the anterior and posterior margins of the tibia that are adjacent to the medial malleolus (Figure 6-79). In external rotation, the tibia superimposes more than one half of the fibula, and the anterior tibial margin is lateral to the posterior margin, superimposing the tibia and closing the medial mortise (Figure 6-80). In internal rotation, the tibia superimposes less than one half of the fibula, and the posterior tibial margin is lateral to the anterior

margin and is superimposed by the talus, and the medial mortise is closed (Figure 6-81).

Tibiotalar Joint Space. The tibiotalar joint is open and the tibia is demonstrated without foreshortening if the patient's lower leg was positioned parallel with the IR and the CR was centered at the level of the tibiotalar joint.

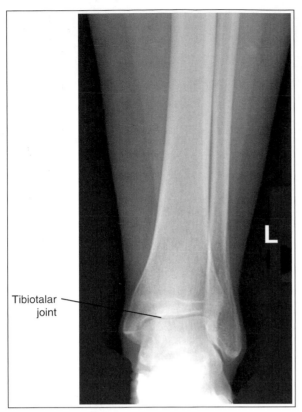

FIGURE 6-82 AP ankle projection taken with the proximal lower leg elevated.

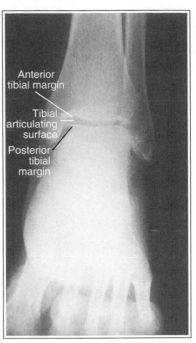

FIGURE 6-83 AP ankle projection taken with the distal lower leg elevated.

Evaluating the Openness of the Tibiotalar Joint.

On an AP ankle projection, determine whether an open joint was obtained and whether the tibia is demonstrated without foreshortening by evaluating the anterior and posterior margins of the distal tibia, adjacent to the joint space. On an AP ankle projection with accurate positioning, the anterior margin is demonstrated approximately 0.125 inch (3 mm) proximal to the posterior margin. If the proximal lower leg was elevated or the CR was centered proximal to the tibiotalar joint, the anterior tibial margin is projected distally, resulting in a narrowed or obscured tibiotalar joint space (Figure 6-82). If the distal lower leg was elevated or the CR was centered distal to the tibiotalar joint, the anterior tibial margin is projected more proximally to the posterior margin than on an AP ankle projection, expanding the tibiotalar joint space and demonstrating the tibial articulating surface (Figure 6-83).

Effect of Foot Positioning on Tibiotalar Joint Visualization.

The position of the foot also determines how well the tibiotalar joint space is demonstrated. The patient's foot should be placed vertically, with its long axis positioned at a 90-degree angle with the lower leg. When the AP ankle projection is taken with the foot dorsiflexed, the trochlear surface of the talus is wedged into the anterior tibial region, resulting in a narrower appearing joint space. If the foot is plantar-flexed, the calcaneus is moved proximally, beneath the body of the talus, resulting in talocalcaneal superimposition and possibly hindering visualization of the talar trochlear surface.

AP Ankle Analysis Practice

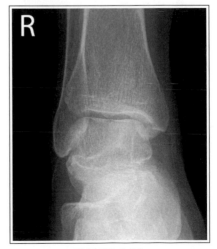

IMAGE 6-16

Analysis. The medial mortise is obscured, the tibia superimposes more than one half of the fibula, and the anterior tibial margin is lateral to the posterior margin. The ankle was externally rotated.

Correction. Internally rotate the ankle.

TABLE 6-11	AP Oblique Ankle Projection	
Image Analysis Guidelines (Figures 6-84 and 6-85)	**Related Positioning Procedures (Figures 6-86 and 6-87)**
• 15- to 20-degree AP oblique (Mortise): • Distal fibula is demonstrated without talar superimposition, demonstrating an open lateral mortise. • Lateral and medial malleoli are in profile. • Tibia superimposes one fourth of the distal fibula. • 45-degree AP oblique: • Lateral mortise is open with differing degrees of mortise narrowing. • Fibula is seen without tibial superimposition. • Tarsi sinus is demonstrated.	• Place the patient in a supine or seated position, with the knee extended. • Center the ankle joint to the IR. • 15- to 20-degree AP oblique (Mortise): Internally rotate the leg and ankle until the intermalleolar plane is parallel with the IR • 45-degree AP oblique: • Internally rotate the leg and ankle until the ankle and foot are at a 45-degree angle with the IR.
• Tibiotalar joint space is open and centered to the exposure field. • Tibia is seen without foreshortening.	• Align the lower leg parallel with the table. • Center a perpendicular CR to the mid-ankle joint, at the level of the medial malleolus.
• Calcaneus is visualized distal to the lateral mortise and fibula.	• Dorsiflex the foot, placing its long axis at a 90-degree angle with the lower leg.
• Distal fourth of the fibula and tibia, the talus, and the surrounding ankle soft tissue are included within the exposure field.	• Longitudinally collimate to include the heel and one fourth of the lower leg. • Transversely collimate to within 0.5 inch (1.25 cm) of the ankle skin line.

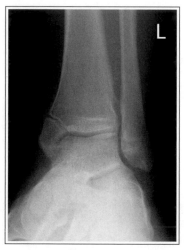

IMAGE 6-17

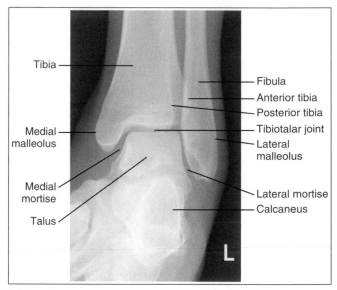

FIGURE 6-84 AP (mortise) oblique ankle projection with accurate positioning.

Analysis. The tibia superimposes less than one half of the fibula, the posterior tibial margin is lateral to the anterior margin and is superimposed by the talus, and the medial mortise is closed. The ankle was internally rotated.

Correction. Externally rotate the ankle.

ANKLE: AP OBLIQUE PROJECTION (MEDIAL ROTATION)

See Table 6-11, (Figures 6-84, 6-85, 6-86, and 6-87).
15- to 20-Degree AP Oblique (Mortise). To obtain the proper degree of rotation for a Mortise position, while viewing the plantar surface of the foot, place your index fingers on the most prominent aspects of the lateral and medial malleoli. Rotate the entire leg internally (medially) until your index fingers and the malleoli are positioned at equal distances from the IR (see Figure 6-87).

This positioning aligns the intermalleolar plane parallel with the IR, rotates the fibula away from the talus to demonstrate an open lateral mortise (talofibular joint), and typically requires 15 to 20 degrees of obliquity. The tibiofibular joint will remain close, as this degree of rotation does not move the fibula from beneath the tibia, nor does it rotate the ankle enough to position the tarsal sinus on end so it is visualized.

Repositioning for Inadequate Rotation. If the leg and foot are internally rotated less than the needed degrees, the tibia superimposes more than one fourth of the fibula, and the lateral and medial mortises are closed (Figure 6-88). If the ankle was internally rotated more than the needed degrees, the tibia will superimpose less

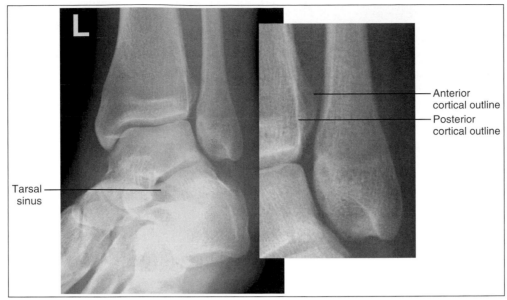

Tarsal
sinus

Anterior
cortical outline
Posterior
cortical outline

FIGURE 6-85 AP (45-degree) oblique ankle projection with accurate positioning.

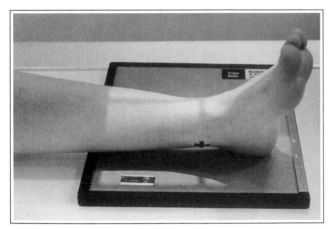

FIGURE 6-86 Proper patient positioning for AP oblique ankle projection.

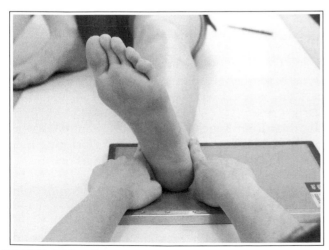

FIGURE 6-87 Aligning the intermalleolar line parallel with IR for AP oblique (mortise) ankle projection.

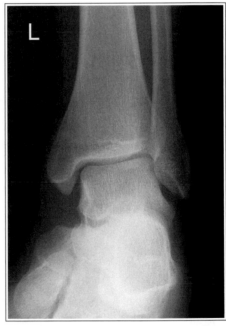

FIGURE 6-88 AP oblique (mortise) ankle projection taken with insufficient obliquity.

than one fourth of the fibula and the lateral mortise will be open (Figure 6-89).

Foot Inversion verus Ankle Rotation. The leg and foot must stay aligned and rotated together for this projection. If the foot is inverted, without leg rotation, the ankle can appear to have been rotated when it has not, and the projection demonstrates a closed lateral mortise (Figure 6-90).

45-Degree AP Oblique. For the 45-degree oblique, the leg and foot are internally rotated until the long axis of the foot is aligned 45 degrees with the IR (Figure 6-91). This rotation moves the fibula from beneath the tibia

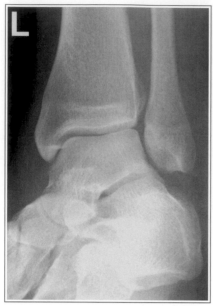

FIGURE 6-89 AP oblique (mortise) ankle projection taken with excessive obliquity.

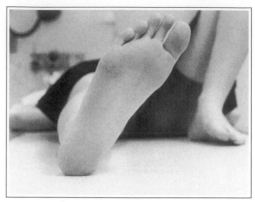

FIGURE 6-91 Proper internal foot rotation: 15 to 20 degrees from vertical.

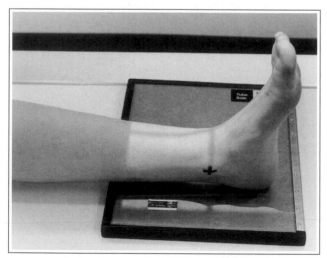

FIGURE 6-90 AP oblique (mortise) ankle projection taken with foot inverted and insufficient obliquity.

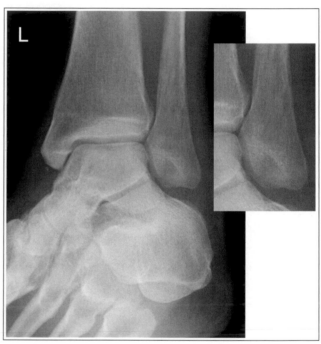

FIGURE 6-92 AP (45-degree) oblique ankle projection with accurate positioning.

and the talus, resulting in open tibiofibular and lateral mortise joint spaces. The narrowness of the lateral mortise differs with a slight degree in obliquity. Compare the superimposition of the anterior and posterior cortical outlines of the lateral tibia and the openness of the tibiotalar joint spaces in Figures 6-85 and 6-92. There are only a few degrees of difference between the amounts of obliquity between the two projections.

Identifying Inadequate Rotation. If the leg and foot are internally rotated less than 45 degrees, the anterior cortical outline of the lateral tibia is lateral to the posterior cortical outline of the lateral tibia (Figures 6-93, 6-94, and 6-95) and the tarsal sinus is poorly

demonstrated. If the leg and foot are internally rotated slightly more than 45 degrees, the anterior cortical outline of the lateral tibia is medial to the posterior cortical outline of the lateral tibia and the sinus tarsi will be clearly seen.

Tibiotalar Joint Space. The tibiotalar joint is open and the tibia is demonstrated without foreshortening if the lower leg is positioned parallel with the IR and the CR is centered at the level of the tibiotalar joint.

Evaluating the Openness of the Tibiotalar Joint. On an AP oblique ankle, determine whether an open tibiotalar joint was obtained and whether the tibia is demonstrated without foreshortening by evaluating the anterior and posterior margins of the distal tibia. And AP oblique ankle with accurate positioning demonstrates

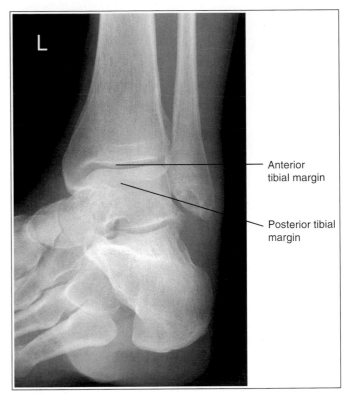

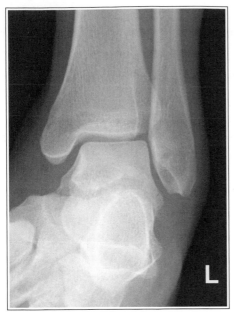

FIGURE 6-93 AP (45-degree) oblique ankle projection taken with insufficient obliquity.

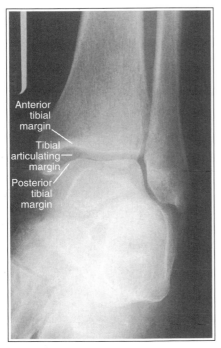

FIGURE 6-94 AP (45-degree) oblique ankle projection taken with insufficient obliquity and with the distal lower leg elevated.

the anterior margin approximately 0.125 inch (3 mm) proximally to the posterior margin. If the proximal lower leg was elevated or the CR was centered proximal to the tibiotalar joint, the anterior tibial margin is projected distally, resulting in a narrowed or obscured tibiotalar joint space. If the distal lower leg was elevated or the CR was centered distal to the tibiotalar joint, the anterior tibial margin is projected more proximally to the posterior margin, expanding the tibiotalar joint space and demonstrating the tibial articulating surface (Figures 6-94 and 6-95).

FIGURE 6-95 AP (45-degree) oblique ankle projection taken with insufficient obliquity and with the distal lower leg elevated.

Calcaneus. To position the calcaneus distal to the lateral mortise and fibula, the foot is dorsiflexed to bring its long axis at a 90-degree angle with the lower leg. If the foot is not dorsiflexed for the AP oblique ankle, the distal aspects of the lateral mortise and distal fibula superimpose the calcaneus and obscure their visualization (Figures 6-96 and 6-97).

AP Oblique Ankle Analysis Practice

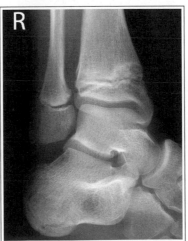

IMAGE 6-18 Mortise oblique.

Analysis. The medial mortise is closed, and there is no tibia superimposition of the fibula. The projection was obtained with more than 15 to 20 degrees of leg and

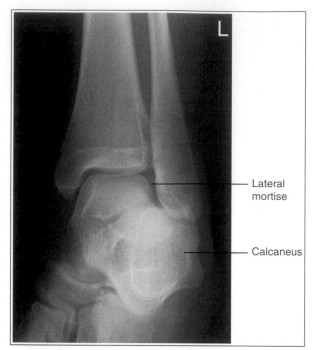

FIGURE 6-96 AP oblique (mortise) ankle projection taken without the foot dorsiflexed.

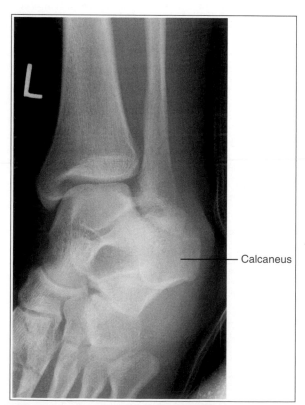

FIGURE 6-97 AP (45-degree) oblique ankle projection taken without the foot dorsiflexed.

ankle obliquity. The tibiotalar joint spaces expanded. The anterior tibial margin has been projected proximal to the posterior margin, and the tibial articulating surface is demonstrated. The distal tibia was elevated.

Correction. Externally rotate the leg and ankle until the medial and lateral malleoli are positioned at equal distances from the IR and depressed the distal tibia or elevate the proximal tibia until the lower leg is placed parallel with the IR.

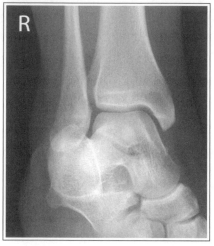

IMAGE 6-19

Analysis. The calcaneus is obscuring the distal aspect of the lateral mortise and distal fibula. The foot was in plantar flexion.

Correction. Dorsiflexed the foot until its long axis forms a 90-degree angle with the lower leg.

ANKLE: LATERAL PROJECTION (MEDIOLATERAL)

See Table 6-12, (Figures 6-98 and 6-99).

Demonstrating the Anterior Pretalar and Posterior Pericapsular Fat Pads. Two soft tissue structures located around the ankle joint that should be demonstrated on AP ankle projections are the anterior pretalar and posterior pericapsular fat pads. The anterior pretalar fat pad is demonstrated anterior to the ankle joint and rests next to the neck of the talus (Figure 6-100). The posterior fat pad is positioned within the indentation formed by the articulation of the posterior tibia and talar bones. Displacement of these pads indicates joint effusion and injury.

Foot Dorsiflexion. Foot plantar flexion results in a forced flattening of the anterior pretalar fat pad, reducing its usefulness in the detection of joint effusion. Dorsiflexing the foot to a 90-degree angle with the lower leg places the tibiotalar joint in a neutral position, more clearly defines the medial longitudinal arch, and prevents foot rotation (Figure 6-101). To obtain a lateral foot on a patient who is unable to dorsiflex, the knee needs to

TABLE 6-12 | Lateral Ankle Projection

Image Analysis Guidelines (Figure 6-98)	Related Positioning Procedures (Figure 6-99)
• Contrast and brightness are adequate to demonstrate the anterior pretalar and posterior pericapsular fat pads.	• Appropriate technique has been set.
• Long axis of the foot is positioned at a 90-degree angle with the lower leg.	• Start with the patient in a supine or standing position. • Dorsiflex the foot, placing its long axis at a 90-degree angle with the lower leg.
• Proximal aspects of the talar domes are aligned. • Tibiotalar joint is open.	• Extend the knee, and align the lower leg parallel with the IR.
• Anterior and posterior aspects of the talar domes are aligned. • Distal fibula is superimposed by the posterior half of the distal tibia. • Tibiotalar joint is at the center of the exposure field.	• Externally rotate the affected leg, and oblique the torso as needed to align the lateral foot surface parallel with the IR (Figure 6-27). • Center the ankle to the IR. • Center a perpendicular CR to the ankle joint at the level of the medial malleolus.
• Talus, 1 inch (2.5 cm) of the fifth MT base, surrounding ankle soft tissue, and the distal fourth of the fibula and tibia are included within the exposure field.	• Longitudinally collimate to include the calcaneus and one fourth of the distal lower leg. • Transversely collimate to include 1 inch (2.5 cm) of the fifth MT base.

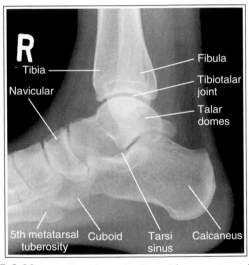

FIGURE 6-98 Lateral ankle projection with accurate positioning.

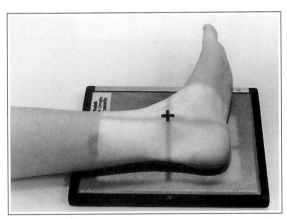

FIGURE 6-99 Lateral ankle projection with proper central ray (CR) centering and collimation.

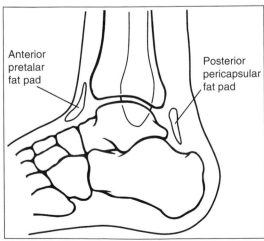

FIGURE 6-100 Location of fat pads.

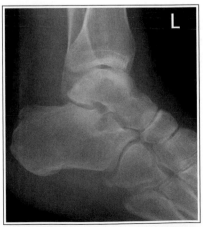

FIGURE 6-101 Lateral ankle projection taken without the foot dorsiflexed.

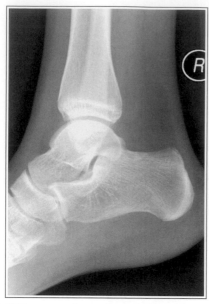

FIGURE 6-102 Accurately positioned lateral ankle projection taken without the foot dorsiflexed.

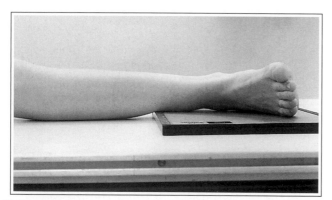

FIGURE 6-103 Proper knee and lower leg positioning for lateral ankle projection.

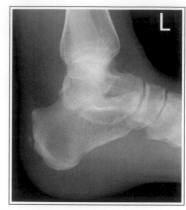

FIGURE 6-104 Lateral ankle projection taken with the proximal lower leg elevated.

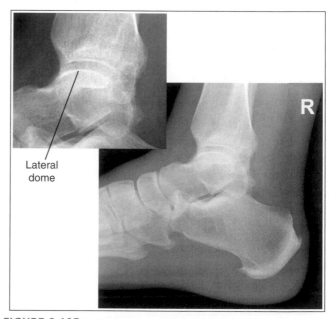

Lateral dome

FIGURE 6-105 Lateral ankle projection taken with the distal lower leg elevated.

be slightly flexed and an immobilization support placed beneath it to elevate it the needed amount to place the plantar surfaces of the heel and forefoot perpendicular with the IR (Figure 6-102).

Medial and Lateral Talar Domes

Proximal Alignment. Correct lower leg positioning for the lateral calcaneus brings the lower leg parallel with the IR and aligns the proximal aspects of the medial and lateral talar dome (Figure 6-103). If the lower leg is not placed parallel with the IR, by keeping the knee extended or by elevating the distal lower leg in a patient with a large upper thigh, the proximal lower leg is positioned farther from the table than the distal lower leg. The resulting projection demonstrates the lateral talar dome proximal to the medial dome, and the height of the medial longitudinal arch appears less than it actually is because the cuboid shifts anteriorly and the navicular bone moves posteriorly in this position (Figure 6-104). The talocalcaneal joint will also be narrowed. If the

distal tibia is positioned farther from the table than the proximal tibia, the medial talar dome is demonstrated proximal to the lateral dome, and the height of the medial arch appears higher than it actually is because the cuboid shifts posteriorly and the navicular bone moves anteriorly in this position (Figure 6-105). The talocalcaneal joint will be wider.

Anterior and Posterior Alignment. To demonstrate accurate anterior and posterior alignment of the talar domes and position the fibula in the posterior half of the tibia, position the lateral surface of the foot parallel with the IR (Figure 6-106). If this surface is not parallel with the IR, the talar domes are demonstrated one anterior to the other and the fibula is not located in the posterior half of the tibia. When the leg is rotated more than needed to place the lateral foot surface parallel with the IR (leg externally rotated), as shown in Figure 6-107, the medial talar dome is demonstrated anterior to the lateral talar dome and the fibula is more posterior on the

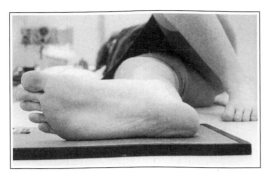

FIGURE 6-106 Proper lateral foot surface positioning for lateral ankle projection.

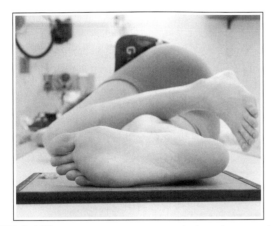

FIGURE 6-107 Poor foot positioning with the calcaneus elevated (leg externally rotated).

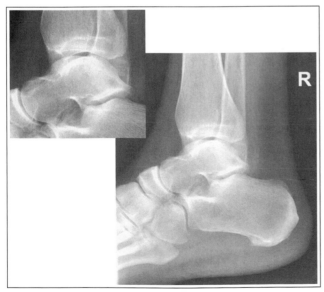

FIGURE 6-108 Lateral ankle projection taken with the leg externally rotated.

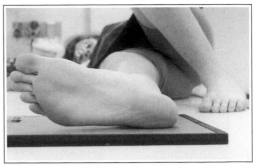

FIGURE 6-109 Poor foot positioning with the calcaneus depressed (leg internally rotated).

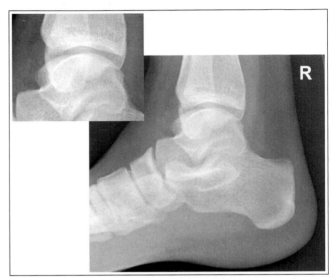

FIGURE 6-110 Lateral ankle projection taken with the leg internally rotated.

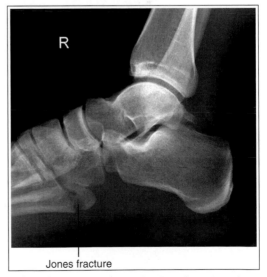

Jones fracture

FIGURE 6-111 Lateral ankle projection demonstrating a Jones fracture.

tibia (Figure 6-108). If the leg is not rotated enough to place the lateral foot surface parallel with the IR (leg internally rotated), as shown in Figure 6-109, the medial talar dome is demonstrated posterior to the lateral talar dome and the fibula will be demonstrated more anteriorly on the tibia (Figure 6-110).

Including the Fifth Metatarsal Base. An inversion injury of the foot and ankle may result in a fracture of the fifth MT base, known as a Jones fracture (Figure 6-111). Including the fifth MT base on the lateral ankle projection allows it to be evaluated for a Jones fracture, eliminating the need for additional projections.

Lateral Ankle Analysis Practice

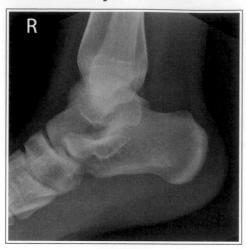

IMAGE 6-20

Analysis. The lateral talar dome is proximal to the medial dome, the height of the medial longitudinal arch appears less than it actually is, and the talocalcaneal joint is narrowed. The proximal lower leg was elevated.

Correction. Extend the knee to position the lower leg parallel with the IR. If the knee was extended for this projection, elevate the lower leg until disposition parallel with the IR.

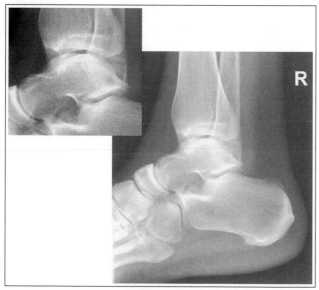

IMAGE 6-21

Analysis. The medial talar dome is positioned anterior to the lateral talar dome, as indicated by the posterior position the fibula on the tibia. The lateral foot surface is not parallel with the IR. The leg was externally rotated.

Correction. Elevate the patient's forefoot, and depress the heel (internally rotate the leg) until the lateral foot surface is parallel with the IR.

TABLE 6-13	AP Lower Leg Projection
Image Analysis Guidelines (Figure 6-112)	**Related Positioning Procedures (Figure 6-113)**
• Image brightness is uniform across the lower leg.	• Position the knee at the cathode end of the tube and the ankle at the anode end of the tube.
• Tibia superimposes about one fourth of the fibular head and about one half of the distal fibula. • Fibular midshaft is free of tibial superimposition.	• Position the patient in a supine or seated position with the knee fully extended. • Dorsiflex the foot to a 90-degree angle with the lower leg and place it at a slight internal rotation (7-10 degrees from vertical), positioning the femoral epicondyles close to parallel with the IR.
• Tibial midshaft is at the center of the exposure field. • Knee and tibiotalar joint spaces are closed.	• Center a perpendicular CR to the midpoint of the lower leg.
• Tibia, fibula, knee, and surrounding lower leg soft tissue are included within the exposure field.	• Center the lower leg to the IR, so the IR extends 1 to 1.5 inches beyond the knee and ankle joints. • Longitudinally collimate until the light field extends just beyond the knee and ankle joints. • Transversely collimate to within 0.5 inch (1.25 cm) of the skin line.

LOWER LEG: AP PROJECTION

See Table 6-13, (Figures 6-112 and 6-113).

Anatomic Position versus AP Projections of the Ankle and Knee. To place the patient in anatomic position, the legs are internally rotated until the femoral epicondyles are aligned parallel with the IR, placing the knees in an AP projection and the ankles in a 15- to 20-degree internal (Mortise) oblique. In this position, the tibia will superimpose about one half of the fibular head (as is expected on an AP knee) and one fourth of the distal fibula (as is expected on a mortise ankle). This is contrary to the AP ankle projection discussed previously, as the leg and foot were not internally rotated for the projection, but remain vertical, and the resulting projection demonstrates the tibia superimposing about one half of the distal fibula. If the lower leg were taken with the ankle in an AP projection, the knee would not be in an AP projection and would demonstrate the fibular head without tibia superimposition (Figure 6-114). Because the ankle and knee joints cannot be demonstrated in a true AP projection at the same time, the image analysis

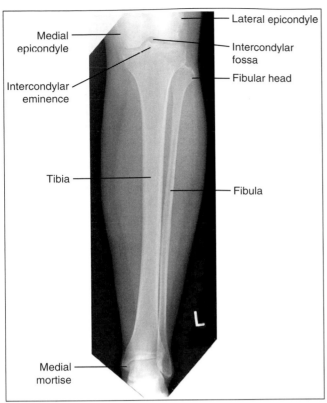

FIGURE 6-112 AP lower leg projection with accurate positioning.

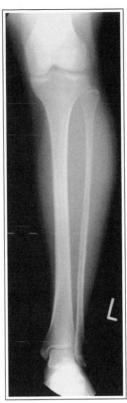

FIGURE 6-114 AP lower leg projection taken with the ankle in a true AP projection and the knee and slight internal rotation.

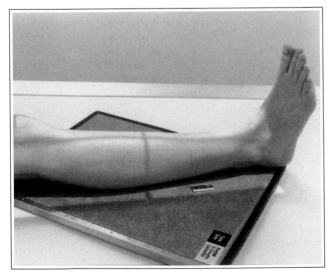

FIGURE 6-113 Proper patient positioning for AP lower leg projection.

guidelines and positioning procedures listed in the preceding are for a projection in which the knee and ankle are placed in slight oblique positions, halfway between the AP knee and AP ankle.

Positioning for Fracture. For a patient with a known or suspected fracture, position the joint closest to the fracture as you would for the AP ankle or knee

projection described previously to provide a true AP projection with which to reference the fracture. If the fracture is situated closer to the distal lower leg, the ankle is positioned using the AP ankle projection described earlier in this book (the foot remains vertical) and the knee will be externally rotation. The resulting projection demonstrates the tibia superimposing about one half of the distal fibula. The amount of proximal tibia and fibular superimposition will depend on the fractures effect on leg rotation (Figure 6-115). If the fracture is situated closer to the proximal lower leg, the knee is positioned using the AP knee projection described earlier in this book and the lower leg will be internally rotated. The resulting projection demonstrates the tibia superimposing about one half of the fibular head. The amount of distal tibia and fibular superimposition will depend on the fractures effect on leg rotation.

Rotation. Rotation of the lower leg can be identified on an AP projection by evaluating the relationship of the fibula to the tibia. When the patient's leg is too externally rotated, the tibia superimposes more than one fourth of the fibular head and more than one half of the distal fibula. Increased external rotation will also cause the tibia to superimpose the fibular midshaft (Figure 6-116). If the leg is too internally rotated, the tibia superimposes less than one fourth of the fibular head and less than one half of the distal fibula.

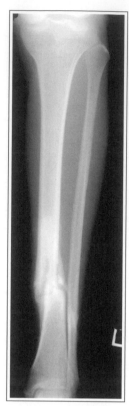

FIGURE 6-115 AP lower leg projection of a patient with a distal lower leg fracture.

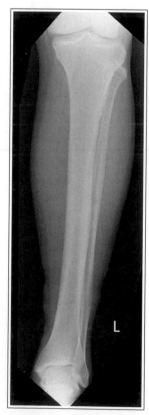

FIGURE 6-116 AP lower leg projection taken with the leg and the sternal rotation.

Knee and Ankle Joint Spaces. The proximal tibia slopes distally from the anterior condylar margin to the posterior condylar margin by approximately 5 degrees. When the lower leg is placed parallel with the IR and the CR is centered to the midshaft of the lower leg, x-rays that diverge in the opposite direction are used to record the projection of the proximal tibia (Figure 6-117). The distal lower leg also slopes distally from the anterior tibial margin to the posterior margin by approximately 3 degrees. Although the x-rays diverge in the same direction as the slope of the distal tibia, they diverge at a greater angle. Because the angle of x-ray divergence is not aligned parallel with either the proximal or distal tibia, the knee and ankle joints are demonstrated as closed spaces on an AP lower leg projection.

Leg and IR Placement. When imaging a long body structure that requires the field size to be open the full length of the IR you must consider the degree of x-ray beam divergence when aligning the leg and IR, as this divergence will project the structures a significant distance from where they are actually placed on the IR (see Figure 6-117). Failing to consider this divergence will result in parts of the structure being clipped from the projection. To ensure that the knee and ankle joints are included on the AP lower leg, the IR must extend 1 to 1.5 inches (2.5-4 cm) beyond each joint. The ankle is located at the level of the medial malleolus, and the knee joint is located 1 inch (2.5 cm) distal to the palpable medial epicondyle.

AP Lower Leg Analysis Practice

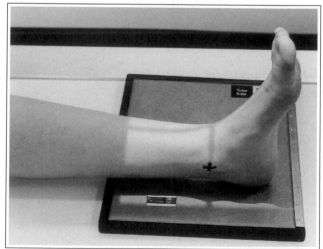

IMAGE 6-22

Analysis. The distal lower leg has been clipped, and the distal and proximal fibula is free of tibial superimposition. The CR and IR were positioned too proximally and the leg was internally rotated.

Correction. Move the CR and IR 1 inch (2.5 cm) distally and externally rotate the leg to an AP projection.

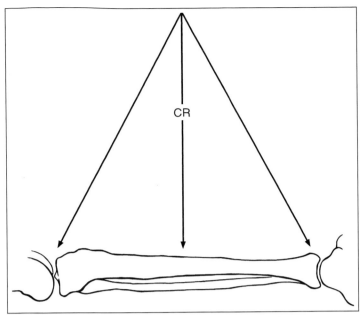

FIGURE 6-117 Effect of x-ray divergence on AP lower leg projection. CR, Central ray.

TABLE 6-14	Lateral Lower Leg Projection
Image Analysis Guidelines (Figures 6-118 and 6-119)	**Related Positioning Procedures (Figure 6-120)**
• Image brightness is uniform across the lower leg.	• Position the knee at the cathode end of the tube and the ankle at the anode end of the tube.
• Tibia superimposes about one half of the fibular head. • Fibular midshaft is demonstrated free of tibial superimposition. • Posterior aspects of the distal tibia and the fibula are aligned.	• Position the patient in a recumbent position with the knee fully extended and the lateral leg surface resting against the IR. • Dorsiflex the foot to a 90-degree angle with the lower leg. • Rotate the patient as needed to position the medial femoral epicondyles slightly anterior (7-10 degrees) to the lateral epicondyle.
• Tibial midshaft is at the center of the exposure field. • Knee and tibiotalar joint spaces are closed.	• Center a perpendicular CR to the midpoint of the lower leg.
• Tibia, fibula, knee, and surrounding lower leg soft tissue are included within the exposure field.	• Center lower leg on the IR so it extends 1 to 1.5 inches beyond the knee and ankle joints. • Longitudinally collimate until the light field extends just beyond the knee and ankle joints. • Transversely collimate to within 0.5 inch (1.25 cm) of the skin line.

LOWER LEG: LATERAL PROJECTION (MEDIOLATERAL)

See Table 6-14, (Figures 6-118, 6-119, and 6-120).
Variation from the True Lateral Knee and Ankle Projections. Because the ankle and knee joints cannot be demonstrated in lateral projections at the same time as explained in the AP lower leg projection, the image analysis guidelines and positioning procedures listed above are for a projection that is in slight internal rotation from the true lateral knee and slight external rotation from the true lateral ankle.

Positioning for Fracture. For a patient with a known or suspected fracture, position the joint closest to the fracture site as you would for a lateral ankle or knee projection to provide a true lateral ankle or knee projection with which to reference the fracture. If the fracture is situated closer to the distal lower leg, the ankle is positioned using the lateral ankle projection described earlier in the text (lateral surface of foot aligned parallel with IR). The resulting projection demonstrates the fibula superimposed by the posterior half of the tibia. The amount of proximal tibia and fibula superimposition will depend on the fractures effect on leg rotation

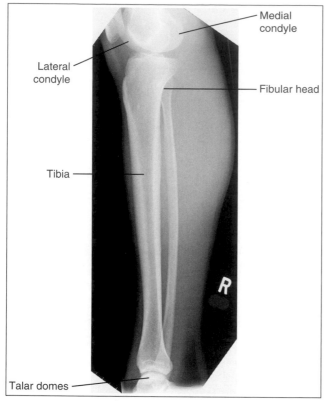

FIGURE 6-118 Lateral lower leg projection with accurate positioning.

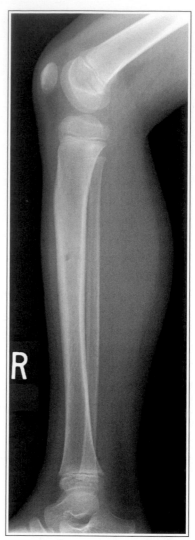

FIGURE 6-119 Pediatric lateral lower leg projection with accurate positioning.

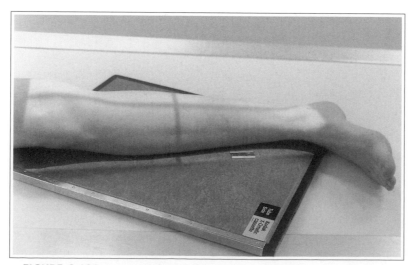

FIGURE 6-120 Proper patient positioning for lateral lower leg projection.

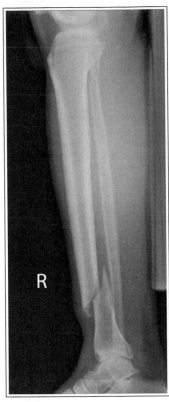

FIGURE 6-121 Lateral lower leg projection of a patient with a distal lower leg fracture.

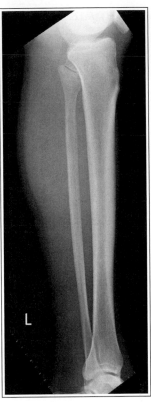

FIGURE 6-122 Lateral lower leg projection taken with excessive external rotation.

(Figure 6-121). If the fracture is situated closer to the proximal lower leg, the knee is positioned using the lateral knee projection described earlier in the text (femoral epicondyles positioned perpendicular with the IR). The resulting projection demonstrates the tibia superimposing about one half of the fibular head. The amount of distal tibia and fibular superimposition will depend on the fracture's effect on leg rotation.

Rotation. Superimposition of the femoral condyles and the talar domes are good indicators of rotation on true lateral knee and ankle projections, but are not reliable for the lateral lower leg, as neither the knee nor the ankle is placed in a true lateral projection, as discussed. The amount of femoral condyle superimposition also depends on the degree of knee flexion and the way in which the diverged x-ray beams are aligned with the medial condyle (see discussion on lateral knee projection). Rotation is then best distinguished by viewing the degree of tibia and fibular head superimposition. If the patient's leg was too externally rotated, the tibia superimposes less than one half of the fibular head (Figure 6-122). If the patient's leg was too internally rotated, the tibia superimposes more than one half of the fibular head, and the posterior aspect of the distal fibula will be anterior to the posterior aspect of the distal tibia (Figure 6-123).

Leg and IR Placement. See AP lower leg.

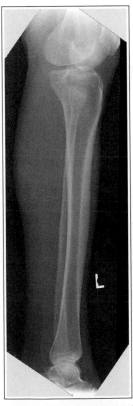

FIGURE 6-123 Lateral lower leg projection taken with insufficient external rotation.

Lateral Lower Leg Analysis Practice

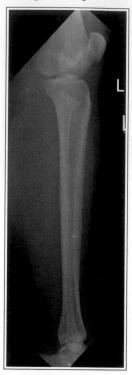

IMAGE 6-23

Analysis. The tibia superimposes more than one half of the fibular head, and the entire fibular midshaft, and posterior aspect of the distal fibula is anterior to the posterior aspect of the distal tibia. The patient's leg was an internal rotation.

Correction. Externally rotate the leg until it is in a lateral projection.

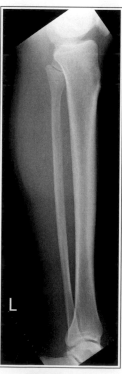

IMAGE 6-24

Analysis. The tibia is superimposing less than one half of the fibular head. The leg was externally rotated more than needed to position it in a lateral projection.
Correction. Internally rotate the leg to a lateral projection.

KNEE: AP PROJECTION

See Table 6-15, (Figures 6-124 and 6-125).
Femoral Epicondyle, and Tibia and Fibular Head Relationship
   Rotation. To place the knee in an AP projection, position the femoral epicondyles parallel with the IR. If the leg is not internally rotated enough to place the epicondyles parallel with the IR, the medial epicondyle is placed closer to the IR than the lateral, and the resulting

TABLE 6-15	AP Knee Projection
Image Analysis Guidelines (Figure 6-124)	**Related Positioning Procedures (Figure 6-125)**
• Femoral epicondyles are in profile and the femoral condyles are symmetric • Intercondylar eminence is centered within the intercondylar fossa • Tibia superimposes one half of the fibular head.	• Position the patient supine with the IR centered beneath the knee joint. • Internally rotate the leg, placing the femoral epicondyles at equidistant and parallel with the IR.
• Patella lies just proximal to the femoral patellar surface and is slightly lateral to the knee midline. • Intercondylar fossa is only partially seen.	• Fully extend the knee.
• Knee (femorotibial) joint space is open. • Anterior and posterior distal tibial margins are aligned. • Fibular head is 0.5 inch (1.25 cm) distal to the tibial plateau.	• Angle the CR to align it parallel with the tibial plateau. • 5 degrees caudal if ASIS to the table measurement is 18 cm or below • perpendicular beam if ASIS to the table measurement is between 19 and 24 cm • 5 degrees cephalic if ASIS to the table measurement is 25 cm and above
• Knee joint (femorotibial) is at the center of the exposure field.	• Center the CR to the midline of the knee at a level 1 inch (2.5 cm) distal to the medial epicondyle.
• One fourth of the distal femur and proximal lower leg and the surrounding knee soft tissue are included within the exposure field	• Longitudinally collimate to include one fourth of the distal femur and proximal lower leg. • Transversely collimate to within 0.5 inch (1.25 cm) of the knee skin line.

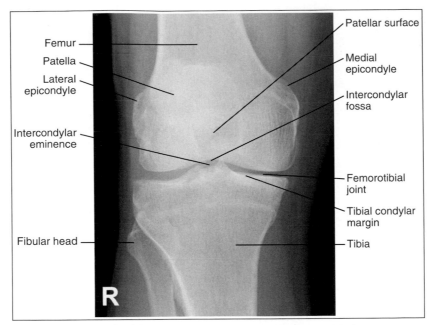

FIGURE 6-124 AP knee projection with accurate positioning.

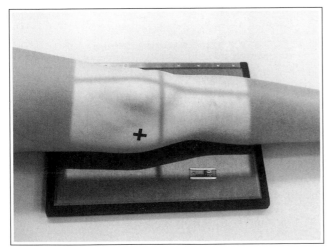

FIGURE 6-125 Proper patient positioning for lateral knee projection.

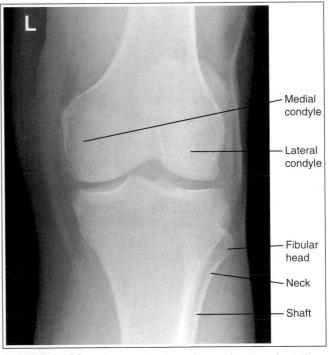

FIGURE 6-126 AP knee projection taken with external rotation.

projection will demonstrate a larger appearing medial femoral condyle when compared with the lateral, and the tibia superimposes more than half of the fibular head (Figure 6-126). If the patient's leg was internally rotated more than needed, the lateral epicondyle will be closer to the IR, and the resulting projection demonstrates a larger appearing lateral condyle, and the tibia superimposes over less than half of the fibular head (Figure 6-127).

Patella and Intercondylar Fossa Demonstration

Effect of Knee Flexion. The placement of the patella on the femur and the degree of intercondylar fossa demonstration are determined by the amount of knee flexion. To visualize the patella and fossa as required, the leg must be in full extension. As the knee is flexed, the patella shifts distally and medially onto the patellar

surface of the femur and then laterally into the intercondylar fossa, duplicating a C-shaped path that is open laterally (Figure 6-128). Thus, the patella is demonstrated at different locations, depending on the degree of knee flexion. Generally, when the knee is flexed 20 degrees, the patella is demonstrated on the patellar surface. With 30 to 70 degrees of knee flexion, the patella is demonstrated between the patellar surface and the intercondylar fossa. At 90 degrees to full knee flexion,

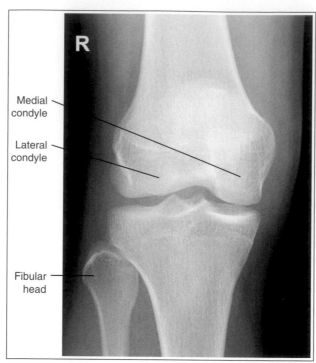

FIGURE 6-127 AP knee projection taken with excessive internal rotation.

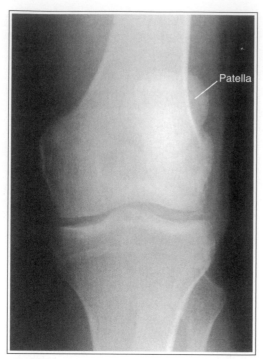

FIGURE 6-129 AP knee projection of patient with patellar subluxation.

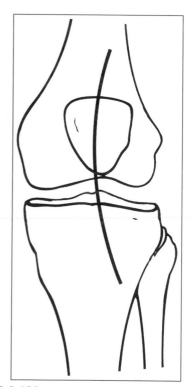

FIGURE 6-128 Movement of patella on knee flexion.

the patella is demonstrated within the intercondylar fossa.

Patellar Subluxation. With patellar subluxation (partial patellar dislocation), the patella may be situated more laterally than normal on an AP knee projection (Figure 6-129). When an AP knee demonstrates a laterally situated patella, evaluate the symmetry of the femoral condyles and the relationship of the tibia and fibular head to rule out external rotation before assuming that the patella is subluxed. External rotation also results in a laterally located patella.

Intercondylar Fossa Visualization with Knee Flexion. The extent of intercondylar fossa demonstration also changes with knee flexion. In full extension, only a slight indentation between the distal medial and lateral femoral condyles indicates the location of the intercondylar fossa. As the knee is flexed, the amount of intercondylar fossa that is demonstrated increases. When the knee is flexed enough to bring the femur to a 60- to 70-degree angle with the table (20 to 30 degrees with CR), the intercondylar fossa is shown in profile (Figure 6-130). When the knee is flexed less or more than this degree, demonstration of the fossa will decrease.

Nonextendable Knee. If the patient is unable to extend the knee fully for an AP knee, an open knee joint can be obtained by completing the following steps.
1. Align the CR perpendicular with the anterior lower leg surface.
2. Decrease the angulation 5 degrees to align the CR parallel with the tibial plateau. For example, if the CR is perpendicular to the anterior lower leg surface when a 15-degree cephalic angulation is used, the angle should be decreased to 10 degrees if the knee cannot be extended.

This setup demonstrates an open knee joint space and the intercondylar fossa. Because the CR is angled to the IR, the distal femur and proximal lower leg will demonstrate some degree of foreshortening distortion. The

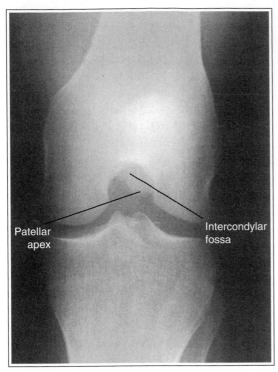

FIGURE 6-130 AP knee projection taken with the knee flexed.

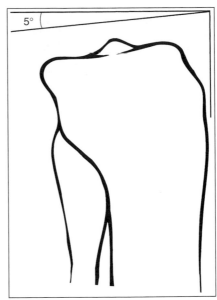

FIGURE 6-131 Slope of the proximal tibia. (Reproduced with permission from Martensen K: Alternative AP knee method assures open joint space, *Radiol Technol* 64:19-23, 1992. Courtesy Radiologic Technology, published by the American Society of Radiologic Technologists.)

amount of the intercondylar fossa that is demonstrated and the severity of the foreshortening distortion will increase with increased CR angulation.

Joint Space and Condylar Margins. The anterior and posterior condylar margins of the tibia are aligned if the correct CR angulation is used, as determined by the patient's upper thigh and buttocks thickness. The tibial plateau slopes distally approximately 3 to 5 degrees from the anterior condylar margin to the posterior condylar margin on both the medial and lateral aspects (Figure 6-131). Only if the CR is aligned parallel with the tibial plateau slope will an open knee joint space and optimal demonstration of the intercondylar eminence and tubercles without foreshortening be obtained.

CR Alignment with Tibial Plateau in the Supine Position. The degree and direction of the CR angulation that is required when the patient is in a supine position depends on the thickness of the patient's upper thigh and buttocks. This thickness determines how the lower leg and the tibial plateau align with the IR. Figure 6-132 shows a guideline that can be used to determine the central ray angulation for different body sizes; it illustrates the relationship of the tibial plateau to the imaging table as the patient's upper thigh thickness increases. Note that a decrease occurs in femoral decline, and a shift occurs in the direction of the tibial plateau slope as the thickness of the thigh decreases. Because of this plateau shift, the central ray angulation must also be adjusted to keep it parallel with the plateau and to

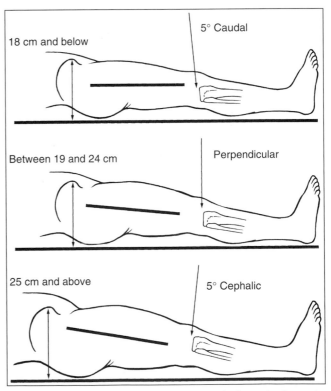

FIGURE 6-132 Determining central ray (CR) angle from the patient's thigh thickness. (Reproduced with permission from Martensen K: Alternative AP knee method assures open joint space, *Radiol Technol* 64:19-23, 1992. Courtesy Radiologic Technology, published by the American Society of Radiologic Technologists.)

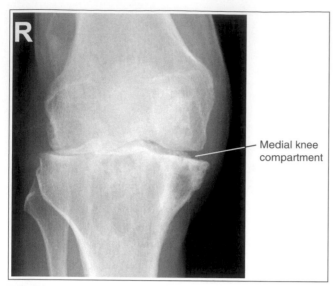

FIGURE 6-133 AP knee projection of a patient with valgus deformity.

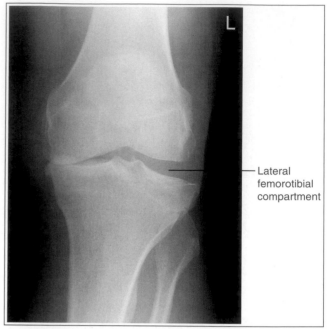

FIGURE 6-134 AP knee projection of a patient with varus deformity

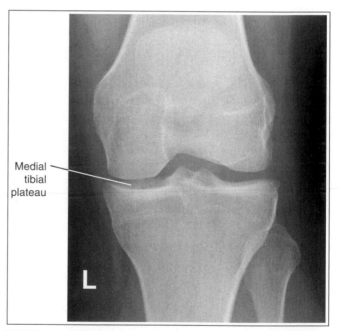

FIGURE 6-135 AP knee projection taken with an excessive cephalic CR angulation.

achieve an open knee joint. For optimal AP knee projections, measure from the patient's anterior superior iliac spine (ASIS) to the imaging table on either side to determine the CR angulation to use for each knee examination. When measuring this distance, do not include the patient's abdominal tissue. Keep the calipers situated laterally next to the ASIS. If the measurement is less than 18 cm, a 5-degree caudal angle should be used. If the measurement is 19 to 24 cm, a perpendicular beam should be used. If the measurement is greater than 24 cm, a 5-degree cephalad angle should be used.

Joint Space Narrowing. On an AP knee with adequate positioning, joint space narrowing is evaluated by measuring the medial and lateral aspects of the knee joint (also referred to as *compartments*). The measurement of each of these compartments is obtained by determining the distance between the most distal femoral condylar surface and the posterior condylar margin of the tibia on each side. Comparison of these measurements with each other, with measurements from previous projections, or with measurements of the other knee determines joint space narrowing or a valgus or varus deformity. In a valgus deformity the lateral compartment is narrower than the medial compartment; in a varus deformity the medial compartment is narrower (Figures 6-133 and 6-134). Precise measurements of the compartments are necessary to ensure early detection of joint space narrowing and are best obtained when the knee joint space is completely open. If an inaccurate CR angulation was used for an AP knee, the knee joint is narrowed or obscured, the intercondylar eminence and tubercles are foreshortened, and the tibial plateau is demonstrated.

Adjusting for Poor CR Angulation. Determine how to adjust for poor CR angulation by judging the shape of the fibular head and its proximity to the tibial plateau. If the fibular head is foreshortened and demonstrated more than 0.5 inch (1.25 cm) distal to the tibial plateau, the cephalad angle was too great (Figure 6-135). If the fibular head is elongated and demonstrated less than 0.5 inch (1.25 cm) distal to the tibial plateau, the caudad angle was too great (Figure 6-136).

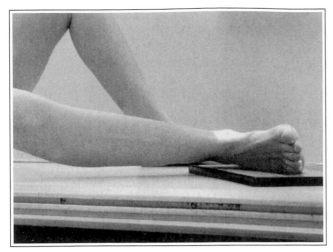

FIGURE 6-136 AP knee projection taken with inadequate cephalic CR angulation.

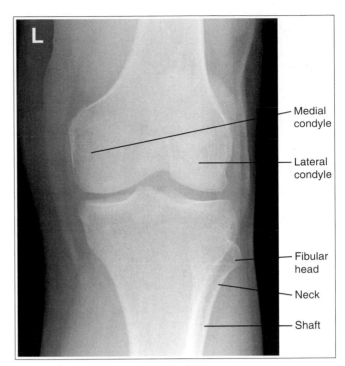

- Medial condyle
- Lateral condyle
- Fibular head
- Neck
- Shaft

IMAGE 6-26

AP Knee Analysis Practice

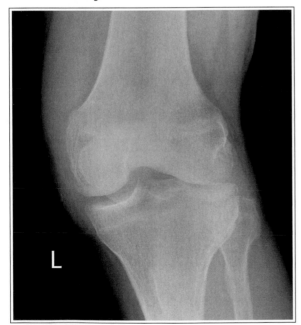

IMAGE 6-25

Analysis. The lateral knee compartment is narrower than the medial knee compartment. The patient's knee demonstrates a valgus deformity. The fibular head is elongated and demonstrated less than 0.5 inch (1.25 cm) distal to the tibial plateau. The CR was angled too caudally.
Correction. Adjust the CR angled cephalically.

Analysis. The femoral epicondyles are not in profile, the medial femoral condyle appears larger than the lateral condyle, and the tibia superimposes more than one half of the fibular head. The leg was externally rotated.
Correction. Internally rotate the leg until the femoral epicondyles are positioned parallel with the IR.

KNEE: AP OBLIQUE PROJECTION (MEDIAL AND LATERAL ROTATION)

See Table 6-16, (Figures 6-137, 6-138, 6-139, and 6-140).
Knee Joint. The anterior and posterior condylar margins of the tibia are superimposed by the use of the correct CR angulation, as determined by the patient's upper thigh and buttocks thickness as explained in the AP knee projection. For optimal AP oblique knee projections, measure each patient from the ASIS to the table after the patient has been accurately positioned to determine the correct CR angulation to use for each examination. When measuring this distance, do not include the patient's abdominal tissue in the measurement (Figure 6-141). Keep the calipers situated laterally, next to the ASIS. It is not uncommon to require a cephalic angle for the AP medial oblique when a perpendicular or caudal angle was used for the AP projection, because the patient's hip is often elevated to accomplish the needed degree of internal obliquity. A caudal CR angle is often needed for the AP lateral oblique, because the patient's pelvis is rotated toward the table to accomplish the external oblique knee and the buttocks do not lift the proximal leg as high off the table.

TABLE 6-16	AP Oblique Knee Projection	
Image Analysis Guidelines (Figures 6-137 and 6-138)		**Related Position Procedures (Figures 6-139 and 6-140)**
• Medial oblique: • Fibular head is seen free of tibial superimposition. • Lateral femoral condyle is in profile without superimposing the medial condyle. • Lateral oblique: • Fibular head is aligned with the anterior edge of the tibia. • Medial femoral condyle is in profile without superimposing the lateral condyle.		• Position the patient supine, with the knee joint centered to the IR. • Medial oblique: Internally rotate the leg until the femoral epicondyles are at a 45-degree angle with IR. • Lateral oblique: Externally rotate the leg until the femoral epicondyles are at a 45-degree angle with IR
• Knee joint space (femorotibial) is open. • The anterior and posterior condylar margins of the tibia are aligned. • Fibular head is approximately 0.5 inch (1.25 cm) distal to the tibial plateau.		• Angle the CR to align it parallel with the tibial plateau. • 5 degrees caudal if ASIS to the table measurement is 18 cm or below • perpendicular beam if ASIS to the table measurement is between 19 and 24 cm • 5 degrees cephalic if ASIS to the table measurement is 25 cm and above
• Knee joint is at the center of the exposure field.		• Center the CR to the midline of the knee at a level 1 inch (2.5 cm) distal to the medial epicondyle.
• One fourth of the distal femur and proximal lower leg and the surrounding knee soft tissue are included within the exposure field.		• Longitudinally collimate to include one fourth of the distal femur and proximal lower leg. • Transversely collimate to within 0.5 inch (1.25 cm) of the knee skin line.

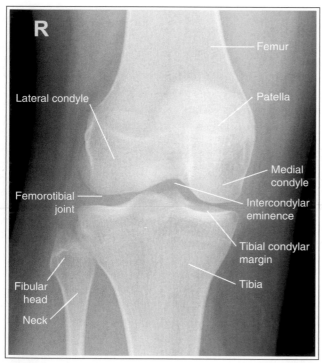

FIGURE 6-137 AP (internal) oblique knee projection with accurate positioning.

Adjusting for Poor CR Angulation. If an inaccurate CR angulation was used for an AP oblique knee, the knee joint space is narrowed or obscured and the anterior and posterior margins of the tibial plateau are not aligned. When evaluating an AP oblique knee projection for which an inaccurate CR angulation was used, you can determine how to adjust the angulation by judging the shape of the fibular head and its proximity to the tibial plateau. If the fibular head is foreshortened and demonstrated more than 0.5 inch (1.25 cm) distal to the tibial plateau (Figure 6-142), the cephalad angle was too great, and if the fibular head is elongated and demonstrated less than 0.5 inch (1.25 cm) distal to the tibial plateau, the caudad angle was too great (Figure 6-143).

Rotation

Medial (Internal) Oblique Position. An accurately positioned AP medial oblique knee projection places the lateral condyle in profile and rotates the fibular head from beneath the tibia, opening the proximal tibiofibular articulation. If the femoral epicondyles are rotated less than 45 degrees with the IR, the tibia is partially superimposed over the fibular head (Figure 6-143). If the femoral epicondyles are rotated more than 45 degrees with the IR, the femoral condyles demonstrate superimposition (Figure 6-144).

Lateral (External) Oblique Position. An accurately positioned AP lateral oblique knee projection places the medial condyle in profile and rotates the tibia onto the fibula, demonstrating alignment of the anterior aspects of the tibia and fibular head on the projection. If the femoral epicondyles are rotated less than 45 degrees with the IR, the fibular head is demonstrated without full tibia superimposition (Figure 6-145). If the femoral epicondyles are rotated more than 45 degrees with the IR, the fibular head is not aligned with the anterior edge of the tibia but is seen posterior to the placement. The more posteriorly situated is the fibula, the farther away from 45 degrees the patient was positioned (Figure 6-146).

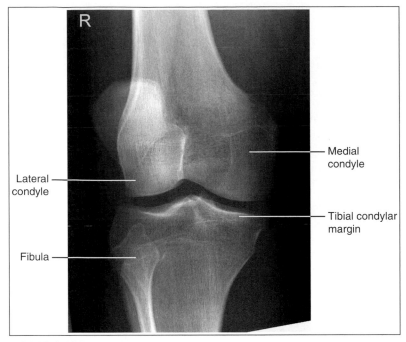

FIGURE 6-138 AP (external) oblique knee projection with accurate positioning.

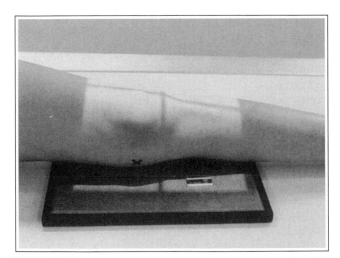

FIGURE 6-139 Proper patient positioning for AP (internal) oblique knee projection.

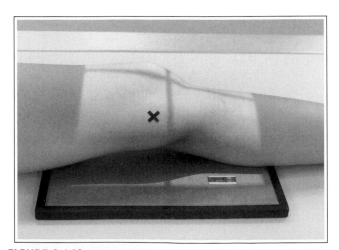

FIGURE 6-140 Proper patient positioning for AP (external) oblique knee projection. X indicates medial femoral epicondyle.

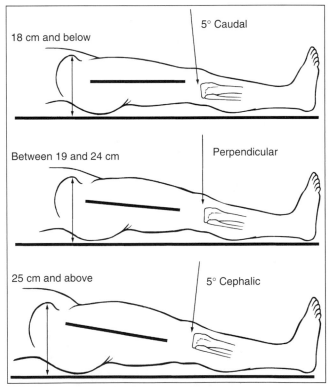

FIGURE 6-141 Determining central ray (CR) angle from the patient's thigh thickness. (Reproduced with permission from Martensen K: Alternative AP knee method assures open joint space, *Radiol Technol* 64:19-23, 1992. Courtesy Radiologic Technology, published by the American Society of Radiologic Technologists.)

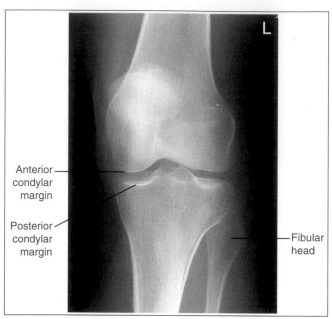

Anterior condylar margin

Posterior condylar margin

Fibular head

FIGURE 6-142 AP medial oblique knee projection taken with excessive cephalic CR angulation.

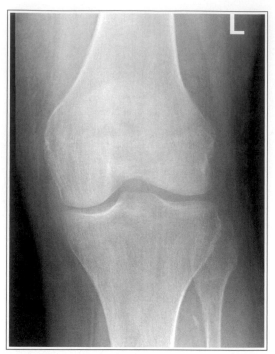

FIGURE 6-143 AP medial oblique knee projection taken with inadequate cephalic CR angulation and with insufficient internal obliquity.

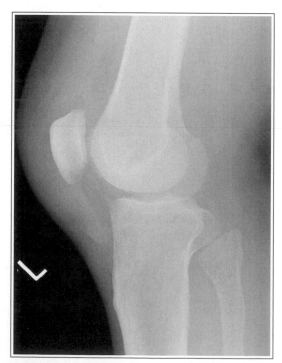

FIGURE 6-144 AP medial oblique knee projection taken with excessive internal obliquity

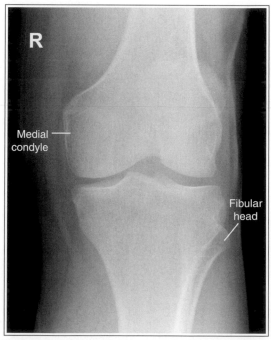

Medial condyle

Fibular head

FIGURE 6-145 AP external oblique knee projection taken with insufficient external obliquity.

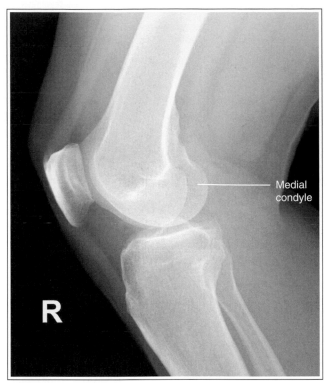

FIGURE 6-146 AP external oblique knee projection taken with excessive external obliquity.

AP Oblique Knee Analysis Practice

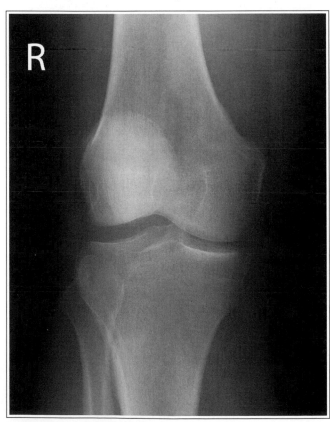

IMAGE 6-27 Medial oblique.

Analysis. The fibular head is demonstrated without full tibia superimposition. The leg was rotated less than 45 degrees with the IR. The knee joint space is obscured, and the fibular head is foreshortened and demonstrated less than 0.5 inch (1.25 cm) distal to the tibial plateau. The CR was angled too caudally.

Correction. Increase the degree of leg rotation until the femoral epicondyles are at a 45-degree angle with the IR and cephalically angle the CR.

KNEE: LATERAL PROJECTION (MEDIOLATERAL)

See Table 6-17, (Figures 6-147, 6-148, and 6-149).

TABLE 6-17	Lateral Knee Projection
Image Analysis Guidelines (Figures 6-147 and 6-148)	**Related Positioning Procedures (Figure 6-149)**
• Contrast resolution is adequate to demonstrate the suprapatellar fat pad.	• Appropriate technique is set.
• Patella is situated proximal to the patellar surface of the femur. • Patellofemoral joint is open.	• Position the patient in a recumbent position with the knee flexed 20 to 30 degrees. • Center the knee joint to the IR.
• Distal margins of the medial and lateral femoral condyles are aligned. • Fibular head is 0.5 inch (1.25 cm) distal to the tibial plateau. • Knee joint space is open.	• Angle the CR 5 to 7 degrees cephalad.
• Anterior and the posterior margins of the medial and lateral femoral condyles are aligned. • Tibia superimposes one half of the fibular head.	• Externally rotate the affected leg, and oblique the torso as needed to align the femoral epicondyles perpendicular to the IR (see Figure 6-27). • Align the CR angle 30-degrees with the long axis of the femur (see Figure 6-87) to project the medial condyle proximoanteriorly.
• Knee joint is at the center of the exposure field.	• Center the CR to the midline of the knee at the level of 1 inch (2.5 cm) distal to the medial epicondyle.
• One fourth of the distal femur and proximal lower leg and the surrounding knee soft tissue are included within the exposure field.	• Longitudinally collimate to include one fourth of the distal femur and proximal lower leg. • Transversely collimate to within 0.5 inch (1.25 cm) of the knee skin line.

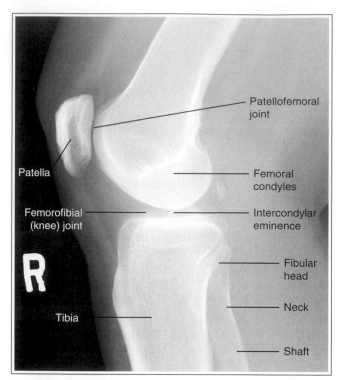

FIGURE 6-147 Lateral (mediolateral) knee projection with accurate positioning.

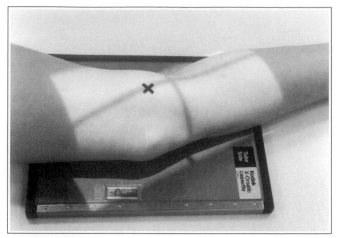

FIGURE 6-149 Proper patient positioning for lateral knee projection. X indicates medial femoral epicondyle.

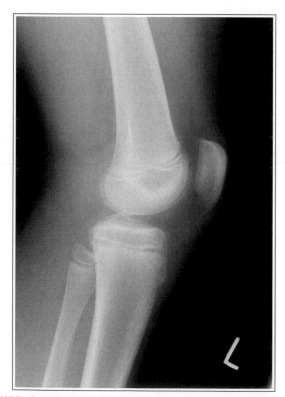

FIGURE 6-148 Pediatric lateral knee projection with accurate positioning.

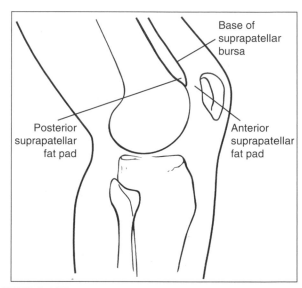

FIGURE 6-150 Location of suprapatellar fat pads. (Reproduced with permission from Martensen K: The knee, *In-Service Reviews in Radiologic Technology,* vol 14, no 7, Birmingham, AL, 1991, In-Service Reviews.)

Patellofemoral Joint and Patella Position

Knee Flexion and Joint Effusion Visualization.

Two soft tissue structures of interest at the knee are used to diagnose joint effusion and knee injury. They are the posterior and anterior suprapatellar fat pads. Both are located anterior to the patellar surface of the distal femur and are separated by the suprapatellar bursa (Figure 6-150). Fluid that collects in the suprapatellar bursa causes the anterior and posterior suprapatellar fat pads to separate. It is a widening of this space that indicates a diagnosis of joint effusion.

If the lateral knee is being obtained to demonstrate fluid in the bursa, knee flexion is best kept at 10 to 15 degrees. With less than 20 degrees of knee flexion, the patella is situated proximal to the patellar surface of the femur, the quadriceps are relaxed, and the patella is fairly

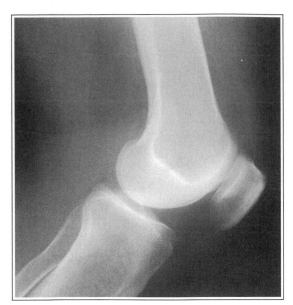

FIGURE 6-151 Lateral knee projection with knee flexed 30-degrees.

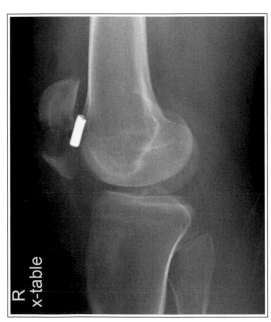

FIGURE 6-152 Cross-table lateral knee projection with fractured patella.

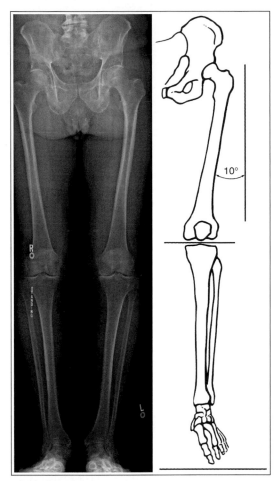

FIGURE 6-153 Femoral inclination in upright position. (Reproduced with permission from Martensen K: The knee, *In-Service Reviews in Radiologic Technology,* vol 14, no 7, Birmingham, AL, 1991, In-Service Reviews.)

mobile. In this patellar position the anterior and posterior suprapatellar fat pads can be easily used to evaluate knee joint effusion. Conversely, when the knee is flexed 20 degrees or more, a tightening of the surrounding knee muscles and tendons is present, the patella comes into contact with the patellar surface of the femur, and the anterior and posterior suprapatellar fat pads are obscured, eliminating their usefulness in diagnosing joint effusion (Figure 6-151).

Positioning for Fracture. If a patellar or other knee fracture is suspected, the knee should remain extended to prevent displacement of bony fragments or vascular injury (Figure 6-152).

Knee Joint Space. When a patient is in an erect position with the legs separated so the knees are situated below the hip joints, the distal margins of the femoral epicondyles are aligned parallel with the surface the patient is standing on and the femoral shafts incline medially approximately 10 to 15 degrees (Figure 6-153). This femoral incline gives the body stability. The amount of inclination a person displays depends on the pelvic width and femoral shaft length. The wider the pelvis and the shorter the femoral shaft length, the more medially the femurs incline. When patients are placed in the recumbent lateral position and rolled onto their side for a lateral knee projection (Figure 6-154), some of this medial femoral inclination is reduced, causing the medial femoral condyle to be situated distal to the lateral condyle. A lateral knee projection is obtained with a perpendicular CR, and this positioning demonstrates the medial condyle distal to the lateral condyle and within the knee joint space, and the fibular head positioned less than 0.5 inch (1.25 cm) from the tibial plateau. The amount of distance demonstrated between the distal margins of the two condyles and fibular head and tibial

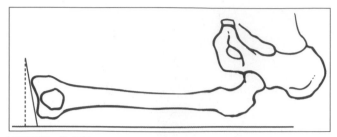

FIGURE 6-154 Reduction in femoral inclination in supine position.

plateau depends on the amount of medial femoral incline reduction that occurred. To project the medial condyle proximally, aligning the distal margins of the condyles and opening the knee joint space the CR is angled 5 to 7 degrees cephalad.

Determining Degree of CR Angulation. Because the degree of femoral inclination varies among patients, so must the degree of needed CR angulation. The wider the pelvis and shorter the femora the greater will be the reduction in femoral inclination. For a patient with a wide pelvis and short femora, a 7-degree cephalic angle is the most reliable angulation to use, with the average patient requiring a 5-degree angle. For a patient with a narrow pelvis and long femora, very little, if any, angulation is required. Although females commonly demonstrate greater pelvic width and femoral inclination and males demonstrate narrower pelvic width and femoral inclination, variations occur in both genders. Each patient's pelvic width and femoral length should be assessed to determine the degree of CR angulation to use before having the patient lie on the table.

Distinguishing Lateral and Medial Condyles. The first step to take when evaluating a poorly positioned lateral knee is to distinguish the lateral and medial condyles. The most reliable method for identifying the medial condyle is to locate the rounded bony tubercle known as the adductor tubercle. It is located posteriorly on the medial aspect of the femur, just superior to the medial condyle. The size and shape of the tubercle are not identical on every patient, although this margin is considerably different from the same margin on the lateral condyle, which is smooth. Once the adductor tubercle is located, the medial condyle is also identified. Another difference between the medial and lateral condyles is evident on their distal articulating surfaces. The distal margin of the medial condyle is convex, and the distal margin of the lateral condyle is flat.

Adjusting for Poor CR Angulation. If an inaccurate CR angulation is used on a lateral knee, the distal articulating margins of the femoral condyles are not aligned, the joint space is narrowed or closed, and the distance from the tibial plateau to the femoral head is more or less than 0.5 inch (1.25 cm). If a patient required a cephalic angulation to project the medial condyle proximally, but no angle was used, the projection demonstrates the distal margin of the medial condyle distal

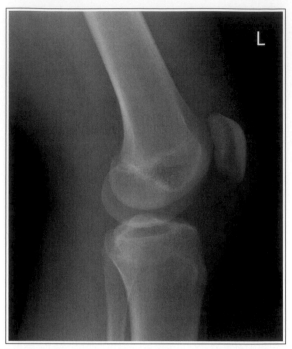

FIGURE 6-155 Lateral knee projection taken without a cephalic CR angulation.

to the distal margin of the lateral condyle and less that 0.5 inch (1.25 cm) of distance is demonstrated between the fibular head and tibial plateau (Figure 6-155). If a patient did not require a cephalic angulation but one was used, or if the angle was too great, the distal margin of the medial condyle is projected proximal to the distal margin of the lateral condyle and more than 0.5 inch (1.25 cm) of distance is demonstrated between the fibular head and the tibial plateau (Figure 6-156).

Anterior and Posterior Alignment of Femoral Condyles. Alignment of the anterior and posterior margins of the femoral condyles is accomplished on a lateral knee by placing the femoral epicondyles perpendicular to the IR and accurately aligning the CR with the femur. As discussed, the medial condyle is positioned distal to the lateral condyle when the patient is placed in the recumbent position. It is also positioned posterior to the lateral condyle when the femoral epicondyles are aligned perpendicular to the IR. To obtain alignment of the anterior and posterior condyle margins, the medial condyle must be projected proximally and anteriorly and is accomplished by aligning the CR with a 30-degree angle with the long axis of the femur, as indicated in Figure 6-157. When aligning the CR think about what you need the angle to do and align it so it does just that; move the medial condyle proximally and anteriorly. This method also more accurately visualizes the tibia superimposing one half of the fibular head, which is 90 degrees from the AP projection (see Figure 6-147).

Alternate Positioning Method. An alternate method of obtaining anterior and posterior alignment of the femoral condyles is to align the femoral epicondyles

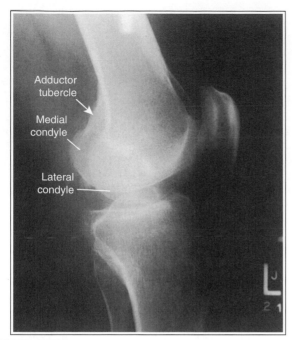

FIGURE 6-156 Lateral knee projection taken with excessive cephalic CR angulation.

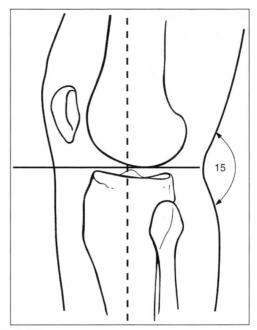

FIGURE 6-158 CR aligned with femur for lateral knee projection. (Reproduced with permission from Martensen K: The knee, *In-Service Reviews in Radiologic Technology,* vol 14, no 7, Birmingham, AL, 1991, In-Service Reviews.)

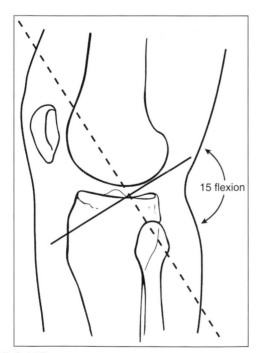

FIGURE 6-157 Proper CR alignment for lateral knee projection. (Reproduced with permission from Martensen K: The knee, *In-Service Reviews in Radiologic Technology,* vol 14, no 7, Birmingham, AL, 1991, In-Service Reviews.)

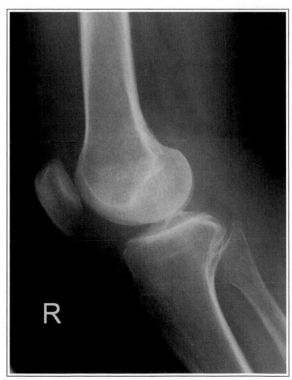

FIGURE 6-159 Alternate CR alignment for lateral knee projection.

perpendicular to the IR, and then roll the patient's patella toward the IR approximately 0.25 inch (0.6 cm) to move the medial condyle anteriorly onto the lateral condyle. Next, align the CR with the long axis of the femur, as shown in Figure 6-158. This CR alignment will move the medial condyle only proximally and demonstrates the fibular head without tibial superimposition (Figure 6-159). Regardless of the method your facility prefers, a

true lateral knee projection has not been obtained unless all aspects of the condyles are superimposed.

Knee Rotation. When a lateral knee is obtained that demonstrates one femoral condyle anterior to the other, the patella must be rolled closer to (leg externally rotated) or farther away from (leg internally rotated) the IR for

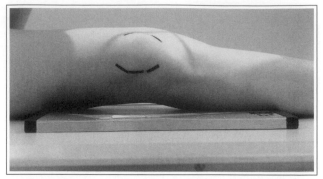

FIGURE 6-160 Poor knee positioning with patella too far from the IR (leg internally rotated).

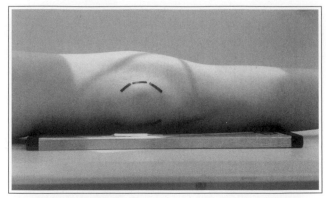

FIGURE 6-162 Poor knee positioning with patella too close to IR (leg externally rotated).

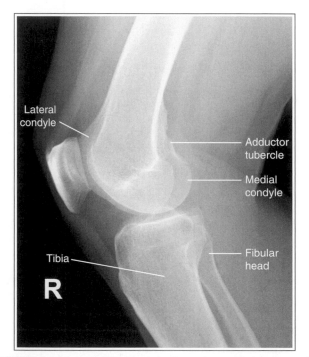

FIGURE 6-161 Lateral knee projection taken with leg internally rotated.

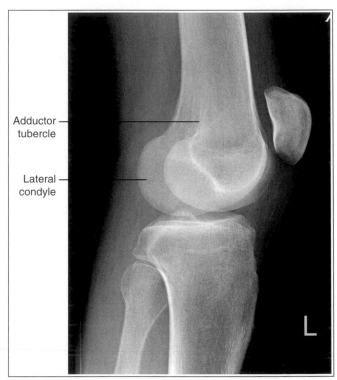

FIGURE 6-163 Lateral knee projection taken with leg externally rotated.

superimposed condyles to be obtained. The first step in determining which way to roll the knee is to distinguish one condyle from the other. As noted, the most reliable method is to locate the adductor tubercle of the medial condyle. When a lateral knee is obtained that demonstrates the adductor tubercle and medial condyle posterior to the lateral condyle, the patella was situated too far from the IR (leg internally rotated) (Figures 6-160 and 6-161). When a lateral knee projection is obtained that demonstrates the medial condyle anterior to the lateral condyle, the patella was situated too close to the IR (leg externally rotated) (Figures 6-162 and 6-163).

Another method used to determine knee rotation is to view the tibiofibular relationship to determine how to reposition for poorly superimposed condyles. If the condyles are not superimposed and the tibia is superimposed over the fibular head, the patella was positioned too far

from the IR (see Figure 6-161). If the fibular head is free of tibial superimposition, the patella was positioned too close to the IR (see Figure 6-163). Although this method is often reliable, the alignment of the CR may affect the results. Figure 6-164 demonstrates such a case. If you use the adductor tubercle and medial condyle to determine how this patient should be repositioned, roll the patient's patella toward the IR (externally rotated leg). If you use the tibiofibular relationship, roll the patient's patella away from the IR (internally rotated leg). The adductor tubercle method is more reliable. This patient's patella needed to be rolled toward the IR to superimpose the condyles.

Knee Flexion. It should also be noted that the tibio-fibular relationship should not be used to determine repositioning when the patient's knee is flexed close to 90 degrees (Figure 6-165). With high degrees of knee flexion, it is proximal and distal femoral elevation and depression that determine the tibiofibular relationship, not leg rotation. To understand this change best, view the skeletal leg in a lateral projection with 90 degrees of leg flexion. Observe how the tibiofibular relationship results in increased tibial superimposition of the fibula when the distal femur is elevated and in decreased tibial superimposition of the fibula when the distal femur is depressed.

Supine (Cross-Table) Lateromedial Knee Projection

Distal Alignment of Femoral Condyles. When a lateromedial knee projection is taken with the patient supine because of trauma or other patient condition, and using a horizontal CR, the cephalad CR angulation described in the preceding is not required, as long as the patient's femoral inclination is not reduced or

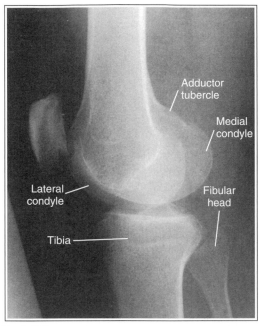

FIGURE 6-164 Lateral knee projection demonstrating medial condyle posteriorly and the fibular head free of tibial superimposition.

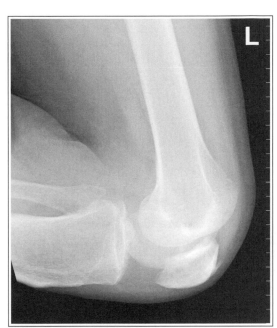

FIGURE 6-165 Lateral knee projection taken with the knee flexed to 90 degrees.

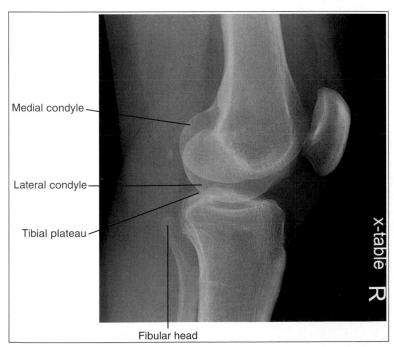

FIGURE 6-166 Crosstable lateromedial knee projection taken with leg adducted or CR directed distally.

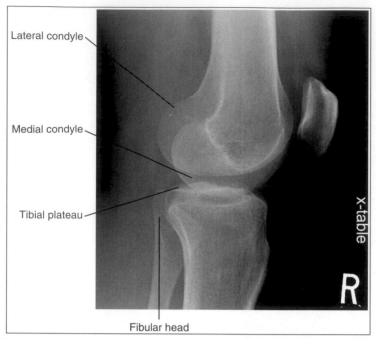

FIGURE 6-167 Crosstable lateromedial knee projection taken with the leg abducted or CR directed proximally.

increased by the distal femur being shifted too laterally or medially, respectively. It should be such that the hip and knee joints are aligned. Figures 6-166 and 6-167 are cross-table lateral knee projections that demonstrate a femoral condyle within the knee joint space because of poor femoral positioning. Figure 6-166 demonstrates the lateral condyle in the joint space, and Figure 6-167 demonstrates the medial condyle. When such a projection is produced, view how far the fibular head is positioned from the tibial plateau. If the distal surfaces of the femoral condyles are accurately superimposed, the fibular head will be positioned about 0.5 inch (1.25 cm) from the tibial plateau. If the CR is directed distally (tube column rotated toward feet) or the leg adducted (moved too medially) for a lateromedial projection of the knee, the lateral condyle will be projected distal to the medial condyle and the fibular head will move farther than 0.5 inch (1.25 cm) from the tibial plateau (see Figure 6-166). If the CR is directed proximally (tube column rotated toward the torso) or the leg abducted (moved too laterally) for a lateromedial projection of the knee, the lateral condyle will be projected proximal to the medial condyle and the fibular head will move closer than 0.5 inch (1.25 cm) from the tibial plateau (see Figure 6-167).

Anterior and Posterior Alignment of Femoral Condyles. If the patient is unable to internally rotate the leg to place the femoral epicondyles perpendicular to the IR the anterior and posterior margins of the femoral condyles will not be aligned. To accomplish this alignment, elevate the leg on a radiolucent sponge and angle the CR anteriorly until it is aligned with the femoral epicondyles. If a grid is used, make certain that the grid is adjusted so that the gridlines are running with the CR

angulation to prevent grid cutoff. Failure to align the CR and epicondyles will result in a projection that demonstrates the medial condyle anterior to the lateral condyle.

Lateral Knee Analysis Practice

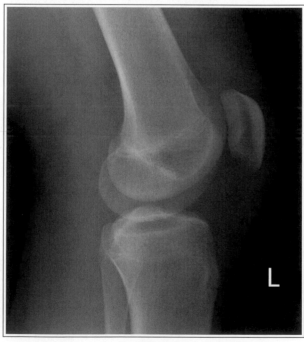

IMAGE 6-28

Analysis. The lateral condyle is proximal to the medial and the fibular head is less than 0.5 inch (1.25 cm) from the tibial plateau. The CR was not angled enough cephalically.

Correction. Angle the CR cephalically.

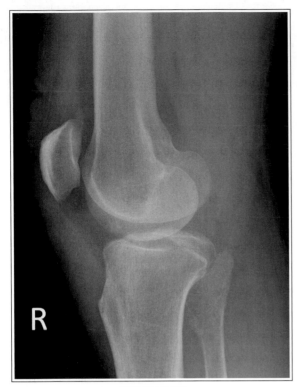

IMAGE 6-29

Analysis. The lateral condyle is proximal to the medial and the fibular head is less than 0.5 inch (1.25 cm) from the tibial plateau. The CR was not angled enough cephalically. Lateral condyle is posterior to the medial condyle and the tibia superimposes less than one half of the fibular head. The leg was externally rotated.
Correction. Angle the CR cephalically and internally rotate the leg.

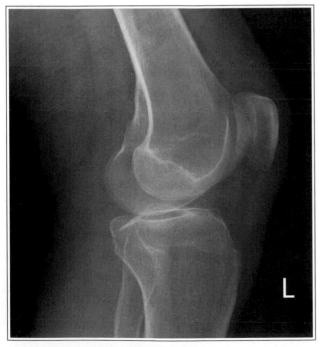

IMAGE 6-30

Analysis. The lateral condyle is proximal to the medial and the fibular head is less than 0.5 inch (1.25 cm) from the tibial plateau. The CR was not angled enough cephalically. The medial condyle is posterior to the lateral condyle and the tibia superimposes more than one half of the fibular head. The leg was internally rotated.
Correction. Angle the CR cephalically and externally rotate the leg.

INTERCONDYLAR FOSSA: PA AXIAL PROJECTION (HOLMBLAD METHOD)

See Table 6-18, (Figures 6-168 and 6-169).
Proximal Intercondylar Fossa Surface and Patella. The proximal surface of the intercondylar fossa is demonstrated in profile when the femoral shaft is placed at a 60- to 70-degree angle with the table or upright IR holder (Figures 6-169 and 6-170). To study this relationship, place a femoral skeleton bone in the PA axial position as described in the preceding and then, while viewing the intercondylar fossa, move the proximal femur closer to and farther away from the imaging table. Note how the anterior and posterior cortical outlines of the proximal fossa are superimposed, demonstrating the proximal surface in profile, when the femur is at a 60- to 70-degree angle with the table, and are not at other degrees.

In this projection, the degree of knee flexion is determined by the degree of femoral shaft angulation with the table or upright IR holder, and as explained in the AP knee projection earlier the degree of knee flexion determines the placement of the patella on the femur. As the degree of knee flexion increases, the patella moves distally onto the patellar surface of the femur and into the intercondylar fossa. The degree of knee flexion achieved when the femur is placed at a 60- to 70-degree angle with the table, situates the patella just proximal to the fossa.

Repositioning for Poor Femur Positioning. If a PA axial projection is obtained that demonstrates the anterior and posterior cortical outlines of the proximal fossa without superimposition, use the placement of the patella on the femur to determine whether the proximal femur was positioned too close to or too far from the table or upright IR holder. If the patellar apex is demonstrated within the fossa, the knee was overflexed (proximal femur positioned too far away from the table; Figure 6-171). If the patella is demonstrated laterally and proximal to the fossa, the knee was underflexed (proximal femur position too close to the table; Figure 6-172).
Knee Joint and Tibial Plateau. To obtain an open knee joint space and demonstrate the tibial plateau and intercondylar eminence and tubercles in profile, dorsiflex the foot and rest the foot on the toes or position the toes at the plane of the front edge of the IR if the patient is standing. Because the tibial plateau slopes downward from the anterior tibial margin to the posterior margin,

TABLE 6-18	PA Axial Knee Projection (Holmblad Method)	
Image Analysis Guidelines (Figure 6-168)	**Related Positioning Procedures (Figure 6-169)**	
• Proximal surface of the intercondylar fossa is in profile. • Patellar apex is demonstrated proximal to the intercondylar fossa.	• Method 1: Stand patient in a PA projection against the upright IR holder, with the knee joint centered to the IR. • Method 2: Kneel the patient on the table, resting on hands and knees, with the knee joint centered to the IR. • Flex the hip and knee until the femur is at a 60- to 70-degree angle with the upright IR holder or table (20 to 30 degrees from CR).	
• Knee joint space is open. • Tibial plateau, intercondylar eminence and the tubercles are in profile. • Fibular head is demonstrated approximately 0.5 inch (1.25 cm) distal to the tibial plateau.	• Dorsiflex the foot. • Method 1: Position toes at the plane of the IR's front edge. • Method 2: Rest the foot on the toes.	
• The medial and the lateral surfaces of the intercondylar fossa and the femoral epicondyles are in profile. • One half of the fibular head superimposes the tibia. • Intercondylar fossa is at the center of the exposure field.	• Adjust knee spacing to align them with the hip joints. • Align the foot's long axis perpendicular to the upright IR holder or table. • Center a perpendicular CR to the midline of the knee, at a level 1 inch (2.5 cm) distal to the medial femoral epicondyle.	
• Distal femur, proximal tibia, and intercondylar fossa eminence and tubercles are included within the exposure field.	• Longitudinally collimate to include the femoral epicondyles. • Transverse collimation to within 0.5 inch (1.25 cm) of the knee skin line.	

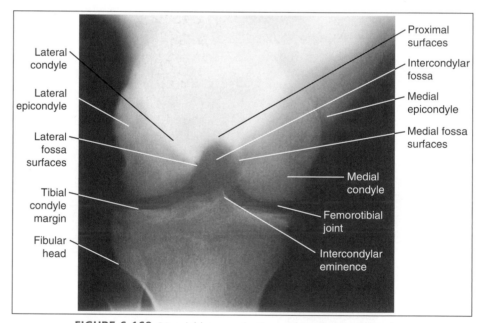

FIGURE 6-168 PA axial knee projection with accurate positioning.

this positioning is necessary to elevate (bring further from table) the distal tibia and align the anterior and the posterior tibial margins and place the tibial plateau in profile. If the foot is not dorsiflexed and resting on the toes, the knee joint space is narrowed or closed and the tibial plateau is demonstrated (Figures 6-172 and 6-173).

Repositioning for Poor Foot Positioning. If a PA axial knee projection is obtained that demonstrates a closed or narrowed knee joint space and the tibial plateau surface, evaluate the proximity of the fibular head to the tibial plateau to determine the needed adjustment. If the

fibular is head is less than 0.5 inch (1.25 cm) from the tibial plateau (see Figure 6-173), the distal lower leg needs to be depressed (brought closer to table). If the fibular head is more than 0.5 inch (1.25 cm) from the tibial plateau (see Figure 6-172), the distal lower leg needs to be elevated. The amount of lower leg adjustment required would be half the distance needed to bring the fibular head to within 0.5 inch (1.25 cm) of the tibial plateau. The small amount of lower leg adjustment that would be needed can be accomplished by varying the degree of foot dorsiflexion or plantar flexion.

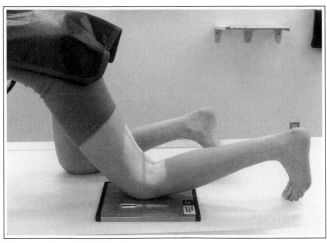

FIGURE 6-169 Proper patient positioning for PA axial knee projection.

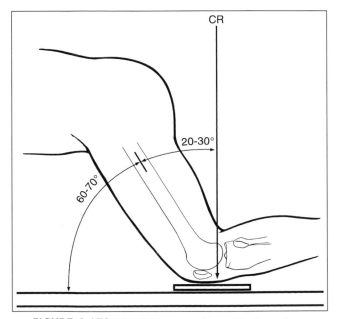

FIGURE 6-170 PA axial knee position. CR, Central ray.

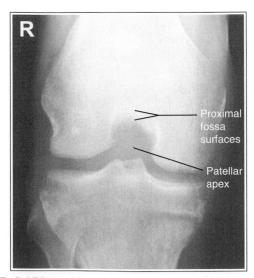

FIGURE 6-171 PA axial knee projection taken with the knee overflexed.

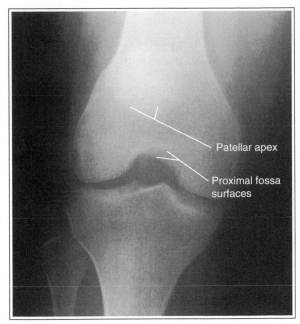

FIGURE 6-172 PA axial knee projection taken with the knee underflexed and the distal lower leg depressed.

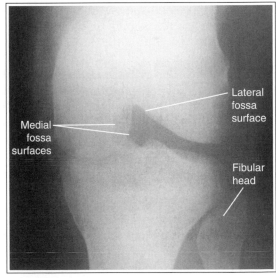

FIGURE 6-173 PA axial knee projection taken with the distal lower leg elevated and the proximal femur position too medially or the heel rotated laterally.

Medial and Lateral Surfaces of the Intercondylar Fossa

Femoral Inclination. As explained in the lateral knee projection, when the knees are accurately aligned with the hip joints the femoral shaft inclines medially approximately 10 to 15 degrees. The amount of inclination the femoral bone displays depends on the length of the femoral shaft and the width of the pelvis from which the femur originated. The longer the femur and the wider the pelvis, the more femoral inclination is demonstrated. To obtain an intercondylar fossa

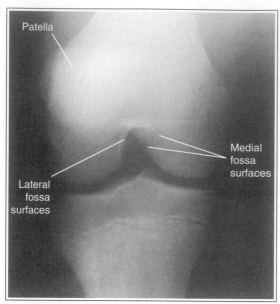

FIGURE 6-174 PA axial knee projection taken with the femur positioned vertically or the heel rotated medially.

projection with the medial and the lateral surfaces superimposed, this inclination should not be offset. If the inclination is offset by shifting the distal femur laterally or the proximal femur medially, causing the femur to be more vertical, the medial and the lateral aspects of the intercondylar fossa are not superimposed, the patella is situated laterally, and more than one half of the fibular head superimposes the tibia (Figure 6-174). If inclination is added to by shifting the distal femur medially or the proximal femur laterally, the medial and the lateral aspects of the fossa are not superimposed, the patella is situated medially, and less than one half of the fibular head superimposes the tibia (see Figure 6-173).

Foot Rotation. Allowing the foot to lean medially or laterally instead of remaining vertical also result in poor medial and lateral fossa superimposition and misalignment of the patella and fibular head and tibia. If the heel is allowed to rotate medially (external foot rotation), the medial and lateral aspects of the intercondylar fossa are not superimposed, the patella is rotated laterally, and more than one half of the fibular head superimposes the tibia (see Figure 6-174). If the heel was rotated laterally (internal foot rotation), the medial and lateral aspects of the intercondylar fossa are not superimposed, the patella is demonstrated medially, and less than one half of the fibular head superimposes the tibia (see Figure 1-173).

PA Axial Knee Analysis Practice

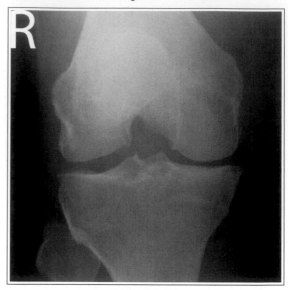

IMAGE 6-31

Analysis. The medial and lateral aspects of the intercondylar fossa are not superimposed, and the patella is situated laterally. Either the proximal femur was positioned vertically or the heel was rotated medially.

Correction. Position the proximal femur laterally allowing the femur to incline naturally and/or align the long axis of the patient's foot perpendicular to the table.

INTERCONDYLAR FOSSA: AP AXIAL PROJECTION (BÉCLÈRE METHOD)

See Table 6-19, (Figures 6-175 and 6-176).

Proximal Intercondylar Fossa Surface. The proximal surface of the intercondylar fossa is place in profile when the CR is aligned parallel with it. This is accomplished on an AP axial projection when the long axis of the femur is placed at a 60-degree angle with the table and the CR is correctly angled and centered to the fossa. With a set CR, poor alignment of the proximal surface of the fossa occurs when the femur is angled more or less than 60 degrees with the table, which also causes the knee to be flexed more or less than 45 degrees, and alters the placement of the patella on the femur. If an AP axial projection is obtained that demonstrates the anterior and posterior cortical margins of the proximal fossa without superimposition, view the patella apex's placement on the femur to determine how femoral elevation and knee flexion would need to be adjusted to obtain accurate positioning and fully demonstrate the intercondylar fossa. As the knee is flexed, the patella shifts distally onto the patellar surface of the femur and then into the intercondylar fossa. Therefore if the long axis of the femur is aligned more than 60 degrees with the table, resulting in increased knee flexion, the patellar apex will be demonstrated within the intercondylar fossa (Figure 6-177). If the long axis of the femur is aligned less than 60

TABLE 6-19	AP Axial Intercondylar Fossa (Béclère Method)
Image Analysis Guidelines (Figure 6-175)	**Related Positioning Procedures (Figure 6-176)**
• Proximal surface of the intercondylar fossa is in profile. • Patellar apex is demonstrated proximal to the intercondylar fossa.	• Place the patient in a supine position. • Elevate the distal femur until the femur is at a 60-degree angle with the table. • Adjust the distal lower leg until the knee is flexed to 45-degrees.
• Knee joint space is open. • Tibial plateau, and intercondylar eminence and tubercles are in profile. • Fibular head is demonstrated approximately 0.5 inch (1.25 cm) distal to the tibial plateau.	• Align the CR perpendicular to the anterior lower leg surface, and then decrease the obtained angulation by 5 degrees. • Place a curved or regular IR under the knee and elevate it on sponges until it is as close to the posterior knee as possible. Center the IR beneath the knee joint
• The medial and the lateral surfaces of the intercondylar fossa, and the femoral epicondyles are in profile. • Tibia superimposes one-half of the fibular head.	• Internally rotate the knee until the femoral epicondyles are aligned parallel with the table.
• Intercondylar fossa is at the center of the exposure field.	• Center the CR to the midline of the knee, at a level 1 inch (2.5 cm) distal to the medial femoral epicondyle.
• Distal femur, proximal tibia, and intercondylar fossa eminence and tubercles are included within the exposure field.	• Longitudinally collimate to include the femoral epicondyles. • Transversely collimate to within 0.5 inch (1.25 cm) of the knee skin line.

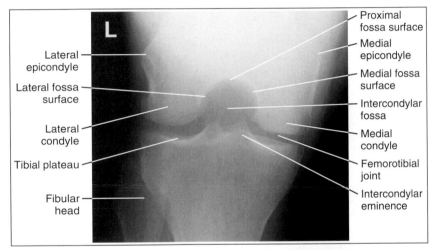

FIGURE 6-175 AP axial knee projection with accurate positioning.

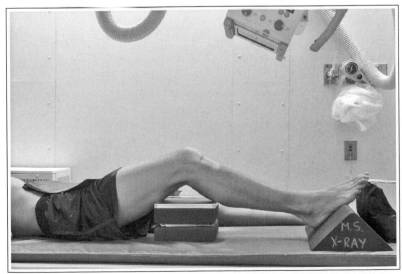

FIGURE 6-176 Proper patient positioning for AP axial (Béclère method) knee projection.

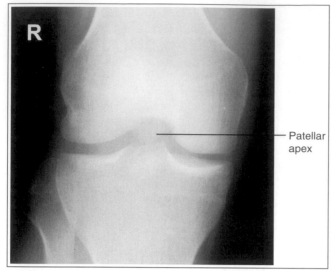

FIGURE 6-177 AP axial (Béclère method) knee projection taken with. Excessive knee flexion.

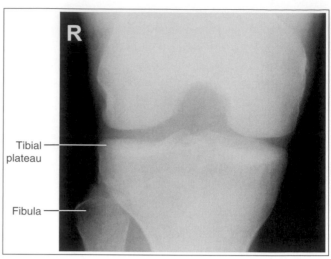

FIGURE 6-179 AP axial (Béclère method) knee projection taken with the distal lower leg elevated or the CR angled too cephalically.

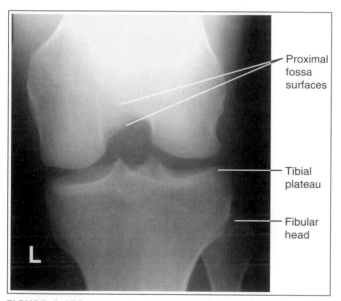

FIGURE 6-178 AP axial (Béclère method) knee projection taken with insufficient knee flexion

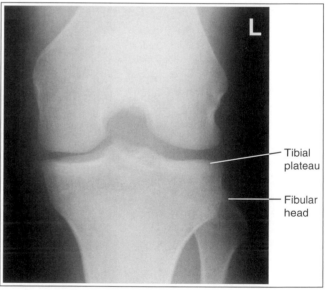

FIGURE 6-180 AP axial (Béclère method) knee projection taken with the distal lower leg depressed or the CR angled too caudally.

degrees with the table, resulting in less knee flexion, the proximal intercondylar fossa surfaces will not be aligned and the patellar apex will be shown above the intercondylar fossa (Figure 6-178).

Knee Joint and Tibial Plateau. To obtain an open knee joint space and demonstrate the tibial plateau, and intercondylar eminence and tubercles in profile, the CR must be aligned parallel with the tibial plateau. This alignment is obtained by first positioning the CR perpendicular with the anterior lower leg surface and then decreasing the obtained angulation by 5 degrees. The 5-degree decrease is needed because the tibial plateau slopes distally by 5 degrees from the anterior condylar margin to

the posterior condylar margin when referenced with the anterior surface of the tibia.

If an AP axial projection demonstrates a closed or narrowed knee joint space and the anterior and posterior condylar margins of the tibial plateau without superimposition, evaluate the proximity of the fibular head to the tibial plateau. If the fibular head is demonstrated more than 0.5 inch (1.25 cm) distal to the tibial plateau, the distal lower leg was elevated too high or the CR was too cephalically angled (Figure 6-179). If the fibular head is demonstrated less than 0.5 inch (1.25 cm) distal to the tibial plateau, the distal lower leg was too depressed or the CR was too caudally angled (Figure 6-180).

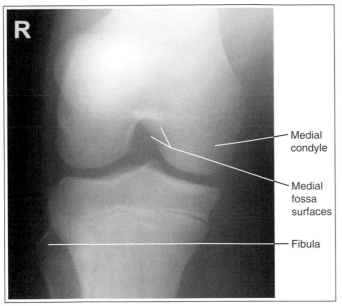

FIGURE 6-181 AP axial (Béclère method) knee projection taken with the knee externally rotated.

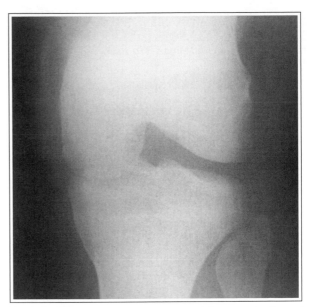

FIGURE 6-182 AP axial (Béclère method) knee projection taken with the knee internally rotated.

The Medial and the Lateral Intercondylar Fossa Surfaces. To fully demonstrate the intercondylar fossa the cortical outlines of the medial and the lateral surfaces of the intercondylar fossa must be in profile. This is accomplished by positioning the femoral epicondyles parallel with the IR. When a projection is obtained that does not demonstrate the lateral and the medial surfaces of the condyle in profile, view the degree of tibial and fibular superimposition and the difference in femoral condylar width to determine the cause of the poor positioning. It the knee was too externally rotated, the medial femoral condyle appears larger than the lateral condyle and the tibia superimposes more than one half of the fibular head (Figure 6-181). If the knee was too internally rotated, the lateral femoral condyle will appear larger than the medial condyle and the tibia will superimpose less than one half of the fibular head (Figure 6-182).

Knee Magnification. The AP axial knee projection demonstrates magnification if a curved cassette is not used and the knee is positioned at an increased OID.

PATELLA AND PATELLOFEMORAL JOINT: TANGENTIAL PROJECTION (MERCHANT METHOD)

See Table 6-20, (Figures 6-183 and 6-184).

Scatter Radiation Control. An optimal 60- to 70-kV technique sufficiently penetrates the bony and soft tissue structures of the knee and provides optimal differential absorption. If it is necessary to increase the kilovoltage above 70 to penetrate a thicker knee, a grid is not needed because of the long OID. When a long OID is used, scatter radiation that would expose the IR when a short OID is used is scattered at a direction away from the IR. Because scatter radiation is not being directed toward the IR, a grid is not needed to absorb the scatter. This is also referred to as the air-gap technique.

Axial Viewer. The AP axial projection method uses an axial viewer knee-supporting device, as shown in Figure 6-184. This freestanding device maintains the knees at a set degree of flexion, provides straps that restrain the patient's legs, and contains an IR holder that keeps the receptor at the proper angle with the CR. The angle of the CR and angle placed on the axial viewer determines what aspect of the femurs anterior surface will be visualized and how well the patellofemoral joint space is demonstrated. Although 45 degrees is the standard angle, the reviewer is capable of supporting the leg at 30-, 60-, or 75-degree angles as well. Each of these angles requires a predetermined CR angulation if an open patellofemoral joint is to be obtained. The easiest way to determine the CR angle to use for the different axial viewer angles is to know that the sum of the CR angle and the axial viewer's angle must equal 105 degrees. For example, if the axial viewer is set at 30 degrees, the CR angulation must be set at 75 degrees (30 + 75 = 105).

Superior Position of Patellae, Femoral Condyles, and Intercondylar Sulci

Rotation. To demonstrate the knees without rotation and to position the patellae, anterior femoral condyles, and intercondylar sulci superiorly, internally rotate the patient's legs until the palpable femoral epicondyles are aligned parallel with the table. This positioning places the distal femurs in an AP projection with the table. Because the lateral condyles are situated anterior to the medial condyles, the lateral condyles demonstrate more height on a tangential (axial) projection if the legs are adequately rotated. If the legs are not sufficiently rotated, the patellae are situated laterally, and either the anterior femoral condyles demonstrate equal height or the medial

TABLE 6-20	Tangential Patella and Patellofemoral Joint Projection (Merchant Method)
Image Analysis Guidelines (Figure 6-183)	**Related Positioning Procedures (Figure 6-184)**
• Magnification of patellae has been kept to minimum. • Patellae, anterior femoral condyles, and intercondylar sulci are seen superiorly. • Lateral femoral condyle demonstrates slightly more height than the medial condyle.	• Set SID at 72 inches. • Set the axial viewer at a 45-degree angle, and position it at the end of the table. • Place the patient in a supine position with the legs positioned between the axial viewer's IR holders. • Internally rotate the legs until the femoral epicondyles are aligned parallel with the IR. • Secure the legs in this position by wrapping the axial viewer's Velcro straps around the patient's calves.
• There is no superimposition of the anterior thigh soft tissue into the joint space. • Patellofemoral joint spaces are open, with no superimposition of the patellae or tibial tuberosities. • A point midway between the patellofemoral joint spaces is at the center of the exposure field.	• Adjust the height of the axial viewer or the table to place the long axis of the femurs parallel with the table. • Position the posterior curves of the knees directly above the bend in the axial viewer. • Place the IR on the ankles so it rests against the viewer's IR holders. • Place a 60-degree caudal angle on the CR. • Center the CR between the knees at the level of the patellofemoral joint spaces.
• Patellae, anterior femoral condyles, and intercondylar sulci are included within the exposure field.	• Longitudinally collimate to include the patellae and the distal femurs. • Transversely collimate to within 0.5 inch (1.25 cm) of the lateral knee skin line.

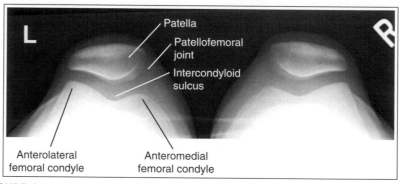

FIGURE 6-183 Tangential (axial) projection knee projection with accurate positioning.

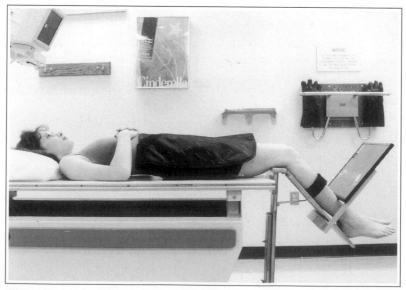

FIGURE 6-184 Proper patient positioning for tangential (axial) projection knee projection.

condyles demonstrate greater height than the lateral condyles (Figure 6-185). Both knees should be evaluates as they may not be rotated equally.

Patellar Subluxation. Because this projection is taken to demonstrate subluxation (partial dislocation) of the patella, the position of the patellae above the intercondylar sulci on an AP axial projection may vary. In a normal knee, the patella is directly above the intercondylar sulcus on an AP axial projection, as shown in Figure 6-183. With patellar subluxation, the patella is lateral to the intercondylar sulcus, as shown in Figure 6-186. Do not mistake a subluxed patella for knee rotation. Although both conditions result in a laterally positioned patella, the rotated knee demonstrates the femoral condyle at the same height or with the medial condyle higher than the lateral condyle, and the nonrotated knee that demonstrates a subluxed patella will demonstrates the lateral condyle higher than the medial condyle.

To demonstrate patellar subluxation, the quadriceps femoris (four muscles that surround the femoral bone) must be in a relaxed position. This is accomplished by instructing the patient to relax the leg muscles, allowing the calf straps to maintain the internal leg rotation. If the patient does not relax the quadriceps muscles, a patella that would be subluxed on relaxation of the muscles may appear normal.

Joint Space Visualization

Anterior Thigh Soft Tissue Projecting into Joint Space. The relationship of the femurs to the table determines how much of the anterior thigh will be exposed and projected into the joint spaces. It is when the femurs are placed parallel with the table that the least amount of tissue will be projected into the joint spaces. Because the distal femurs are typically lower than the proximal femurs when the patient is supine the height of the axial

viewer needs to be elevated or the table lowered to bring the long axis of the femur parallel with the table.

If the distal femurs are positioned closer to the table than the proximal femurs for an AP axial knee, the angled CR traverses the anterior thigh soft tissue, projecting it into the patellofemoral joint space (Figures 6-187 and 6-188). Although the patellofemoral joint space remains open on such a projection, the space is often underexposed.

Patellae and Tibial Tuberosities in Joint Space. The relationship of the posterior knee curves to the bend of the axial viewer determines whether the CR will be parallel with the patellofemoral joint spaces. To demonstrate open patellofemoral joint spaces, position the posterior curves of the knees directly above the bend in the axial viewer, as shown in Figure 6-189. If the posterior curves of the knees are situated at or below the bend of the axial viewer (causing the knees to be flexed more than the degree that is set on the axial viewer), the CR is not parallel with the patellofemoral joint space, and the patellae will rest against the intercondylar sulci (Figures 6-190 and 6-191). If the posterior curves of the knees are situated too far above the bend of the axial viewer (causing the knees to be extended more than the degree set on the axial viewer), the tibial tuberosities are demonstrated within the patellofemoral joint space (Figures 6-192 and 6-193).

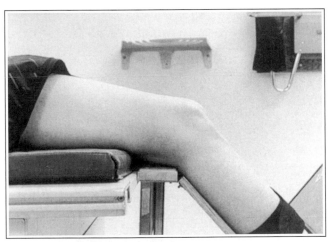

FIGURE 6-187 Poor femur positioning.

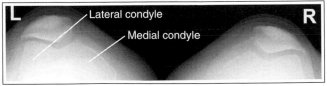

FIGURE 6-185 Tangential (Merchant) patella projection taken without internal leg rotation

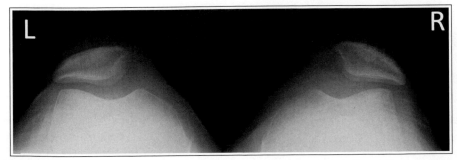

FIGURE 6-186 Tangential (Merchant) patella projection of a patient with patellar subluxation.

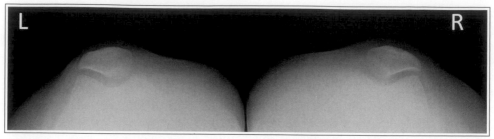

FIGURE 6-188 Tangential (Merchant) patella projection taken with the distal femurs depressed.

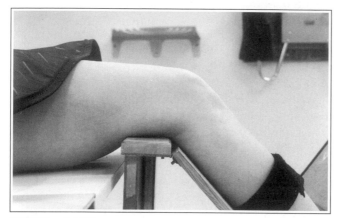

FIGURE 6-189 Proper posterior knee and axial viewer positioning.

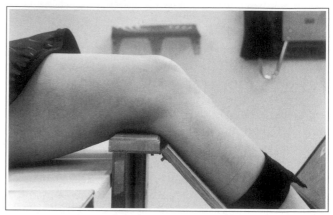

FIGURE 6-192 Posterior knee curve situated above bend in axial viewer.

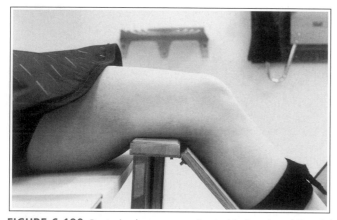

FIGURE 6-190 Posterior knee curve situated below bend in axial viewer.

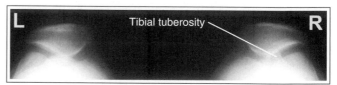

FIGURE 6-193 Tangential (Merchant) patella projection taken with the knees extended more than the degree that is set on the axial viewer.

Positioning for Large Calves. The tibial tuberosities may also be demonstrated within the patellofemoral joint spaces in a patient with thick calves, even when the posterior knee curves have been accurately positioned to the bend of the axial viewer. The thick calves cause the lower leg to be elevated from the viewer and the knee to not be bent as much as is indicated on the axial viewer degree. For such patients, the axial viewer's angulation should be decreased until the knees are flexed 45 degrees or the CR angulation can be increased (5 to 10 degrees) to better align with the joint space.

Light Field Silhouette Indicates Accurate Positioning. Evaluate the silhouette of the knees that is created on the IR when the collimation light is on before exposing the IR. When the patient's legs have been accurately positioned, these silhouettes will display oval shadows with indentations on each side that outline the patellae (Figure 6-194).

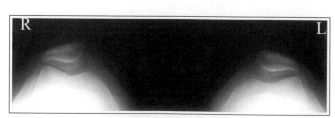

FIGURE 6-191 Tangential (Merchant) patella projection taken with the knees flexed more than the degree that is set on the axial viewer.

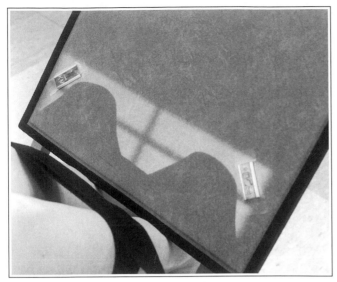

FIGURE 6-194 Proper knee silhouettes and CR centering.

Tangential (Merchant) Patella Analysis Practice

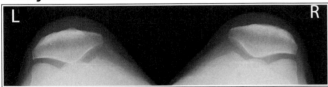

IMAGE 6-32

Analysis. The tibial tuberosities are demonstrated within the patellofemoral joint spaces. The posterior knee curve was positioned too far above the axial viewer's bend. The patellae are demonstrated directly above the intercondylar sulci and are rotated laterally. The medial femoral condyles demonstrate more height than the lateral condyles. The legs were externally rotated.

Correction. Slide the knees toward the axial viewer until the posterior knee curvature is just superior to the bend on the viewer and internally rotate the legs until the patella are situated superiorly.

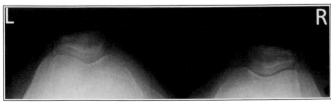

IMAGE 6-33

Analysis. The patellae are resting against the intercondylar sulci, obscuring the patellofemoral joint spaces. The patient's posterior knee curve is positioned at or below the bend on the axial viewer.

Correction. Slide the knees away from the axial viewer until the patient's posterior knee curvature is just superior to the bend of the viewer.

FEMUR: AP PROJECTION

See Table 6-21, (Figures 6-195 and 6-196).

Distal Femur

Epicondyles and Femoral Condyle Shape. Internally rotating the leg until the femoral epicondyles are at equal distances from the IR determines whether an AP projection has been obtained. If the leg was too externally (laterally) rotated, the epicondyles are not in profile, the medial femoral condyle is larger than the lateral condyle, and the tibia is superimposes more than half of the fibular head (Figure 6-197). If the leg was too internally (medially) rotated, the epicondyles are not demonstrated in profile, the lateral femoral condyle is larger than the

TABLE 6-21	AP Distal Femur Projection
Image Analysis Guideline (Figure 6-195)	**Related Positioning Procedures (Figure 6-196)**
• Image brightness is uniform across the femur.	• Position the proximal femur at the cathode end of the tube and the distal femur at the end of the tube.
• Femoral epicondyles are in profile. • Femoral condyles are symmetric in shape. • Tibia superimposes one half of the fibular head.	• Position the patient in a supine position, with the knee fully extended. • Place the lower edge of the IR and grid 2 inches (5 cm) below the knee joint. • Internally rotate the leg until the femoral epicondyles are aligned parallel with IR.
• Long axis of the femoral shaft is aligned with the long axis of the collimated field.	• Center the midfemur to the IR.
• Distal femoral shaft is at the center of the exposure field.	• Center a perpendicular CR to the midfemur and the IR.
• Distal femoral shaft and surrounding femoral soft tissue, the knee joint, and 1 inch (2.5 cm) of the lower leg are included within the exposure field. • Any orthopedic apparatus located in the distal femur is included in its entirety. • 2 inches (5 cm) of overlap with the proximal AP femur projection is evident if the entire femur is imaged.	• Longitudinally collimate to a 17 inch (43 cm) field size. • Transversely collimate to within 0.5 inch (1.25 cm) of the lateral femoral skin line.

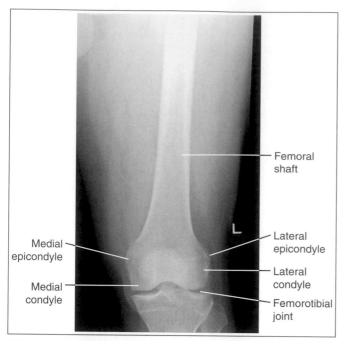

FIGURE 6-195 AP distal femur projection with accurate positioning.

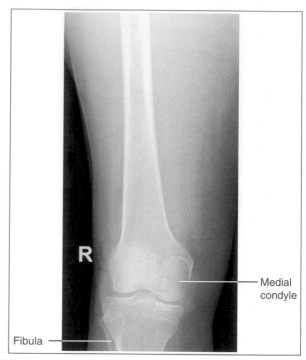

FIGURE 6-197 AP distal femur projection taken with external rotation.

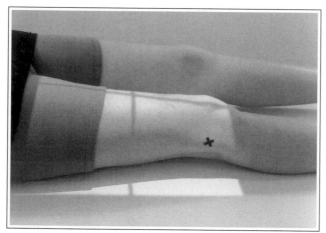

FIGURE 6-196 Proper patient positioning for AP distal femur projection. X indicates lateral femoral epicondyle.

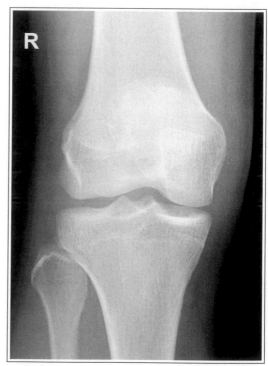

FIGURE 6-198 AP distal femur projection taken with internal rotation.

medial condyle, and the tibia superimposes less than half of the fibular head (Figure 6-198).

Positioning for Fracture. When a fractured femur is in question, the leg should not be internally rotated, but left as is. Forced internal rotation of a fractured femur may injure the blood vessels and nerves that surround the injured area. Because the leg is not internally rotated when a fracture is in question, the distal femur commonly demonstrates external rotation.

Femoral Shaft Overlap. When a femur is ordered, projections of the distal and proximal femur are obtained. These projections should demonstrate at least 2 inches (5 cm) of femoral shaft overlap. If longitudinal

collimation is decreased from the full IR length for one of the projections to reduce exposure and prevent greater than a 2-inch (5 cm) femoral shaft overlap, make certain that the overlapped area is not located at the section where a fracture or disease process is demonstrated.

TABLE 6-22	AP Proximal Femur Projection	
Image Analysis Guidelines (Figure 6-199)		**Related Positioning Procedures (Figure 6-200)**
• Image brightness is uniform across the femur.		• Position the proximal femur at the cathode end of the tube and the distal femur at the anode end.
• Ischial spine is aligned with the pelvic brim. • Obturator foramen is open.		• Place the patient in a supine position, with the knee extended. • Position the ASISs at equal distances from the table. • Place the upper edge of the IR and grid at the level of the affected ASIS.
• Femoral neck is demonstrated without foreshortening. • Greater trochanter is in profile laterally. • Lesser trochanter is completely superimposed by the proximal femur.		• Internally rotate the leg until the femoral epicondyles are aligned parallel to the IR.
• Long axis of the femoral shaft is aligned with the long axis of the exposure field.		• Center the midfemur to the IR.
• Proximal femoral shaft is at the center of the exposure field. • Proximal femoral shaft, hip, and surrounding femoral soft tissue are included within the exposure field. • Any orthopedic apparatus located in the proximal femur or hip is included in its entirety. • 2 inches (5 cm) of overlap is evident with distal AP femur projection if the entire femur is imaged.		• Center a perpendicular CR to the midfemur and the IR. • Longitudinally collimate to a 17 inch (43 cm) field size. • Transversely collimate to within 0.5 inch (1.25 cm) of the lateral femoral skin line.

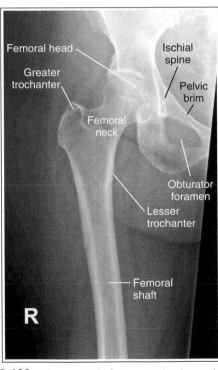

FIGURE 6-199 AP proximal femur projection with accurate positioning.

Proximal Femur

See Table 6-22, (Figures 6-199 and 6-200).

Pelvis Rotation. Rotation of the pelvis on an AP proximal femur projection is detected by evaluating the relationship of the ischial spine and the pelvic brim and visualization of the obturator foramen. When the pelvis has been rotated toward the affected femur, the ischial spine is demonstrated without pelvic brim superimposition and visualization of the obturator foramen is

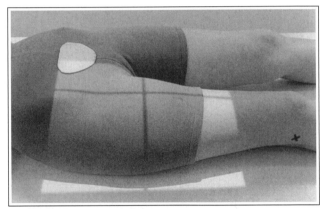

FIGURE 6-200 Proper patient positioning for AP proximal femur projection.

decreased (Figure 6-201). When the pelvis has been rotated away from the affected femur, the ischial spine is not aligned with the pelvic brim but is demonstrated closer to the acetabulum, and demonstration of the obturator foramen is increased (Figure 6-202).

Femoral Neck and Trochanters. For an AP femur projection, which shows the femoral neck without foreshortening and the greater trochanter in profile, the leg is internally rotated until the foot is tilted 15 to 20 degrees from vertical and the femoral epicondyles are positioned parallel with the table (Figure 6-203). Generally, when a patient is relaxed, the legs and feet are externally rotated. On external rotation, the femoral neck inclines posteriorly (toward the table) and is foreshortened on an AP femoral projection. Increased external rotation increases the degree of posterior decline and foreshortening of the femoral neck on the projection. If the leg was externally rotated enough to position the foot at a 45-degree angle and an imaginary line connecting

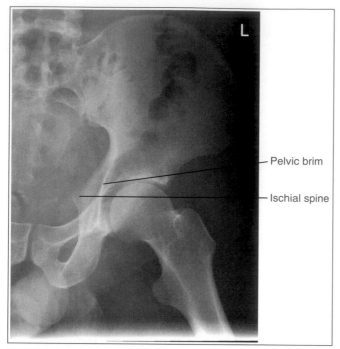

FIGURE 6-201 AP proximal femur projection taken with the pelvis rotated from the affected femur and leg externally rotated.

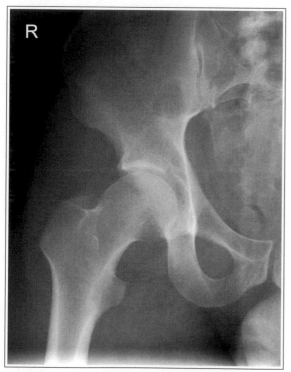

FIGURE 6-202 AP proximal femur projection taken with the pelvis rotated away from the affected femur and leg externally rotated.

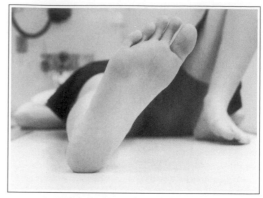

FIGURE 6-203 Proper foot rotation.

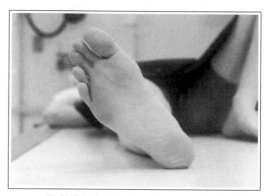

FIGURE 6-204 Poor foot rotation.

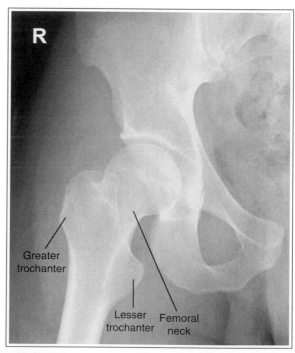

FIGURE 6-205 AP proximal femur projection taken with the leg externally rotated and the foot positioned at 45 degrees with the table.

the femoral epicondyles at a 60- to 65-degree angle with the table, the femoral neck declines posteriorly enough to nearly position it on end, demonstrating maximum femoral neck foreshortening and the lesser trochanter in profile (Figures 6-204 and 6-205). If the leg is positioned with the foot placed vertically and an imaginary line connecting the femoral epicondyles at approximately a 15- to 20-degree angle with the table, the femoral neck is only partially foreshortened and the lesser trochanter is demonstrated in partial profile (Figure 6-206).

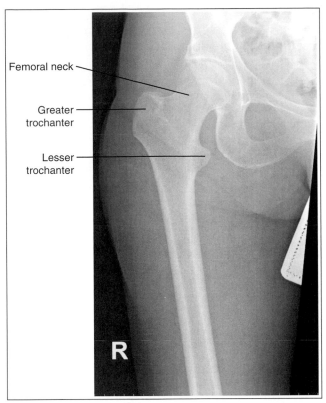

FIGURE 6-206 AP proximal femur projection taken with the foot positioned vertically.

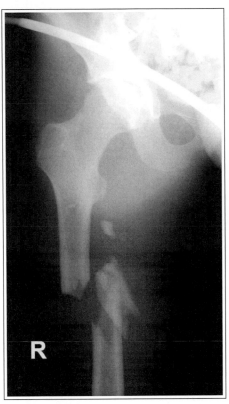

FIGURE 6-207 AP proximal femur projection demonstrating a fracture.

Positioning for Fracture. When a fracture of the femur is suspected, the leg should not be rotated, but left as is. Forced rotation of a fractured proximal femur may injure the blood vessels and nerves that surround the injured area. Because the leg is not internally rotated when a fracture is in question, such an AP femoral projection demonstrates the femoral neck with some degree of foreshortening and the lesser trochanter without femoral shaft superimposition (Figure 6-207).

Soft Tissue. The surrounding femoral soft tissue should be included to allow detection of subcutaneous air and hematomas.

AP Femur Analysis Practice

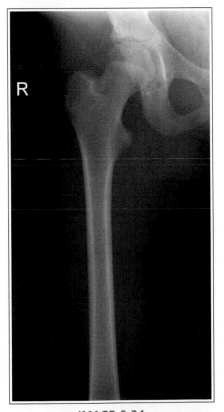

IMAGE 6-34

Analysis. The lesser trochanter is demonstrated in profile. The patient's leg was externally rotated.

TABLE 6-23	Distal Femur: Lateral Distal Femur Projection
Image Analysis Guidelines (Figure 6-208)	**Related Positioning Procedures (Figure 6-209)**
• Image brightness is uniform across the femur.	• Position the proximal femur at the cathode end of the tube and the knee at the anode end of the tube.
• Anterior and the posterior margins of the medial and lateral femoral condyles are aligned. • Femoral shaft is seen without foreshortening, with medial femoral condyle projected 0.5 inch (1.25 cm) distal to the lateral femoral condyle.	• Place the patient in a recumbent position with the affected leg against the table. • Position the lower edge of the IR and grid 2 inch below the knee joint. • Flex the affected knee 45-degrees and rotate the patient as needed to position the femoral epicondyles perpendicular to the IR.
• Long axis of the femoral shaft is aligned with the long axis of the collimated field.	• Center the midfemur to the midline of the IR.
• Distal femoral shaft is at the center of the exposure field. • Unaffected leg is not demonstrated on the projection.	• Center a perpendicular CR to the midfemur and the IR. • Draw the unaffected leg posteriorly and support it or flex the knee and draw it anteriorly across the proximal femur of the affected leg, supporting it as needed to maintain femoral epicondyle positioning.
• Distal femoral shaft, surrounding femoral soft tissue, knee joint, and 1 inch (2.5 cm) of the lower leg are included within the exposure field. • Any orthopedic apparatus located in the distal femur is included in its entirety. • 2 inches (5 cm) of overlap is evident with proximal lateral femur projection if the entire femur is imaged.	• Longitudinally collimate to a 17 inch (43 cm) field size • Transversely collimate to within 0.5 inch (1.25 cm) of the lateral femoral skin line.

Correction. Internally rotate the leg until the foot is tilted 15 to 20 degrees from vertical and the femoral epicondyles are positioned parallel with the table.

FEMUR: LATERAL PROJECTION (MEDIOLATERAL)

See Table 6-23, (Figures 6-208 and 6-209).
Femoral Condyles
Anterior and Posterior Femoral Condyle Alignment. If the femoral epicondyles are not positioned perpendicular to the IR, the lateral projection demonstrates one femoral condyle anterior to the other condyle. The patient's patella must be rolled closer to or farther from the IR by adjusting patient rotation to align the condylar margins. The first step in determining which way to roll the patient's knee is to distinguish one condyle from the other. Because the CR is centered proximal to the knee joint for a lateral femur, x-ray divergence will cause the medial condyle to project distal to the lateral condyle about 0.5 inches (1.25 cm) when the mediolateral projection is obtained. Consequently the distal condyle will be the medial condyle. If a lateral distal femur is obtained that demonstrates the medial condyle posterior to the lateral condyle, the patient's patella was situated too far away from the IR (leg internally rotated; Figure 6-210). If a lateral distal knee projection is obtained that demonstrates the medial condyle anterior to the lateral condyle, the patient's patella was situated too close to the IR (leg externally rotated; Figure 6-211).

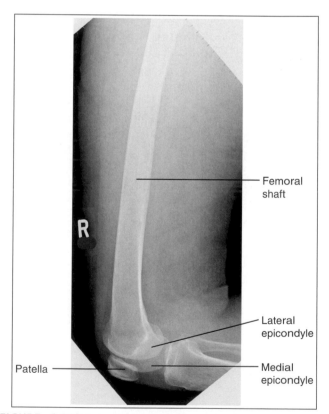

FIGURE 6-208 Lateral distal femur projection with accurate positioning.

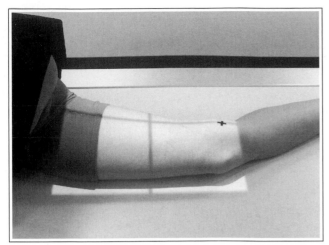

FIGURE 6-209 Proper patient positioning for lateral distal femur projection. X indicates medial femoral epicondyle.

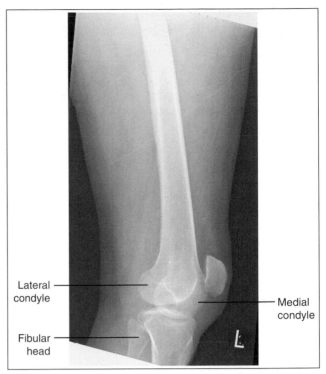

FIGURE 6-211 Lateral distal femur projection taken with the leg externally rotated

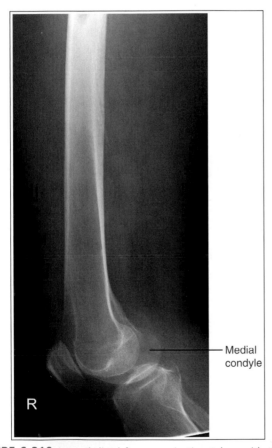

FIGURE 6-210 Lateral distal femur projection taken with the leg internally rotated.

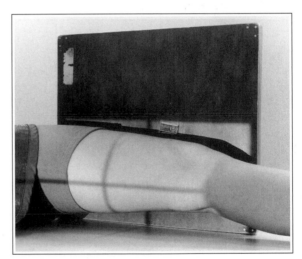

FIGURE 6-212 Proper patient positioning for crosstable mediolateral distal femur projection.

Positioning for Fracture. When a fracture of the femur is suspected, the leg should not be internally rotated, but left as is. Forced rotation of a fractured proximal femur may injure the blood vessels and nerves that surround the injured area. In such cases, cross-table lateromedial knee projections are commonly performed, with the patient remaining in the supine position (Figure 6-212). To obtain a projection that demonstrates alignment of the anterior and posterior margins of the femoral condyles and the femur without rotation, elevate the leg on a radiolucent sponge and angle the CR anteriorly until it is aligned with the femoral epicondyles. If a grid is used, make certain that the grid is adjusted so that the gridlines are running with the CR angulation to prevent grid cutoff. Failure to align the CR and epicondyles will result in a projection that demonstrates the medial condyle anterior to the lateral condyle.

If a lateromedial projection is obtained, to prevent femoral foreshortening the IR or femur should be adjusted to align them parallel with each other. This

TABLE 6-24	**Proximal Lateral Femur Projection**
Image Analysis Guidelines (Figure 6-213)	**Related Positioning Procedures (Figure 6-214)**
• Image brightness is uniform across the femur.	• Position the proximal femur at the cathode end of the tube and the distal femur at the anode end
• Lesser trochanter is in profile medially. • Femoral neck and head are superimposed over the greater trochanter.	• Place the patient in a recumbent AP oblique projection, with the affected side closest to IR. • Flex the affected knee as needed for support and draw the unaffected leg posteriorly. • Externally rotate the leg, and rotate the pelvis toward the affected femur as needed to place the femoral epicondyles perpendicular to the IR.
• Femoral shaft is seen without foreshortening. • Femoral neck is demonstrated on end. • Greater trochanter is demonstrated at the same transverse level as the femoral head. • Long axis of the femoral shaft is aligned with the long axis of the collimated field.	• Ensure that the distal femur is not elevated and that the entire femur is placed against the table. • Place the upper edge of IR and grid at the level of the affected ASIS. • Center the midfemur to the midline of the IR.
• Proximal femoral shaft is at the center of the exposure field. • Proximal femoral shaft, hip joint, and surrounding femoral soft tissue are included within the collimated field. • Any orthopedic apparatus located in the proximal femur or hip are included in its entirety. • 2 inches (5 cm) of overlap is evident with distal lateral femur projection if the entire femur is imaged.	• Center a perpendicular CR to the midfemur and the IR. • Longitudinally collimate to a 17 inch (43 cm) field size. • Transversely collimate to within 0.5 inch (1.25 cm) of the lateral femoral skin line.

parallelism is identified by the lateral condyle being projected about 0.5 inches (1.25 cm) distal to the medial condyle on the image. If the knee is placed too close to the IR, the lateral condyle will demonstrate more than 0.5 inch (1.25 cm) distally, and if the knee is placed too far from the IR, the lateral condyle will be closer than 0.5 inch (1.25 cm) to the medial condyle.
Femoral Shaft Overlap. See AP distal femur.

Proximal Femur

See Table 6-24, (Figures 6-213 and 6-214).
Greater and Lesser Trochanter. Accurate leg and help rotation aligns the femoral epicondyles perpendicular to the IR on the lateral femur. This rotation causes the greater trochanter to move beneath the femoral neck and head and brings the lesser trochanter in profile medially. If the leg and health are not rotated enough to place the femoral epicondyles perpendicular, the greater trochanter is not positioned beneath the neck and head but is partially demonstrated laterally and the lateral trochanter is partially demonstrated medially (Figure 6-215). If the leg and pelvis are rotated too much, positioning the medial epicondyles anterior to the lateral, the greater trochanter is partially in profile medially and the lesser trochanter will be obscured (Figure 6-216).
Effect of Femur Abduction. The femoral shaft is demonstrated without foreshortening, the femoral neck is demonstrated on end, and the greater trochanter is demonstrated at the same transverse level as the femoral head when the femur is positioned flat against the table. To

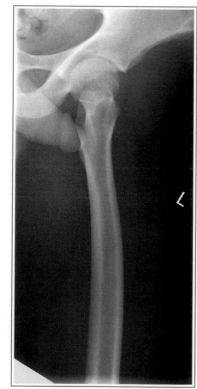

FIGURE 6-213 Lateral proximal femur projection with accurate positioning.

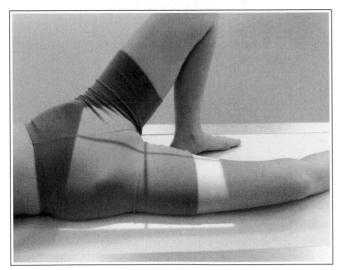

FIGURE 6-214 Proper patient positioning for lateral proximal femur projection.

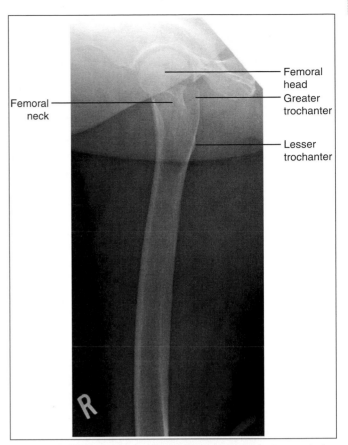

FIGURE 6-216 Lateral proximal femur projection taken with the leg and pelvis excessively rotated.

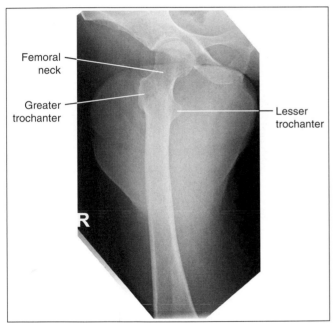

FIGURE 6-215 Lateral proximal femur projection taken with the leg and pelvis insufficiently rotated to place the femoral epicondyles perpendicular to the IR.

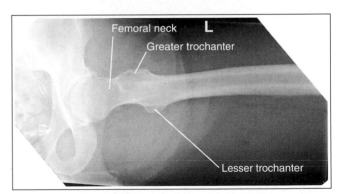

FIGURE 6-217 Lateral proximal femur projection taken with the distal femur is elevated.

understand the relationship between the femoral shaft and neck, study a femoral skeletal bone placed in a lateral projection. Note that when the femur rests against a flat surface in a lateral projection, the femoral neck is on end. With this position, the femoral neck is completely foreshortened. Because of this foreshortening, the femoral neck cannot be evaluated on a projection taken in this manner. If instead of being positioned flat against the table the distal femur is elevated for the projection, the femoral shaft is shown with increased foreshortening, the femoral neck is shown with decreased foreshortening, and the greater trochanter will be at a transverse level distal to the femoral head (Figure 6-217). The

higher the distal femur is elevated the greater will be the changes.

Midfemur and Grid Midline Alignment. If the femur cannot be brought into alignment with the grid midline, increased transverse collimation can be obtained by rotating the collimator head until one of its axes is aligned with the long axis of the femur (Figure 6-218).

Positioning for Fracture. For a patient with a suspected or known fracture, rotating, flexing, or abducting the affected leg or rolling the patient onto the affected side may cause further soft tissue and bony injury. Therefore, an axiolateral projection of the proximal femur should be used (Figures 6-219, 6-220, and 6-221). For

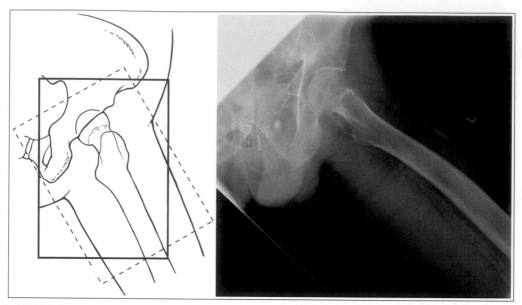

FIGURE 6-218 CR centering for proximal femur projection. Dotted line rectangle indicates area covered if collimator head is turned.

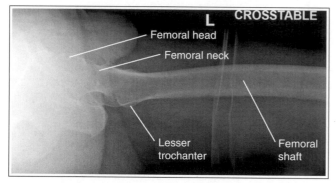

FIGURE 6-219 Crosstable lateral proximal femur projection with accurate positioning.

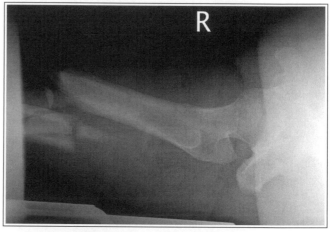

FIGURE 6-220 Proximal femur projection with fracture.

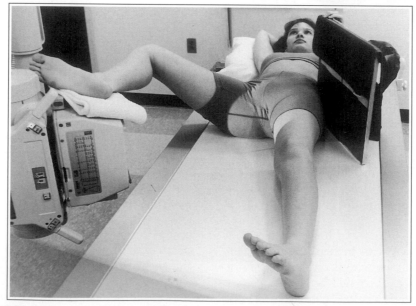

FIGURE 6-221 Proper patient positioning for crosstable lateral proximal femur projection.

this projection, the patient remains in a supine position, the IR is placed against the medial aspect of the femur, and a horizontal beam is directed perpendicular to the IR. Refer to the axiolateral hip projection in Chapter 7 for image analysis guidelines and related positioning procedures for the projection.

Lateral Femur Image Analysis Practice

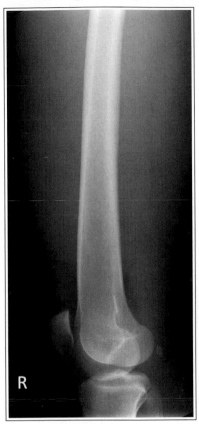

IMAGE 6-35

Analysis. The medial condyle is positioned anterior to the lateral condyle. The patient's patella was situated too close to the IR (leg externally rotated).

Correction. Internally rotate the leg until the femoral epicondyles are positioned perpendicular to the IR.

Pelvis, Hip, and Sacroiliac Joints

OUTLINE

Pelvis: AP Projection, 366
  AP Pelvis Analysis
    Practice, 370
Pelvis: AP Frog-Leg Projection
  (Modified Cleaves Method), 370
  AP Frog-Leg Pelvis Analysis
    Practice, 374
Hip: AP Projection, 374
  AP Hip Analysis Practice, 377

Hip: AP Frog-Leg (Mediolateral)
  Projection (Modified Cleaves
  Method), 378
  AP Frog-Leg Hip Analysis
    Practice, 382
Hip: Axiolateral (Inferosuperior)
  Projection (Danelius-Miller
  Method), 382
  Axiolateral Analysis Practice, 386

Sacroiliac (SI) Joints: AP Axial
  Projection, 386
  AP Axial SI Joints Analysis
    Practice, 387
Sacroiliac Joints: AP Oblique
  Projection (Left and Right
  Posterior Oblique Positions), 388
  AP Oblique SI Joint Analysis
    Practice, 389

OBJECTIVES

After completion of this chapter, you should be able to do the following:

- Identify the required anatomy on projections of the hip, pelvis, and sacroiliac (SI) joints.
- Describe how to position the patient, image receptor (IR), and central ray (CR) properly for hip, pelvic, and SI joint projections.
- List the requirements for accurate positioning for hip, pelvic, and SI joint projections.
- State how to reposition the patient properly when hip, pelvic, and SI joint projections with poor positioning are produced.
- Discuss how to determine the amount of patient or CR adjustment is required to improve hip, pelvic, and SI joint projections with poor positioning.
- List the soft tissue fat planes demonstrated on AP hip and pelvic projections, and describe their locations.

- Explain how leg rotation affects which anatomic structures of the proximal femur are demonstrated.
- Discuss why the leg of a patient with a proximal femoral fracture should never be rotated to obtain AP and lateral projections, and state how these projections should be taken.
- Define the differences demonstrated between the pelvic bones of female and male patients.
- Describe how the anatomic structures of the proximal femur are demonstrated differently for frog-leg hip and pelvic projections when the distal femur is abducted at different angles to the imaging table.
- Describe how to localize the femoral neck for an axiolateral hip projection.
- State which SI joint is of interest when the patient is rotated for oblique SI joint projections.

KEY TERMS

gluteal fat plane
iliopsoas fat plane

obturator internus fat plane

pericapsular fat plane

IMAGE ANALYSIS GUIDELINES

Technical Data. When the technical data in Table 7-1 are followed, or adjusted as needed for additive and destructive patient conditions (see Table 2-6), along with the best practices discussed in Chapters 1 and 2, all hip and pelvic projections will demonstrate the image analysis guidelines in Box 7-1 unless otherwise indicated.

PELVIS: AP PROJECTION

See Table 7-2, (Figures 7-1, 7-2, and 7-3).
Fat Planes. When evaluating pelvic projections, the reviewer not only analyzes the bony structures but also studies the placement of the soft tissue fat planes. Four fat planes are of interest on AP hip projections, and their visualization aids in the detection of intra-articular

TABLE 7-1	Hip and Pelvis Technical Data					
Projection	**kV**	**Grid**	**AEC**		**mAs**	**SID**
AP, pelvis	80-85	Grid	Both outside			40-48 inches (100-120 cm)
AP frog-leg, pelvis	80-85	Grid	Both outside			40-48 inches (100-120 cm)
AP, hip	80-85	Grid	Center			40-48 inches (100-120 cm)
AP frog-leg, hip	80-85	Grid	Center			40-48 inches (100-120 cm)
Axiolateral (inferosuperior), hip	80-85	Grid			60	40-48 inches (100-120 cm)
AP axial, sacroiliac joints	80-85	Grid	Center			40-48 inches (100-120 cm)
AP oblique, sacroiliac joints	80-85	Grid	Center			40-48 inches (100-120 cm)
Pediatric	65-75	Grid			3-5	40-48 inches (100-120 cm)

Use grid if part thickness measures 4 inches (10 cm) or more and adjust mAs per grid ratio requirement.

TABLE 7-2	AP Pelvis Projection

Image Analysis Guidelines (Figures 7-1 and 7-2)	Related Positioning Procedures (Figure 7-3)
• Contrast and density are adequate to demonstrate the pericapsular gluteal, iliopsoas, and obturator fat planes.	• Set appropriate technical factors.
• Sacrum and coccyx are aligned with the symphysis pubis. • Obturator foramina are open and uniform in size and shape. • Iliac wings are symmetrical.	• Place the patient in a supine AP projection with the knees extended. • Position the midsagittal plane of the body to the midline of the IR. • Position the ASISs equidistant from the IR, aligning the midcoronal plane parallel with the IR.
• Femoral necks are demonstrated without foreshortening. • Greater trochanters are in profile laterally. • Lesser trochanters are superimposed by the femoral necks.	• Internally rotate the legs until the femoral epicondyles are aligned parallel with the table.
• Inferior sacrum is at the center of the exposure field.	• Center a perpendicular CR to the midsagittal plane at a level halfway between the symphysis pubis and the midpoint of an imaginary line connecting the ASISs.
• Iliac wings, symphysis pubis, ischia, acetabula, femoral necks and heads, and greater and lesser trochanters are included within the exposure field.	• Center the IR and grid to the CR. • Longitudinally collimate to approximately 5 inches (12.5 cm) below the symphysis pubis or to a 14-inch (35 cm) field size. • Transversely collimate to within 0.5 inch (1.25 cm) of the lateral skin line or to a 17-inch (43 cm) field size.
• Any orthopedic apparatuses located at the hip(s) are included in their entirety.	• If an orthopedic apparatus is present, adjust the CR centering more inferior to include the apparatus(s).

BOX 7-1	Hip and Pelvis Imaging Analysis Guidelines

- The facility's identification requirements are visible.
- A right or left marker identifying the correct side of the patient is present on the projection and is not superimposed over the VOI.
- Good radiation protection practices are evident.
- Bony trabecular patterns and cortical outlines of the anatomical structures are sharply defined.

- Contrast resolution is adequate to demonstrate the surrounding soft tissue, bony trabecular patterns, and cortical outlines.
- No quantum mottle or saturation is present.
- Scatter radiation has been kept to a minimum.
- There is no evidence of removable artifacts.

and periarticular disease: the obturator internus fat plane, which lies within the pelvic inlet next to the medial brim; the iliopsoas fat plane, which lies medial to the lesser trochanter; the pericapsular fat plane, which is found superior to the femoral neck; and the gluteal fat plane, which lies superior to the pericapsular fat plane (Figure 7-4).

Differences Between Male and Female Pelves. Be aware of the bony architectural differences that exist between the male and female pelves (Table 7-3). These

differences are the result of the need for the female pelvis to accommodate fetal growth during pregnancy and fetal passage during delivery.

Pelvis Rotation. Nonrotated pelvis projections demonstrate symmetrical iliac wings and obturator foramina, and the sacrum and coccyx aligned with the symphysis pubis. If the pelvis is rotated into a left posterior oblique (LPO) position, the left iliac wing is wider than the right, the left obturator foramen is narrower than the right, and the sacrum and coccyx are not aligned with the

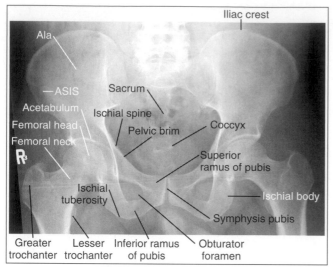

FIGURE 7-1 AP male pelvis projection with accurate positioning.

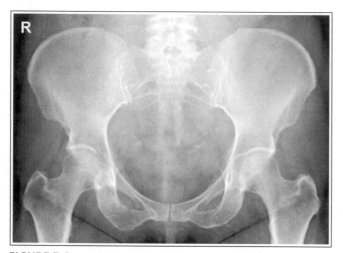

FIGURE 7-2 AP female pelvis projection with accurate positioning.

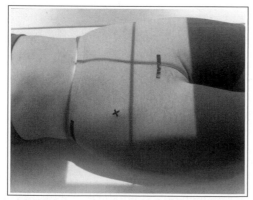

FIGURE 7-3 Proper patient positioning for AP pelvis projection.

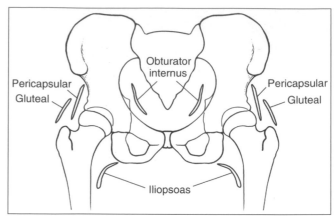

FIGURE 7-4 Location of fat planes.

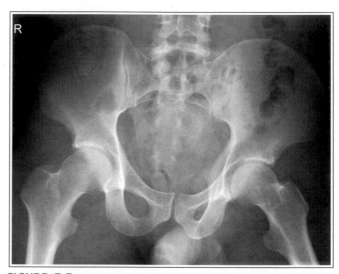

FIGURE 7-5 AP pelvis projection taken with the pelvis rotated toward the left side positioned closer to the IR.

TABLE 7-3	Male and Female Pelvic Differences	
Parameter	Male	Female
Overall Shape	Bulkier, deeper, narrower	Smaller, shallower, and wider
Ala (iliac wing)	Narrower, nonflared	Wider, flared
Pubic arch angle	Acute angle	Obtuse angle
Inlet shape	Smaller, heart shaped	Larger, rounded shape
Obturator foramen	Larger	Smaller

Femoral Neck and Greater and Lesser Trochanter Visualization. To demonstrate the femoral necks without foreshortening and the greater trochanters in profile on an AP pelvis projection, the patient's leg should be internally rotated until the feet are angled 15 to 20 degrees from vertical and the femoral epicondyles are positioned parallel with the table (Figure 7-6; see Figure 7-1). Sandbags or tape may be needed to help maintain this internal leg rotation. A pelvic projection may not demonstrate the proximal femurs with exactly the same

symphysis pubis but are rotated toward the right hip (Figure 7-5). If the patient was rotated into a right posterior oblique (RPO) position, the opposite is true. The right iliac wing is wider than the left, the right obturator foramen is narrower than the left, and the sacrum and coccyx are rotated toward the left hip.

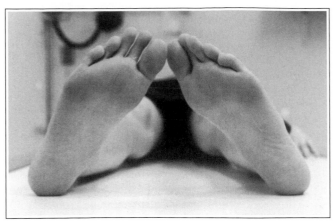

FIGURE 7-6 Proper internal foot positioning (15 to 20 degrees from vertical).

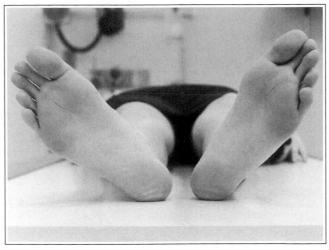

FIGURE 7-7 Poor foot positioning.

degree of internal rotation. How each proximal femur appears will depend on the degree of internal rotation placed on that leg.

Detecting Poor Leg Positioning. The relationship of the patient's entire leg to the table determines how the femoral necks and trochanters are shown on an AP pelvis projection. In general, when patients are relaxed their legs and feet are externally rotated. On external rotation the femoral necks decline posteriorly (toward the table) and are foreshortened on an AP pelvis projection. Greater external rotation increases the posterior decline and fore-shortening of the femoral necks. If the patient's legs are externally rotated enough to position the feet at a 45-degree angle, with an imaginary line connecting the femoral epicondyles at a 60- to 65-degree angle with the imaging table, the femoral necks are demonstrated on end and the lesser trochanters are demonstrated in profile (Figures 7-7 and 7-8). If the patient's legs are positioned with the feet placed vertically, with an imaginary line connecting the femoral epicondyles at approximately a 15- to 20-degree angle with the table, the lesser trochan-ter is demonstrated in partial profile and the femoral neck is only partially foreshortened (Figure 7-9).

Positioning for Femoral Neck or Proximal Femoral Fracture or Hip Dislocation. Often, when a fracture of the femoral neck or proximal femur is suspected, a pelvic projection is ordered instead of an AP projection of the affected hip. This is because pelvic fractures are fre-quently associated with proximal femur fractures. If a patient has a suspected femur fracture or hip dislocation, the leg should not be internally rotated but should be left as is. Because the leg is not internally rotated when a fracture or dislocation is in question, such a pelvic projection demonstrates the affected femoral neck with some degree of foreshortening and the lesser trochanter without femoral shaft superimposition (Figure 7-10).

CR Centering for Analysis of Hip Joint Mobil-ity. When an AP pelvis projection is being taken specifi-cally to evaluate hip joint mobility, the CR should be centered to the midsagittal plane at a level 1-inch (2.5 cm)

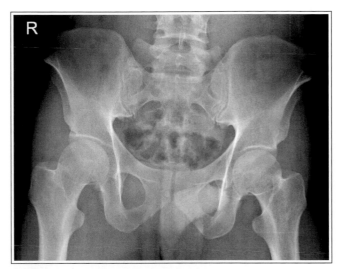

FIGURE 7-8 AP pelvis projection taken with the legs externally rotated enough to position the feet at a 45-degree angle with the table.

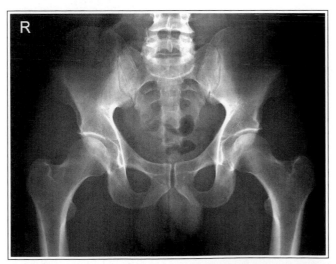

FIGURE 7-9 AP pelvis projection taken with the feet placed vertical and the femoral epicondyles at a 60- to 65-degree angle with the table.

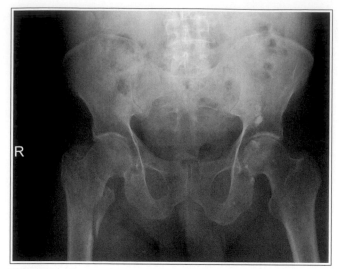

FIGURE 7-10 AP pelvis projection of a patient with a right femoral neck fracture.

superior to the symphysis pubis. Such positioning centers the hip joints on the projection but may result in clipping of the superior ilia.

AP Pelvis Analysis Practice

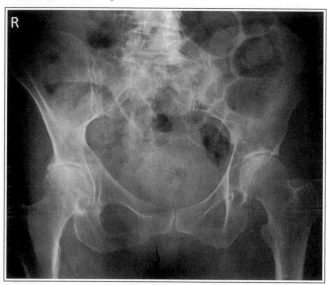

IMAGE 7-1

Analysis. The left obturator foramen is narrower than the right foramen, the left iliac wing is wider than the right, and the sacrum and coccyx are rotated toward the right hip. The left side lesser trochanter is demonstrated medially and the femoral neck is foreshortened. The pelvis was rotated onto the left side (LPO) and the left leg was externally rotated.

Correction. Rotate the patient toward the right hip until the anterior superior iliac spines (ASISs) are positioned at equal distances from the IR and internally rotate the left leg until the foot is angled 15 to 20 degrees from vertical and the femoral epicondyles are positioned parallel with the table.

PELVIS: AP FROG-LEG PROJECTION (MODIFIED CLEAVES METHOD)

See Table 7-4, (Figures 7-11 and 7-12).

Pelvis Rotation. The obturator foramen and iliac wings are symmetrical, and the sacrum and coccyx are aligned with the symphysis pubis on a nonrotated pelvis. If the pelvis is rotated into an LPO position, the left ilium is wider than the right, the left obturator foramen is narrower than the right, and the sacrum and coccyx are not aligned with the symphysis pubis but are rotated toward the right hip (Figure 7-13). If the patient is rotated into an RPO position, the opposite is true. The right ilium is wider than the left, the right obturator foramen is narrower than the left, and the sacrum and coccyx are rotated toward the left hip.

Lesser and Greater Trochanter Visualization. For an AP frog-leg pelvis projection, the medial and lateral placement of the greater and lesser trochanters is determined when the patient flexes the knee and hip. To position the greater trochanter accurately beneath the proximal femur and position the lesser trochanter in profile, flex the patient's knee and hip until the femur is angled at 60 to 70 degrees with the table (20 to 30 degrees from vertical) (Figure 7-14).

Identifying Poor Knee and Hip Flexion. For an AP frog-leg pelvis projection, the relationship of the greater and the lesser trochanters with the proximal femurs is determined when the patient flexes the knees and hips. If the knees and hips are not flexed enough to place the femur at a 60- to 70-degree angle with the table, the greater trochanters are demonstrated laterally, as with an AP projection (Figure 7-15). If the knees and hips are flexed too much, placing the femurs at an angle greater than 60 to 70 degrees with the table, the greater trochanters are demonstrated medially (see Figure 7-39).

Femoral Neck and Greater Trochanter Visualization. The degree of femoral abduction determines the amount of femoral neck foreshortening and the transverse level at which the greater trochanters are demonstrated between the femoral heads and lesser trochanters. If the femoral shafts are abducted to 20 to 30 degrees from vertical (60- to 70-degree angle from the table; Figure 7-16), the femoral necks are demonstrated without foreshortening and the proximal greater trochanters are at the same transverse level as the lesser trochanters on a AP frog-leg pelvis projection (Figure 7-17). If the femoral shafts are abducted to a 45-degree angle from vertical and the table (Figure 7-18), the femoral necks are partially foreshortened and the proximal greater trochanters are at a transverse level halfway between the femoral heads and the lesser trochanters (see Figure 7-11). If the femoral shafts are abducted until they are placed next to the table (Figure 7-19), the proximal femoral shafts are demonstrated without foreshortening, the proximal greater trochanters are at the same

TABLE 7-4	AP Frog-leg Pelvis Projection
Image Analysis Guidelines (Figure 7-11)	**Related Positioning Procedures (Figure 7-12)**
• Contrast and density are adequate to demonstrate the pericapsular gluteal, iliopsoas, and obturator fat planes.	• Set appropriate technical factors.
• Sacrum and coccyx are aligned with the symphysis pubis.	• Place the patient in a supine position.
• Obturator foramina are open and uniform in size and shape.	• Position the midsagittal plane of the body to the midline of the IR.
• Iliac wings are symmetrical.	• Position the ASISs equidistant from the IR, aligning the midcoronal plane parallel with the IR.
• Lesser trochanters are in profile medially.	
• Femoral necks are superimposed over the adjacent greater trochanters.	• Flex the knees and hips until the femurs are angled at 60 to 70 degrees with the table (20 to 30 degrees from vertical).
• Femoral necks are partially foreshortened.	Abduct the femoral shaft to a 45-degree angle with the table.
• Proximal greater trochanters are demonstrated at a transverse level halfway between the femoral heads and lesser trochanters.	
• Inferior sacrum is at the center of the exposure field.	• Center a perpendicular CR to the midsagittal plane at a level 1-inch (2.5 cm) superior to the symphysis pubis.
• Ilia, symphysis pubis, ischia, acetabula, femoral necks and heads, and greater and lesser trochanters are included within the exposure field.	• Center the IR and grid to the CR. • Longitudinally collimate to approximately 5 inches (12.5 cm) below the symphysis pubis or to a 14-inch (35 cm) field size. • Transversely collimate to within 0.5 inch (1.25 cm) of the lateral skin line or to a 17-inch (43 cm) field size.

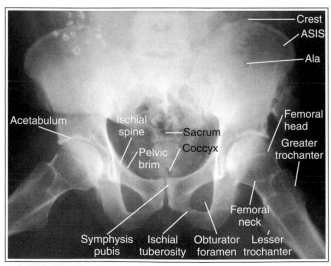

FIGURE 7-11 AP frog-leg pelvis projection with accurate positioning.

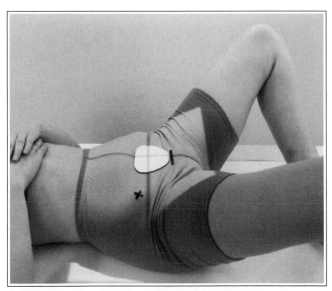

FIGURE 7-12 Proper patient positioning for AP frog-leg pelvis projection.

transverse level as the femoral heads, and the femoral necks are demonstrated on end on an AP frog-leg pelvis projection (Figure 7-20).

Importance of Symmetrical Femoral Abduction. An AP frog-leg projection may not demonstrate the proximal femurs with exactly the same degree of femoral abduction. How each proximal femur appears depends on the degree of femoral abduction placed on that leg. As a standard, unless the projection is ordered to evaluate hip mobility, both femurs should be abducted equally for the projection. This symmetrical abduction helps prevent pelvic rotation. It may be necessary to position an angled sponge beneath the femurs to maintain the desired femoral abduction.

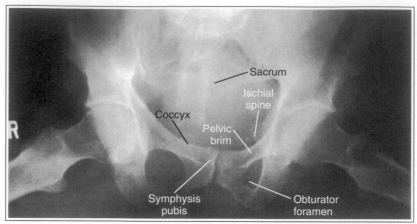

FIGURE 7-13 AP frog-leg pelvis projection taken with the left side of the pelvis rotated toward the IR.

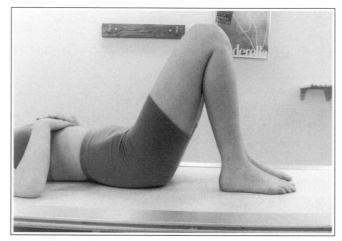

FIGURE 7-14 Proper knee and hip flexion (60 to 70 degrees from table).

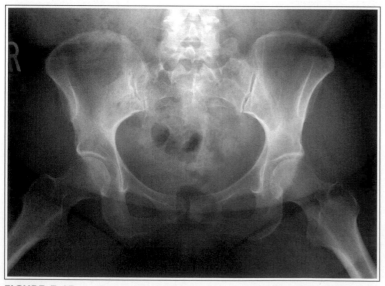

FIGURE 7-15 Insufficient knee and hip flexion (less than 60 degrees from table).

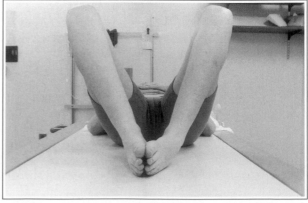

FIGURE 7-16 Femurs in only slight abduction (20 degrees from vertical).

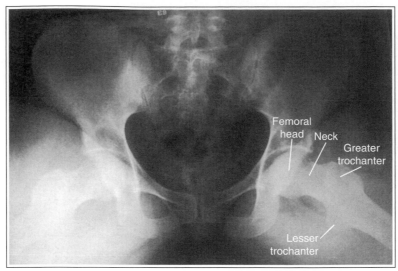

FIGURE 7-17 AP frog-leg pelvis projection taken with the femoral shafts abducted to a 60- to 70-degree angle with the table.

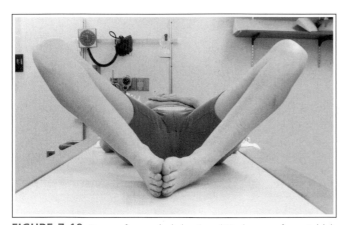

FIGURE 7-18 Proper femoral abduction (45 degrees from table).

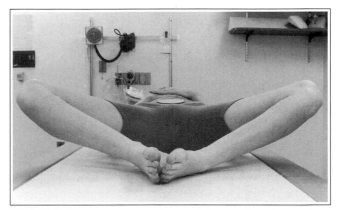

FIGURE 7-19 Femurs in maximum abduction (20 degrees from table).

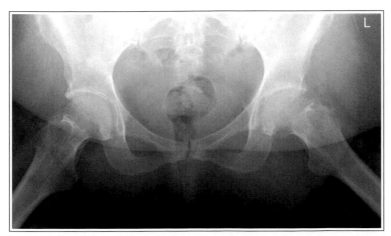

FIGURE 7-20 AP frog-leg pelvis projection taken with the femoral shafts abducted to a 20-degree angle with the table.

AP Frog-Leg Pelvis Analysis Practice

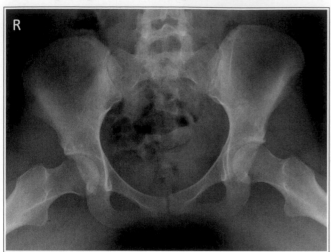

IMAGE 7-2

Analysis. The femoral necks are demonstrated without foreshortening and the proximal greater trochanter and lesser trochanter are demonstrated at approximately the same transverse level. The femurs were in only slight abduction, at an approximately 70-degree angle with the IR.

Correction. Decrease the degree of femoral abduction.

HIP: AP PROJECTION

See Table 7-5, (Figures 7-21 and 7-22).

Pelvis Rotation. To ensure that the pelvis is not rotated when positioning for an AP hip projection, judge the distances from the ASISs to the IR. The distances on each side should be equal. This positioning aligns the ischial spine with the pelvic brim, and the sacrum and coccyx with the symphysis pubis.

Identifying Rotation. Rotation on an AP hip projection is initially detected by evaluating the relationship of the ischial spine and the pelvic brim, the alignment of the sacrum and coccyx with the symphysis pubis, and the degree of obturator foramen demonstration. If the patient was rotated toward the affected hip, the ischial spine is demonstrated without pelvic brim superimposition, the sacrum and coccyx are not aligned with the symphysis pubis but are rotated away from the affected hip, and the obturator foramen is narrowed (Figure 7-23). If the patient has been rotated away from the affected hip, the ischial spine is not aligned with the pelvic brim but is demonstrated closer to the acetabulum, the sacrum and coccyx are not aligned with the symphysis pubis but are rotated toward the affected hip, and the obturator foramen is widened (Figure 7-24).

Femoral Neck. To demonstrate an AP hip projection with the femoral neck shown without foreshortening and the greater trochanter in profile, the patient's leg is internally rotated until the foot is angled 15 to 20 degrees

TABLE 7-5	AP Hip Projection
Image Analysis Guidelines (Figure 7-21)	**Related Positioning Procedures (Figure 7-22)**
• Contrast and density are adequate to demonstrate the pericapsular gluteal, iliopsoas, and obturator fat planes.	• Set appropriate technique factors.
• Ischial spine is aligned with the pelvic brim. • Sacrum and coccyx are aligned with the symphysis pubis. • Obturator foramen is open.	• Place the patient in a supine AP projection with the knee extended. • Position the ASISs at equidistant from the IR, aligning the midcoronal plane parallel with the IR.
• Femoral neck is demonstrated without foreshortening. • Greater trochanter is in profile laterally. • Lesser trochanter is superimposed by the femoral neck.	• Internally rotate the leg until the femoral epicondyles are aligned parallel with the table.
• Femoral head or the femoral neck is at the center of the exposure field.	• Center a perpendicular CR to femoral head or femoral neck.
• Acetabulum, greater and lesser trochanters, femoral head and neck, and one-half of the sacrum, coccyx, and symphysis pubis are included within the exposure field.	• Center the IR and grid to the CR. • Longitudinally collimate to include the ASIS. • Transversely collimate to the midsagittal plane and within 0.5 inch (1.25 cm) of the lateral hip skin line or to a 10-inch (25 cm) field size.
• Any orthopedic apparatus located at the hip are included in their entirety.	• If an orthopedic apparatus is present, adjust the CR centering more inferior and open the longitudinally collimated field to include the apparatus.

from vertical and the femoral epicondyles are positioned parallel with the table (Figures 7-21 and 7-25). A sandbag or tape may be needed to help the patient maintain this internal leg rotation.

Identifying Poor Leg Rotation. The relationship of the patient's leg to the table determines how the femoral neck and trochanters are shown on an AP hip projection. In general, when patients are relaxed their legs and feet are externally rotated. On external rotation the femoral neck declines posteriorly (toward the table) and is foreshortened on an AP hip projection. Increased external rotation increases the degree of posterior decline and foreshortening of the femoral neck on the projection. If

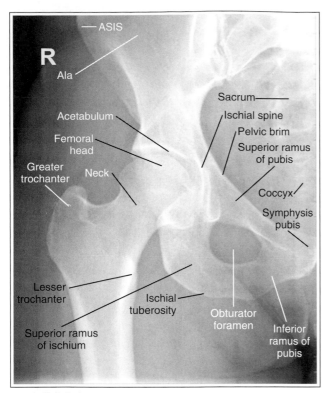

FIGURE 7-21 AP hip projection with accurate positioning.

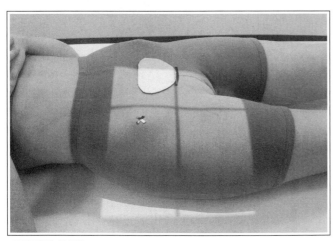

FIGURE 7-22 Proper patient positioning for AP hip projection.

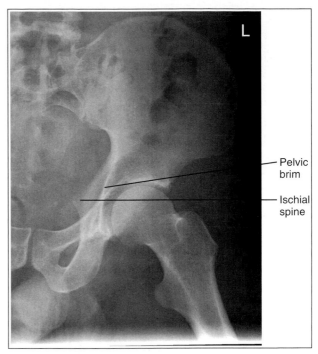

FIGURE 7-23 AP hip projection taken with the patient rotated toward the affected hip.

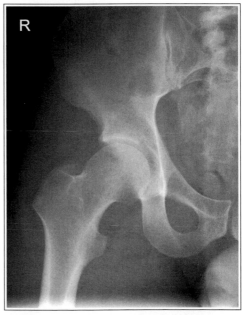

FIGURE 7-24 AP hip projection taken with the patient rotated away from the affected hip.

the patient's leg is externally rotated enough to position the foot at a 45-degree angle, with an imaginary line connecting the femoral epicondyles at a 60- to 65-degree angle with the table, the femoral neck is demonstrated on end and the lesser trochanter is demonstrated in profile (Figures 7-26 and 7-27). If the patient's leg is positioned with the foot placed vertically, with an imaginary line connecting the femoral epicondyles at approximately a 15- to 20-degree angle with the table, the lesser trochanter is demonstrated in partial profile and the femoral neck is only partially foreshortened (Figure 7-28).

Positioning for Dislocated Hip, or Fractured Femoral Neck or Proximal Femur. When a patient has a dislocated hip or a fracture of the femoral neck or proximal femur, the leg should not be internally rotated but left as is. Forced internal rotation of a dislocated hip or fractured femur may injure the blood supply and nerves that surround the injured area. Because the leg is not internally rotated when a dislocation or fracture is suspected, the resulting AP hip

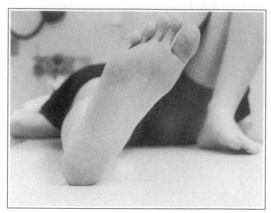

FIGURE 7-25 Proper internal foot rotation (15 to 20 degrees from vertical).

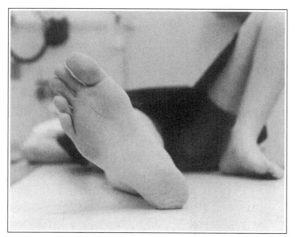

FIGURE 7-26 Poor foot rotation.

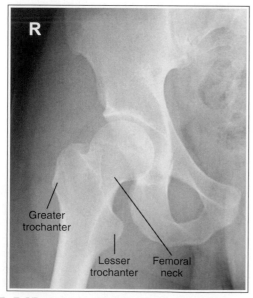

FIGURE 7-27 AP hip projection taken with the leg externally rotated to position the foot at a 45-degree angle with table.

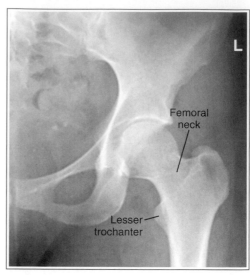

FIGURE 7-28 AP hip projection taken with the foot placed vertically and the femoral epicondyles at a 15- to 20-degree angle with the table.

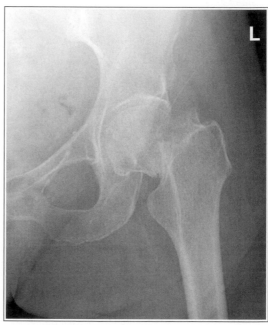

FIGURE 7-29 AP hip projection taken of a patient with a femoral neck fracture.

projection may demonstrate the femoral neck with some degree of foreshortening and the lesser trochanter without femoral shaft superimposition (Figure 7-29).

CR Centering

Localizing the Femoral Head and Neck. Two methods are used to localize the femoral head and neck for hip projections, with the second method being the preferred method when imaging the obese patient. To use the first method to place the femoral head in the center of the exposure field, center the CR 1.5 inches (4 cm) distal to the midpoint of a line connecting the ASIS and symphysis pubis (Figure 7-30). To place the femoral neck in the center of the exposure field, center

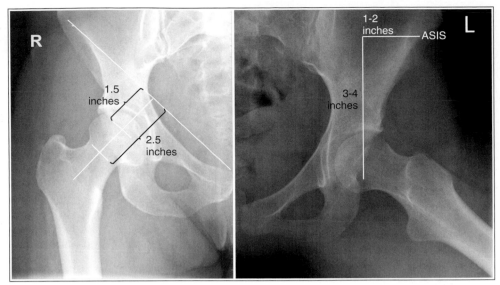

FIGURE 7-30 Localization of hip joint and femoral neck.

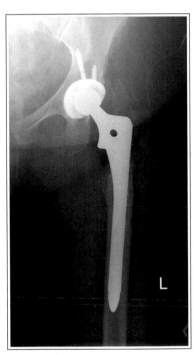

FIGURE 7-31 AP hip with metal apparatus.

AP Hip Analysis Practice

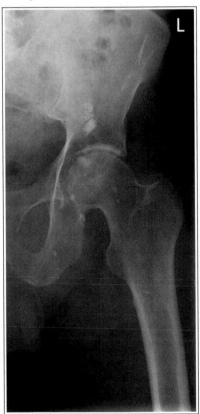

IMAGE 7-3

the CR 2.5 inches (6.25 cm) distal to the midline of a line connecting the ASIS and symphysis pubis. For the second method, position the CR 1 to 2 inches (2.5-5 cm) medial and 3 to 4 inches (9-10 cm) distal to the ASIS (see Figure 7-30).

Including Orthopedic Apparatuses. To include long orthopedic apparatuses, such as a total hip prosthesis, use a larger computed radiography IR cassette, or for DR increase the longitudinal collimation and move the CR centering point more distal on the femur to include the entire apparatus and any surrounding attachment materials (Figure 7-31).

Analysis. The femoral neck is partially foreshortened, and the lesser trochanter is demonstrated in profile. The leg was externally rotated, bringing the foot vertical and the femoral epicondyles to an approximately 15- to 20-degree angle with the table.

Correction. Internally rotate the leg until the foot is angled 15 to 20 degrees from vertical and the femoral epicondyles are positioned parallel with the table.

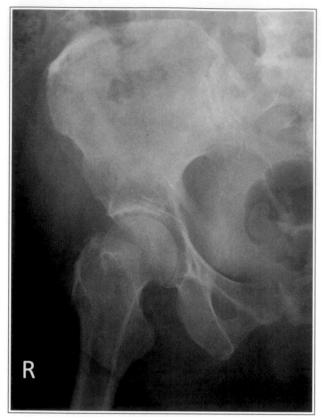

IMAGE 7-4

Analysis. The ischial spine is demonstrated without pelvic brim superimposition, the sacrum and coccyx are not aligned with the symphysis pubis but are rotated away from the affected hip, and the obturator foramen is narrowed. The patient was rotated toward the affected hip. The femoral neck is foreshortened, and the lesser trochanter is demonstrated in profile. The leg was externally rotated.

Correction. Rotate the patient away from the affected hip until the ASISs are positioned at equal distances from the IR. Internally rotate the leg until the foot is angled 15 to 20 degrees from vertical and the femoral epicondyles are positioned parallel with the table.

HIP: AP FROG-LEG (MEDIOLATERAL) PROJECTION (MODIFIED CLEAVES METHOD)

See Table 7-6, (Figures 7-32 and 7-33).

Pelvis Rotation. Equal alignment of the ASISs to the table produces the required AP pelvis without rotation and demonstrates alignment of the ischial spine and pelvic brim and sacrum and coccyx and symphysis pubis on the AP frog-leg hip projection. If instead the patient was rotated toward the affected hip for the AP frog-leg, the ischial spine is demonstrated without pelvic brim superimposition, the sacrum and coccyx are not aligned with the symphysis pubis but are rotated away from the

TABLE 7-6	AP Frog-leg (Mediolateral) Hip Projection	
Image Analysis Guidelines (Figure 7-32)	**Related Positioning Procedures (Figure 7-33)**
• Ischial spine is aligned with the pelvic brim. • Sacrum and coccyx are aligned with the symphysis pubis. • Obturator foramen is open.	• Place the patient in a supine AP projection with the knee extended. • Position the ASISs at equidistant from the IR, aligning the midcoronal plane parallel with the IR.
• Lesser trochanter is in profile medially. • Femoral neck is superimposed over the greater trochanter.	• Flex the knee and hip until the femur is angled at 60 to 70 degrees with the table.
• Femoral neck is partially foreshortened. • Proximal greater trochanter is demonstrated at a transverse level halfway between the femoral head and the lesser trochanter.	• Abduct the femoral shaft to a 45-degree angle with the table.
• Femoral neck is at the center of the exposure field.	• Center a perpendicular CR 2.5 inches (6.25 cm) distal to the midpoint of the line connecting the ASIS and symphysis pubis.
• Acetabulum, greater and lesser trochanters, femoral head and neck, and one-half of the sacrum, coccyx, and symphysis pubis are included within the exposure field.	• Center the IR and grid to the CR. • Longitudinally collimate to include the ASIS. • Transversely collimate to the patient's midsagittal plane and within 0.5 inch (1.25 cm) of the lateral hip skin line or to a 10-inch (25 cm) field size.

affected hip, and demonstration of the obturator foramen is decreased (Figure 7-34). If the patient was rotated away from the affected hip, the ischial spine is not aligned with the pelvic brim but is demonstrated closer to the acetabulum, the sacrum and coccyx are not aligned with the symphysis pubis but are rotated toward the affected hip, and demonstration of the obturator foramen is increased (Figure 7-35).

Lauenstein and Hickey Methods. The Lauenstein and Hickey methods are modifications of the frog-leg hip projection. For these methods, the patient is positioned as described for the AP frog-leg projection with the femur flexed and abducted, except that the pelvis is rotated toward the affected hip as needed to position the femur flat against the table (Figure 7-36).

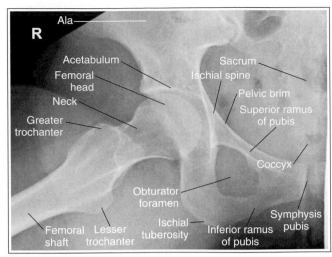

FIGURE 7-32 AP frog-leg hip projection with accurate positioning.

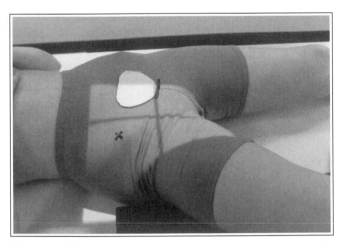

FIGURE 7-33 Proper patient positioning for AP frog-leg hip projection.

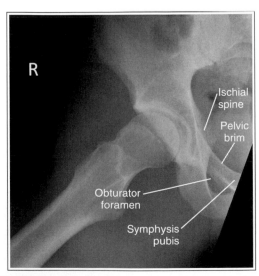

FIGURE 7-34 AP frog-leg hip projection taken with the patient rotated toward the affected hip.

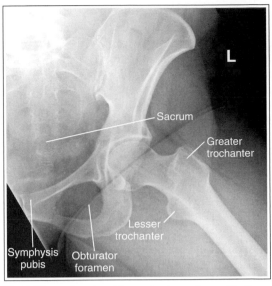

FIGURE 7-35 AP frog-leg hip projection taken with the patient rotated away from the affected hip and the knee and hip flexed less than needed to position the femur at a 60- to 70-degree angle with the table.

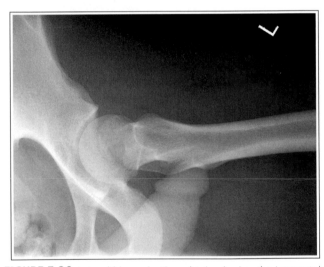

FIGURE 7-36 Lateral hip projection obtained using the Lauenstein and Hickey methods.

Lesser and Greater Trochanter. For an AP frog-leg hip projection, the medial and lateral placement of the greater and lesser trochanters is determined when the patient flexes the knee and hip. Use a femoral skeletal bone for a better understanding of how the relationship of the greater and lesser trochanters to the proximal femur changes as the distal femur is elevated with knee and hip flexion. Begin by placing the femoral bone on a flat surface in an AP projection. While slowly elevating the distal femur, observe how the greater trochanter rotates around the proximal femur. First, the greater trochanter moves beneath the proximal femur; then, as elevation of the distal femur continues, it moves from beneath the proximal femur and is demonstrated on the medial side of the femur. To position the greater trochanter accurately beneath the proximal femur and position the lesser trochanter in profile, flex the knee and hip until the femur is angled at 60 to 70 degrees with the table (20 to 30 degrees from vertical) (Figure 7-37).

Poor Knee and Hip Flexion. If the knee and hip are not flexed enough to place the femur at a 60- to 70-degree angle with the table, the greater trochanter is demonstrated laterally, as it is on an AP projection (Figures 7-35 and 7-38). If the knee and hip are flexed too much, placing the femur at an angle greater than 60 to 70 degrees with the table, the greater trochanter is demonstrated medially (Figure 7-39). The greater trochanter is also demonstrated medially, as shown in Figure 7-39, when the foot and ankle of the affected leg are elevated and placed on top of the unaffected leg. This positioning causes the femur to rotate externally. The foot of the affected leg should remain resting on the table.

Femoral Neck and Greater Trochanter Visualization. The degree of femoral abduction determines the amount of femoral neck foreshortening and the transverse level at which the proximal greater trochanter is demonstrated between the femoral head and lesser trochanter. Accurate positioning has been obtained for a mediolateral hip when the proximal femur demonstrates only partial foreshortening and the proximal greater trochanter is at the transverse level halfway between the femoral head and lesser trochanter. This positioning is obtained when the femoral shaft is at a 45-degree angle from vertical (Figures 7-38 and 7-40).

Use a femoral skeleton bone to understand how leg abduction determines the visualization of the femoral neck and the position of the greater trochanter. Place the femoral bone on a flat surface in an AP projection, with the distal femur elevated until the greater trochanter is positioned beneath the proximal femur and the lesser trochanter is in profile (20 to 30 degrees from vertical or 60 to 70 degrees from flat surface). From this position, abduct the femoral bone (move

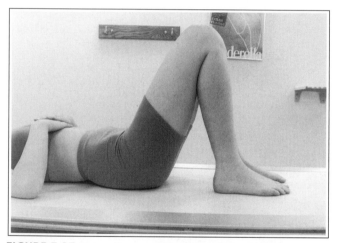

FIGURE 7-37 Proper knee and hip flexion (60 to 70 degrees from table).

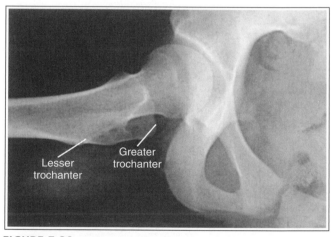

FIGURE 7-39 AP frog-leg hip projection taken with the knee and hip flexed more than needed to position the femur at a 60- to 70-degree angle with the table.

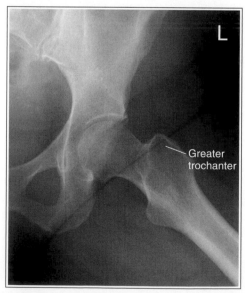

FIGURE 7-38 AP frog-leg hip projection taken with the knee and hip flexed less than needed to position the femur at a 60- to 70-degree angle with the table, and with proper leg abduction.

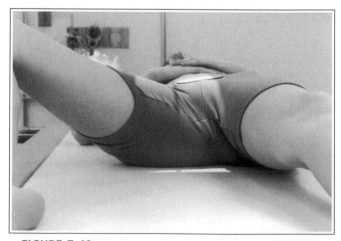

FIGURE 7-40 Proper leg abduction, 45 degrees from table.

the lateral surface of the femoral bone toward the flat surface). As the bone moves toward the flat surface, observe how the femoral neck is positioned more on end and the greater trochanter moves proximally (toward the femoral head).

Poor Leg Abduction. If the femoral shaft is abducted 20 to 30 degrees from vertical (60- to 70-degree angle with the table; Figure 7-41) the femoral neck is demonstrated without foreshortening and the proximal greater trochanter is at the same transverse level as the lesser trochanter (Figure 7-42). If the femoral shaft is abducted to the table (Figure 7-43), the proximal femoral shaft is demonstrated without foreshortening, the proximal greater trochanter is at the same transverse level as the femoral head, and the femoral neck is demonstrated on end (Figure 7-44).

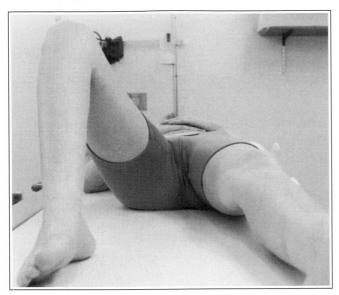

FIGURE 7-41 Femur in only slight abduction, 20 degrees from vertical (70 degrees from table).

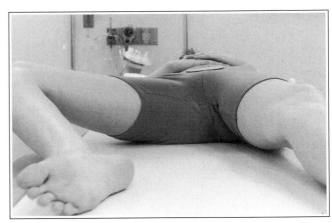

FIGURE 7-43 Femur in maximum abduction (20 degrees from table).

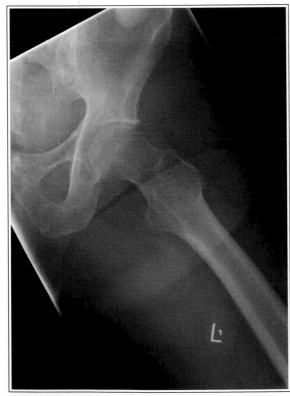

FIGURE 7-42 AP frog-leg hip projection taken with the leg abducted to bring femur at a 60- to 70-degree angle with the table.

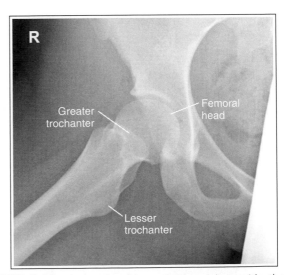

FIGURE 7-44 AP frog-leg hip projection taken with the leg abducted to bring femur at a 20-degree angle with the table.

AP Frog-Leg Hip Analysis Practice

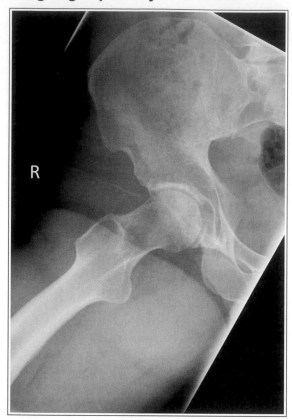

IMAGE 7-5

Analysis. The ischial spine is demonstrated without pelvic brim superimposition, the sacrum and coccyx are not aligned with the symphysis pubis but are rotated away from the affected hip, and the obturator foramen is narrow. The greater trochanter is partially demonstrated laterally, indicating that the leg was flexed less than the needed 60 to 70 degrees from the IR.

Correction. Rotate the patient away from the affected hip until the ASISs are positioned at equal distances from the IR and increase the degree of knee and hip flexion until the femur is positioned at a 60- to 70-degree angle with the IR.

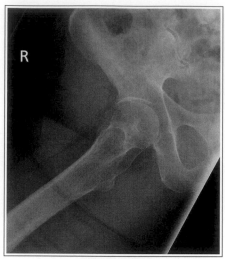

IMAGE 7-6

Analysis. The ischial spine is not aligned with the pelvic brim but is demonstrated closer to the acetabulum, the sacrum and coccyx are not aligned with the symphysis pubis but are rotated toward the affected hip, and the obturator foramen is wide. The patient was rotated away from the affected hip. The femoral neck is demonstrated on end and is entirely foreshortened and the proximal greater trochanter is demonstrated on the same transverse level as the femoral head. The femur was abducted until it was positioned flat against the table.

Correction. Rotate the patient toward the affected hip until the ASISs are positioned at equal distances from the IR and decrease the degree of femoral abduction until the femur is at a 45-degree angle with the IR.

HIP: AXIOLATERAL (INFEROSUPERIOR) PROJECTION (DANELIUS-MILLER METHOD)

See Table 7-7, (Figures 7-45 and 7-46).

Unaffected Leg Position. Flexion and abduction of the unaffected leg move its bony and soft tissue structures away from the affected hip. Inadequate flexion or abduction of the unaffected leg results in superimposition of soft tissue onto the affected hip, preventing its visualization (Figure 7-47).

Femoral Neck Visualization and Greater and Lesser Trochanter Alignment. To obtain an axiolateral hip projection that demonstrates the femoral neck without foreshortening, the CR must be aligned perpendicular to it. This alignment is accomplished by localizing the femoral neck by first finding the center of an imaginary line drawn between the symphysis pubis and the ASIS, and then bisecting that line by drawing a perpendicular line distally (Figure 7-48). This imaginary line parallels the long axis of the femoral neck as long as the leg is not abducted. Once the long axis of the femoral neck has been located, align the CR perpendicular to it and the IR parallel with it.

TABLE 7-7	Axiolateral Hip Projection	
Image Analysis Guidelines (Figure 7-45)	**Related Positioning Procedures (Figure 7-46)**
• Soft tissue from the unaffected thigh does not superimpose the femoral head or neck.	• Place the patient in a supine position with the affected hip positioned next to the lateral edge of the table. • Flex the unaffected leg until the femur is as close to vertical as patient can tolerate, support the leg position by using a specially designed leg holder or suitable support. • Abduct the unaffected leg as far as the patient will allow.
• Femoral neck is demonstrated without foreshortening. • Greater and lesser trochanters are demonstrated at approximately the same transverse level.	• Center a horizontal CR to the patient's midthigh, at the level of the femoral neck, located at a level 2.5 inches (6.25 cm) distal to the midpoint of a line connecting the ASIS and symphysis pubis.
• Lesser trochanter is in profile posteriorly. • Greater trochanter is superimposed by the femoral shaft.	• Internally rotate the affected leg until the femoral epicondyles are aligned parallel with the table.
• Femoral neck is at the center of the exposure field. • Acetabulum, greater and lesser trochanters, femoral head and neck, and ischial tuberosity are included within the exposure field. • Any orthopedic apparatus located at the hip are included in their entirety.	• Position the upper edge of the IR and grid firmly in the crease formed at the patient's waist, just superior to the iliac crest. • Align the IR and grid parallel with the femoral neck and perpendicular to the CR. • Longitudinally collimate to a 12-inch (30 cm) field size. • Transversely collimate to within 0.5 inch (1.25 cm) of the proximal femoral skin line or to a 10-inch (25 cm) field size.
• Excessive scatter radiation is not present.	• Tightly collimate and place a flat lead contact strip or the straight edge of a lead apron over the top, unused portion of the IR.

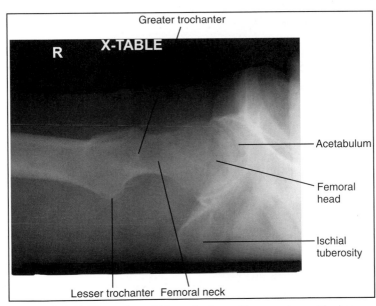

FIGURE 7-45 Axiolateral hip projection with accurate positioning.

Effect of CR and Femoral Neck Misalignment. Misalignment of the CR with the femoral neck results in femoral neck foreshortening and a shift in the transverse level at which the greater trochanter is located. If the angle formed between the femur and the CR is too large, the proximal greater trochanter is demonstrated proximal to the transverse level of the lesser trochanter and is superimposed by a portion of the femoral neck (Figure 7-49). If the angle between the femur and the CR is too small, the proximal greater trochanter is demonstrated distal to the transverse level of the lesser trochanter. This mispositioning seldom occurs, because the table and x-ray tube alignment possibilities make such an angle difficult to obtain.

Lesser and Greater Trochanter. Rotation of the affected leg determines the relationship of the lesser and greater trochanter to the proximal femur on an axiolateral hip projection. In general, when a patient is placed on the table and the affected leg is allowed to rotate freely, it is externally rotated. To position the

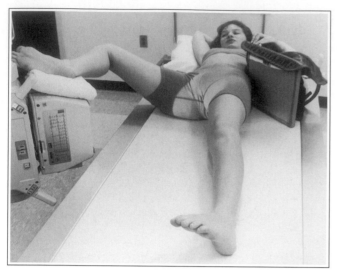

FIGURE 7-46 Proper patient positioning for axiolateral hip projection.

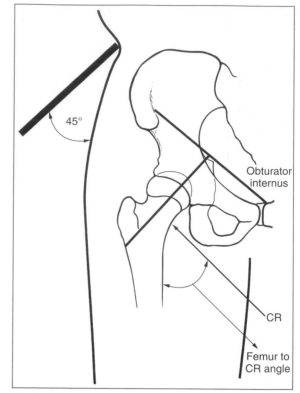

FIGURE 7-48 Locating the femoral neck and proper IR placement for small and average patients.

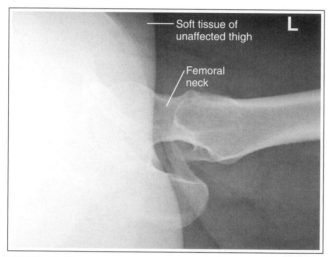

FIGURE 7-47 Axiolateral hip projection taken with insufficient flexion and abduction of the unaffected leg.

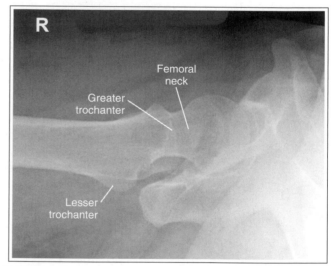

FIGURE 7-49 Axiolateral hip projection taken with the too large of a femur to CR angulation.

proximal femur in a lateral projection, demonstrating the lesser trochanter in profile posteriorly and superimposing the greater trochanter by the femoral shaft, the affected leg must be internally rotated until an imaginary line drawn between the femoral epicondyles is positioned parallel with the table. This places the foot at a 15- to 20-degree internal rotation from the vertical position (Figure 7-50).

   Identifying Poor Leg Rotation. If the affected leg is not rotated internally, the greater trochanter is demonstrated posteriorly and the lesser trochanter is superimposed over the femoral shaft (Figure 7-51). How much of the greater trochanter is demonstrated without femoral shaft superimposition depends on the degree of external rotation. Greater external rotation increases the amount of greater trochanter shown.

   Hip Dislocation or Fractured Femoral Neck or Proximal Femur. When a patient has a dislocated hip

or a suspected or known femoral fracture, the leg should not be internally rotated but left as is. Because the patient's leg is not internally rotated in such cases, it is acceptable for the greater trochanter to be demonstrated posteriorly and the lesser trochanter to be superimposed over the femoral shaft (Figure 7-52).

Including Acetabulum and Femoral Head. Once the leg has been positioned, place the upper edge of the IR and grid against the affected side at the level of the iliac crest (see Figure 7-46). This placement positions the IR so the acetabulum, femoral head and neck, and proximal femur are included on the axiolateral hip when the CR is centered to the IR. To demonstrate the femoral neck without distortion, move the lower edge of the IR and grid away from the patient's leg until it is aligned parallel with the femoral neck and perpendicular to the CR.

Obese Patient. For patients with ample lateral soft tissue thickness, the upper edge of the IR and grid needs to be positioned superior to the iliac crest (Figure 7-53). This superior positioning will result in magnification because of the increase in the object–image receptor distance (OID) but is necessary if the acetabulum and femoral head are to be included on the axiolateral hip projection.

CR Centering

Including Orthopedic Apparatuses. To include long orthopedic apparatuses, such as a total hip prosthesis, use a larger IR length and lower the CR centering point to include the entire apparatus and any surrounding attachment materials (Figure 7-54).

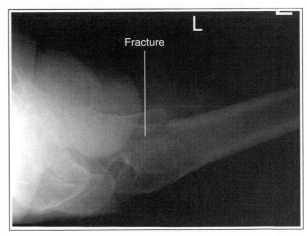

FIGURE 7-52 Axiolateral hip projection demonstrating a fractured femoral neck.

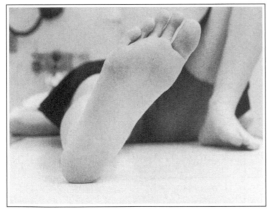

FIGURE 7-50 Proper foot position 15 to 20 degrees from vertical.

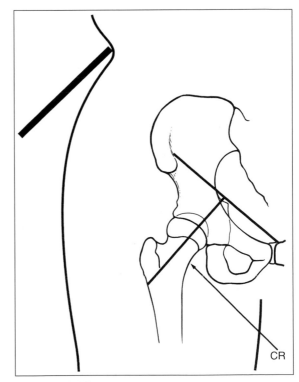

FIGURE 7-53 Proper IR placement for large patients.

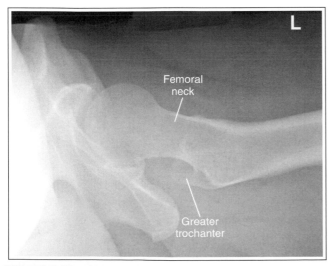

FIGURE 7-51 Axiolateral hip projection taken with the leg externally rotated.

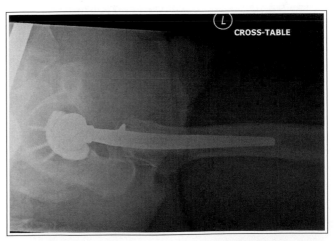

FIGURE 7-54 Lateral hip with metal apparatus.

Axiolateral Analysis Practice

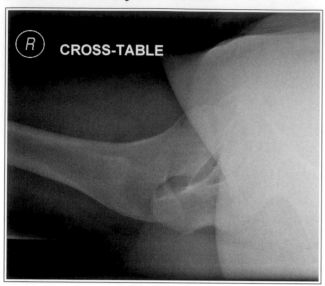

IMAGE 7-7

Analysis. Soft tissue from the unaffected thigh is superimposing the acetabulum and femoral head of the affected hip. The unaffected hip was not adequately flexed and abducted to draw superior to the acetabulum. The greater trochanter is demonstrated posteriorly, and the lesser trochanter is superimposed over the femoral shaft. The affected leg was in external rotation.

Correction. Flex and abduct the unaffected leg, drawing it away from the affected acetabulum and femoral head, and internally rotate the leg until the femoral epicondyles are aligned parallel with the IR and the foot is angled internally 15 to 20 degrees from vertical.

SACROILIAC (SI) JOINTS: AP AXIAL PROJECTION

See Table 7-8, (Figures 7-55 and 7-56).
Median Sacral Crest and Symphysis Pubis and Sacrum and Pelvic Brim Alignment. An AP axial projection of the sacroiliac joints is demonstrated when the patient's ASISs are placed at equal distances from the IR and are demonstrated when the median sacral crest is aligned with the symphysis pubis and the sacrum is at an equal distance from the lateral wall of the pelvic brim on both sides.

Detecting Sacroiliac Joint Rotation. Rotation is detected on an AP axial sacroiliac joint projection by evaluating the alignment of the long axis of the median sacral crest with the symphysis pubis and the distance from the sacrum to the lateral pelvic brim. When the patient is rotated away from the AP projection, the sacrum moves in a direction opposite from the movement of the symphysis pubis and is positioned next to the lateral pelvic brim situated farther from the IR. If the patient is rotated into an LPO position, the sacrum is rotated toward the patient's right pelvic brim. If the

TABLE 7-8	AP Axial Sacroiliac Joints Projection
Image Analysis Guidelines (Figure 7-55)	**Related Positioning Procedures (Figure 7-56)**
• Median sacral crest is aligned with the symphysis pubis. • Sacrum is at equal distance from the lateral wall of the pelvic brim on both sides.	• Place the patient in a supine AP projection with the knees extended. • Position the ASISs at equidistant from the IR, aligning the midcoronal plane parallel with IR.
• Sacroiliac joints are demonstrated without foreshortening. • Sacrum is elongated. • Symphysis pubis superimposes the inferior sacral segments.	• Place a 30-degree cephalic angle on the CR for a male patient and a 35-degree cephalic angle on the CR for a female patient.
• Long axis of the median sacral crest is aligned with the long axis of the collimated field.	• Position the midsagittal plane of the body to the midline of the IR.
• Second sacral segment is at the center of the exposure field.	• Center the CR to the patient's midsagittal plane at a level 1.5 inches (3 cm) superior to the symphysis pubis.
• Sacroiliac joints and the first through fourth sacral segments are included within the exposure field.	• Center the IR and grid to the CR. • Open the longitudinal collimation to include the symphysis pubis. • Transversely collimate to approximately a 9-inch (22-cm) field size.

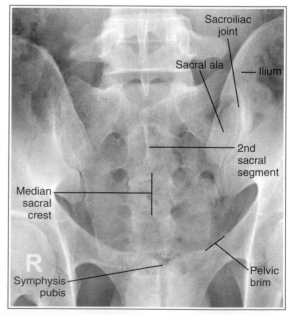

FIGURE 7-55 AP axial sacroiliac joint projection with accurate positioning.

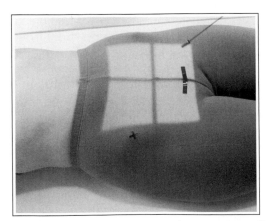

FIGURE 7-56 Proper patient positioning for AP axial sacroiliac joint projection.

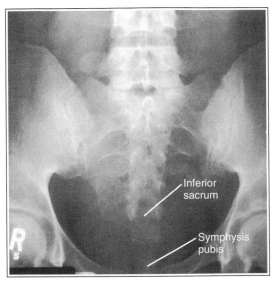

Inferior sacrum

Symphysis pubis

FIGURE 7-57 AP axial sacroiliac joint projection taken with insufficient cephalic angulation.

patient is rotated into an RPO position, the sacrum rotates toward the patient's left pelvic brim.

Visualizing the Sacroiliac Joints Without Distortion. When the patient is placed in a supine AP projection, with the legs extended, the lumbosacral curve causes the proximal sacrum and SI joints to be angled 30 to 35 degrees with the table and IR.

Adjusting CR Angulation for Patient Variations. To demonstrate the SI joints without foreshortening, a 30-degree cephalic angle should be used for male patients and a 35-degree cephalic angle for female patients. Patients with less or greater lumbosacral curvature will require a decrease or increase, respectively, in cephalic angulation to maintain the 30- to 35-degree alignment of the CR and SI joints.

Identifying Poor CR Angulation. If an AP axial SI joint projection is taken with a perpendicular CR or without enough cephalad angulation, the SI joints and the first through third sacral segments are foreshortened (Figure 7-57). If the AP axial SI joint projection is taken with too much cephalic angulation, the sacrum and SI joints demonstrate elongation and the symphysis pubis

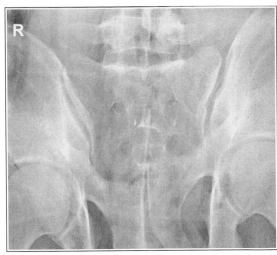

FIGURE 7-58 AP axial sacroiliac joint projection taken with excessive cephalic angulation.

is superimposed over the inferior aspects of the sacrum and SI joints (Figure 7-58).

Sacral Alignment and CR Centering. Aligning the long axis of the median sacral crest with the long axis of the exposure field allows for tight collimation and ensures that the CR is angled properly into the SI joints. To obtain proper alignment, find the point halfway between the patient's palpable ASISs and then align this point and the palpable symphysis pubis with the center of the collimator's longitudinal light line.

AP Axial SI Joint Analysis Practice

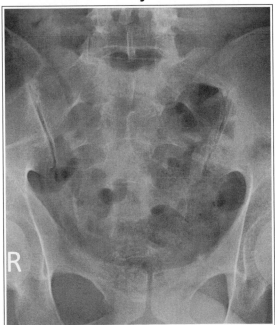

IMAGE 7-8

Analysis. The SI joints are foreshortened, and the inferior sacrum is demonstrated without symphysis pubis superimposition. The CR was inadequately angled.

Correction. Angle the CR 30 to 35 degrees cephalad.

SACROILIAC JOINTS: AP OBLIQUE PROJECTION LEFT AND RIGHT POSTERIOR OBLIQUE POSITIONS

See Table 7-9, (Figures 7-59 and 7-60).

Alternate Marking. Because the SI joint of interest is situated farther from the IR when AP oblique projections are taken, the marker used identifies the SI joint situated farther from the IR. This differs from the way most oblique projections are marked; routinely, the side marked is the one positioned closer to the IR, but is necessary to label the joint being imaged. It is important to position the marker as far laterally as possible to avoid the confusion that placing it medially may cause.

Ilium and Sacrum. When AP oblique SI projections are taken, the elevated sacroiliac joint is the joint of interest and its associated sacral ala and ilia are positioned in profile with accurate patient obliquity. The accuracy of an AP oblique SI joint is determined by evaluating the lack of ilium and sacral superimposition. The degree of separation or cavity demonstrated between the ilium and sacrum, which represents the SI joint, varies from patient to patient. The ilia and sacrum fit very snugly together and in older patients the joint spaces between them may be smaller or even nonexistent because of fibrous adhesions or synostosis. If the patient was not rotated enough to place the ilium and sacral ala in profile, the inferior and superior sacral aspects of the ala are demonstrated without ilium superimposition, whereas the lateral sacral ala is superimposed over the iliac tuberosity (Figure 7-61). The lateral sacrum is also demonstrated without ilium superimposition. If the patient was rotated more than needed to position the ilium and sacral ala in profile, the ilium is superimposed over the lateral sacral ala and the inferior sacrum (Figure 7-62).

TABLE 7-9	AP Oblique Sacroiliac Joints Guidelines	
Image Analysis Guidelines (Figure 7-59)	**Related Positioning Procedures (Figure 7-60)**
• A right or left marker identifying the sacroiliac joint positioned farther from the IR is present on the projection and is not superimposed over the anatomy of interest.	• Place marker to identify the sacroiliac joint situated farther from the IR, as it is the joint of interest. This differs from the routine marking guidelines.
• Ilium and sacrum are demonstrated without superimposition. • Sacroiliac joint is open.	• Start with the patient in a supine AP projection, with the knees extended. • Rotate the patient toward the unaffected side until the midcoronal plane is at a 25- to 30-degree angle with the table. • Place a radiolucent support beneath the elevated hip and thorax to help maintain the position.
• Long axis of the sacroiliac joint is aligned with the long axis of the collimated field.	• Align the long axis of the sacroiliac joint with the midline of the IR.
• Sacroiliac joint of interest is at the center of the exposure field.	• Center a perpendicular CR 1 inch (2.5 cm) medial to the elevated ASIS.
• Sacroiliac joint, sacral ala, and ilium are included within the exposure field.	• Center the IR and grid to the CR. • Longitudinally collimate to the elevated iliac crest. • Transversely collimate to the elevate ASIS.

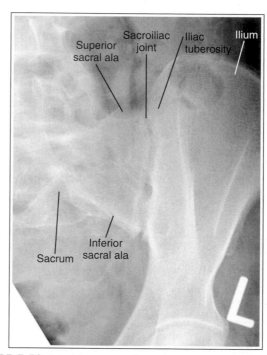

FIGURE 7-59 AP oblique sacroiliac joint projection with accurate positioning.

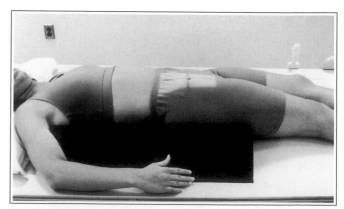

FIGURE 7-60 Proper patient positioning for AP oblique sacroiliac joint projection.

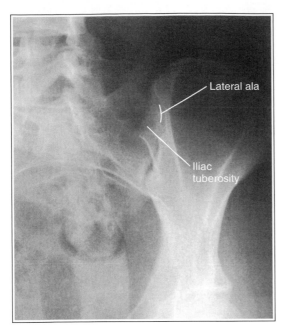

FIGURE 7-61 AP oblique sacroiliac joint taken with insufficient pelvic obliquity.

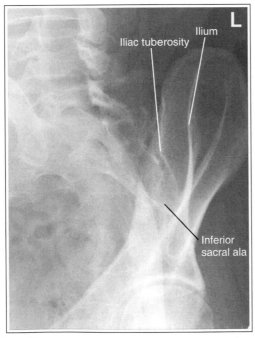

FIGURE 7-62 AP oblique sacroiliac joint taken with excessive pelvic obliquity.

AP Oblique SI Joint Analysis Practice

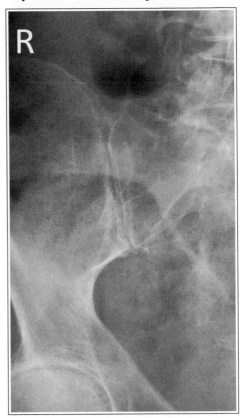

IMAGE 7-9

Analysis. The SI joint is closed. The superior and inferior sacral alae are demonstrated without iliac superimposition, and the lateral sacral ala is superimposed over the iliac tuberosity. The patient was insufficiently rotated. **Correction.** Increase the pelvic obliquity.

Cervical and Thoracic Vertebrae

OUTLINE

Cervical Vertebrae: AP Axial
 Projection, 391
  AP Cervical Vertebrae Analysis
  Practice, 396
Cervical Atlas and Axis: AP
 Projection (Open-Mouth
 Position), 396
  AP Cervical Atlas and Axis
  Analysis Practice, 400
Cervical Vertebrae: Lateral
 Projection, 400

Lateral Cervical Vertebrae
 Analysis Practice, 406
Cervical Vertebrae: PA or AP Axial
 Oblique Projection (Anterior and
 Posterior Oblique Positions), 406
  PA Axial Oblique Cervical
  Vertebrae Analysis
  Practice, 411
Cervicothoracic Vertebrae: Lateral
 Projection (Twining Method;
 Swimmer's Technique), 412

Lateral Cervicothoracic
 Vertebrae Analysis
 Practice, 414
Thoracic Vertebrae: AP
 Projection, 414
  AP Thoracic Vertebrae Analysis
  Practice, 418
Thoracic Vertebrae: Lateral
 Projection, 418
  Lateral Thoracic Vertebrae
  Analysis Practice, 422

OBJECTIVES

After completion of this chapter, you should be able to do the following:

- Identify the required anatomy on cervical and thoracic vertebral projections.
- Describe how to position the patient, image receptor (IR), and central ray (CR) properly for cervical and thoracic vertebral projections.
- List the image analysis guidelines for cervical and thoracic vertebral projections with accurate positioning.
- State how to reposition the patient properly when cervical and thoracic vertebral projections with poor positioning are produced.
- Discuss how to determine the amount of patient or CR adjustment required to improve cervical and thoracic vertebral projections with poor positioning.
- State the technical factors routinely used for cervical and thoracic vertebral projections, and describe which anatomic structures are demonstrated when the correct technique factors are used.
- Describe how the upper and lower cervical vertebrae can move simultaneously and independently.
- Explain how a patient with a suspected subluxation or fracture of the cervical vertebral column is positioned for cervical projections.
- Discuss the curvature of the cervical vertebrae, and explain how the intervertebral disk spaces slant.

- Describe why a 5-degree cephalic CR angulation is often required for an AP open-mouth projection of the atlas and axis.
- State how the relationship between the dens and atlas's lateral masses changes when the head is rotated.
- Describe how the prevertebral fat stripe is used as a diagnostic tool.
- Explain how the patient is positioned to demonstrate AP cervical mobility.
- Discuss the procedures that are taken if C7 is not demonstrated on a lateral cervical projection.
- Describe the positioning and analysis differences that exist between AP and PA oblique cervical projections.
- Discuss when it is necessary to achieve a lateral cervicothoracic projection of the cervical vertebrae.
- Describe the curvature of the thoracic vertebrae.
- List two methods used to obtain uniform image density on an AP thoracic vertebral projection.
- Discuss how scoliosis is differentiated from rotation on AP and lateral thoracic projections.
- Explain the breathing methods used to demonstrate the thoracic vertebrae on a lateral thoracic projection.
- Describe two methods that are used to offset the sagging of the lower thoracic column that results when the patient is in a lateral projection.

IMAGE ANALYSIS GUIDELINES

Technical Data. When the technical data in Table 8-1 are followed, or adjusted as needed for additive and destructive patient conditions (see Table 2-6), along with the best practices discussed in Chapters 1 and 2, all cervical and thoracic vertebral projections will demonstrate the image analysis guidelines in Box 8-1 unless otherwise indicated.

CERVICAL VERTEBRAE: AP AXIAL PROJECTION

See Table 8-2, (Figures 8-1 and 8-2).
Rotation. When the patient and cervical vertebrae are rotated away from the AP axial projection, the vertebral bodies move toward the side positioned closer to the IR,

and the spinous processes move toward the side positioned farther from the IR. The upper (C1-C4) and lower (C5-C7) cervical vertebrae can demonstrate rotation independently or simultaneously, depending on which part of the body is rotated. If the head is rotated but the thorax remains in an AP projection, the upper cervical vertebrae demonstrate rotation as C1 rotates on C2, and the lower cervical vertebrae remain in an AP projection. If the thorax is rotated but the head remains in a forward position, the lower cervical vertebrae demonstrate rotation and the upper cervical vertebrae remain in an AP projection (Figure 8-3). If the patient's head and thorax are rotated simultaneously, the entire cervical column demonstrates rotation.

Rotation is present on an AP axial projection in the following situations: (1) if the mandibular angles and mastoid tips are not demonstrated at equal distances from the cervical vertebrae; (2) if the spinous processes are not demonstrated in the midline of the cervical bodies; (3) if the pedicles and articular pillars are not symmetrically demonstrated lateral to the vertebral bodies; and (4) if the medial ends of the clavicles are not demonstrated at equal distances from the vertebral column. The side of the patient positioned closer to the IR and toward which the mandible is rotated is the side that the vertebral bodies are rotated toward and demonstrates fewer articular pillars and less clavicular and vertebral column superimposition.

CR and Intervertebral Disk Alignment. The cervical vertebral column demonstrates a lordotic curvature. This curvature and the shape of the vertebral bodies cause the disk-articulating surfaces of the vertebral bodies to slant upward anteriorly to posteriorly. To obtain open intervertebral disk spaces and undistorted vertebral bodies, the CR must be angled in the same direction as the slope

BOX 8-1	Cervical and Thoracic Vertebrae Imaging Analysis Guidelines

- The facility's identification requirements are visible.
- A right or left marker identifying the correct side of the patient is present on the projection and is not superimposed over the VOI.
- Good radiation protection practices are evident.
- Bony trabecular patterns and cortical outlines of the anatomical structures are sharply defined.
- Contrast resolution is adequate to demonstrate the surrounding soft tissue, air-filled trachea, bony trabecular patterns, and cortical outlines.
- No quantum mottle or saturation is present.
- Scatter radiation has been kept to a minimum.
- There is no evidence of removable artifacts.

TABLE 8-1	Cervical and Thoracic Vertebrae Technical Data					
Projection	**kV**	**Grid**	**AEC**	**mAs**	**SID**	
AP axial, cervical vertebrae	75-85	Grid	Center		40-48 inches (100-120 cm)	
AP, open-mouth, C1 and C2	75-85	Grid		5	40-48 inches (100-120 cm)	
Lateral, cervical vertebrae	75-85	Grid*	Center		72 inches (150-180 cm)	
PA or AP axial oblique, cervical vertebrae	75-85	Grid*	Center		72 inches (150-180 cm)	
Lateral (Twining method), cervicothoracic vertebrae	80-95	Grid	Center		40-48 inches (100-120 cm)	
AP, thoracic vertebrae	80-90	Grid	Center		40-48 inches (100-120 cm)	
Lateral, thoracic vertebrae	80-90	Grid	Center		40-48 inches (100-120 cm)	
Pediatric	65-75	Grid		2-3	40-48 inches (100-120 cm)	

*Optional because of air-gap.

TABLE 8-2	AP Axial Cervical Vertebrae Projection	
Image Analysis Guidelines (Figure 8-1)	**Related Positioning Procedures (Figure 8-2)**	
• Spinous processes are aligned with the midline of the cervical bodies. • Mandibular angles and mastoid tips are at equal distances from the cervical vertebrae. • Articular pillars and pedicles are symmetrically visualized lateral to the cervical bodies. • Distances from the vertebral column to the medial clavicular ends are equal.	• Position the patient in a supine or upright AP projection. • Place the shoulders at equal distances from the IR, aligning the midcoronal plane parallel with the IR. • Position the face forward, placing the mandibular angles and mastoid tips at equal distances from the IR.	
• Intervertebral disk spaces are open. • Vertebral bodies are demonstrated without distortion. • Each vertebra's spinous process is visualized at the level of its inferior intervertebral disk space.	• Erect position: Angle the CR 20-degree cephalad. • Supine position: Angle the CR 15-degree cephalad.	
• Third cervical vertebra is demonstrated in its entirety. • Occipital base and mandibular mentum are superimposed. • Long axis of the cervical column is aligned with the long axis of the exposure field.	• Align the lower surface of upper incisors and the tip of the mastoid process perpendicular to the IR. • Align the midline of the neck with the midline of the IR and grid.	
• Fourth cervical vertebra is at the center of the exposure field.	• Center the CR to the midsagittal plane at a level halfway between the external auditory meatus (EAM) and the jugular notch.	
• Second through seventh cervical vertebrae and the surrounding soft tissue are included within the exposure field.	• Center the IR and grid to the CR. • Open the longitudinal collimation to the EAM and the jugular notch. • Transversely collimate to within 0.5 inch (1.25 cm) of the lateral neck skin line.	

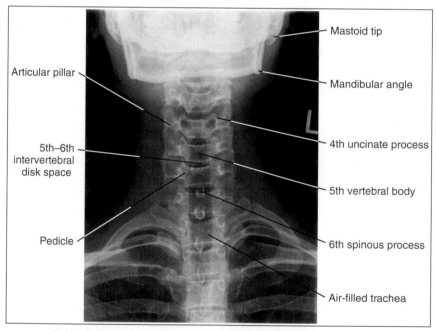

FIGURE 8-1 AP axial cervical projection with accurate positioning.

of the vertebral bodies. This can be easily discerned by viewing the lateral cervical projection in Figure 8-4. Studying this lateral cervical projection, you can see that when the correct CR angulation is used, each vertebra's spinous process is located within its inferior intervertebral disk space. The degree of CR angulation needed to obtain open intervertebral disk spaces and to align the spinous processes within them accurately depends on the degree of cervical lordotic curvature.

Upright versus Supine Position. If the AP axial projection is performed with the patient in an upright position, the cervical vertebrae demonstrate more lordotic curvature than if the examination is performed with the patient supine. In a supine position, the gravitational pull placed on the middle cervical vertebrae results in straightening of the cervical curvature. Figure 8-4 demonstrates a lateral cervical projection taken with the patient in an upright position and Figure 8-5

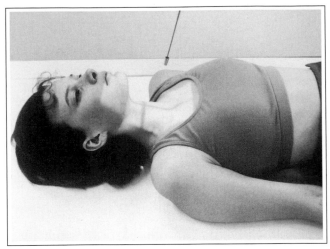

FIGURE 8-2 Proper patient positioning for AP axial cervical projection.

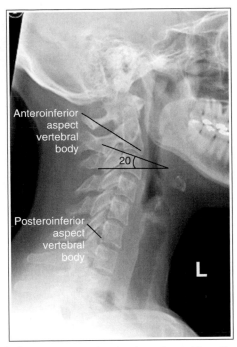

FIGURE 8-4 Lateral cervical projection taken with patient upright.

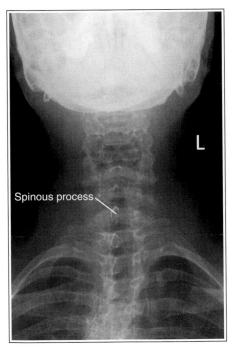

FIGURE 8-3 AP axial cervical projection taken with thorax rotated toward the patient's left side.

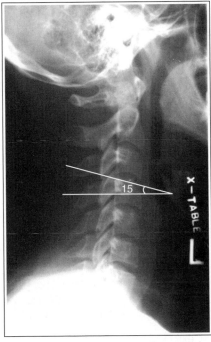

FIGURE 8-5 Lateral cervical projection taken with patient supine.

demonstrates a lateral cervical projection taken with the patient supine. Note the difference in lordotic curvature between these two projections. Because of this difference, the CR angulation is varied when an AP axial projection is taken with the patient erect rather than supine. In the erect position, a 20-degree cephalad CR angulation is needed to align the CR parallel with the intervertebral disk spaces, and in the supine position, a 15-degree cephalad CR angulation sufficiently aligns the CR parallel with the intervertebral disk spaces.

Kyphotic Patient. The kyphotic patient demonstrates an exaggerated kyphotic curvature of the thoracic vertebrae that will cause excessive lordotic curvature of the cervical vertebrae. To demonstrate the cervical

vertebrae with open intervertebral spaces for an upright AP axial projection, it will be necessary to adjust the degree of CR angulation above that routinely needed for a patient without kyphosis, depending on the severity of the condition. Figure 8-6 demonstrates a kyphotic patient requiring a 30-degree CR angulation to demonstrate open intervertebral disk spaces. If the AP axial projection is taken with the kyphotic patient in a supine position, a radiolucent sponge should be placed beneath the

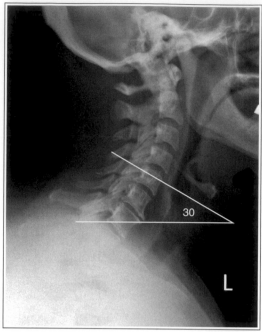

FIGURE 8-6 Lateral cervical projection taken on a kyphotic patient.

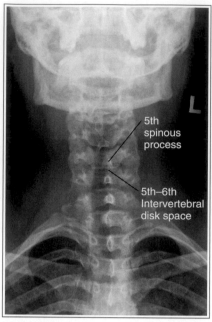

FIGURE 8-8 AP axial cervical projection taken with insufficient cephalic CR angulation.

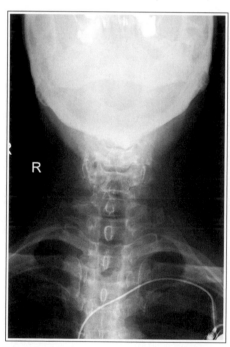

FIGURE 8-7 AP axial cervical projection taken of a kyphotic patient.

patient's head to prevent the upper cervical vertebrae from extending toward the table and from superimposing the occipital base on the projection (Figure 8-7).

Effect of CR Misalignment. Misalignment of the CR and intervertebral disk spaces results in closed disk spaces, distorted vertebral bodies, and projection of the spinous processes into the vertebral bodies. If a cephalic CR angulation is not used or is insufficiently angled, the resulting projection demonstrates closed intervertebral

disk spaces, and each vertebra's spinous process is demonstrated within its vertebral body (see Figures 8-3 and 8-8). This anatomic relationship also results if the patient's head and upper cervical vertebrae are tilted (anteriorly) toward the x-ray tube for the examination. If the CR is angled more than needed to align the CR parallel with the intervertebral disk spaces, or if the patient's cervical vertebral column was extended posteriorly for the examination as with a kyphotic patient, the resulting projection demonstrates closed intervertebral disk spaces, with each vertebra's spinous process demonstrated within the inferior adjoining vertebral body, and elongated uncinate processes (see Figures 8-7 and 8-9).

Occipital Base and Mandibular Mentum Positioning. Accurate positioning of the occiput and mandibular mentum is achieved when the lower surface of the upper incisors and the tip of the mastoid process is aligned perpendicular to the IR (see Figure 8-2). With this position, you might expect the mandible to be superimposed over the upper cervical vertebrae, but this will not be the case because the cephalad CR angulation used will project the mandible superiorly.

Effect of Occiput-Mentum Mispositioning. Mispositioning of the occiput and mentum results in a projection demonstrating an obstructed upper cervical vertebrae. If the mandibular mentum is positioned superior to the occipital base (head tilted too far backward), the upper cervical vertebrae are superimposed over the occiput (Figure 8-10). If the mandibular mentum is positioned inferior to the occipital base (chin tucked too far downward), it is superimposed over the superior cervical vertebrae (Figure 8-11).

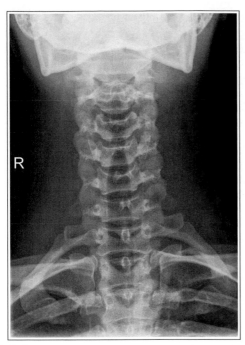

FIGURE 8-9 AP axial cervical projection taken with excessive cephalic CR angulation.

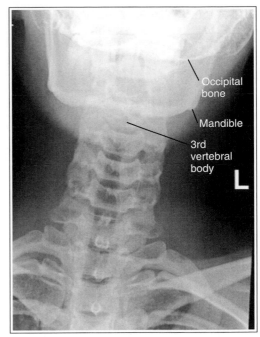

FIGURE 8-11 AP axial cervical projection taken with the chin tucked too far downward to align the upper incisors and mastoid tip perpendicular to the IR, and without the vertebral column aligned with the long axis of the IR.

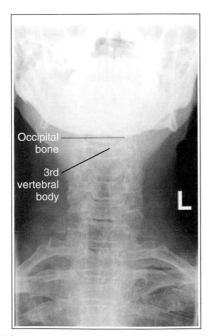

FIGURE 8-10 AP axial cervical projection taken with the head tilted too far backward to align the upper incisors and mastoid tip perpendicular to the IR.

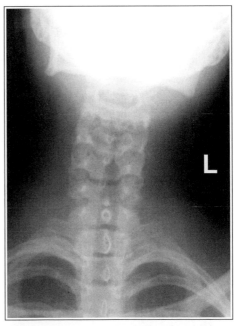

FIGURE 8-12 AP axial cervical projection taken with lateral flexion of the cervical column.

Cervical Column and Exposure Field Alignment.
Aligning the long axis of the cervical column with the long axis of the collimated field ensures that no lateral flexion of the cervical column is present (Figure 8-12) and allows for tight collimation (see Figure 8-11).

Trauma. When cervical vertebral projections are exposed on a trauma patient with suspected subluxation or fracture, obtain the AP axial projection with the patient positioned as is. Do not attempt to remove the cervical collar or adjust the head or body rotation, mandible position, or cervical column tilting. Such movement may result in greater injury to the vertebrae or spinal cord. Spinal cord injuries may occur from mishandling the patient after the initial injury has taken place.

AP Cervical Vertebrae Analysis Practice

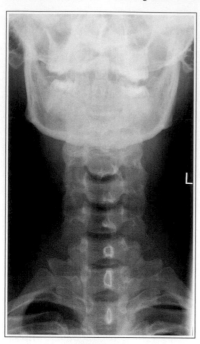

IMAGE 8-1

Analysis. The anteroinferior aspects of the cervical bodies are obscuring the intervertebral disk spaces, and each vertebra's spinous process is demonstrated within its vertebral body. The CR angulation was insufficient to align it parallel with the intervertebral disk spaces. The mandible is superimposing the third cervical vertebrae. The chin was tucked too far downward.
Correction. Increase the degree of CR angulation and elevate the chin until the lower surface of the upper incisors and the mastoid tip is aligned perpendicular with the IR.

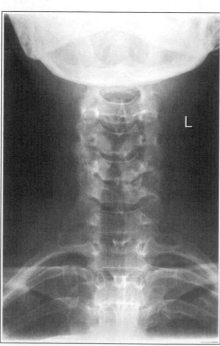

IMAGE 8-2

Analysis. The posteroinferior aspects of the cervical bodies are obscuring the intervertebral disk spaces, the uncinate processes are elongated, and each vertebra's spinous process is demonstrated within the inferior adjoining vertebral body. The CR was angled too cephalically.
Correction. Decrease the degree of cephalic CR angulation.

CERVICAL ATLAS AND AXIS: AP PROJECTION (OPEN-MOUTH POSITION)

See Table 8-3, (Figures 8-13 and 8-14).
Rotation. Rotation of the atlas and axis occurs when the head is turned away from an AP projection. On head rotation, the atlas pivots around the dens so that the lateral mass located on the side from which the face is turned is displaced anteriorly and the mass located on the side toward which the face is turned is displaced

TABLE 8-3	AP Cervical Atlas and Axis Projection
Image Analysis Guidelines (Figure 8-13)	**Related Positioning Procedures (Figure 8-14)**
• Atlas is symmetrically seated on the axis, with the atlas's lateral masses at equal distances from the dens. • Spinous process of the axis is aligned with the midline of the axis's body. • Mandibular rami are visualized at equal distances from the lateral masses.	• Position the patient in a supine or upright AP projection. • Place the shoulders at equal distances from the IR, aligning the midcoronal plane parallel with the IR. • Place the face forward, aligning the mandibular angles and mastoid tips at equal distances from the IR.
• Upper incisors and occipital base are seen superior to the dens and the atlantoaxial joint. • Atlantoaxial joint is open.	• Instruct the patient to open the mouth as widely as possible. • Tuck the chin until a line connecting the lower edge of the upper incisors and tip of the mastoid process is aligned perpendicular to the IR. • Angle the CR 5 degrees cephalically.
• Dens is at the center of the exposure field.	• Center the CR to the midsagittal plane and midpoint of the open mouth.
• Atlantoaxial and occipitoatlantal joints, the atlas's lateral masses and transverse processes, and the axis's dens and body are included within the exposure field.	• Center the IR and grid to the CR. • Open the longitudinal collimation to the EAM. • Transversely collimate to a 5-inch (12.5-cm) field size.

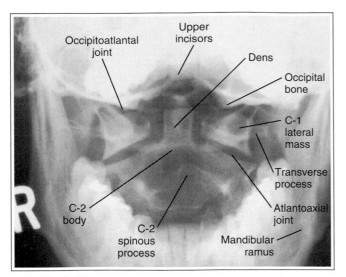

FIGURE 8-13 AP atlas and axis projection with accurate positioning.

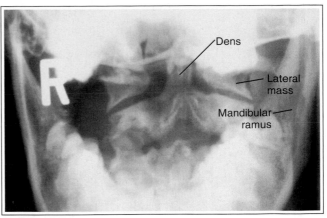

FIGURE 8-15 AP atlas and axis projection taken with the face rotated toward the patient's right side.

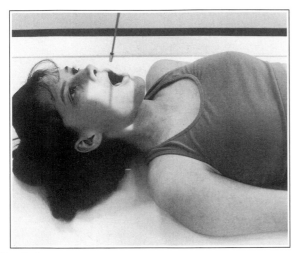

FIGURE 8-14 Proper patient positioning for AP atlas and axis projection.

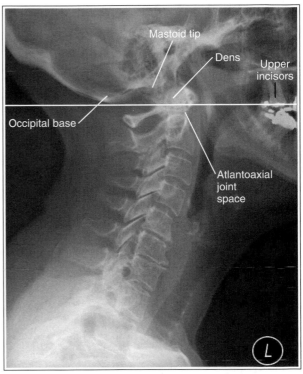

FIGURE 8-16 Lateral cervical projection demonstrating upper incisor, dens, atlantoaxial joint space, and posterior occiput relationship.

posteriorly. This displacement causes the space between the lateral mass and dens to narrow on the side from which the face is turned and to enlarge on the side toward which the face is turned (Figure 8-15). As the amount of head rotation increases, the axis rotates in the same direction as the atlas, resulting in a shift in the position of its spinous process in the direction opposite that in which the patient's face is turned.

Detecting Direction of Rotation. To determine how the patient's face was turned, judge the distance between the mandibular rami and lateral masses. The side that demonstrates the greater distance is the side toward which the face was rotated.

Upper Incisor, Occipital Base, and CR Positioning. The dens and the atlantoaxial joint are located at the midsagittal plane, at a level 0.5 inch (1.25 cm) inferior to an imaginary line connecting the mastoid tips. The goal of the AP open-mouth projection is to demonstrate the dens and atlantoaxial joint without occiput or

without upper incisor (top teeth) superimposition. To accomplish this goal the patient's chin is tucked until an imaginary line connecting the lower surface of the upper incisors and the tip of the mastoid process is aligned perpendicular to the IR and the patient's mouth is open as widely as possible. It may be necessary to position a small angled sponge beneath the head to maintain accurate head positioning, especially if the chin has to be tucked so much that it is difficult to open the mouth adequately. The sponge causes the upper incisors and mastoid tip to align perpendicularly without requiring as much chin-tucking. The lateral cervical projection in Figure 8-16 demonstrates how the upper incisors and occipital base are aligned when the incisors and mastoid

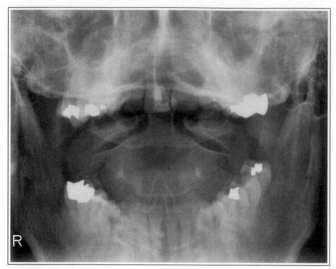

FIGURE 8-17 AP atlas and axis projection taken with the upper incisors and mastoid tip aligned perpendicular to the IR and the CR angled 5 degrees cephalically.

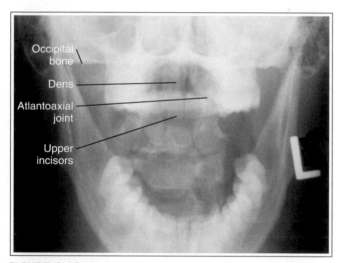

FIGURE 8-18 AP atlas and axis projection taken with the upper incisors and mastoid tip aligned perpendicular to the IR and a perpendicular CR.

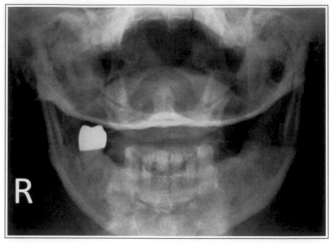

FIGURE 8-19 AP atlas and axis projection taken with the head tilted too far backward to align the upper incisors and mastoid tip perpendicular to the IR.

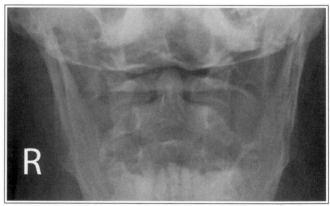

FIGURE 8-20 AP atlas and axis projection taken with the CR angled too cephalically.

tip are aligned perpendicular to the IR. By studying this projection, you might conclude that this positioning, with a perpendicular CR, would demonstrate the atlantoaxial joint space free of upper incisor and occiput superimposition, but the tip of the dens would be obscured, as shown in Figure 8-17. However, because the upper incisors are positioned at a long object–image receptor distance (OID), their magnification must be considered. In most patients, when the upper incisors and mastoid tip are aligned perpendicularly, magnification will cause the upper incisors to be demonstrated as much as 1 inch (2.5 cm) inferior to the occipital base (Figure 8-18). For these magnified incisors to be projected superior to the dens, a 5-degree cephalic angle may be placed on the CR. If, instead of adjusting the CR angulation, the chin were tilted upward in an attempt to shift the upper incisors superiorly, the occipital base

would simultaneously be shifted inferiorly, causing the dens and atlantoaxial joint to superimpose it (Figure 8-19). If the occiput is positioned accurately superior to the dens, but the atlantoaxial joint is closed and the upper incisors are positioned too superiorly, the cervical spine was extended as shown in Figure 8-21 or the CR was angled too cephalically. This positioning will also demonstrate the spinous process of the axis at the level of the third vertebral body (Figure 8-20).

Positioning for Trauma. For the dens and atlantoaxial joint to be demonstrated without incisor or occiput superimposition when imaging a trauma patient, the direction of the CR must be changed from the standard position. A trauma patient's head and neck cannot be adjusted until the initial projections have been cleared by the radiologist, because of the potential of this movement to cause increased injury, and the cervical collar worn by these patients tilts the chin upward. In this position, the line connecting the incisors and mastoid tip is at about a 10-degree caudal angulation and the upper incisors are at an angle with the CR that will result in

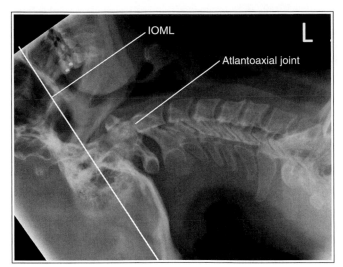

FIGURE 8-21 Lateral cervical projection to visualize IOML, dens, and atlantoaxial joint alignment for trauma AP atlas and axis projection.

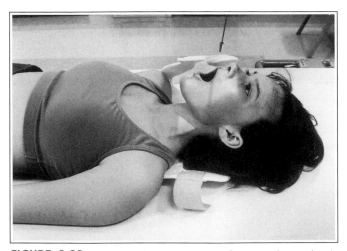

FIGURE 8-22 Proper patient positioning for AP atlas and axis projection taken to evaluate trauma.

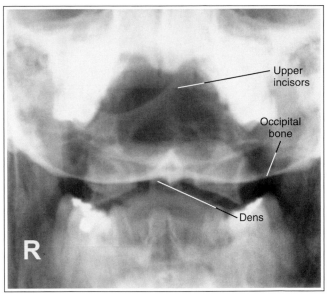

FIGURE 8-23 AP atlas and axis projection taken with insufficient caudal CR angulation.

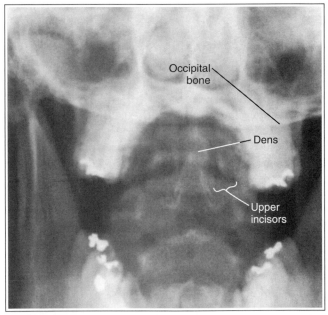

FIGURE 8-24 AP atlas and axis projection taken with excessive caudal CR angulation.

less magnification of them, because of foreshortening, on the resulting projection. Because of this upper chin tilting, the occipital base is positioned directly beneath the dens and atlantoaxial joint space and they will superimpose it if the CR is not angled caudally to project them inferiorly (Figure 8-21). The infraorbitomeatal line (line connecting the inferior orbital rim and the external ear opening; IOML) is easy to access in a patient wearing a cervical collar and when the CR is aligned it can be used to determine the needed angulation. Once the CR is aligned with the IOML, attempt to get the patient to drop the lower jaw. Do not adjust head rotation or tilting. If the cervical collar allows the lower jaw to move without elevating the upper jaw, instruct the patient to drop the lower jaw. If the cervical collar prevents lower jaw movement without elevating the upper jaw, instruct the patient about the importance of holding the head and neck perfectly still; then have the ordering physician remove the front of the cervical collar so that the patient

can drop the jaw without adjusting the head or neck position (Figure 8-22). After the jaw is dropped, align the CR to the midsagittal plane at a level 0.5 inch (1.25 cm) inferior to the lower surface of the upper incisors. Immediately after the projection is taken, the physician should return the front of the cervical collar to its proper position. For trauma positioning, insufficient caudal angulation causes the upper incisors to be demonstrated superior to the dens and the dens to be superimposed over the occipital base (Figure 8-23). If the CR was angled too caudally, the occipital base is demonstrated superior to the dens and the upper incisors are superimposed over the dens (Figure 8-24).

AP Cervical Atlas and Axis Analysis Practice

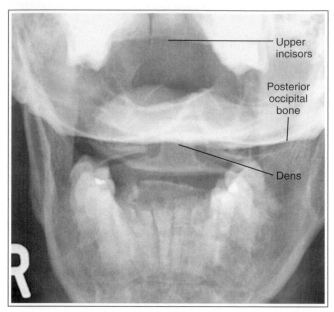

IMAGE 8-3

Analysis. The dens is superimposed over the occipital base and the upper incisors are demonstrated superior to the occipital base. The chin was elevated. The distances from the atlas's lateral masses to the dens and from the mandibular rami to the dens are narrower on the left side than on the right side. The face was rotated toward the right side.

Correction. Lower the upper incisors until the lower edge of the upper incisors and mastoid tip is aligned perpendicular with the IR and rotate the face toward the left side until it is forward.

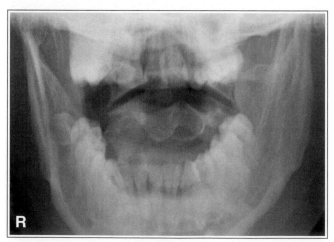

IMAGE 8-4

Analysis. The distances from the atlas's lateral masses to the dens and from the mandibular rami to the dens are narrower on the left side than on the right side. The face was rotated toward the right side. The upper incisors are demonstrated inferior to the occipital base, obscuring the dens and atlantoaxial joint space. The CR was not angled 5 degrees cephalically.

Correction. Rotate the face toward the left side until it is forward and angle the CR 5 degrees cephalically.

CERVICAL VERTEBRAE: LATERAL PROJECTION

See Table 8-4, (Figures 8-25 and 8-26).

Prevertebral Fat Stripe Visualization. The soft tissue structure of interest on a lateral cervical projection is the prevertebral fat stripe. It is located anterior to the cervical vertebrae and is visible on correctly exposed lateral cervical projections with accurate positioning (Figure 8-27). The reviewer evaluates the distance between the anterior surface of the cervical vertebrae and the prevertebral fat stripe. Abnormal widening of this space is used for the detection and localization of fractures, masses, and inflammation.

Rotation. Rotation can be detected on a lateral cervical projection by evaluating each vertebra for anterior and posterior pillar superimposition and for zygapophyseal joint superimposition. When the patient is rotated, the pillars and zygapophyseal joints on one side of the vertebra move anterior to those on the other side (Figures 8-28 and 8-29). Because the two sides of the vertebrae are mirror images, it is very difficult to determine from a rotated lateral cervical projection which side of the patient is rotated anteriorly and which is rotated posteriorly. The magnification of the side situated farther from the IR may provide a moderately reliable clue at the articular pillar regions.

Head Positioning. Accurate positioning of the head accomplishes four goals: (1) alignment of the cervical vertebral column parallel with the IR; (2) demonstration of C1 and C2 without occiput or mandibular superimposition; (3) superimposition of the anterior, posterior, superior, and inferior aspects of the cranial and mandibular cortices, and (4) superimposition of the superior and inferior aspects of the right and left articular pillars and zygapophyseal joints.

Effect of Mandibular Rotation and Elevation on C1 and C2 Visualization. The position of the mandible and demonstration of C1 and C2 on a lateral projection are affected by head positioning. The posterior cortices of the mandibular rami are superimposed when the head's midsagittal plane was aligned parallel with the IR. If the posterior cortices of the mandibular rami are not superimposed on a lateral projection, one mandibular ramus is situated anteriorly to the other (Figures 8-30 and 8-31). If the chin was elevated adequately to place the acanthiomeatal line (AML; line connecting acanthion and external auditory meatus [EAM]) parallel with the floor, the mandibular rami are demonstrated anterior to the vertebral column. If the chin was not

TABLE 8-4 | Lateral Cervical Vertebrae Projection

Image Analysis Guidelines (Figure 8-25)	Related Positioning Procedures (Figure 8-26)
• Contrast resolution is adequate to visualize the prevertebral fat stripe.	• Use the appropriate technical factors.
• Anterior and posterior aspects of the right and left articular pillars and the right and left zygapophyseal joints of each cervical vertebra are superimposed. • Spinous processes are in profile.	• Place the patient in an upright lateral position, with the midsagittal plane aligned parallel with the IR. • Position the shoulders, the mastoid tips, and the mandibular rami directly on top of each other, aligning the midcoronal plane perpendicular to the IR.
• Posterior arch of C1 and spinous process of C2 are in profile without occipital base superimposition. • The bodies of C1 and C2 are seen without mandibular superimposition, and the cranial cortices and the mandibular rami are superimposed. • Superior and inferior aspects of the right and left articular pillars and zygapophyseal joints of each cervical vertebra are superimposed. • Intervertebral disk spaces are open.	• Place the head in a lateral position. • Elevate the chin, positioning the AML parallel with the floor. • Align the IPL perpendicular to the IR. • Position the shoulders on the same horizontal plane.
• Long axis of the cervical vertebral column is aligned with the long axis of the exposure field. • Fourth cervical vertebra is at the center of the exposure field.	• Align the long axis of the cervical vertebral column with the long axis of the IR. • Center the CR to the midcoronal plane at a level halfway between the EAM and the jugular notch.
• Sella turcica, clivus, first through seventh cervical vertebrae, and superior half of the first thoracic vertebra and the surrounding soft tissue are included within the exposure field.	• Center the IR and grid when used to the CR. • Open the longitudinal and transverse collimation fields enough to include the clivus and sella turcica, which are at the level 0.75 inch (2 cm) anterosuperior to the EAM.

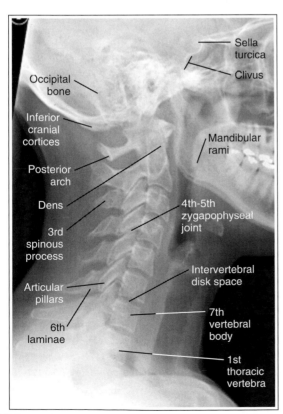

FIGURE 8-25 Lateral cervical projection with accurate positioning.

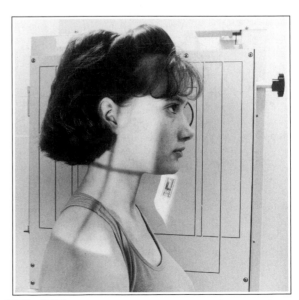

FIGURE 8-26 Proper patient positioning for lateral cervical projection.

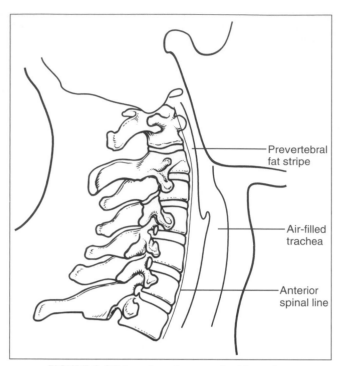

FIGURE 8-27 Location of prevertebral fat stripe.

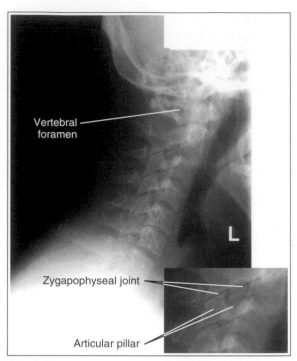

FIGURE 8-29 Lateral cervical projection taken with the patient rotated.

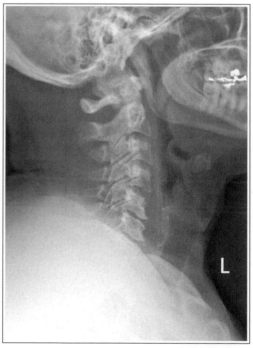

FIGURE 8-28 Lateral cervical projection taken with the patient's right side rotated slightly posteriorly.

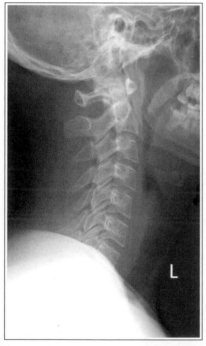

FIGURE 8-30 Lateral cervical projection taken without the chin elevated enough to place the acanthiomeatal line parallel with the floor and the shoulders not positioned on the same horizontal plane.

adequately elevated, one or both of the mandibular rami are superimposed over the bodies of C1 and/or C2 (see Figure 8-30).

Detecting Lateral Head and Shoulder Tilting That Causes Lateral Cervical Flexion. If the patient's head is tilted toward or away from the IR enough to flex the upper cervical column laterally, or the shoulders are not placed on the same plane but are tilted enough to flex the lower cervical column laterally, the lateral projection will demonstrate a superoinferior separation between the right and left articular pillars and zygapophyseal joints of the flexed vertebrae (Figures 8-30, 8-31, and 8-32).

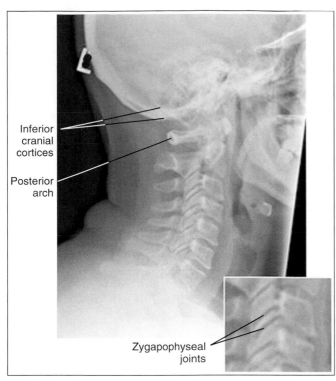

FIGURE 8-31 Lateral cervical projection taken with the head and upper cervical vertebral column tilted away from the IR and without the chin elevated enough to place the AML parallel with the floor.

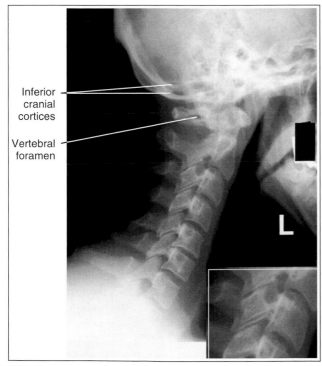

FIGURE 8-32 Lateral cervical projection taken with the head and upper cervical vertebral column tilted toward the IR.

Head-tilting will also result in a superoinferior separation between the cranial cortices and between the mandibular rami; this can be avoided by positioning the interpupillary line (IPL; line connecting the outer corners of the eyelids) parallel with the floor and the shoulders on the same horizontal plane. If the head and upper cervical vertebral column were tilted away from the IR, there is a separation between the right and left articular pillars and zygapophyseal joints of the upper cervical vertebrae, the inferior cortices of the cranium and the mandibular rami are demonstrated without superimposition, and the posterior arch of C1 remains in profile (see Figure 8-31). If the head was tilted toward the IR, there is a separation between the right and left articular pillars and zygapophyseal joints of the upper cervical vertebrae, the inferior cortices of the cranium and the mandibular rami are demonstrated without superimposition, and the vertebral foramen of C1 is demonstrated (see Figure 8-32). When the shoulders are not positioned on the same horizontal plane, there is a separation between the right and left articular pillars and zygapophyseal joints of the lower cervical vertebrae (see Figure 8-30). It is not possible to determine whether the right or left shoulder was positioned lower when such a projection has been obtained, but it is most common for the shoulder positioned adjacent to the IR to be the lower one as the patient leans toward the IR.

Cervical Column and Exposure Field Alignment. Aligning the long axis of the cervical vertebral column with the long axis of the exposure field ensures against AP flexion or extension of the cervical column and allows for tight collimation. This alignment is obtained by positioning the neck vertically in a neutral position and aligning the midline of the neck with the collimator's longitudinal light line; it places the cervical column in a neutral position.

Lateral Flexion and Extension Projections to Evaluate AP Cervical Vertebral Mobility. Flexion and extension lateral projections are obtained to evaluate AP vertebral mobility. For hyperflexion, instruct the patient to tuck the chin into the chest as far as possible (Figure 8-33). For patients who demonstrate extreme degrees of flexion, it may be necessary to place the IR crosswise to include the entire cervical column on the same projection. Such a projection should meet all the analysis requirements listed for a neutral lateral projection, except that the long axis demonstrates forward bending (Figure 8-34). For hyperextension, instruct the patient to extend the chin up and backward as far as possible (Figure 8-35). Such a projection should meet all the analysis requirements listed for a neutral lateral projection, except that the long axis demonstrates backward bending (Figure 8-36). If the lateral projection is used with the patient in flexion or extension, an arrow pointing in the direction the neck is moving or a flexion or extension marker should be included to indicate the direction of neck movement.

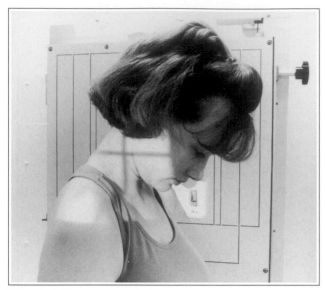

FIGURE 8-33 Patient positioning for lateral cervical projection with hyperflexion.

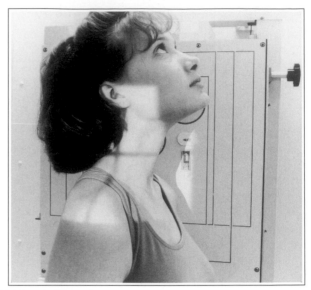

FIGURE 8-35 Patient positioning for lateral cervical projection with hyperextension.

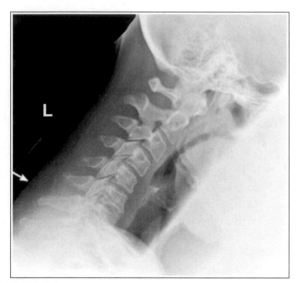

FIGURE 8-34 Lateral cervical projection taken with the patient in hyperflexion.

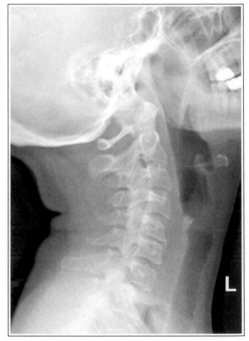

FIGURE 8-36 Lateral cervical projection taken with the patient in hyperextension.

Importance of Including the Clivus. The clivus, a slanted structure that extends posteriorly off the sella turcica, and the dens, are used to determine cervical injury. A line drawn along the clivus should point to the tip of the dens on the normal upper lateral cervical vertebral projection.

Demonstration of C7 and T1 Vertebrae. The seventh cervical vertebra and first thoracic vertebra are located at the level of the shoulders. This location makes it difficult to demonstrate them because of the great difference in lateral thickness between the neck and the shoulders. The best method to demonstrate C7 is to have the patient hold 5- or 10-lb weights on each arm to depress the shoulders and attempt to move them inferior to C7. Weights are best placed on each arm rather than in each hand, because sometimes the shoulders will elevate when weights are placed in the hands. Without weights, it is often difficult to demonstrate more than six cervical vertebrae (Figures 8-28 and 8-37). Taking the projection on expiration also aids in lowering the shoulders.

In Trauma or Recumbency. For trauma or recumbent patients who do not have upper extremity or

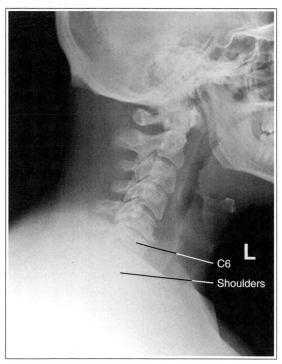

FIGURE 8-37 Lateral cervical projection taken without adequate shoulder depression.

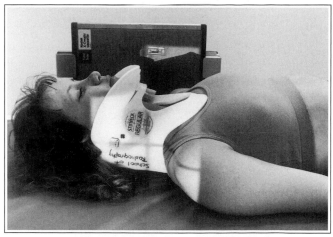

FIGURE 8-38 Proper patient positioning for lateral cervical projection taken to evaluate trauma.

requirements listed for a nontrauma lateral projection as possible without moving the patient.

Lateral Cervical Vertebrae Analysis Practice

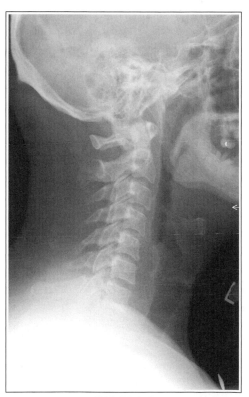

IMAGE 8-5

shoulder injuries, depress the shoulders by having a qualified assistant, with the consent of a physician, pull down on the patient's arms while the projection is taken. To accomplish this, instruct an assistant to wear a protection apron and stand at the end of the imaging table or stretcher, with the patient's feet resting against the assistant's abdomen and the assistant's hands wrapped around the patient's wrists. The assistant should slowly pull on the patient's arms until the shoulders are moved inferiorly as much as possible.

Lateral Cervicothoracic Projection (Twining Method). If even after using weights to depress the shoulders C7 cannot be demonstrated in its entirety, a special projection known as the lateral cervicothoracic projection (Twining method) should be taken and is described later in this chapter.

Trauma. When cervical vertebral projections are taken of a trauma patient with suspected subluxation or fracture, take the lateral projection with the patient's position left as is. Do not attempt to remove the cervical collar or adjust head or body rotation, mandible position, or vertebral tilting. This might result in increased injury to the vertebrae or spinal cord. A trauma lateral cervical vertebral projection is obtained by placing a lengthwise IR against the patient's shoulder and directing a horizontal beam to the cervical vertebrae (Figure 8-38). Such a projection should meet as many of the analysis

Analysis. The articular pillars and zygapophyseal joints on one side of the patient are situated anterior to those on the other side. The patient was rotated.

Correction. Rotate the patient until the midcoronal plane is aligned perpendicular to the IR.

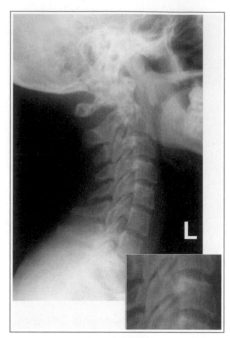

IMAGE 8-6

Analysis. The articular pillars and zygapophyseal joints on one side of the patient are situated anterior to those on the other side. The patient was rotated. The cranial and mandibular cortices are accurately aligned, and the mandibular rami are superimposed over the body of C2. The patient's chin was not adequately elevated.

Correction. Rotate the patient until the midcoronal plane is aligned perpendicular to the IR and elevate the chin until the AML is aligned parallel with the floor.

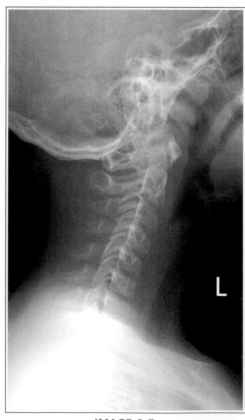

IMAGE 8-7

Analysis. The inferior cortices of the cranium and mandible are demonstrated without superimposition, the vertebral foramen of C1 is visualized, and the right and left articular pillars and zygapophyseal joints demonstrate a superoinferior separation. The patient's head and upper cervical vertebrae were tilted toward the IR.

Correction. Tilt the head away from the IR until the IPL is aligned perpendicular to the IR.

CERVICAL VERTEBRAE: PA OR AP AXIAL OBLIQUE PROJECTION (ANTERIOR AND POSTERIOR OBLIQUE POSITIONS)

See Table 8-5, (Figures 8-39, 8-40, 8-41, and 8-42).

Midcoronal Plane Rotation. When PA axial oblique projections (see Figure 8-41) are obtained with adequate midcoronal plane obliquity, the foramina and pedicles situated closer to the IR are demonstrated, whereas AP axial oblique projections (see Figure 8-42) demonstrate the foramina and pedicles situated farther from the IR.

Effect of Incorrect Rotation. If the cervical vertebral rotation is less than 45 degrees, the intervertebral foramina are narrowed or obscured and the pedicles of interest are foreshortened (Figure 8-43). If the cervical vertebrae are rotated more than 45 degrees, the pedicles of interest are partially foreshortened and the opposite pedicles are aligned with the midline of the vertebral bodies, and the zygapophyseal joints that are demonstrated without vertebral body superimposition are demonstrated in profile (Figure 8-44). Because it is possible for the upper and lower cervical vertebrae to be rotated to different degrees on the same projection, one needs to evaluate the entire cervical vertebrae for proper rotation (Figure 8-45).

CR and Intervertebral Disk Space Alignment. The cervical vertebral column demonstrates a lordotic curvature. This curvature, along with the shape of the cervical bodies, causes the disk-articulating surfaces of the vertebral bodies to slant downward posteriorly to anteriorly. To obtain open intervertebral disk spaces, undistorted and uniformly shaped vertebral bodies, the upper vertebral column must be aligned parallel with the IR, and the CR angled in the same direction as the slope of the vertebral bodies. This is accomplished by angling the CR 15 to 20 degrees caudally for PA axial oblique projections and 15 to 20 degrees cephalically for AP axial oblique projections. The larger degree is used on patients with higher degrees of lordotic cervical curvature.

Identifying Inaccurate Vertebral Column Alignment with the IR and CR Angulation. If the cervical vertebral column is tilted or if the CR is inaccurately angled with the intervertebral disk spaces, the disk spaces will be obscured and the cervical bodies are not seen as distinct individual structures. The upper and lower cervical vertebrae should be evaluated separately when a poorly positioned axial oblique projection has been obtained, as cervical vertebral column tilting of the upper cervical

TABLE 8-5	PA and AP Axial Oblique Cervical Vertebrae Projection
Image Analysis Guidelines (Figures 8-39 and 8-40)	**Related Positioning Procedures (Figures 8-41 and 8-42)**
• Second through seventh intervertebral foramina are open, demonstrating uniform size and shape. • LPO and RAO: Right pedicles are shown in profile and left pedicles are aligned with the anterior vertebral bodies. • RPO and LAO: left pedicles are shown in profile and right pedicles are aligned with the anterior vertebral bodies.	• Begin with the patient in a recumbent or upright PA or AP projection. • Rotate the patient until the midcoronal plane is at a 45-degree angle to the IR. • To demonstrate the foramina and pedicles on both sides of the cervical vertebrae, right and left oblique projections are taken.
• Inferior outline of the outer cranial cortices demonstrate about 0.25 inch (0.6 cm) between them. • Inferior mandibular rami demonstrate about 0.5 inch (1.25 cm) between them. • Posterior arch of the atlas and vertebral foramen are seen. • Intervertebral disk spaces are open. • Cervical bodies are seen as individual structures and are uniform in shape.	• Position the IPL parallel with the floor. • Align the cervical vertebral column parallel with the IR. • PA axial oblique projection: Angle the CR 15 to 20 degrees caudally. • AP axial oblique projection: Angle the CR 15 to 20 degrees cephalically.
• Oblique head: The upper cervical vertebrae are seen with occipital and mandibular superimposition. • Lateral head: The upper cervical vertebrae are seen without occipital or mandibular superimposition, and the right and left posterior cortices of the cranium and the mandible are aligned.	• Oblique head: Rotate the head 45 degrees with the body. • Lateral head: Turn the face away from the side of interest until the head's midsagittal plane is aligned parallel with the IR. • Elevate the chin until the AML is aligned parallel with the floor.
• Fourth cervical vertebra is at the center of the exposure field.	• Center the CR to the midsagittal plane, halfway between the EAM and jugular notch.
• First through seventh cervical vertebrae, the first thoracic vertebra, and the surrounding soft tissue are included within the exposure field.	• Center the IR and grid when used to the CR. • Open the longitudinally collimated field to the EAM and jugular notch and transversely collimate to within 0.5 inch (1.25 cm) of the skin line.

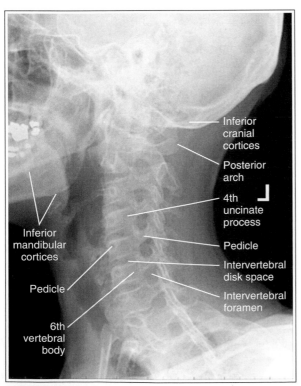

FIGURE 8-39 PA axial oblique cervical projection with cranium in lateral projection and accurate positioning.

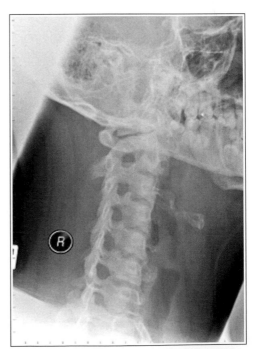

FIGURE 8-40 PA axial oblique cervical projection with cranium in PA oblique projection and accurate positioning.

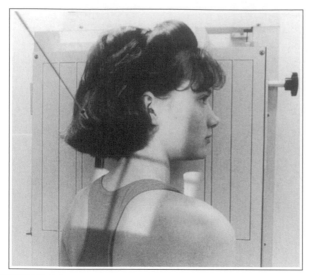

FIGURE 8-41 Proper patient positioning for PA axial oblique cervical projection.

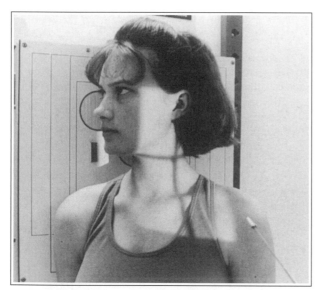

FIGURE 8-42 Proper patient positioning for AP axial oblique cervical projection.

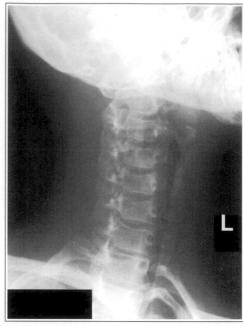

FIGURE 8-43 PA axial oblique cervical projection taken with the patient insufficiently rotated.

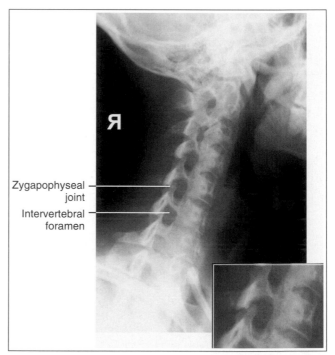

Zygapophyseal
joint

Intervertebral
foramen

FIGURE 8-44 PA axial oblique cervical projection taken with the patient excessively rotated.

vertebrae is caused by the head being positioned too close or far away from the IR (poor IPL positioning) and lower cervical vertebrae tilting is caused by the upper thorax being tilted anteriorly. Also, because this examination can be performed using anterior or posterior oblique positions that require differing CR angulations, and the typical cervical vertebral series requires the radiographer to change angle directions several times, radiographers should be able to identify a projection that was taken with an incorrect CR angle.

The PA axial oblique projections in Figures 8-46 and 8-47 were taken with the cervical vertebral column tilted anteriorly (vertebrae leaning toward the IR) or with the CR angled too cephalically to align with the intervertebral disk spaces. Note that the intervertebral disk spaces are closed, the cervical bodies are distorted, and zygapophyseal joint spaces are demonstrated. Figure 8-47

demonstrates more tilting or an increase in cephalic CR angulation than Figure 8-46, as indicated by the transverse process being seen in the intervertebral foramen. If this same analysis was for an AP projection, the cervical vertebral column would have been tilted anteriorly or the CR angulation would have been positioned too caudally.

Positioning for Kyphosis. In patients with severe kyphosis, the lower cervical vertebrae are angled toward

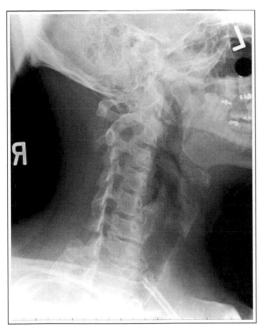

FIGURE 8-45 PA axial oblique cervical projection taken with the upper cervical vertebrae adequately rotated and the lower cervical vertebrae excessively rotated.

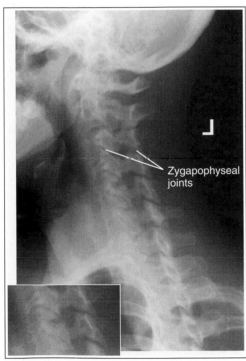

FIGURE 8-46 PA axial oblique cervical projection taken with the cervical vertebral column and the patient's head tilted toward the IR.

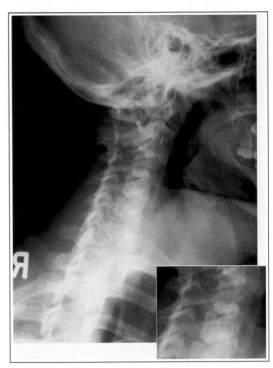

FIGURE 8-47 PA axial oblique cervical projection taken with the cervical vertebral column tilted toward the IR and the patient's head tilted away from the IR.

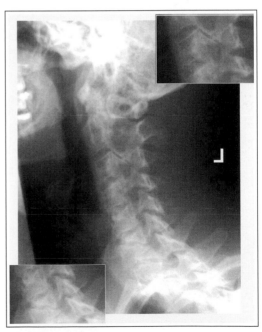

FIGURE 8-48 PA axial oblique cervical projection of a patient with kyphosis.

the IR because of the greater lordotic curvature of this area. To demonstrate the lower cervical vertebrae with open intervertebral disk spaces and undistorted cervical bodies on a patient with this condition, the CR will need to be angled more than the suggested 15 to 20 degrees for the oblique projections. The projection in Figure 8-48 was taken on a patient with kyphosis without the increase in CR angulation. Note the difference in the intervertebral disk space openness, vertebral body distortion, and the demonstration of the zygapophyseal joints between the upper and lower cervical regions.

Interpupillary Line Positioning. The distances demonstrated between the inferior cortical outlines of the cranium and the mandibular rami are a result of the angulation placed on the CR. On PA axial oblique projections, the caudal angle projects the cranial cortex situated farther from the IR approximately 0.25 inch (0.6 cm) inferiorly and the mandibular ramus situated farther from the IR approximately 0.5 inch (1.25 cm) inferiorly. The ramus is projected farther inferiorly because it is located at a larger OID than the cranial cortex. On AP axial oblique projections, the cephalic CR angle projects the cranial cortex and mandibular rami situated farther from the IR superiorly. The distance between these two cortical outlines will be increased or decreased if the patient's head is allowed to tilt toward or away from the IR. Such tilting also causes the upper cervical vertebrae to lean toward or away from the IR. To avoid head and upper cervical column tilting, position the IPL parallel with the floor.

Detecting Poor Interpupillary Line Positioning.

On oblique projections, if the head and upper cervical column are allowed to tilt, the atlas and its posterior arch are distorted. From such a projection, one can determine whether the head and upper cervical vertebrae were tilted toward or away from the IR by evaluating the distance demonstrated between the inferior cranial cortices and the inferior mandibular rami and the openness of the atlas's vertebral foramen. For PA oblique projections these distances are increased and the foramen is open, when the head and upper cervical vertebrae are tilted away from the IR (Figures 8-47 and 8-49). If these distances are decreased and the foramen is not demonstrated, the head and upper cervical vertebrae were tilted toward the IR (see Figure 8-46). For AP oblique projections when the head and upper cervical vertebrae are tilted away from the IR the distances will increase and

the foramen is not demonstrated and when they are tilted toward IR the distances will decrease and the foramen is demonstrated.

Head Positioning. The desired position of the head for an AP axial oblique projection varies among facilities. If an oblique head is desired, rotate the patient's head 45 degrees with the body. If a lateral head is desired, turn the face away from the side of interest until the head's midsagittal plane is aligned parallel with the IR. To demonstrate the upper cervical vertebrae without mandibular superimposition and aligned right and left cranial and mandibular cortices on an AP axial oblique projection, place the patient's cranium in a lateral projection and adjust chin elevation until the AML is aligned parallel with the floor. If the chin is not properly elevated and/or the patient's head is rotated, the mandibular rami are superimposed over C1 and C2 (Figure 8-50).

Trauma. When imaging the cervical vertebrae of a trauma patient with suspected subluxation or fracture, obtain the trauma AP axial lateral projections and lateral position and have them evaluated before the patient is moved for the AP axial oblique projection. The trauma AP axial oblique projection of the cervical vertebrae is accomplished by elevating the supine patient's head, neck, and thorax enough to place a lengthwise IR beneath the neck. If the right vertebral foramina and pedicles are of interest, the IR should be shifted to the left enough to align the left mastoid tip with the longitudinal axis of the IR and inferior enough to position the right gonion (angle of jaw when head is in neutral position; C3) with the transverse axis of the IR. Angle the CR 45 degrees medially to the right side of the patient's neck and rotate the tube 15 degrees cephalically, and then center the CR

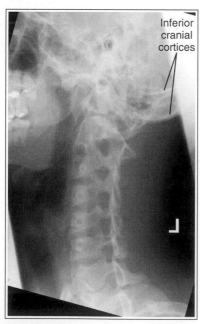

FIGURE 8-49 PA axial oblique cervical projection taken with the patient's head tilted away from the IR.

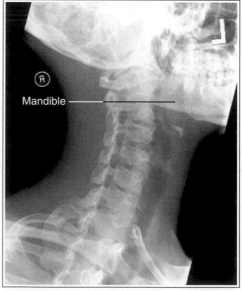

FIGURE 8-50 PA axial oblique cervical projection taken with the head in and oblique position.

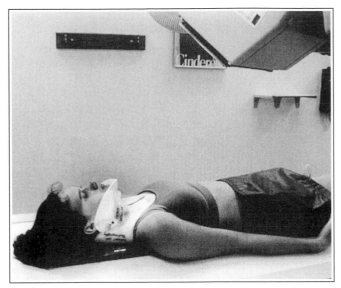

FIGURE 8-51 Proper patient positioning for AP axial oblique cervical projection taken to evaluate trauma.

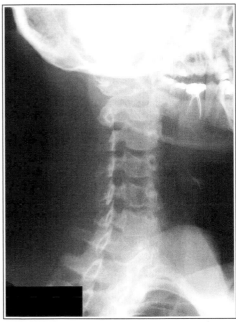

FIGURE 8-52 AP axial oblique cervical projection with accurate positioning taken to evaluate trauma.

halfway between the anterior and posterior surfaces of the neck at the level of the thyroid cartilage (C4) (Figure 8-51). If the left vertebral foramina and pedicles are of interest, shift the IR to the right enough to align the right mastoid tip with the longitudinal axis of the IR and inferior enough to position the left gonion with the transverse axis of the IR. The CR should be angled and centered as described earlier, except that it should be directed to the left side of the patient's neck. A trauma AP axial oblique cervical projection should meet all the analysis requirements listed for a regular AP axial oblique cervical projection; the cranium will be in an oblique position (Figure 8-52).

PA Axial Oblique Cervical Vertebrae Analysis Practice

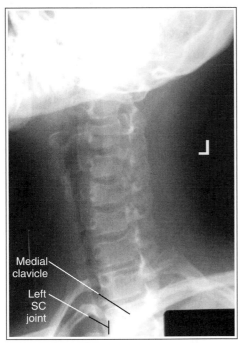

IMAGE 8-8 PA axial oblique.

Analysis. The pedicles and intervertebral foramina are obscured, and portions of the left sternoclavicular joint and medial clavicular and are superimposed by the vertebral column. The patient was not rotated the required 45 degrees.

Correction. Increase the patient obliquity until the midcoronal plane is placed at a 45-degree angle with the IR.

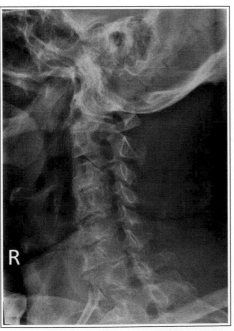

IMAGE 8-9 PA axial oblique.

Analysis. The intervertebral disk spaces are closed, the cervical bodies are distorted, and zygapophyseal joint spaces are demonstrated. The cervical vertebral column was tilted anteriorly or the CR angled too close to perpendicular (too cephalically).

Correction. Posteriorly tilt the cervical vertebral column until it is parallel with the IR or adjust the CR angle caudally until it is aligned with the intervertebral disk spaces.

CERVICOTHORACIC VERTEBRAE: LATERAL PROJECTION (TWINING METHOD; SWIMMER'S TECHNIQUE)

See Table 8-6, (Figures 8-53 and 8-54).

Exam Indication. This examination is performed when the routine lateral cervical projection does not adequately demonstrate the seventh cervical vertebra or when the routine lateral thoracic projection does not demonstrate the first through third thoracic vertebrae.

Rotation. If the patient is rotated for the cervicothoracic vertebrae projection, the right-side articular pillars, posterior ribs, zygapophyseal joints, and humeri move away from the left side, obscuring the pedicles and distorting the vertebral bodies. When rotation is demonstrated on a lateral projection, determine which side was rotated anteriorly and which side was rotated posteriorly by evaluating the location of the humerus that was positioned closer to the IR, which can be identified by its placement by the patient's head. If this humerus was rotated anteriorly, the shoulder positioned closest to the IR was positioned anteriorly (Figure 8-55). If this humerus was rotated posteriorly, the shoulder positioned closest to the IR was positioned posteriorly (Figure 8-56).

IPL and Midsagittal Plane Positioning. To obtain open disk spaces and undistorted vertebral bodies, position the head in a lateral projection, with the IPL perpendicular to and the midsagittal plane parallel with the IR. If the patient is in a recumbent position, it may be necessary to elevate the head on a sponge to place it in a lateral position and prevent cervical column tilting (Figure 8-57).

Trauma. When routine cervical projections are obtained in a trauma patient with suspected subluxation or fracture and the seventh lateral cervical vertebra is not demonstrated, obtain the lateral cervicothoracic projection with the patient's head, neck, and body trunk left as is. Instruct the patient to elevate the arm farther from the x-ray tube and depress the arm closer to the tube. Then place the IR and grid against the lateral body surface, centering its transverse axis at a level 1 inch (2.5 cm) superior to the jugular notch (Figure 8-58). Position the CR horizontal to the posterior neck surface and the center of the IR and grid. If the shoulder closer to the CR is not well-depressed, a 5-degree caudal angulation is recommended.

Identifying C7. The seventh cervical vertebra can be identified on a lateral cervicothoracic projection by locating the elevated clavicle, which is normally shown traversing the seventh cervical vertebra.

TABLE 8-6	**Lateral Cervicothoracic Vertebrae Projection**
Image Analysis Guidelines (Figure 8-53)	**Related Positioning Procedures (Figure 8-54)**
• Right and left cervical zygapophyseal joints, the articular pillars, and the posterior ribs are superimposed.	• Position the patient in an upright or a recumbent lateral projection. • Recumbent: Flex the knees and hips for support. • Upright: Distribute patient's weight on both feet equally. • Position the shoulders, the posterior ribs, and the ASISs on top of each other, aligning the midcoronal plane perpendicular with the IR.
• Humerus elevated above the patient's head is aligned with the vertebral column. • Fifth through seventh cervical vertebrae are demonstrated without shoulder superimposition.	• Elevate the arm positioned closer to the IR above the patient's head as high as the patient can allow. • Place the other arm against the patient's side, and instruct the patient to depress the shoulder. Use a 5-degree caudal CR angulation if patient is unable to depress the shoulder. • Take the exposure on expiration.
• Intervertebral disk spaces are open. • Vertebral bodies are demonstrated without distortion.	• Place the head in a lateral position, with the IPL perpendicular to and the midsagittal plane parallel with the IR. • Supine: Elevate head on a sponge if needed to obtain position.
• First thoracic vertebra is at the center of the exposure field.	• Center a perpendicular CR to the midcoronal plane at a level 1 inch (2.5 cm) superior to the jugular notch or at the level of the vertebral prominens.
• Fifth through seventh cervical vertebrae and first through third thoracic vertebrae are included within the exposure field.	• Center the IR and grid to the CR. • Open the longitudinally collimated field to the patient's mandibular angle. • Transversely collimate to within 0.5 inch (1.25 cm) of the skin line.

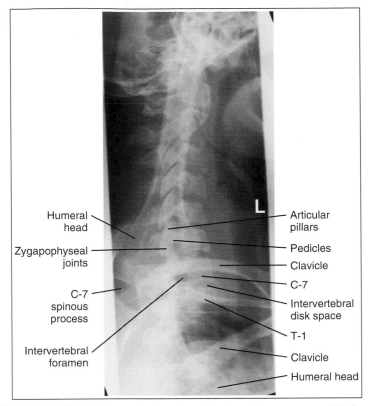

Humeral head

Zygapophyseal joints

C-7 spinous process

Intervertebral foramen

Articular pillars

Pedicles

Clavicle

C-7

Intervertebral disk space

T-1

Clavicle

Humeral head

FIGURE 8-53 Lateral cervicothoracic projection with accurate positioning.

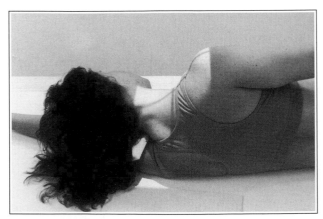

FIGURE 8-54 Proper patient positioning for recumbent lateral cervicothoracic projection.

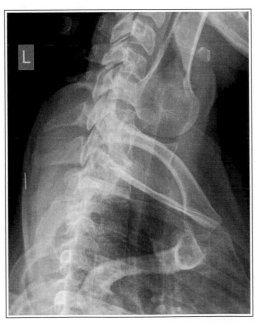

FIGURE 8-55 Lateral cervicothoracic projection taken with the left shoulder positioned anteriorly.

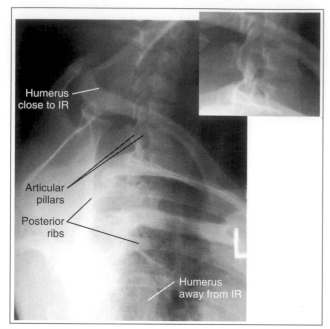

FIGURE 8-56 Lateral cervicothoracic projection taken with the left shoulder positioned posteriorly.

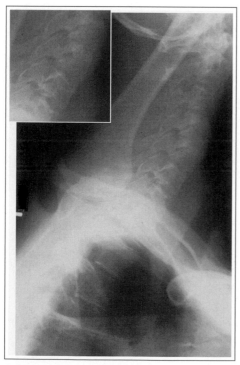

FIGURE 8-57 Lateral cervicothoracic projection taken with the head and upper cervical vertebrae tilted toward the IR.

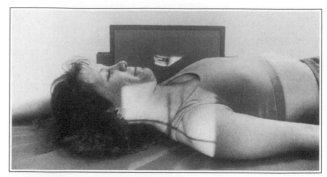

FIGURE 8-58 Proper patient positioning for lateral cervicothoracic projection taken to evaluate trauma.

Lateral Cervicothoracic Vertebrae Analysis Practice

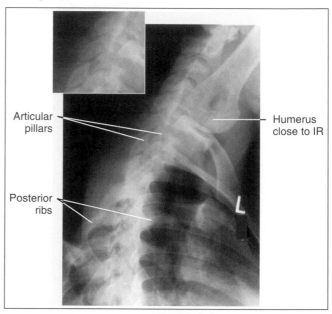

IMAGE 8-10

Analysis. The right and left articular pillars, zygapophyseal joints, and the posterior ribs are demonstrated without superimposition. The left thorax was rotated anteriorly.

Correction. Rotate the right thorax anteriorly until the midcoronal plane is perpendicular to the IR.

THORACIC VERTEBRAE: AP PROJECTION

See Table 8-7, (Figures 8-59 and 8-60).
Obtaining Uniform Brightness Across Thoracic Vertebrae

Anode Heel Effect. The anode heel effect decreases the number of photons reaching the upper thoracic vertebrae and results in decreased brightness in this area. This method works sufficiently in patients who have very little difference in AP body thickness between their upper and lower thoracic vertebrae but does not provide an

TABLE 8-7	AP Thoracic Vertebrae Projection	
Image Analysis Guidelines (Figure 8-59)	**Related Positioning Procedures (Figure 8-60)**	
• There is uniform brightness across the thoracic vertebrae.	• Use the appropriate technical factors. • Position the upper thoracic vertebrae at the anode end of the tube and the lower thoracic vertebrae at the cathode end.	
• Spinous processes are aligned with the midline of the vertebral bodies. • Distances from the vertebral column to the sternal clavicular ends and from the pedicles to the spinous processes are equal on the two sides. • Intervertebral disk spaces are open. • Vertebral bodies are seen without distortion. • Seventh thoracic vertebra is at the center of the exposure field.	• Position the patient in a supine or upright AP projection. • Place the shoulders, the posterior ribs, and the ASISs at equal distances from the IR, aligning the midcoronal plane parallel with the IR. • Supine: Flex the hips and knees until the lower back rests firmly against the table. • Center the CR to the midsagittal plane at the level halfway between the jugular notch and the xiphoid.	
• Seventh cervical vertebra, first through twelfth thoracic vertebrae, first lumbar vertebra, and 2.5 inches (6.25 cm) of the posterior ribs and mediastinum on each side of the vertebral column are included within the collimated field. • No more than 9 posterior ribs are demonstrated above the diaphragm.	• Center the IR and grid to the CR. • Open the longitudinal collimation to a 17-inch (43 cm) field size for adult patients. • Transversely collimate to about an 8-inch (20-cm) field size. • Take the exposure after a full suspended expiration.	

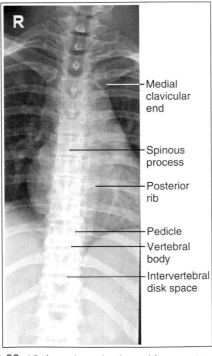

Medial clavicular end

Spinous process

Posterior rib

Pedicle
Vertebral body

Intervertebral disk space

FIGURE 8-59 AP thoracic projection with accurate positioning.

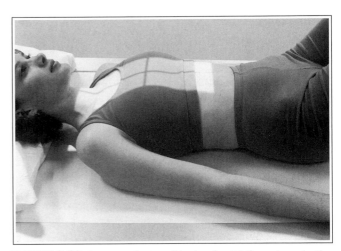

FIGURE 8-60 Proper patient positioning for AP thoracic projection without compensating filter.

adequate density decrease in patients with larger thickness differences. To use the anode heel effect, position the patient's head and upper thoracic vertebrae at the anode end of the tube and the feet and lower thoracic vertebrae at the cathode end. Then set an exposure (mAs) that adequately demonstrates the middle thoracic vertebrae. Because the anode will absorb some of the photons aimed at the anode end of the IR, the upper thoracic vertebrae will receive less exposure than the lower vertebrae.

Expiration Versus Inspiration. Patient respiration determines the amount of brightness and contrast resolution demonstrated between the mediastinum and vertebral column. These differences are a result of the variation in atomic density that exists between the thoracic cavity and the vertebrae. The thoracic cavity is largely composed of air, which contains very few atoms in a given area; the same area of bone, as in the vertebrae, contains many compacted atoms. As radiation goes through the patient's body, fewer photons are absorbed in the thoracic cavity than in the vertebral column, because fewer atoms with which the photons can interact are present in the thoracic cavity. Consequently, more photons will penetrate the thoracic cavity to expose the IR than will penetrate the vertebral column. Taking the exposure on full suspended expiration reduces the air volume and

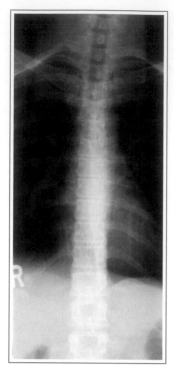

FIGURE 8-61 AP thoracic projection taken after full inspiration.

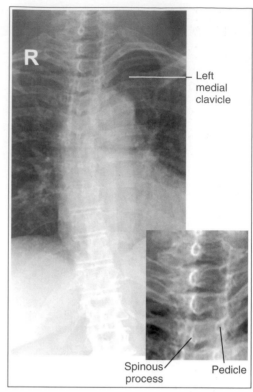

FIGURE 8-62 AP thoracic projection taken with the left side of the upper thorax positioned closer to the IR.

compresses the tissue in this area, allowing better visualization of the posterior ribs and mediastinum region (compare Figures 8-59 and 8-61). It should be noted, however, that the contrast created on an AP thoracic vertebral projection taken on inspiration can be valuable in detecting thoracic tumors or disease.

Rotation. The upper and lower thoracic vertebrae can demonstrate rotation independently or simultaneously, depending on which section of the body is rotated. If the patient's shoulders and upper thorax were rotated and the pelvis and lower thorax remained supine, the upper thoracic vertebrae demonstrate rotation. If the patient's pelvis and lower thorax were rotated and the thorax and shoulders remained supine, the lower thoracic vertebrae demonstrate rotation. If the patient's thorax and pelvis were rotated simultaneously, the entire thoracic column demonstrates rotation.

Rotation is effectively detected on an AP thoracic projection by comparing the distances between pedicles and spinous processes on the same vertebra and the distances between the vertebral column and medial ends of the clavicles. When no rotation is present, the comparable distances are equal. If one side demonstrates a larger distance, vertebral rotation is present. The side demonstrating a larger distance is the side of the patient positioned closer to the IR (Figure 8-62).

Distinguishing Rotation From Scoliosis. In patients with spinal scoliosis, the thoracic bodies may appear rotated because of the lateral twisting of the vertebrae. Scoliosis of the vertebral column can be very severe, demonstrating a large amount of lateral deviation, or it

can be subtle, demonstrating only a small amount of deviation (Figure 8-63). Severe scoliosis is very obvious and is seldom mistaken for patient rotation, whereas subtle scoliotic changes may be easily mistaken for rotation. Although both conditions demonstrate unequal distances between the pedicles and spinous processes, certain clues can be used to distinguish subtle scoliosis from rotation. The long axis of a rotated vertebral column remains straight, whereas the scoliotic vertebral column demonstrates lateral deviation. When the thoracic vertebrae demonstrate rotation, it has been caused by the rotation of the upper or lower torso. Rotation of the middle thoracolumbar vertebrae does not occur unless the upper and lower thoracic vertebrae also demonstrate rotation. On an AP projection of a patient with scoliosis, the thoracolumbar vertebrae may demonstrate rotation without corresponding upper or lower vertebral rotation. Familiarity with the difference between a rotated thoracic vertebral column and a scoliotic one prevents unnecessarily repeated procedures in patients with spinal scoliosis.

CR and Intervertebral Disk Space Alignment. The thoracic vertebral column demonstrates a kyphotic curvature. Because the thoracic vertebrae have very limited flexion and extension movements, it is difficult to achieve a significant reduction of this curvature. A small reduction can be obtained by placing the patient's head on a thin pillow or sponge and flexing the hips and knees until the lower back rests firmly against the table. Both

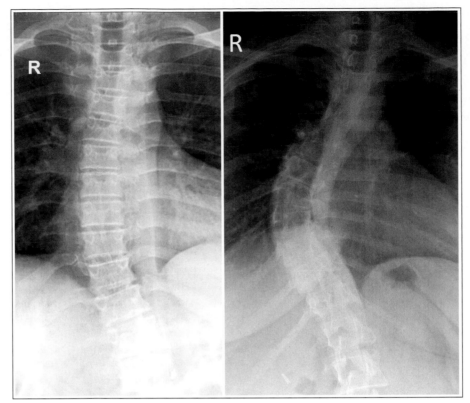

FIGURE 8-63 AP thoracic projection demonstrating spinal scoliosis.

procedures improve the relationship of the upper and lower vertebral disk spaces and bodies with the x-ray beam. The head position reduces the upper vertebral curvature, and the hip and knee position reduces the lower vertebral curvature. If the CR and intervertebral disk spaces are not aligned, it is difficult for the reviewer to evaluate the height of the disk spaces and vertebral bodies (Figure 8-64).

Positioning for Kyphosis. To demonstrate open disk spaces and undistorted vertebral bodies in a patient with excessive spinal kyphosis, it may be necessary to angle the CR until it is perpendicular to the vertebral area of interest, which may vary between the upper and lower thoracic regions. Because it is painful for such a patient to lie supine on the table, it is best to perform the examination with the patient upright, or in a lateral recumbent position with use of a horizontal beam.

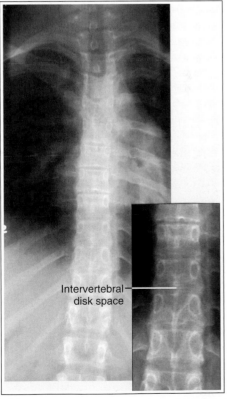

FIGURE 8-64 AP thoracic projection taken with the patient's legs extended.

AP Thoracic Vertebrae Analysis Practice

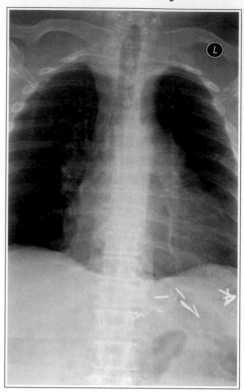

IMAGE 8-11

Analysis. The upper thoracic intervertebral disk spaces are closed and the CR was centered too inferiorly. This CR and upper thoracic disk spaces were not parallel.

Correction. Center the CR halfway between the jugular notch and xiphoid.

THORACIC VERTEBRAE: LATERAL PROJECTION

See Table 8-8, (Figures 8-65 and 8-66).

Breathing Technique. The thoracic vertebrae have many overlying structures, including the axillary ribs and lungs. Using a long exposure time (3-4 seconds) and requiring the patient to breathe shallowly (costal breathing) during the exposure forces a slow and steady, upward and outward movement of the ribs and lungs. This technique is often referred to as *breathing technique*. This movement causes blurring of the ribs and lung markings on the projection, providing greater thoracic vertebral demonstration (Figure 8-65). Deep breathing, which requires movement (elevation) of the sternum and a faster and expanded upward and outward movement of the ribs and lungs, should be avoided during the breathing technique, because deep breathing results in motion of the thoracic cavity and vertebrae (Figure 8-67). If patient motion cannot be avoided when using the extended 3 to 4 seconds for breathing

TABLE 8-8	Lateral Thoracic Vertebrae Projection
Image Analysis Guidelines (Figure 8-65)	**Related Positioning Procedures (Figure 8-66)**
• Thoracic vertebrae are seen through overlying lung and rib structures.	• Breathing technique: Use a long exposure time (3-4 seconds) and require the patient to costal breathe (shallow breathing) during the exposure. • Suspended respiration: Use if patient motion cannot be avoided for breathing technique.
• Intervertebral foramina are clearly demonstrated. • Pedicles are in profile. • Posterior surfaces of each vertebral body are superimposed. • No more than 1/2 inch (1.25 cm) of space is demonstrated between the posterior ribs.	• Position patient in a recumbent or upright left lateral position. • Place the shoulders, the posterior ribs, and the ASISs directly on top of one another, aligning the midcoronal plane perpendicular to the IR. • Recumbent: Flex the knees and hips, and position a pillow or sponge between the knees that is thick enough to maintain lateral position.
• Humeri or their soft tissue are not obscuring vertebrae.	• Abduct the arms to a 90-degree angle with the body.
• Intervertebral disk spaces are open. • Vertebral bodies are demonstrated without distortion.	• Align the thoracic vertebral column parallel with the IR. • Recumbent: Tuck a radiolucent sponge between the lateral body surface and table just superior to the iliac crest, if needed to maintain alignment.
• Seventh thoracic vertebra is at the center of the exposure field.	• Center a perpendicular CR to the inferior scapular angle.
• Seventh cervical vertebra, first through twelfth thoracic vertebrae, and first lumbar vertebra are included within the exposure field.	• Center the IR and grid to the CR. • Open the longitudinal collimation field to a 17-inch (43-cm) field size for adult patients. • Transversely collimate to an 8-inch (20-cm) field size.

technique, take the projection on suspended respiration to reduce the air volume within the thoracic cavity (Figure 8-68).

Rotation. The upper and lower thoracic vertebrae can demonstrate rotation independently or simultaneously, depending on which section of the torso was rotated. If the shoulders were not placed on top of each other but the ASISs were aligned, the upper thoracic vertebrae demonstrate rotation and the lower thoracic vertebrae demonstrate a lateral projection. If the ASISs

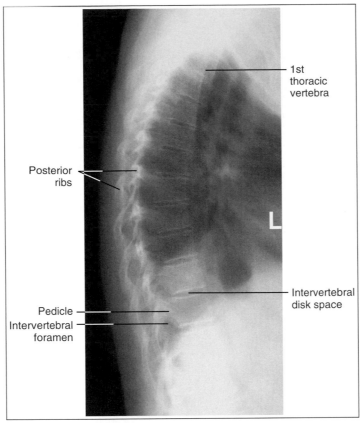

FIGURE 8-65 Lateral thoracic projection with accurate positioning.

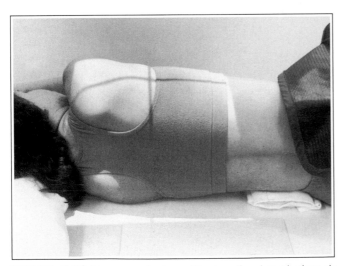

FIGURE 8-66 Proper patient positioning for lateral thoracic projection.

were rotated but the shoulders were placed on top of each other, the lower thoracic vertebrae demonstrate rotation and the upper vertebrae demonstrate a lateral projection.

Rotation can be detected on a lateral thoracic projection by evaluating the superimposition of the right and left posterior surfaces of the vertebral bodies and the amount of posterior rib superimposition. On a nonrotated lateral projection, the posterior surfaces are superimposed and the posterior ribs are almost superimposed.

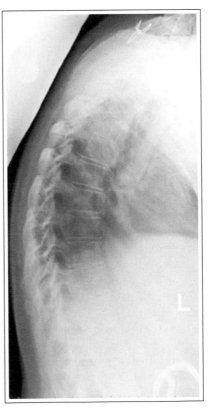

FIGURE 8-67 Lateral thoracic projection taken with patient breathing deeply and with the lower thoracic vertebrae positioned closer to the IR than the upper thoracic vertebrae.

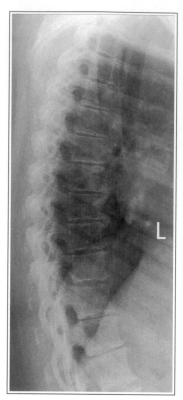

FIGURE 8-68 Lateral thoracic projection taken with suspended respiration.

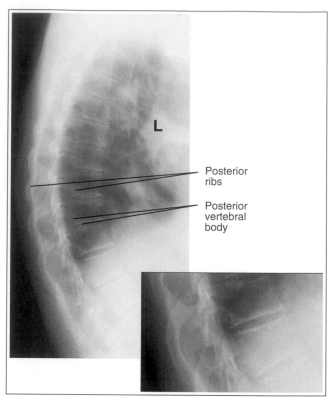

Posterior ribs

Posterior vertebral body

FIGURE 8-69 Lateral thoracic projection taken with the right side rotated posteriorly.

Because the posterior ribs positioned farther from the IR were placed at a greater OID than the other side, they demonstrate more magnification. This magnification prevents the posterior ribs from being directly superimposed but positions them approximately ½ inch (2.5 cm) apart. This distance is based on a 40-inch (102-cm) SID. If a longer SID is used, the distance between the posterior ribs is decreased and, if a shorter SID is used, the distance is increased. On rotation, the right and left posterior surfaces of the vertebral bodies are demonstrated one anterior to the other on a lateral projection. Because the two sides of the thorax and vertebrae are mirror images, it is very difficult to determine from a rotated lateral projection which side of the patient was rotated anteriorly and which posteriorly. If the patient was only slightly rotated, one way of determining which way the patient was rotated is to evaluate the amount of posterior rib superimposition. If the patient's elevated side was rotated posteriorly, the posterior ribs demonstrate more than 1 inch (2.5 cm) of space between them (Figures 8-69 and 8-70). If the patient's elevated side was rotated anteriorly, the posterior ribs are superimposed on slight rotation (Figure 8-71) and demonstrate greater separation as rotation of the patient increases. Another method is to view the scapulae and humeral heads when visible. The scapula and humeral head demonstrating the greatest magnification will be the ones situated farthest from the IR (see Figure 8-70).

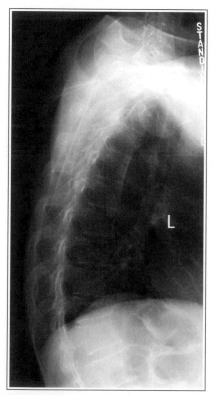

FIGURE 8-70 Lateral thoracic projection taken with the right side rotated posteriorly.

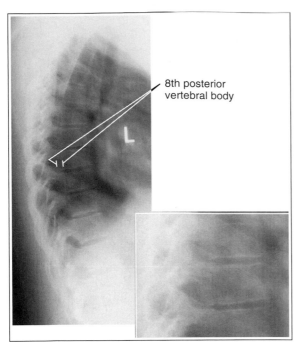

FIGURE 8-71 Lateral thoracic projection taken with the right side rotated anteriorly.

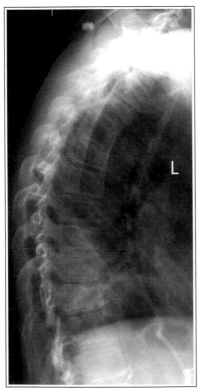

FIGURE 8-72 Lateral thoracic projection of a patient with spinal scoliosis.

Distinguishing Rotation From Scoliosis. On the lateral projection of a patient with spinal scoliosis, the lung field may appear rotated because of the lateral deviation of the vertebral column (Figure 8-72). On such a projection, the posterior ribs demonstrate differing degrees of separation depending on the severity of the

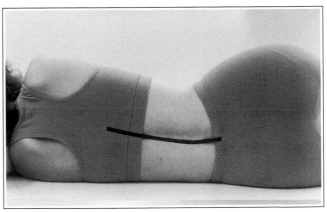

FIGURE 8-73 Poor alignment of vertebral column with table.

scoliosis. View the accompanying AP thoracic projection (see Figure 8-63) to confirm this patient condition.

CR Intervertebral Disk Space Alignment. The thoracic and lumbar vertebral columns are capable of lateral flexion. When the patient is placed in a lateral recumbent position, the vertebral column may not be aligned parallel with the table and IR but may sag at the level of the lower thoracic and lumbar vertebrae region, especially in a patient who has broad shoulders and narrow hips or wide hips and a narrow waist (Figure 8-73). This sagging results in the thoracic column being tilted with the IR. If the thoracic column is allowed to tilt with the IR, the x-ray beams will not be aligned parallel with the intervertebral disk spaces and perpendicular with the vertebral bodies. Tilting on a lateral thoracic projection is most evident at the lower thoracic vertebral region, where it causes the intervertebral disk spaces to be closed and the vertebral bodies to be distorted (Figures 8-67 and 8-74). For a patient who has a tilting thoracic column, it may be necessary to tuck an immobilization device between the lateral body surface and table just superior to the iliac crest, elevating the sagging area. The radiolucent sponge should be thick enough to bring the thoracic vertebral column parallel with the table and IR (see Figure 8-66).

An alternative method of obtaining open intervertebral disk spaces and undistorted thoracic bodies in a patient whose thoracic column is tilted with the IR is to cephalically angle the CR until it is aligned perpendicular with the vertebral column.

Scoliotic Patient. A scoliotic patient should be placed on the side (right or left) that will allow the CR to be directed into the spinal curve to obtain open into vertebral disk spaces and undistorted vertebral bodies.

Locating T7. With the patient's arm positioned at a 90-degree angle with the body, the inferior scapular angle is placed over the seventh thoracic vertebra.

Verifying Inclusion of All Thoracic Vertebrae. When viewing a lateral thoracic projection, you can be sure that the twelfth thoracic vertebra has been included by locating the vertebra that has the last rib attached to it. This is the twelfth vertebra. To confirm this finding,

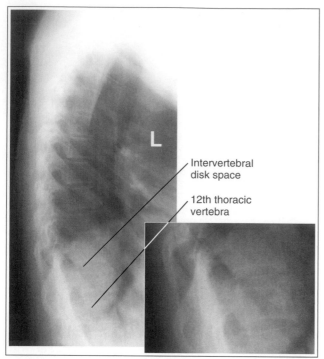

FIGURE 8-74 Lateral thoracic projection taken with the lower thoracic vertebrae positioned closer to the IR than the upper thoracic vertebrae.

follow the posterior vertebral bodies of the lower thoracic and upper lumbar vertebrae, watching for the subtle change in curvature from kyphotic to lordotic. The twelfth thoracic vertebra is located just above it. The first thoracic vertebra can be identified on a lateral thoracic projection by counting up from the twelfth thoracic vertebra or by locating the seventh cervical vertebral prominens. The first thoracic vertebra is at the same level as this prominens.

Lateral Cervicothoracic (Twining Method) Projection. Because of shoulder thickness and the superimposition of the shoulders over the first through third thoracic vertebrae, it may be necessary to take a supplementary projection of this area to demonstrate the thoracic vertebrae. Refer to the description of this projection presented earlier in this chapter.

Lateral Thoracic Vertebrae Analysis Practice

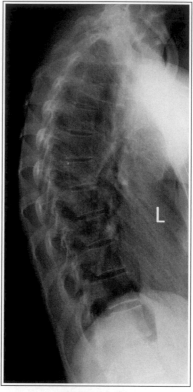

IMAGE 8-12

Analysis. The posterior ribs demonstrate more than 0.5 inch (1.25 cm) of space between them. The right thorax was rotated posteriorly.

Correction. Rotate the right thorax anteriorly until the mid-coronal plane is perpendicular with the IR.

Lumbar, Sacral, and Coccygeal Vertebrae

OUTLINE

Lumbar Vertebrae: AP
Projection, 424
  AP Lumbar Analysis
  Practice, 428
Lumbar Vertebrae: AP Oblique
Projection (Right and Left
Posterior Oblique Positions), 428
  AP Oblique Lumbar Analysis
  Practice, 430

Lumbar Vertebrae: Lateral
Projection, 430
  Lateral Lumbar Vertebrae
  Analysis Practice, 435
L5-S1 Lumbosacral Junction:
Lateral Projection, 436
  Lateral L5-S1 Analysis
  Practice, 438
Sacrum: AP Axial Projection, 438

AP Sacrum Analysis
Practice, 440
Sacrum: Lateral Projection, 440
  Lateral Sacrum Analysis
  Practice, 442
Coccyx: AP Axial Projection, 443
  AP Coccyx Analysis Practice, 444
Coccyx: Lateral Projection, 444

OBJECTIVES

After completion of this chapter, you should be able to do the following:

- Identify the required anatomy on lumbar, sacral, and coccygeal projections.
- Describe how to position the patient, image receptor (IR), and central ray (CR) properly for lumbar, sacral, and coccygeal projections.
- State how to mark and display lumbar, sacral, and coccygeal projections properly.
- List the typical artifacts that are found on lumbar, sacral, and coccygeal projections.
- List the image analysis guidelines for lumbar, sacral, and coccygeal projections with accurate positioning.
- State how to reposition the patient properly when lumbar, sacral, and coccygeal projections with poor positioning are produced.
- Discuss how to determine the amount of patient or CR adjustment required to improve lumbar, sacral, and coccygeal projections with poor positioning.

- State the curvature of the lumbar vertebrae, sacrum, and coccyx.
- State which zygapophyseal joints are demonstrated when posterior and anterior oblique lumbar projections are produced.
- List the anatomic structures that make up the parts of the "Scottie dogs" demonstrated on an oblique lumbar image with accurate positioning.
- Explain which procedures are used to produce lateral lumbar, L5-S1 spot, sacral, and coccygeal projections with the least amount of scatter radiation reaching the IR.
- State two methods of positioning the long axis of the lumbar column parallel with the long axis of the table for a lateral lumbar projection.
- Describe how the patient is positioned to demonstrate AP mobility of the lumbar vertebral column.
- State why the patient is instructed to empty the bladder and colon before an AP sacral or coccygeal projection is taken.

KEY TERM

interiliac line

IMAGE ANALYSIS GUIDELINES

Technical Data. When the technical data in Table 9-1 are followed, or adjusted as needed for additive and destructive patient conditions (see Table 2-6), along with the best practices discussed in Chapters 1 and 2, all upper extremity projections will demonstrate the image analysis guidelines in Box 9-1 unless otherwise indicated.

LUMBAR VERTEBRAE: AP PROJECTION

See Table 9-2, (Figures 9-1 and 9-2).

Psoas Muscle Demonstration. The soft tissue structures that are visualized on AP lumbar vertebral projections are the psoas muscles. They are located laterally to the lumbar vertebrae, originating at the first lumbar vertebra on each side and extending to the corresponding side's lesser trochanter. They are used in lateral flexion

BOX 9-1	Lumbar Vertebrae, Sacrum, and Coccyx Imaging Analysis Guidelines

- The facility's identification requirements are visible.
- A right or left marker identifying the correct side of the patient is present on the projection and is not superimposed over the VOI.
- Good radiation protection practices are evident.
- Bony trabecular patterns and cortical outlines of the anatomic structures are sharply defined.
- Contrast resolution is adequate to demonstrate the soft tissue, bony trabecular patterns, and cortical outlines.
- No quantum mottle or saturation is present.
- Scatter radiation has been kept to a minimum.
- There is no evidence of removable artifacts.

TABLE 9-1	Lumbar Vertebrae, Sacrum and Coccyx Technical Data				
Projection	**kV**	**Grid**	**AEC**	**mAs**	**SID**
AP, lumber vertebrae	85-95	Grid	Center		40-48 inches (100-120 cm)
AP oblique, lumbar vertebrae	85-95	Grid	Center		40-48 inches (100-120 cm)
Lateral, lumbar vertebrae	90-100	Grid	Center		40-48 inches (100-120 cm)
Lateral, L5-S1 lumbosacral junction	90-100	Grid	Center		40-48 inches (100-120 cm)
AP axial, sacrum	85-90	Grid	Center		40-48 inches (100-120 cm)
Lateral, sacrum	90-100	Grid	Center		40-48 inches (100-120 cm)
AP axial, coccyx	80-85	Grid	Center		40-48 inches (100-120 cm)
Lateral, coccyx	85-90	Grid	Center		40-48 inches (100-120 cm)
Pediatric	65-75	Grid*		3-4	40-48 inches (100-120 cm)

*Use grid if part thickness measures 4 inches (10 cm) or more and adjust mAs per grid ratio requirement.

TABLE 9-2	AP Lumbar Vertebrae Projection

Image Analysis Guidelines (Figure 9-1)	Related Positioning Procedures (Figure 9-2)
<ul><li>Psoas muscles are demonstrated.</li><li>Spinous processes are aligned with the midline of the vertebral bodies, with equal distances from the pedicles to the spinous processes on both sides.</li><li>Sacrum and coccyx are centered within the inlet pelvis.</li><li>Intervertebral disk spaces are open.</li><li>Vertebral bodies are seen without distortion.</li><li>Long axis of the lumbar column is aligned with the long axis of the exposure field.</li><li>The L3 vertebra is at the center of the exposure field.</li><li>8 × 17 inch (20 × 43 cm) field size: 12th thoracic vertebra, 1st through 5th lumbar vertebrae, sacroiliac joints, sacrum, coccyx and psoas muscles are included within the exposure field.</li><li>8 × 14 inch (20 × 35 cm) field size: 12th thoracic vertebra, 1st through 5th lumbar vertebrae, sacroiliac joints, and psoas muscles are included in the exposure field.</li></ul>	<ul><li>Position the patient in a supine or upright AP projection.</li><li>Place the shoulders and ASISs at equal distances from the table, aligning the mid-coronal plane parallel with the IR.</li><li>Flex the knees and hips, resting the lower back against the table.</li><li>Align the midsagittal plane with the longitudinal light field.</li><li>Center a perpendicular CR to the midsagittal plane at a level 1-1.5 inches (2.5-4 cm) superior to the iliac crest.</li><li>Center the IR and grid to the CR.</li><li>Open the longitudinal collimation the desired 17-inch (43-cm) or 14-inch (35-cm) field size.</li><li>Transversely collimate to an 8-inch (20-cm) field size.</li></ul>

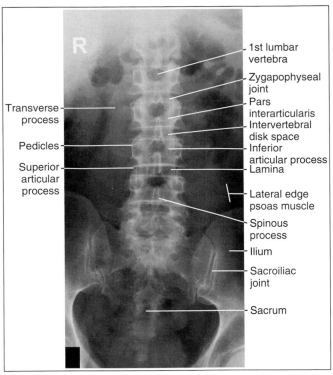

Transverse process

Pedicles

Superior articular process

1st lumbar vertebra

Zygapophyseal joint

Pars interarticularis

Intervertebral disk space

Inferior articular process

Lamina

Lateral edge psoas muscle

Spinous process

Ilium

Sacroiliac joint

Sacrum

FIGURE 9-1 AP lumbar vertebral projection with accurate positioning.

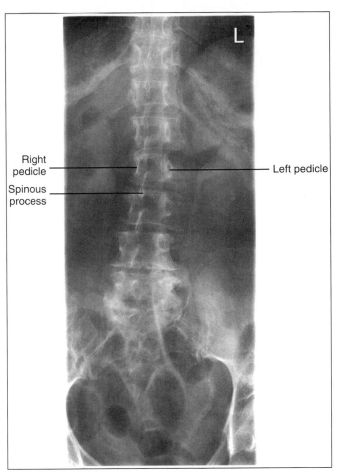

Right pedicle

Spinous process

Left pedicle

FIGURE 9-3 AP lumbar projection taken with patient's right side closer to IR than left side.

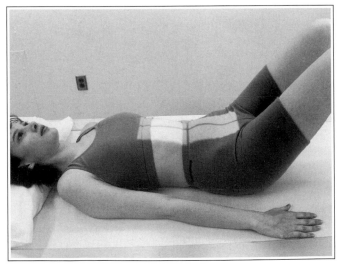

FIGURE 9-2 Proper patient positioning for AP lumbar vertebral projection.

and rotation of the thigh and in flexion of the vertebral column. On an AP lumbar projection, they are visible on each side of the vertebral bodies as long, triangular soft tissue shadows.

Rotation. The upper and lower lumbar vertebrae can demonstrate rotation independently or simultaneously, depending on which section of the body is rotated. If the patient's thorax was rotated and the pelvis remained supine, the upper lumbar vertebrae demonstrate

rotation. If the patient's pelvis was rotated and the thorax remained supine, the lower lumbar vertebrae demonstrate rotation. If the patient's thorax and pelvis were rotated simultaneously, the entire lumbar column demonstrates rotation.

Rotation is effectively detected on an AP lumbar projection by evaluating the alignment of the spinous processes in the vertebral body. If no rotation is present, the spinous processes are aligned with the midline of the vertebral bodies, positioning them at equal distances from the pedicles. On rotation the spinous processes move away from the midline and closer to the pedicles on one side and away from the corresponding pedicles, resulting in different distances between the spinous processes and pedicles (Figure 9-3). The side toward which the spinous processes rotate and that demonstrates the least distance from the spinous processes to the pedicles is the side of the patient positioned farther from the table and IR. Lower lumbar rotation can also be detected by evaluating the position of the sacrum and coccyx within the pelvic inlet. If no rotation was present, they are centered within the pelvic inlet. On rotation, the sacrum and coccyx rotate toward the side of the pelvic inlet positioned farther from the IR.

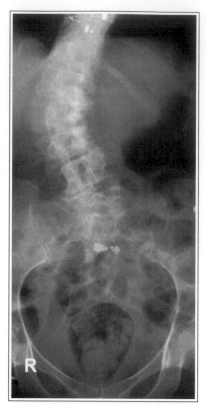

FIGURE 9-4 AP lumbar projection taken of a patient with severe scoliosis.

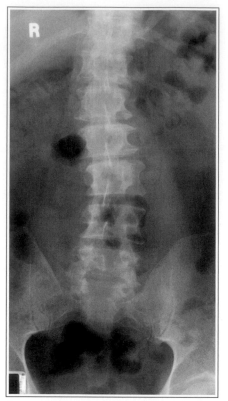

FIGURE 9-5 AP lumbar projection taken of a patient with subtle scoliosis.

Distinguishing Rotation From Scoliosis. In patients with spinal scoliosis, the lumbar bodies may appear rotated because of the lateral twisting of the vertebrae. Severe scoliosis is very obvious and is seldom mistaken for patient rotation (Figure 9-4), whereas subtle scoliotic changes can be easily mistaken for rotation (Figure 9-5). Although both conditions demonstrate unequal distances between the pedicles and spinous processes, certain clues can be used to distinguish subtle scoliosis from rotation. The long axis of a rotated vertebral column remains straight, whereas the scoliotic vertebral column demonstrates lateral deviation. If the lumbar vertebrae demonstrate rotation, it has been caused by the rotation of the upper or lower torso. Rotation of the middle lumbar vertebrae (L3 and L4) does not occur unless the lower thoracic or upper or lower lumbar vertebrae also demonstrate rotation. On a scoliotic projection, the middle lumbar vertebrae may demonstrate rotation without corresponding upper or lower vertebral rotation.

CR Alignment with Intervertebral Disk Spaces. When the patient is in a supine position with the legs extended, the lumbar vertebrae have an exaggerated lordotic curvature (Figure 9-6). Obtaining an AP lumbar projection with the patient in this position results in the lower vertebrae (L4 and L5) demonstrating closed intervertebral disk spaces and distorted vertebral bodies because of how the x-ray beams are directed at the disk spaces and vertebral bodies (Figure 9-7). To straighten the lumbar vertebral column and better align the intervertebral disk spaces parallel with and the vertebral bodies perpendicular to the CR, flex the knees and hips until the lower back rests against the table (Figure 9-8).

Effect of Lordotic Curvature. On an AP lumbar projection, determine how well the CR parallels the intervertebral disk spaces by evaluating the openness of the T12 through L3 intervertebral disk spaces, the foreshortening of the sacrum, and the distance of the sacrum from the symphysis pubis. If the lordotic curvature was adequately reduced, these disk spaces are open and the sacrum demonstrates less foreshortening and is positioned close to the symphysis pubis. If the lordotic curvature was not adequately reduced, the intervertebral disk spaces are closed, and the sacrum is foreshortened and is positioned farther from the symphysis pubis (Figures 9-6 and 9-9).

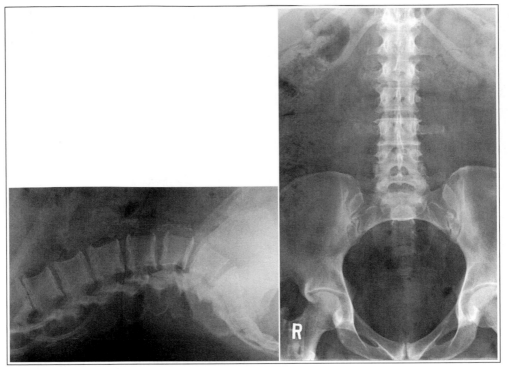

FIGURE 9-6 Lateral and AP lumbar projections taken on the same patient demonstrating intervertebral disk space alignment.

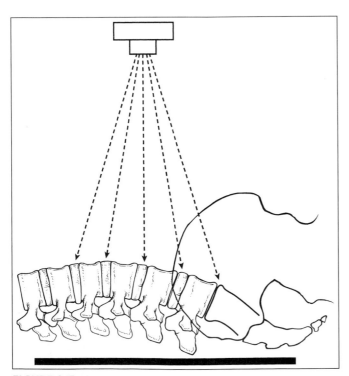

FIGURE 9-7 Alignment of CR and lumbar vertebrae when legs are not flexed.

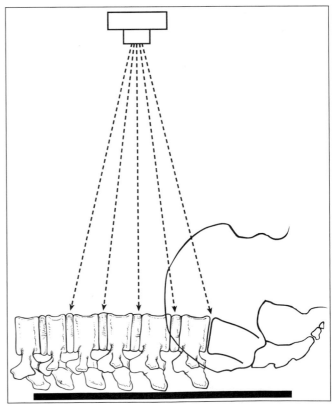

FIGURE 9-8 Alignment of CR and lumbar vertebrae when legs are flexed.

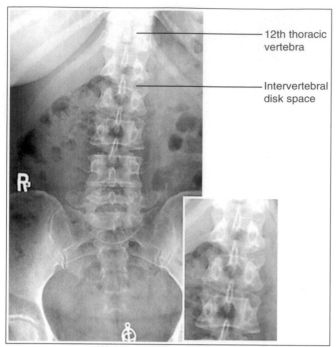

— 12th thoracic vertebra

— Intervertebral disk space

FIGURE 9-9 AP lumbar projection taken without knees and hips flexed.

AP Lumbar Analysis Practice

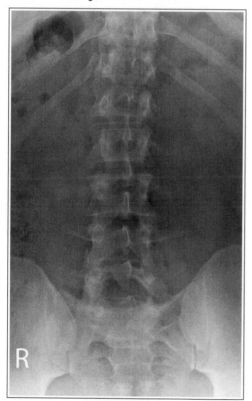

IMAGE 9-1

Analysis. The distance from the left pedicles to the spinous process is narrower than the same distance from the right pedicles to the spinous process. The patient was rotated toward the right side (RPO rotation).

TABLE 9-3	AP Oblique Lumbar Vertebrae Projection	
Image Analysis Guidelines (Figure 9-10)	**Related Positioning Procedures (Figure 9-11)**
• Superior and inferior articular processes are in profile. • Zygapophyseal joints are demonstrated. • Pedicles are seen halfway between the midpoint of the vertebral bodies and the lateral border of the vertebral bodies.	• Start with patient positioned in a supine or upright AP projection. • Rotate the patient until the midcoronal plane is at a 45-degree angle with the IR. • Supine: Support patient obliquity with a radiolucent sponge. • Both right and left AP oblique projections are taken.
• 3rd lumbar vertebra is at the center of the exposure field.	• Center a perpendicular CR 2 inches (5 cm) medial to the elevated ASISs, at a level 1.5 inches (4 cm) superior to the iliac crest.
• 12th thoracic vertebra, 1st through 5th lumbar vertebrae, 1st and 2nd sacral segments, and sacroiliac joints are included within the exposure field.	• Center the IR and grid to the CR. • Open the longitudinally collimated field to a 14-inch (35-cm) field size. • Transversely collimate to an 8-inch (20-cm) field size.

Correction. Rotate the patient toward the left side until the mid-coronal plane is aligned parallel with the IR.

LUMBAR VERTEBRAE: AP OBLIQUE PROJECTION (RIGHT AND LEFT POSTERIOR OBLIQUE POSITIONS)

See Table 9-3, (Figures 9-10 and 9-11).

AP or PA Projection. This examination can be performed using an AP or PA oblique projection. In the AP oblique projection (right posterior oblique [RPO] and left posterior oblique [LPO] positions; see Figure 9-11) the zygapophyseal joints of interest are placed closer to the IR. In the PA oblique projection (right anterior oblique [RAO] and left anterior oblique [LAO] positions), the zygapophyseal joints of interest are positioned farther from the IR, resulting in greater magnification.

Rotation. The articular processes are placed in profile by rotating the thorax until the midcoronal plane is at a 45-degree angle with the IR (see Figure 9-11). To demonstrate the right and left articular processes and zygapophyseal joints of each vertebra, both right and left AP oblique projections must be taken.

Scottie Dogs and Accurate Lumbar Obliquity. The accuracy of an AP oblique projection is often judged by the demonstration of five Scottie dogs stacked on top of

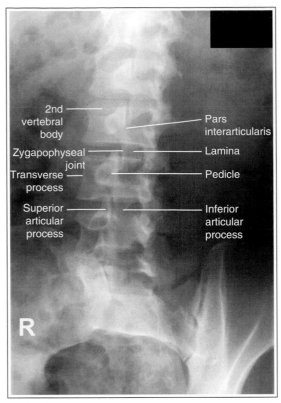

FIGURE 9-10 AP oblique lumbar vertebral projection with accurate positioning.

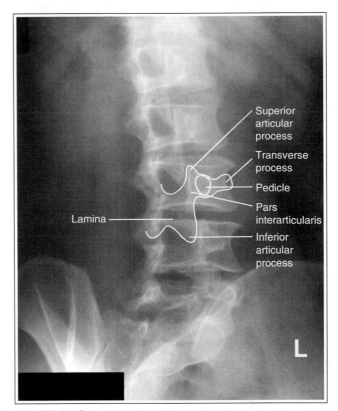

FIGURE 9-12 Identifying "Scottie dogs" and lumbar anatomy.

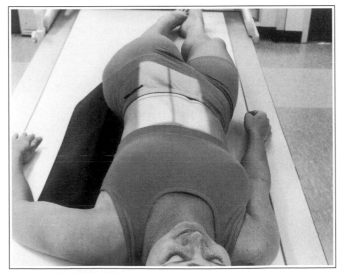

FIGURE 9-11 Proper patient positioning for AP (posterior) oblique lumbar vertebral projection.

one another. Figure 9-12 is a close-up of an accurately positioned oblique lumbar vertebra with the Scottie dog parts outlined and labeled. It should be noted that the Scottie dogs can be identified even on oblique projections with poor positioning. Judge the openness of each zygapophyseal joint to determine whether the lumbar vertebrae have been adequately rotated.

Identifying Poor Obliquity. If a lumbar vertebra was insufficiently rotated to position the superior and inferior articular processes (ear and front leg of Scottie dog) in profile, the corresponding zygapophyseal joint is closed, the pedicle (eye of Scottie dog) is situated closer to the lateral vertebral body border, and more of the lamina (body of Scottie dog) is demonstrated (Figure 9-13). If a lumbar vertebra was rotated more than needed to position the superior and inferior articular processes in profile, the corresponding zygapophyseal joint is closed, the pedicles are demonstrated closer to the vertebral body midline, and less of the lamina is demonstrated (Figure 9-14).

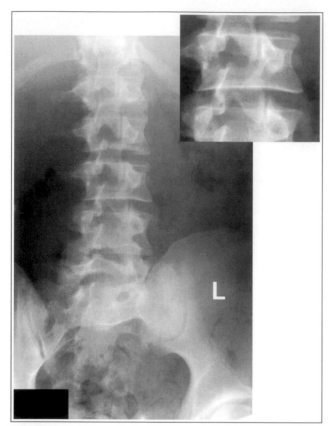

FIGURE 9-13 AP oblique lumbar projection taken with insufficient patient rotation.

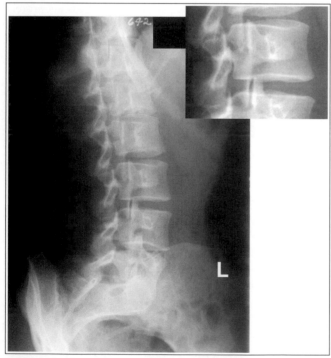

FIGURE 9-14 AP oblique lumbar projection taken with excessive patient rotation.

AP Oblique Lumbar Analysis Practice

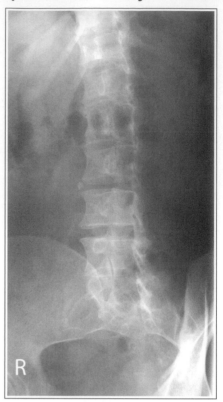

IMAGE 9-2

Analysis. The superior and inferior articular processes are not in profile, the corresponding zygapophyseal joints are closed, and the pedicles are demonstrated closer to the vertebral body midline. The patient was rotated more than 45 degrees.

Correction. Decrease the degree of rotation until the midcoronal plane is at a 45-degree angle with the IR.

LUMBAR VERTEBRAE: LATERAL PROJECTION

See Table 9-4, (Figures 9-15 and 9-16).

Rotation

Effect of Rotation. The upper and lower lumbar vertebrae can demonstrate rotation independently or simultaneously, depending on which section of the torso is rotated. If the thorax was rotated but the pelvis remained in a lateral position, the upper lumbar vertebrae demonstrate rotation. If the pelvis was rotated but the thorax remained in a lateral position, the lower lumbar vertebrae demonstrate rotation.

Detecting Rotation. Rotation can be detected on a lateral lumbar projection by evaluating the superimposition of the right and left posterior surfaces of the vertebral bodies. On a nonrotated lateral lumbar image, these posterior surfaces are superimposed, appearing as one. On rotation, these posterior surfaces are not

TABLE 9-4	Lateral Lumbar Vertebrae Projection
Image Analysis Guidelines (Figure 9-15)	**Related Positioning Procedures (Figure 9-16)**
• Intervertebral foramina are demonstrated and the spinous processes are in profile. • Right and left pedicles and the posterior surfaces of each vertebral body are superimposed.	• Position the patient in an upright or recumbent left lateral position. • Place the shoulders, the posterior ribs, and the ASISs directly on top of one another, aligning the midcoronal plane perpendicular to the IR. • Recumbent: Flex the knees and hips, and place a pillow or sponge between the knees that is thick enough to prevent spinal rotation.
• Intervertebral disk spaces are open. • Vertebral bodies are seen without distortion. • Lumbar vertebral column is in a neutral position, without AP flexion or extension. • Long axis of the lumbar vertebral column is aligned with the long axis of the exposure field. • 8 × 14 inch (20 × 35 cm) field size: L3 vertebra is at the center of the exposure field. • 8 × 17 inch (20 × 43 cm) field size: L4 vertebra and iliac crest are at the center of the exposure field.	• Align the midsagittal plane parallel with the IR. • Position the midcoronal plane with the long axis of the IR, aligning the thoracic and pelvic regions. • Align the long axis of the lumbar vertebral column with the collimator's longitudinal light line. • 8 × 14 inch (20 × 35 cm) field size: Center a perpendicular CR to the coronal plane located halfway between the elevated ASIS and posterior wing at the level 1.5 inches (4 cm) superior to the iliac crest. • 8 × 17 inch (20 × 43 cm) field size: Center a perpendicular CR to the coronal plane located halfway between the elevated ASIS and posterior wing at the level of the iliac crest.
• 8 × 14 inch (20 × 35 cm) field size: 12th thoracic vertebra, 1st through 5th vertebrae, and L5-S1 intervertebral disk space are included in the exposure field. • 8 × 17 inch (20 × 43 cm) field size: 11th and 12th thoracic vertebra, 1st through 5th lumbar vertebrae, and sacrum are included within the exposure field.	• Center the IR and grid to the CR. • Open the longitudinal collimation to the desired 14-inch (35-cm) or 17-inch (43-cm) field size. • Transversely collimate to an 8-inch (20-cm) field size.

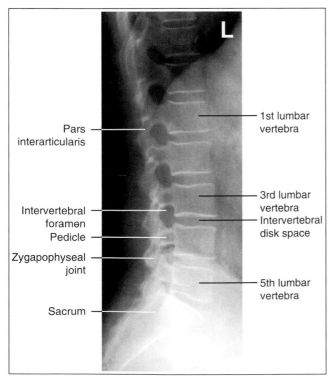

FIGURE 9-15 Lateral lumbar vertebral projection with accurate positioning.

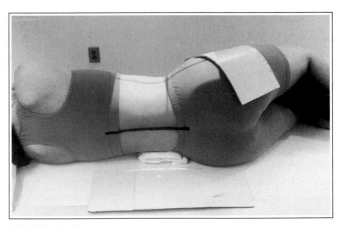

FIGURE 9-16 Proper patient positioning for lateral lumbar vertebral projection.

superimposed, but one is demonstrated anterior to the other (Figure 9-17). Because the two sides of the vertebrae, thorax, and pelvis are mirror images, it is very difficult to determine from a rotated lateral lumbar projection which side of the patient was rotated anteriorly and which posteriorly, unless the twelfth posterior ribs are demonstrated. The twelfth posterior rib that demonstrates the greatest magnification and is situated inferiorly is adjacent to the side of the patient positioned farther from the IR.

CR Alignment with Intervertebral Disk Spaces. When the patient is placed in a lateral recumbent position, the

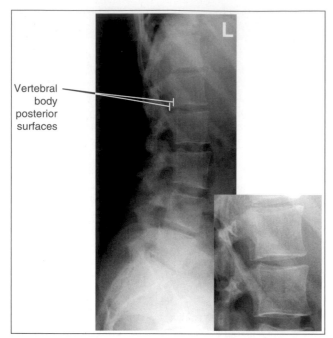

FIGURE 9-17 Lateral lumbar vertebral projection taken with right side rotated posteriorly.

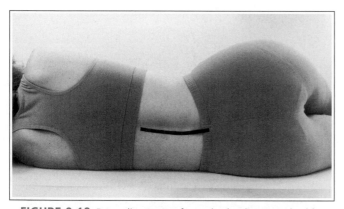

FIGURE 9-18 Poor alignment of vertebral column and table.

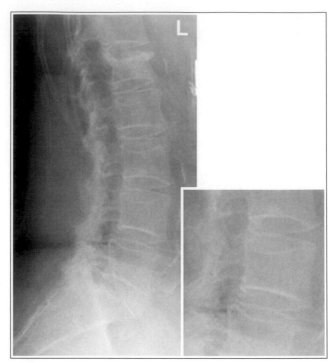

FIGURE 9-19 Lateral lumbar projection taken with vertebral column tilted with IR.

center of the lumbar vertebral column may sag toward the IR (Figure 9-18) because of lateral flexion, or may be straight but tilted at an angle with the IR. This will most often occur when imaging patients with broad shoulders and narrow hips or wide hips and a narrow waist. A slight bit of sagging is acceptable and will actually help to better align the x-ray beams with the intervertebral disk spaces. If the lumbar column demonstrates excessive sagging or tilting, the diverging x-ray beams will not be aligned parallel with the intervertebral disk spaces and perpendicular to the vertebral bodies and the resulting projection will demonstrate closed disk spaces and distorted vertebral bodies (Figure 9-19). For a patient who has excessive lumbar column sagging, it may be necessary to tuck a radiolucent sponge between the lateral body surface and table just superior to the iliac crest, elevating the sagging area. The sponge should be thick enough to bring the lumbar vertebral column close to parallel with the table and IR (see Figure 9-16). For

a patient whose lumbar column is tilted with the IR, open disk spaces and undistorted vertebral bodies can be obtained by angling the CR as needed to align it perpendicular to the lumbar vertebral column.

Scoliotic Patient. Whether the patient is lying on the right or left side is insignificant, although left-side positioning is often easier for the technologist. One exception to this guideline is the scoliotic patient, who should be placed on the table so that the CR is directed into the spinal curve (Figure 9-20) to better demonstrate open intervertebral disk spaces. Determine how the patient's curve is directed by viewing the patient's back and following the curve of the vertebral column and evaluating the AP projection. Figure 9-21 demonstrates AP and lateral projections taken on a patient with a scoliotic lumbar column that curves toward the right side of the patient.

Evaluating AP Mobility of Lumbar Vertebrae. If the lumbar vertebrae are being imaged in the lateral projection to demonstrate AP vertebral mobility, two laterals are taken, one with the patient in maximum flexion and one in maximum extension. The x-ray order can be for an upright or supine position. For maximum flexion, instruct the patient to flex the shoulders, upper thorax, and knees anteriorly, rolling into a tight ball (Figure 9-22). The resulting projection should meet all the requirements listed for a lateral projection with accurate positioning, except that the lumbar vertebral column demonstrates a very straight longitudinal axis without lordotic curvature (Figure 9-23). For maximum extension, instruct the patient to arch the back by extending

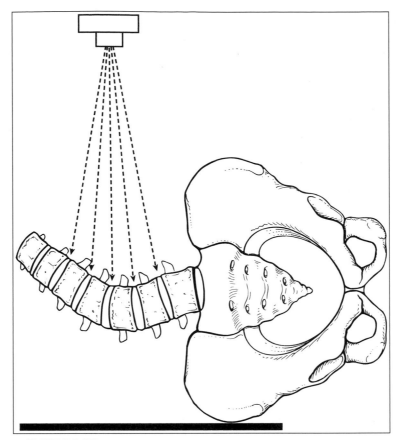

FIGURE 9-20 Alignment of CR and scoliotic lumbar vertebral column.

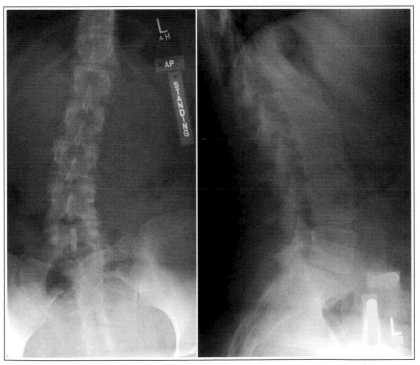

FIGURE 9-21 AP and lateral lumbar vertebrae projections of patient with scoliosis with CR entering on right side for the lateral.

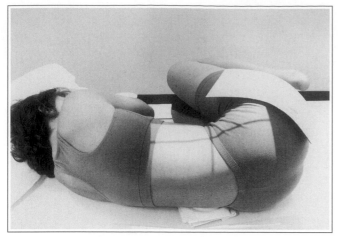

FIGURE 9-22 Proper patient positioning for lateral (flexion) lumbar vertebral projection.

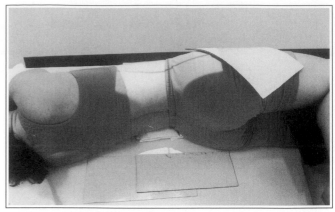

FIGURE 9-24 Proper patient positioning for lateral (extension) lumbar vertebral projection.

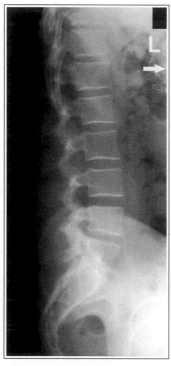

FIGURE 9-23 Lateral lumbar projection taken with patient in flexion.

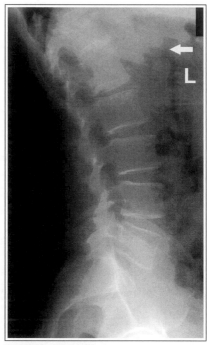

FIGURE 9-25 Lateral lumbar projection taken with patient in an extension.

the shoulders, upper thorax, and legs as far posteriorly as possible (Figure 9-24). The resulting projection should meet all the requirements listed for a lateral projection with accurate positioning, except that the lumbar vertebral column demonstrates an increased lordotic curvature (Figure 9-25).

Lumbar Vertebrae and IR Center Alignment. Aligning the long axis of the lumbar vertebral column with the collimator's longitudinal light line allows tight collimation, which will reduce patient dose and is necessary to reduce the production of scatter radiation. The lumbar vertebrae are located in the posterior half of the torso. Their exact posterior location can be determined by palpating the ASIS and posterior iliac wing (at the level of

the sacroiliac joint) of the side of the patient situated farther from the IR. The long axis of the lumbar vertebral column is aligned with the coronal plane that is situated halfway between these two structures (Figure 9-26).

Supplementary Projection of the L5-S1 Lumbar Region. A coned-down projection of the L5-S1 lumbar region is required when a lateral lumbar projection is obtained that demonstrates insufficient contrast resolution in this area or the L5-S1 joint space is closed. In patients with wide hips, it is often difficult to set exposure factors that adequately demonstrate the upper and lower lumbar regions concurrently. For these patients, set exposure factors that adequately demonstrate the upper lumbar region. Then obtain a tightly collimated lateral projection of the L5-S1 lumbar region to demonstrate the lower lumbar area. See the description for the

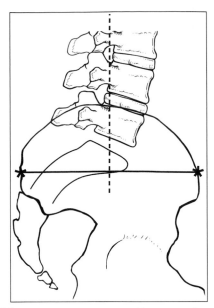

FIGURE 9-26 Proper CR centering and long axis placement. Asterisks identify the posterior iliac wing and anterior superior iliac spines.

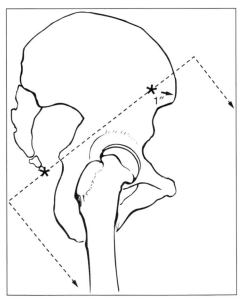

FIGURE 9-27 Gonadal shielding for lateral vertebral, sacral, and coccygeal projections.

lateral projection of the L5-S1 lumbosacral junction later in this chapter.

Gonadal Shielding. Gonadal protection shielding may be used for this procedure without covering needed anatomical structures. Begin by palpating the patient's coccyx and elevated ASIS. Next, draw an imaginary line connecting the coccyx with a point 1 inch posterior to the ASIS, and position the longitudinal edge of a large flat contact shield or lead half-apron anteriorly against this imaginary line (Figure 9-27). This shielding method can also be safely used for patients being imaged for lateral sacral and coccygeal projections without fear of obscuring areas of interest (Figure 9-28).

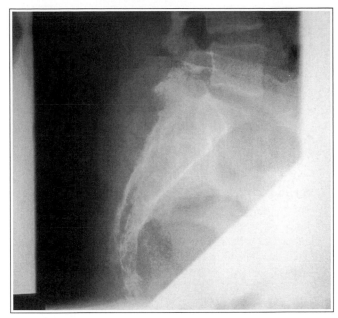

FIGURE 9-28 Proper gonadal shielding for lateral vertebral, sacral, and coccygeal projections.

Lateral Lumbar Vertebrae Analysis Practice

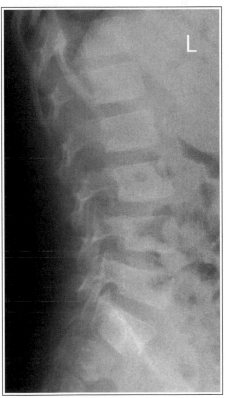

IMAGE 9-3

Analysis. The posterior surfaces of the vertebral bodies are not superimposed. The right side of the patient was rotated anteriorly.

Correction. Rotate the right side of the patient posteriorly until the midcoronal plane is aligned perpendicular with the IR.

TABLE 9-5	Lateral L5-S1 Lumbosacral Junction Projection	
Image Analysis Guidelines (Figure 9-29)	**Related Positioning Procedures (Figure 9-30)**	
• L5-S1 Intervertebral foramen is demonstrated. • Right and left pedicles are superimposed and in profile. • Greater sciatic notches are nearly superimposed.	• Position the patient in a recumbent or upright left lateral position. • Place the shoulders, the posterior ribs, and the ASISs directly on top of one another, aligning the midcoronal plane perpendicular to the IR. • Recumbent: Flex the knees and hips, and place a pillow or sponge between the knees that is thick enough to prevent vertebral rotation.	
• L5-S1 intervertebral disk space is open. • L5 vertebral body and sacrum are demonstrated without distortion. • Pelvic alae are nearly superimposed.	• Position the vertebral column parallel with the IR and the interiliac line perpendicular to the IR.	
• L5-S1 lumbosacral disk space is at the center of the exposure field. • 5th lumbar vertebra and 1st and 2nd sacral segments are included within the exposure field.	• Center a perpendicular CR to a point 2 inches (5 cm) posterior to the elevated ASIS and 1.5 inches (4 cm) inferior to the iliac crest. • Center the IR and grid to the CR. • Longitudinally collimate 1 inch (2.5 cm) superior to the iliac crest. • Transversely collimate to an 8-inch (20-cm) field size.	

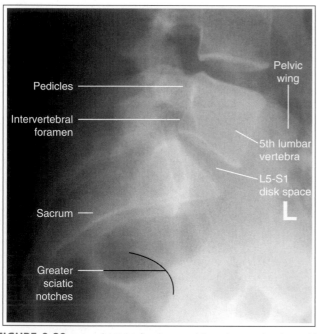

Pedicles

Intervertebral foramen

Sacrum

Greater sciatic notches

Pelvic wing

5th lumbar vertebra

L5-S1 disk space

L

FIGURE 9-29 Lateral L5-S1 lumbosacral junction projection with accurate positioning.

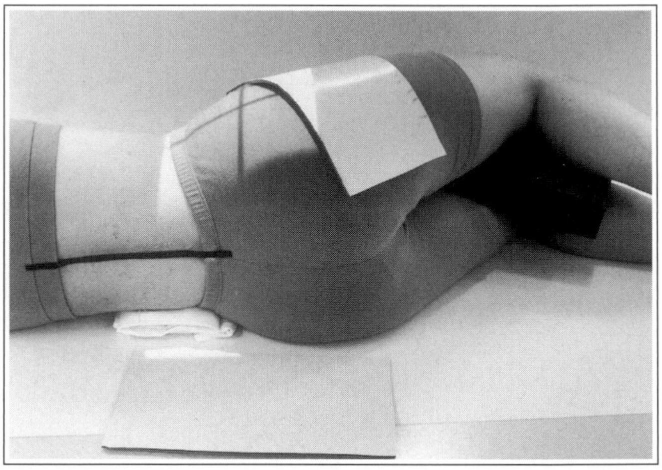

L5-S1 LUMBOSACRAL JUNCTION: LATERAL PROJECTION

See Table 9-5, (Figures 9-29 and 9-30).

Rotation. Rotation can be detected on a lateral L5-S1 projection by evaluating the openness of the intervertebral foramen and the superimposition of the greater sciatic notches and alignment of the femoral heads, when seen. On a nonrotated lateral L5-S1 projection, the intervertebral foramen is open, and the greater sciatic notches are superimposed and the femoral heads are aligned. On rotation, neither the greater sciatic notches are superimposed nor are the femoral heads aligned, but they are demonstrated one anterior to the other (Figure 9-31).

FIGURE 9-30 Proper lateral L5-S1 lumbosacral junction positioning.

Because the two sides of the pelvis are mirror images, it is difficult to determine which side of the patient was rotated anteriorly and which posteriorly on a lateral L5-S1 lumbosacral junction projection with poor positioning. When rotation has occurred, it is most common for the side of the patient situated farther from the IR to be rotated anteriorly, because of the gravitational forward and downward pull on this side's arm and leg, if a sponge is not placed between the patient's knees. If the patient's femoral heads are visible on the projection, they may be used to determine rotation as long as the vertebral column was not sagging and the L5-S1 disk space is open. The femoral head that is projected more inferiorly and demonstrates the greatest magnification is the one situated farther from the IR.

Central Ray and L5-S1 Disk Space Alignment. To obtain an open L5-S1 intervertebral disk space and demonstrate the L5 vertebral body and sacrum without

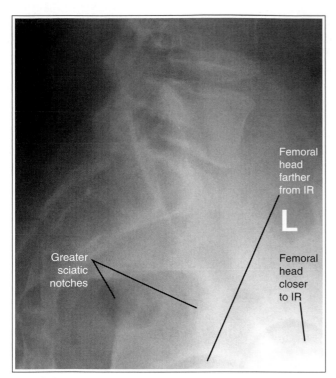

FIGURE 9-31 L5-S1 lateral lumbosacral junction projection taken with right side positioned posteriorly.

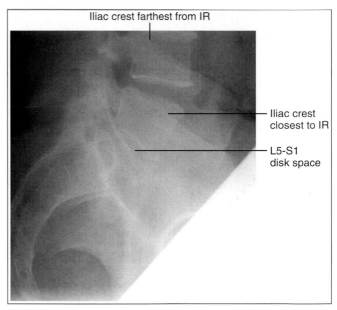

FIGURE 9-32 L5-S1 lateral lumbosacral junction projection taken without the vertebral column aligned parallel with the IR.

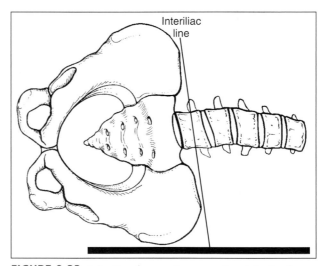

FIGURE 9-33 Adjusting for sagging curved vertebral column.

distortion, the vertebral column is aligned parallel with the table, the interiliac line is aligned perpendicular to the table, and a perpendicular CR is used.

Detecting Lateral Lumbar Flexion. The lumbar vertebral column is capable of lateral flexion (see discussion in lateral lumbar projection, see Figure 9-18). If this flexion is not considered during positioning, the diverging x-ray beams will not be aligned parallel with the L5-S1 disk space and perpendicular to L5 or the long axis of the sacrum. Lateral lumbar flexion can be detected on an L5-S1 projection by evaluating the superimposition of the pelvic alae and the openness of the L5-S1 disk space. A laterally flexed projection demonstrates the pelvic alae without superoinferior alignment and a closed L5-S1 disk space (Figure 9-32).

Adjusting for the Sagging Vertebral Column. Two methods may be used to overcome the sagging vertebral column:

1. Place a radiolucent sponge between the patient's lateral body surface and table just superior to the iliac crest to elevate the vertebral column, aligning it parallel with the table (see Figure 9-30); use a perpendicular CR.

2. Leave the patient positioned as is and angle the CR caudally until it parallels the interiliac line (Figure 9-33).

Scoliotic Patient. One exception to this guideline is the scoliotic patient, who should be placed on the table so that the CR is directed into the spinal curve to better obtain open intervertebral joint spaces. Determine how the patient's curve is directed by viewing the patient's back and following the curve of the vertebral column and evaluating the AP projection.

Lateral L5-S1 Analysis Practice

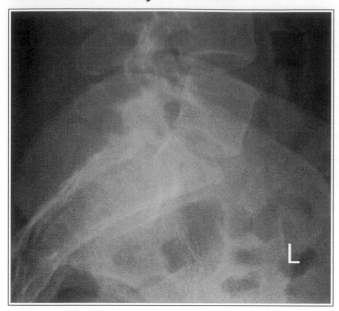

IMAGE 9-4

Analysis. The L5-S1 intervertebral disk space is closed and the L5 vertebral body is distorted. The lumbar vertebral column was sagging toward the table.

Correction. Place a radiolucent sponge between the patient's lateral body surface and table to align the vertebral column parallel with the table or angle the CR caudally until it parallels the interiliac line.

SACRUM

SACRUM: AP AXIAL PROJECTION

See Table 9-6, (Figures 9-34 and 9-35).

Emptying Bladder and Rectum. The patient's urinary bladder should be emptied before the procedure. It is also recommended that the colon be free of gas and fecal material. Elimination of urine, gas, and fecal material from the area superimposed over the sacrum improves its demonstration (Figure 9-36).

Rotation. Rotation is effectively detected on an AP axial sacral projection by comparing the amount of iliac spine demonstrated without pelvic brim superimposition and by evaluating the alignment of the median sacral

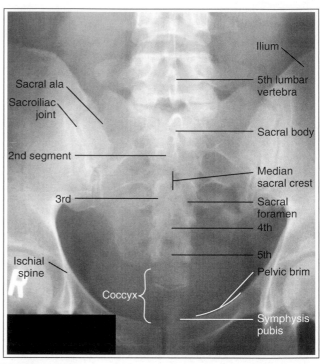

FIGURE 9-34 AP axial sacral projection with accurate positioning.

TABLE 9-6	**AP Axial Sacral Projection**
Image Analysis Guidelines (Figure 9-34)	**Related Positioning Procedures (Figure 9-35)**
• No evidence of urine, gas, or fecal material superimposing the sacrum.	• Have the patient empty urinary bladder and bowels before the procedure.
• Ischial spines are equally demonstrated and are aligned with the pelvic brim. • Median sacral crest and coccyx are aligned with the symphysis pubis. • 1st through 5th sacral segments are seen without foreshortening. • Sacral foramina demonstrate equal spacing. • Symphysis pubis is not superimposed over any portion of the sacrum.	• Place the patient in a supine AP projection on the table with the legs extended. • Place the shoulders and ASIS at equal distances from the table, aligning the mid-coronal plane parallel with the IR. • Angle the CR 15 degrees cephalad.
• 3rd sacral segment is at the center of the exposure field.	• Center the CR to the midsagittal plane at a level 2 inches (5 cm) superior to the symphysis pubis (2 inches inferior to the ASIS).
• 5th lumbar vertebra, 1st through 5th sacral segments, 1st coccygeal vertebra, symphysis pubis, and sacroiliac joints are included within the collimated field.	• Center the IR and grid to the CR. • Open the longitudinally collimated field to the symphysis pubis. • Transversely collimate to an 8-inch (20-cm) field size.

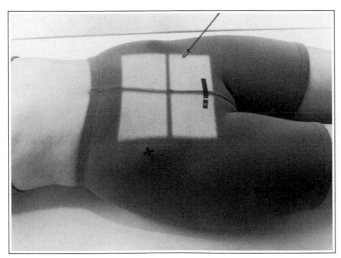

FIGURE 9-35 Proper patient positioning for AP axial sacral projection.

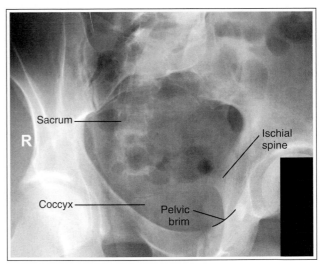

FIGURE 9-37 AP axial sacral projection taken with patient rotated onto the left side.

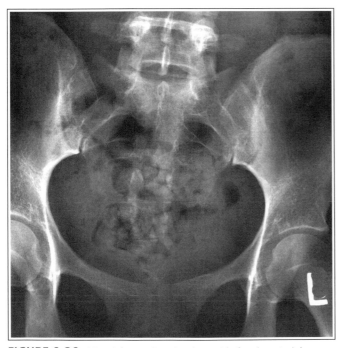

FIGURE 9-36 AP axial sacral projection with fecal material superimposing the sacrum.

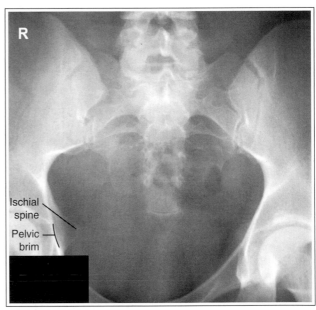

FIGURE 9-38 AP axial sacral projection taken with the patient rotated onto the right side and insufficient cephalic CR angulation.

crest and coccyx with the symphysis pubis. If the patient was rotated away from the AP projection, the sacrum shifts toward the side positioned farther from the table and IR, and the pelvic brim and symphysis shift toward the side positioned closer to the table and IR. If the patient was rotated into an LPO position, the left ischial spine is demonstrated without pelvic brim superimposition, and the median sacral crest and coccyx are not aligned with the symphysis pubis but are rotated toward

the right side (Figure 9-37). If the patient is rotated into an RPO position, the opposite is true—the right ischial spine is demonstrated without pelvic brim superimposition, and the median sacral crest and coccyx are rotated toward the left side (Figure 9-38).

CR and Sacral Alignment. When the patient is in a supine position with the legs extended, the lumbar vertebral column demonstrates a lordotic curvature and the sacrum demonstrates a kyphotic curvature (Figure 9-39).

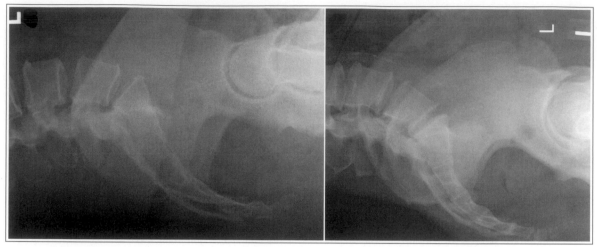

FIGURE 9-39 Two lateral sacrum projections demonstrating different degrees of lordotic curvature of the lumbar vertebral column.

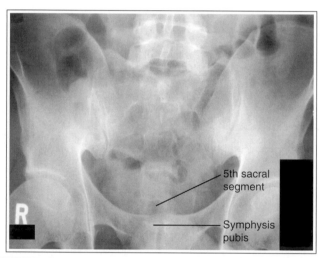

FIGURE 9-40 AP axial sacral projection taken with excessive cephalic CR angulation.

To demonstrate the sacrum without foreshortening, the CR needs to be aligned perpendicular to its long axis, which for most patients requires a 15-degree cephalad CR angulation.

Effect of CR and Sacral Misalignment. Because the degree of lumbar lordotic curvature can vary between patients and the pelvis and the sacrum tilt more with the IR as the lumbar lordotic curvature increases, the CR angle may need to be adjusted to best demonstrate the AP sacrum without foreshortening. If an AP axial sacral projection was taken with an insufficient CR angulation, the first, second, and third sacral segments are foreshortened (see Figure 9-38). If the projection was taken with excessive CR angulation, the sacrum will be elongated and the symphysis pubis will superimpose the inferior sacral segments (Figure 9-40).

AP Sacrum Analysis Practice

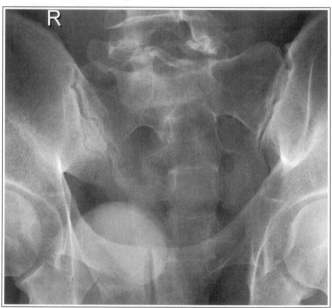

IMAGE 9-5

Analysis. The patient was rotated toward the right side (RPO rotation) and the cephalic CR angulation was excessive.

Correction. Rotate the patient toward the left side until the midcoronal plane is parallel with the IR and slightly decrease the degree of cephalic CR angulation.

SACRUM: LATERAL PROJECTION

See Table 9-7, (Figures 9-41 and 9-42).

Rotation. Rotation can be detected on a lateral sacral projection by evaluating the openness of the L5-S1

TABLE 9-7 | Lateral Sacral Projection

Image Analysis Guidelines (Figure 9-41)	Related Positioning Procedures (Figure 9-42)
• L5-S1 Intervertebral foramen is open. • Median sacral crest is in profile. • Greater sciatic notches are superimposed. • Femoral heads are aligned.	• Place the patient in a recumbent or upright left lateral position. • Place the shoulders, the posterior ribs, and the ASISs directly on top of one another, aligning the midcoronal plane perpendicular to the IR. • Recumbent: Flex the patient's knees and hips for support, and place a pillow or sponge between the knees that is thick enough to prevent anterior rotation.
• L5-S1 intervertebral disk space is open. • L5 vertebral body and sacrum are demonstrated without distortion. • Pelvic alae are nearly superimposed.	• Position the vertebral column parallel with the IR and the interiliac line perpendicular to the IR.
• 3rd sacral segment is at the center of the exposure field.	• Center a perpendicular CR to the coronal plane located 3-4 inches (7.5-10 cm) posterior to the elevated ASIS.
• 5th lumbar vertebra, 1st through 5th sacral segments, promontory, and first coccygeal vertebra are included within the exposure field.	• Center the IR and grid to the CR. • Open the longitudinal collimation to include the iliac crest and coccyx. • Transversely collimate to an 8-inch (20-cm) field size.

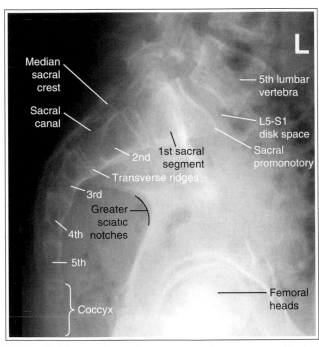

FIGURE 9-41 Lateral sacral projection with accurate positioning.

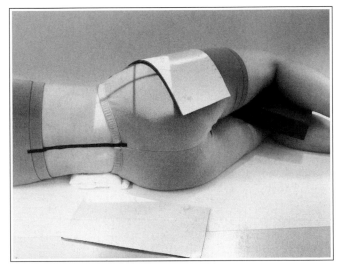

FIGURE 9-42 Proper patient positioning for lateral sacral projection.

intervertebral foramen and the superimposition of the greater sciatic notches and the femoral heads, when seen. On a nonrotated lateral sacral projection, the intervertebral foramen is open, the greater sciatic notches are superimposed, and the femoral heads are aligned. On rotation, the intervertebral foramen closes and the greater sciatic notches and the femoral heads are demonstrated one anterior to the other (see Figure 9-43). Because the two sides of the pelvis are mirror images, it is difficult to determine which side of the patient was rotated anteriorly and which posteriorly on a lateral sacral projection with poor positioning. When rotation has occurred, it is most common for the side of the patient situated farther from the IR to be rotated anteriorly because of the gravitational forward and downward pull on this side's arm and leg, if a sponge is not placed between the patient's knees. When visible, the patient's femoral heads may be used to determine rotation. The femoral head that is projected more inferiorly and demonstrates the greater magnification is the one situated farther from the IR.

CR and L5-S1 Disk Space and Sacral Alignment

Detecting Lateral Lumbar Flexion. If the lateral vertebral column is allowed to flex laterally, causing it to sag for the lateral sacral projection, the resulting projection demonstrates the greater sciatic notches without superoinferior alignment and a closed L5-S1 disk space (Figure 9-44) (see discussion in lateral lumbar projection, Figure 9-18).

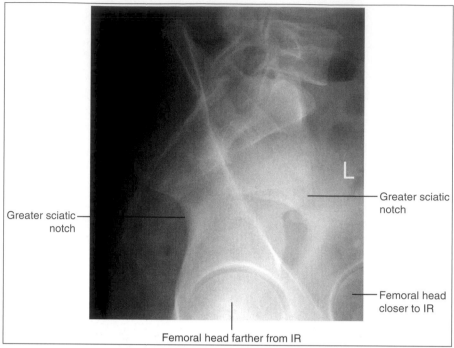

Greater sciatic notch

L

Greater sciatic notch

Femoral head closer to IR

Femoral head farther from IR

FIGURE 9-43 Lateral sacral projection taken with the right side rotated posteriorly.

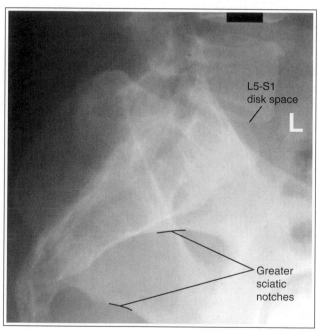

L5-S1 disk space

L

Greater sciatic notches

FIGURE 9-44 Lateral sacral projection taken without the vertebral column and sacrum aligned parallel with the IR.

Adjusting for the Sagging Vertebral Column. Two methods may be used to overcome the sagging vertebral column:

1. Place a radiolucent sponge between the patient's lateral body surface and table just superior to the iliac crest to elevate the vertebral column, aligning it parallel with the table (see Figure 9-30); use a perpendicular CR.

2. Leave the patient positioned as is and angle the CR caudally until it parallels the interiliac line (see Figure 9-33).

Lateral Sacrum Analysis Practice

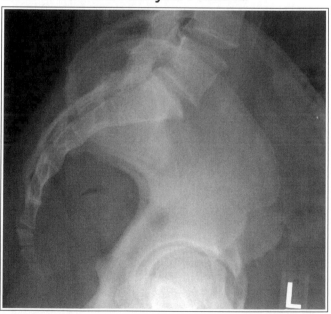

L

IMAGE 9-6

Analysis. The L5-S1 intervertebral disk space is closed and the L5 vertebral body and sacrum are distorted. The lumbar vertebral column was sagging toward the table. **Correction.** Place a radiolucent sponge between the patient's lateral body surface and table to align the vertebral column parallel with the table or angle the CR caudally until it parallels the interiliac line.

TABLE 9-8	**AP Axial Coccygeal Projection**
Image Analysis Guidelines (Figure 9-45)	**Related Positioning Procedures (Figure 9-46)**
• No evidence of urine, gas, or fecal material is superimposed over the coccyx. • Coccyx is aligned with the symphysis pubis and is at equal distances from the lateral walls of the inlet pelvis.	• Have the patient empty urinary bladder and bowels before the procedure. • Position the patient on the table in a supine AP projection with the legs extended. • Place the shoulders and ASISs at equal distances from the table, aligning the midcoronal plane parallel with the IR.
• 1st through 3rd coccygeal vertebrae are seen without foreshortening and without symphysis pubis superimposition. • Coccyx is at the center of the exposure field.	• Angle the CR 10 degrees caudally. • Center the CR to the midsagittal plane at a level 2 inches (5 cm) superior to the symphysis pubis (2 inches inferior to the ASIS).
• 5th sacral segment, three coccygeal vertebrae, symphysis pubis, and pelvic brim are included within the collimated field.	• Center the IR and grid to the CR. • Open the longitudinal collimation to the symphysis pubis. • Transversely collimate to a 6-inch (15-cm) field size.

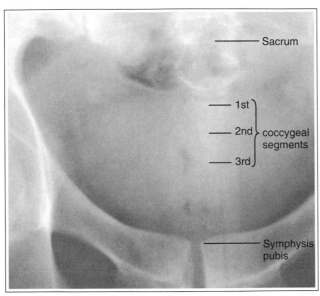

FIGURE 9-45 AP axial coccygeal projection with accurate positioning.

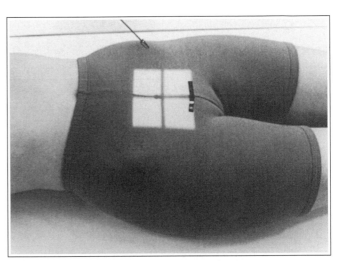

FIGURE 9-46 Proper patient positioning for AP axial coccygeal projection.

COCCYX: AP AXIAL PROJECTION

See Table 9-8, (Figures 9-45 and 9-46).

Emptying Bladder and Rectum. The patient's urinary bladder should be emptied before the procedure. It is also suggested that the colon be free of gas and fecal material. Both procedures will prevent overlap of these materials onto the coccyx, thereby improving its visualization (Figures 9-47 and 9-48).

Rotation. Rotation is detected on an AP coccyx projection by evaluating the alignment of the long axis of the coccyx with the symphysis pubis and by comparing the distances from the coccyx to the lateral walls of the inlet pelvis. If the patient was rotated away from the supine position, the coccyx moves in a direction opposite the direction of the symphysis pubis and is positioned closer to the lateral pelvic wall situated farther from the table and IR. If the patient was rotated into an LPO position,

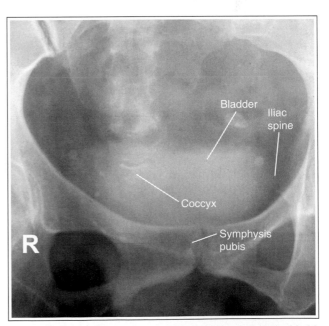

FIGURE 9-47 AP axial coccyx projection taken without the bladder emptied and with the patient rotated onto the left side.

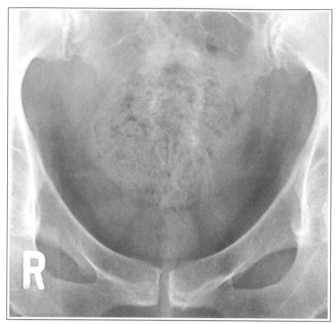

FIGURE 9-48 AP axial coccyx projection demonstrating fecal matter superimposed over the coccyx.

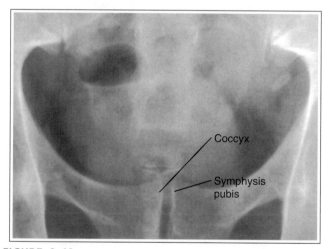

FIGURE 9-49 AP axial coccyx projection demonstrating insufficient caudal CR angulation.

the coccyx is rotated toward the right side (see Figure 9-47). If the patient was rotated into an RPO position, the coccyx is rotated toward the left side.

CR and Coccyx Alignment. When the patient is in an AP projection with the legs extended, the coccyx curves anteriorly and is located beneath the symphysis pubis. To demonstrate the coccyx without foreshortening and without overlap by the symphysis pubis, a 10-degree caudal CR angulation is used. This angle aligns the CR perpendicular to the coccyx and projects the symphysis pubis inferiorly. If the AP projection of the coccyx is taken with an insufficient caudal CR angle, the second and third coccygeal vertebrae Iure foreshortened and are superimposed by the symphysis pubis (Figure 9-49).

AP Coccyx Analysis Practice

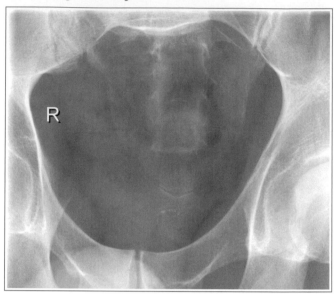

IMAGE 9-7

Analysis. The patient was rotated toward the right side (RPO rotation) and the cephalic CR angulation was slightly insufficient.

Correction. Rotate the patient toward the left side until the midcoronal plane is parallel with the IR and slightly increase the degree of caudal CR angulation.

COCCYX: LATERAL PROJECTION

See Table 9-9, (Figures 9-50 and 9-51).

Rotation. Rotation can be detected on a lateral coccyx projection by evaluating the superimposition of the greater sciatic notches. On a nonrotated lateral coccygeal projection, the greater sciatic notches are superimposed. On rotation the greater sciatic notches are not superimposed but are demonstrated one anterior to the other, and the coccyx and posteriorly situated ischium are almost superimposed on slight rotation and truly superimposed on severe rotation (Figure 9-52). Because the two sides of the pelvis are mirror images, it is difficult to determine which side of the patient was rotated anteriorly and which posteriorly on a lateral coccygeal projection with poor positioning. When rotation has occurred, it is most common for the side of the patient situated farther from the IR to have been rotated anteriorly if a sponge was not placed between the patient's knees, because of the gravitational forward and downward pull on this side's arm and leg.

CR and Vertebral Column

   Detecting Lateral Lumbar Flexion. If the lateral vertebral column is allowed to flex laterally, causing it to sag for the lateral sacral projection, the resulting projection demonstrates a foreshortened coccyx (see discussion in lateral lumbar projection, Figure 9-18).

TABLE 9-9	Lateral Coccygeal Projection
Image Analysis Guidelines (Figure 9-50)	**Related Positioning Procedures (Figure 9-51)**
• Median sacral crest is in profile. • Greater sciatic notches are superimposed.	• Place the patient in a recumbent or upright left lateral position. • Place the shoulders, the posterior ribs, and the ASISs directly on top of one another, aligning the midcoronal plane perpendicular to the IR. • Recumbent: Flex the patient's knees and hips for support, and position a pillow or sponge between the knees that is thick enough to prevent anterior rotation.
• Coccyx is seen without foreshortening.	• Align the vertebral column parallel with the table and place the interiliac line perpendicular to the table.
• Coccyx is at the center of the exposure field.	• Center a perpendicular CR 3.5 inches (9 cm) posterior and 2 inches (5 cm) inferior to the elevated ASIS.
• 5th sacral segment, 1st through 3rd coccygeal vertebrae, and inferior median sacral crest are included within the exposure field.	• Center the IR and grid to the CR. • Longitudinally and transversely collimate to a 4-inch (10-cm) field size.

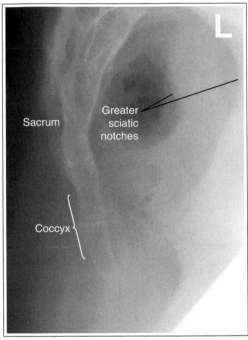

FIGURE 9-50 Lateral coccygeal projection with accurate positioning.

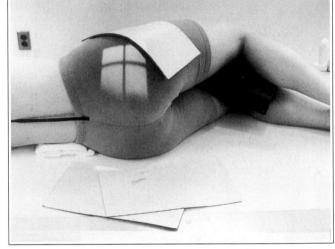

FIGURE 9-51 Proper patient positioning for lateral coccygeal projection.

Adjusting for the Sagging Vertebral Column. Two methods may be used to overcome the sagging vertebral column:

1. Place a radiolucent sponge between the patient's lateral body surface and table just superior to the iliac crest to elevate the vertebral column, aligning it parallel with the table (see Figure 9-30); use a perpendicular CR.
2. Leave the patient positioned as is and angle the CR caudally until it parallels the interiliac line (Figure 9-33).

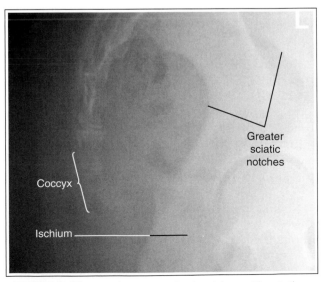

FIGURE 9-52 Lateral coccyx projection taken with rotation.

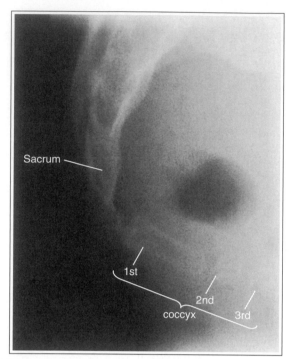

FIGURE 9-53 Lateral coccyx projection taken with excessive collimation.

Collimation. Because tight collimation is essential to obtain optimal recorded detail visibility, collimate longitudinally and transversely to a 4-inch (10-cm) field. The third coccygeal vertebra is situated slightly more anteriorly than the first coccygeal vertebra. With injury, this anterior position may be increased, causing the coccyx to align transversely (see Figure 9-53). When this condition is suspected, transverse collimation should not be too tight.

Sternum and Ribs

OUTLINE

Sternum: PA Oblique Projection
(Right Anterior Oblique
Position), 447
Sternum: Lateral
Projection, 450

Ribs: AP or PA Projection
(Above or Below
Diaphragm), 453
AP/PA Rib Projection
Analysis Practice, 457

Ribs: AP Oblique Projection
(Right and Left Posterior
Oblique Positions), 457
AP/PA Oblique Rib Projection
Analysis Practice, 460

OBJECTIVES

*After completion of this chapter, you should be able to do
the following:*

- Identify the required anatomy on sternal and rib
projections.
- Describe how to properly position the patient, image
receptor (IR), and central ray (CR) on sternal and rib
projections.
- List the image analysis requirements for sternal and rib
projections with accurate positioning and state how to
reposition the patient when less than optimal
projections are produced.
- Describe how the patient is positioned to achieve
homogeneous density on PA oblique sternal
projections.

- Explain why a 30-inch (76 cm) source–image receptor
distance (SID) is used on PA oblique sternal projections.
- Define costal breathing, and discuss the advantages of
using it for PA oblique sternal projections.
- Describe how thoracic thickness affects how far the
sternum is positioned from the vertebral column when
the patient is rotated.
- List ways of reducing the amount of scatter radiation
that reaches the IR when the sternum is imaged in the
lateral projection.
- Discuss when it is appropriate to take an AP projection
of the ribs rather than a PA projection and why the AP
oblique projection is preferred over the PA oblique
projection when the axillary ribs are imaged.

STERNUM

IMAGE ANALYSIS GUIDELINES

Technical Data. When the technical data in Table 10-1
are followed or adjusted as needed for additive and
destructive patient conditions (see Table 2-6), along
with the best practices discussed in Chapters 1 and 2,
all upper extremity projections will demonstrate the
image analysis guidelines in Box 10-1 unless otherwise
indicated.

STERNUM: PA OBLIQUE PROJECTION (RIGHT ANTERIOR OBLIQUE POSITION)

See Table 10-2, (Figures 10-1 and 10-2).
Why the RAO Position? The right AP oblique projection (RAO position) is used to rotate the sternum from
beneath the thoracic vertebrae. It is chosen over the left
anterior oblique (LAO) position because the RAO position superimposes the heart shadow over the sternum
(Figure 10-3). Because the air-filled lungs and heart

shadow have different atomic densities, they demonstrate distinctly different degrees of brightness on the
resulting projection using the same exposure factors.
The air-filled lungs demonstrate less brightness than the
heart shadow. Positioning the sternum in the heart
shadow ensures homogeneous brightness across the
entire sternum. Any portion of the sternum positioned
outside the heart shadow demonstrates less brightness
than the portion positioned within the heart shadow.
Blurring Overlying Sternal Structures. In the PA
oblique projection, the sternum has many overlying
structures—the posterior ribs, lung markings, heart
shadow, and left inferior scapula. Specific positioning
techniques should be followed to show a sharply defined
sternum while magnifying and blurring these overlying
structures. The SID recommended for the PA oblique
sternum varies among positioning textbooks. It ranges
from 30 to 40 inches (76-100 cm). A short (30-inch) SID
provides increased magnification and blurring of the posterior ribs and left scapula but also results in a higher
patient entrance skin dosage. Facility protocol dictates
the SID that is used. Using a breathing technique, which

TABLE 10-1	Sternum and Ribs Technical Data					
Projection	kV	Grid	AEC	mAs	SID	
PA oblique (RAO position), sternum	70-80	Grid	Center		30-40 inches (75-100 cm)	
Lateral, sternum	75-80	Grid		50	72 inches (180 cm)	
AP or PA, above diaphragm	75-85	Grid	Center		40-48 inches (100-120 cm)	
AP or PA, below diaphragm	80-90	Grid	Center		40-48 inches (100-120 cm)	
PA oblique, above diaphragm	75-85	Grid	Center		40-48 inches (100-120 cm)	
PA oblique, below diaphragm	80-90	Grid	Center		40-48 inches (100-120 cm)	

TABLE 10-2	PA Oblique Sternum Projection
Image Analysis Guidelines (Figure 10-1)	**Related Positioning Procedures (Figure 10-2)**
• Sternum demonstrates homogeneous brightness. • Manubrium, SC joints, sternal body, and xiphoid process are demonstrated within the heart shadow without vertebral superimposition. • Midsternum is at the center of the exposure field.	• Place the patient in a recumbent or upright right PA oblique projection. • Rotate the patient until the midcoronal plane is angled 15 to 20 degrees with the table. • Align the midsternum to the midline of the longitudinal light field line (3 inches to the left of the thoracic spinous processes). • Position the top of the IR 1.5 inches (3.75 cm) superior to the jugular notch. • Center a perpendicular CR to the IR and grid.
• Sternum is demonstrated without motion or distortion. • Ribs and lung markings are blurred. • Posterior ribs and left scapula are magnified. • Jugular notch, SC joints, sternal body, and xiphoid process are included within the exposure field.	• Use a 30- to 40-inch (76-100 cm) SID. • Have patient costal (shallow) breathe while using a long exposure time (3 to 4 seconds). • Open the longitudinal collimation to a 12-inch (30 cm) field size. • Transversely collimate to the thoracic spinous processes and left inferior scapular angle.

SC, Sternoclavicular.

BOX 10-1	Sternum and Ribs Technical Data Imaging Analysis Guidelines

- The facility's identification requirements are visible.
- A right or left marker identifying the correct side of the patient is present on the projection and is not superimposed over the VOI.
- Good radiation protection practices are evident.
- Bony trabecular patterns and cortical outlines of the anatomic structures are sharply defined.
- Contrast resolution is adequate to demonstrate the surrounding soft tissue, bony trabecular patterns, and cortical outlines.
- No quantum mottle or saturation is present.
- Scattered radiation has been kept to a minimum.
- There is no evidence of removable artifacts.

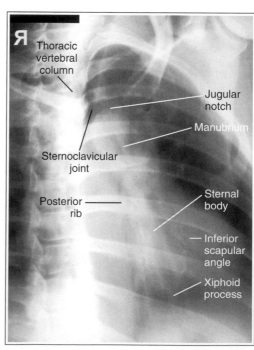

FIGURE 10-1 PA oblique sternum projection (RAO position) with accurate positioning.

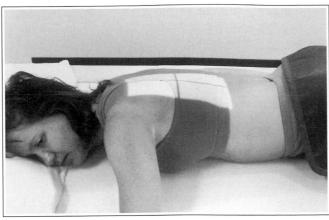

FIGURE 10-2 Proper patient positioning for PA oblique sternum projection (RAO position).

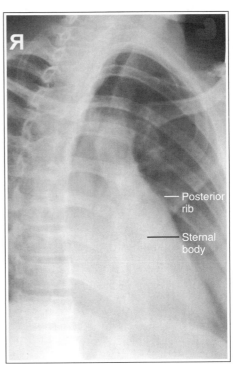

FIGURE 10-4 PA oblique sternum projection taken with the patient breathing deeply instead of shallowly, causing the sternum to move and blur.

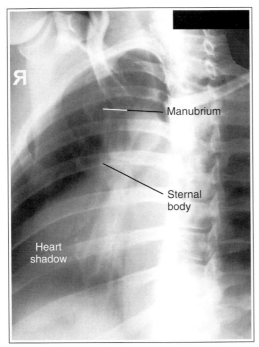

FIGURE 10-3 PA oblique sternal projection taken with the patient in an LAO position.

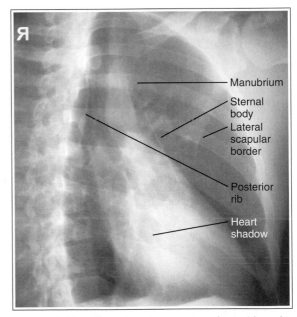

FIGURE 10-5 PA oblique sternal projection taken without breathing technique and with excessive patient obliquity.

requires a long exposure time (3 to 4 seconds) and requires the patient to breathe shallowly (costal breathing) during the exposure, forces upward and outward and downward and inward movements of the ribs and lungs, thus blurring the posterior ribs and lung markings on the projection. Deep breathing requires movement (elevation) of the sternum to provide deep lung expansion and should be avoided during breathing technique because this sternal motion would blur the sternum on the projection (Figure 10-4). If breathing technique is not used, the details and cortical outlines of the posterior ribs, left scapula, and lung markings are sharply defined, and the increased recorded detail obscures the details of the sternum (Figure 10-5).

Patient Obliquity. Rotating the patient until the mid-coronal plane is angled 15 to 20 degrees to the IR draws the sternum from beneath the thoracic vertebrae (see Figure 10-2). This degree of obliquity provides you with a PA oblique projection of the sternum with only a small amount of rotation. To evaluate an anatomic structure sufficiently, two projections of the area of interest, taken 90 degrees from each other, are obtained. The PA oblique (RAO) and lateral projections are obtained to fulfill this requirement for the sternum. Although these are not exactly 90 degrees from each other, it is necessary to rotate the patient slightly for the PA oblique projection to demonstrate the sternum without vertebral superimposition.

Determining the Required Obliquity. To determine the exact obliquity needed to rotate the sternum away from the thoracic vertebral column on a prone patient, place the fingertips of one hand on the right sternoclavicular (SC) joint and the fingertips of the other hand on the spinous processes of the upper thoracic vertebrae. Rotate the patient until your fingers on the SC joint are positioned just to the left of the fingers on the spinous processes.

Evaluating Accuracy of Obliquity. When evaluating a PA oblique sternal projection, note that patient obliquity was sufficient when the sternum is located within the heart shadow and the manubrium and right SC joint are shown without vertebral superimposition. If the patient was not adequately rotated, the right SC joint and manubrium are positioned beneath the vertebral column (Figure 10-6). If patient obliquity was excessive, the sternum is rotated to the left of the heart shadow and the sternum demonstrates excessive transverse foreshortening (see Figure 10-5).

Field Size. The field size used for a PA oblique sternum projection depends on the age and gender of the patient. The adult male sternum is approximately 7 inches (18 cm) long, but the female sternum is considerably shorter. A 10 × 12 inch (24 × 30 cm) field size should sufficiently accommodate male and female adult patients. Because chest depth from the thoracic vertebrae to the

manubrium is less than from the thoracic vertebrae to the xiphoid process, the manubrium remains closer to the thoracic vertebrae than the xiphoid process when the patient is rotated. The sternum, then, is not aligned with the longitudinal plane but is slightly tilted. Because of this sternal tilt, the transverse collimation should be confined to the thoracic spinous processes and the left inferior angle of the scapula.

STERNUM: LATERAL PROJECTION

See Table 10-3, (Figures 10-7 and 10-8).

Positioning for Homogeneous Brightness. Homogeneous brightness over the entire sternum region is difficult to obtain because the lower sternum is superimposed by the pectoral (chest) muscles or by the female breast tissue, whereas the upper sternum is free of this

TABLE 10-3	Lateral Sternum Projection
Image Analysis Guidelines (Figure 10-7)	**Related Positioning Procedures (Figure 10-8)**
• Sternum demonstrates homogeneous brightness.	• Control scatter radiation by tight collimation, using a grid, and placing a lead sheet anterior to the sternum close to the patient's skin line.
• Manubrium, sternal body, and xiphoid process are in profile. • Anterior ribs are not superimposed over the sternum.	• Place the patient upright with the right or left side against the IR in a lateral projection. • Position the shoulders, the posterior ribs, and the ASISs directly on top of each other, aligning the midcoronal plane perpendicular to the IR. • Take exposure after deep suspended inspiration.
• No superimposition of humeral soft tissue over the sternum is present. • Midsternum is at the center of the exposure field.	• Extend the arms behind the back with the hands clasped. • Place the top edge of the IR 1.5 inches (4 cm) above the jugular notch. • Align the sternum to the midline of the longitudinal light field line. • Set the SID at 72 inches (180 cm). • Center a horizontal CR to the IR and grid.
• Jugular notch, sternal body, and xiphoid process are included within the exposure field.	• Collimate longitudinally and transversely to within 0.5 inch (1.25 cm) of the sternum.

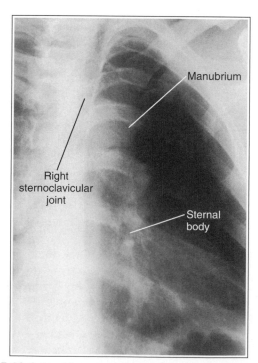

FIGURE 10-6 PA oblique sternal projection taken with insufficient patient obliquity.

Manubrium

Right sternoclavicular joint

Sternal body

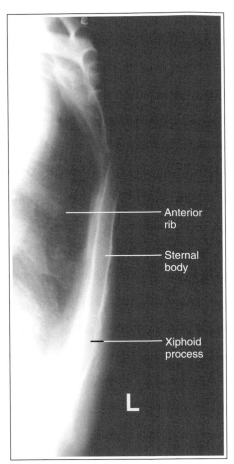

FIGURE 10-7 Lateral sternum projection with accurate positioning.

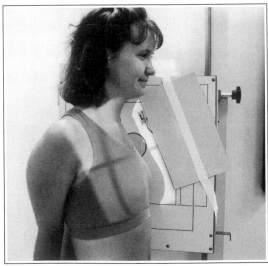

FIGURE 10-8 Proper patient positioning for lateral sternum projection.

superimposition. The amount of brightness difference between the two halves of the sternum depends on the development of the patient's pectoral muscles and the amount of female breast tissue. Enlargement of either tissue requires an increase in exposure to demonstrate the sternum through them. This increase may overexpose

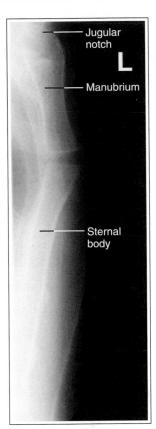

FIGURE 10-9 Lateral sternum projection of superior sternum with accurate positioning.

the upper sternum region on the projection, requiring an additional projection to be taken with a lower exposure so the entire sternum can be demonstrated (Figure 10-9).

Reducing Scatter Radiation. A remarkable amount of scatter radiation is evident on a lateral sternal projection anterior to the sternum. One can be certain that if scatter is demonstrated here, it is also overlying the projection of the sternum, decreasing the overall contrast resolution. To eliminate some of this scatter radiation and produce higher contrast, tightly collimate, use a grid, and place a lead sheet anterior to the sternum close to the patient's skin line (see Figure 10-8). For the upright patient the lead sheet may be taped to the upright IR.

Rotation. Rotation is effectively detected on a lateral sternum projection by evaluating the degree of anterior rib and sternal superimposition. If a lateral sternum projection demonstrates rotation, the right and left anterior ribs are not superimposed; one side is positioned anterior to the sternum and the other side is positioned posterior to the sternum. Determine how to reposition after obtaining a rotated lateral sternal projection by using the heart shadow to identify the right and left anterior ribs. Because the heart shadow is located in the left chest cavity and extends anteroinferiorly, outlining the superior border of the heart shadow enables recognition of the left side of the chest. If the left lung and ribs were

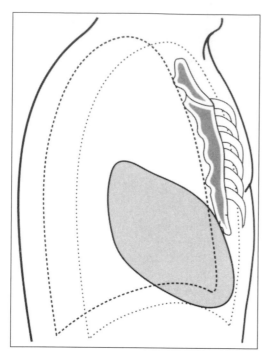

FIGURE 10-10 Rotation—left lung anterior.

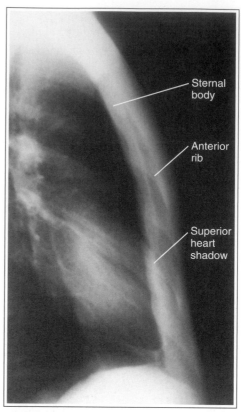

FIGURE 10-11 Lateral sternal projection taken with the left thorax rotated anteriorly.

positioned anterior to the sternum, as shown in Figure 10-10, the outline of the superior heart shadow continues beyond the sternum and into the anteriorly located lung (Figure 10-11). If the right lung and ribs were positioned anterior to the sternum, as shown in Figure 10-12, the superior heart shadow does not continue into the anteriorly situated lung, but ends at the sternum (Figure 10-13). Once the right and left sides of the chest have been identified, reposition the patient by rotating the thorax. If the left lung and ribs were anteriorly positioned, rotate the left thorax posteriorly. If the right lung and ribs were anteriorly positioned, rotate the right thorax posteriorly.

Respiration. Elevation of the sternum, resulting from deep suspended inspiration, aids in better sternal demonstration by drawing the sternum away from the anterior ribs.

Humerus Positioning. Extending the patient's arms behind the back with the hands clasped positions the humeral soft tissue away from the sternum.

The Supine Patient. If the patient is unable to be positioned upright, a lateral sternum projection can be obtained with the patient supine. In this position, rest the patient's arms against the sides, position a grid cassette vertically against the patient's arm, and use a horizontal beam. All other positioning and analysis requirements are the same as for an upright projection.

Source-Image Distance. A 72-inch (180 cm) source-image distance (SID) is used to minimize the sternal magnification that would result because of the long sternum to IR distance.

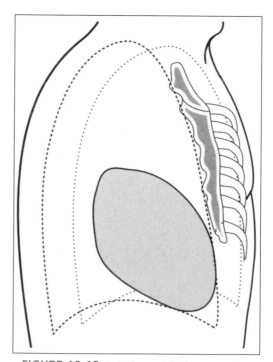

FIGURE 10-12 Rotation—right lung anterior.

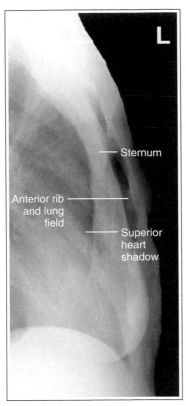

FIGURE 10-13 Lateral sternal projection taken with the right thorax rotated anteriorly.

RIBS

RIBS: AP OR PA PROJECTION (ABOVE OR BELOW DIAPHRAGM)

See Table 10-4, (Figures 10-14, 10-15, 10-16, and 10-17). **Soft Tissue Structures of Interest.** The demonstration of the soft tissue structures that surround the ribs is very important. When an upper rib fracture is suspected, the surrounding upper thorax, axillary, and neck soft tissues and vascular lung markings are carefully studied for signs (e.g., hematoma, presence of air) that indicate associated lung pathology (e.g., pneumothorax, interstitial emphysema) or rupture of the trachea, bronchus, or aorta. When a lower rib fracture is suspected, the upper abdominal tissue is examined for signs of associated injury to the kidney, liver, spleen, or diaphragm.

AP versus PA Projection. When the patient complains of anterior rib pain, take a PA projection to place the anterior ribs closer to the IR. When the posterior ribs are the affected ribs, take an AP projection to place the posterior ribs closer to the IR. Compare the difference in posterior rib detail sharpness in Figures 10-14 and 10-15. Figure 10-14 was obtained in an AP projection and Figure 10-15 in a PA projection. Note how the posterior ribs in Figure 10-15 are magnified, demonstrating

TABLE 10-4	AP or PA Rib Projection	
Image Analysis Guidelines (Figures 10-14 and 10-15)	**Related Positioning Procedures (Figures 10-16 and 10-17)**
• Rib magnification is kept to a minimum.	• *Anterior ribs:* Place the patient in a prone or upright PA projection. • *Posterior ribs:* Place the patient in a supine or upright AP projection.
• A rib marker is present.	• Tape a rib marker on the patient's skin near the area where the ribs are tender to pinpoint the location of potential injury.
• Thoracic vertebrae–rib head articulations are demonstrated. • Sternum and vertebral column are superimposed. • Distances from the vertebral column to the sternal ends of the clavicles, when seen, are equal. • Distances from the spinous processes to the pedicles on each side are equal.	• Position the shoulders, the posterior ribs, and the ASISs at equal distances from the IR, aligning the midcoronal plane parallel with the IR.
Above Diaphragm • Scapula is outside the lung field.	**Above Diaphragm** • *AP projection:* Abduct the arm and internally rotate the elbows and shoulders anteriorly. • *PA projection:* Abduct and slightly flex the arms and rotate them internally. • Elevate the chin.
• 8 posterior ribs are seen above the diaphragm. • 7th posterior rib is at the center of the exposure field.	• Take the exposure after deep suspended inspiration. • *AP projection:* Center a perpendicular CR halfway between the midsagittal plane and the affected lateral rib surface, at the level halfway between the jugular notch and xiphoid process. • *PA projection:* Center a perpendicular CR halfway between the midsagittal plane and the affected lateral rib surface, at the level of the inferior scapular angle.

Continued

TABLE 10-4	AP or PA Ribs Projection—cont'd	
Image Analysis Guidelines (Figures 10-14 and 10-15)		**Related Positioning Procedures (Figures 10-16 and 10-17)**
• Affected side's 1st through 9th ribs and vertebral column are included within the exposure field.		• Center the IR and grid to the CR. • Open the longitudinal collimation to a 17-inch (43 cm) field. • Transversely collimate to the thoracic vertebral column and the patient's lateral skin line.
Below Diaphragm • 8th through 12th posterior ribs are demonstrated below the diaphragm.		**Below Diaphragm** • Take the exposure after full expiration.
• 10th posterior rib is at the center of the exposure field.		• Place the lower edge of the IR at the level of the iliac crest. • Center the IR's long axis halfway between the midsagittal plane and the affected lateral rib surface. • Center a perpendicular CR to the IR and grid.
• Part of the thoracic and lumbar vertebral column and the 8th through 12th ribs of the affected side of the patient are included within the exposure field.		• Open the longitudinal collimation to a 17-inch (43 cm) field size. • Transversely collimate to the vertebral column and within 0.5 inch (1.25 cm) of the lateral skin line.

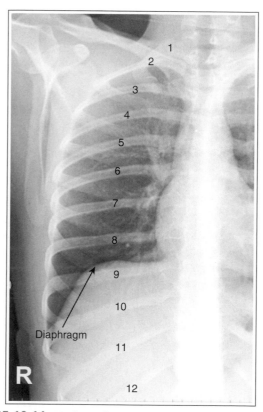

FIGURE 10-14 AP above-diaphragm rib projection with accurate positioning.

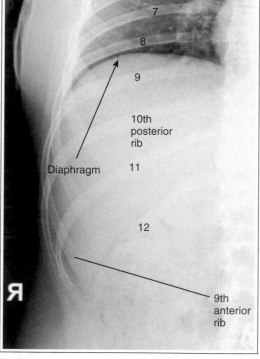

FIGURE 10-15 PA below-diaphragm rib projection with accurate positioning.

less detail sharpness than the posterior ribs in Figure 10-14, which were positioned closer to the IR for the projection.

Rotation. Rotation is effectively detected on an AP or PA rib projection by evaluating the sternum and vertebral column superimposition and by comparing the distances between the vertebral column and the sternal ends of the clavicles and the distances from the pedicles to the spinous processes. When a projection of the ribs demonstrates rotation and the patient was in an AP projection, the side of the patient positioned closer to the IR demonstrates the sternum and SC joint without vertebral column superimposition, and the greatest spinous process to pedicle distance (Figure 10-18). The opposite is true for a PA projection—the side of the chest positioned farther from the IR demonstrates the sternum and the

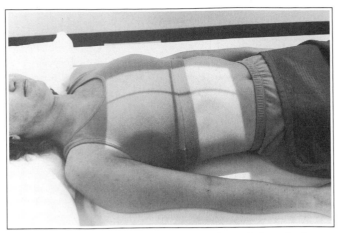

FIGURE 10-16 Proper patient positioning for AP below-diaphragm rib projection.

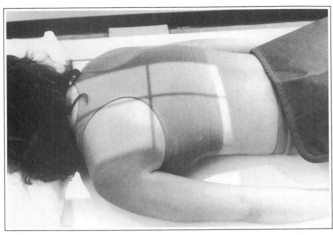

FIGURE 10-17 Proper patient positioning for PA above-diaphragm rib projection.

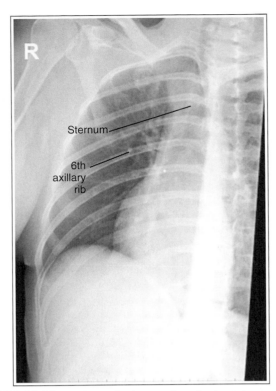

FIGURE 10-18 AP above-diaphragm rib projection taken with the patient rotated toward the right side.

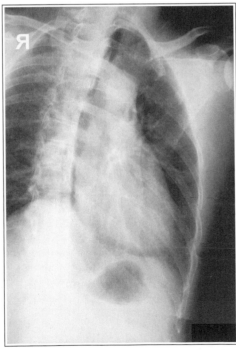

FIGURE 10-19 PA above-diaphragm rib projection taken with the patient rotated toward the right side.

SC joint without vertebral column superimposition and the greatest spinous process to pedicle distance (Figure 10-19).

Scoliosis versus Rotation. In projections of patients with spinal scoliosis, the ribs and vertebral column will appear rotated because of the lateral deviation of the vertebrae (Figure 10-20). Become familiar with this condition to prevent unnecessarily repeated procedures on these patients.

Respiration. The number of ribs located above or below the diaphragm is determined by the depth of patient inspiration. In full suspended inspiration, up to 10 axillary ribs may be demonstrated above the diaphragm. In expiration, only seven or eight axillary ribs are clearly visible above the diaphragm, and four or five ribs are demonstrated below the diaphragm. When the above-diaphragm ribs are imaged, take the exposure on full inspiration to maximize the number of ribs located above the diaphragm. Any ribs situated below the diaphragm will not be well demonstrated because the increase in exposure would be needed to demonstrate the abdominal tissue they surround. When below-diaphragm ribs are imaged, it is necessary to use a higher kV and exposure than needed for the above-diaphragm ribs to penetrate the denser abdominal tissue. Any ribs situated above the diaphragm for this projection may have

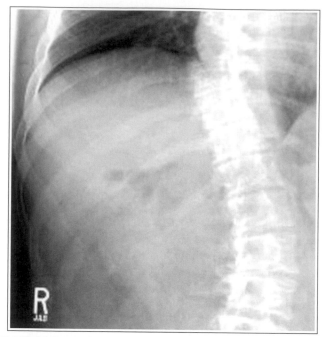

FIGURE 10-20 AP above-diaphragm rib projection taken of a patient with spinal scoliosis.

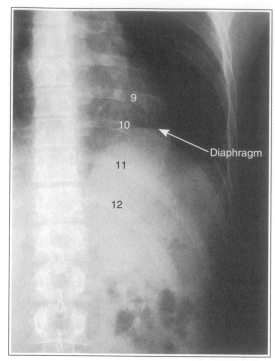

FIGURE 10-21 PA below-diaphragm rib projection taken after full inspiration.

insufficient brightness to evaluate (Figure 10-21). To maximize the number of ribs located below the diaphragm, take the exposure on full suspended expiration.

Locating the Inferior Scapula to Center the CR in a PA Projection and Remove Scapula from Exposure Field. Palpate the inferior scapular angle with the arm next to the patient's body. After accurate centering has been accomplished, abduct the arm to position it out of the collimated field. Abducting the arm shifts the inferior scapular angle laterally and inferiorly, so centering should be accomplished before arm abduction. Internally rotating the arm places the elbows and shoulders anteriorly and positions the scapula outside the lung field (Figure 10-22).

CR Positioning When Both Sides of the Rib Are Examined on One Projection. It should be noted that some positioning textbooks suggest that PA or AP above- and below-diaphragm rib projections be taken to include both sides of the ribs on the same projection. For this positioning, the CR is centered to the midsagittal plane instead of halfway between the midsagittal plane and lateral rib surface transfers fields size is increased to 17 inches (43 cm).

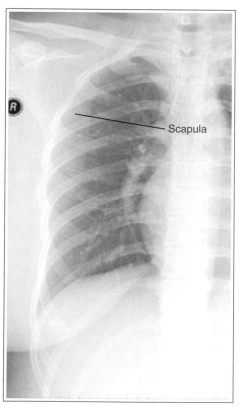

FIGURE 10-22 AP above-diaphragm rib projection taken without the right elbow and shoulder anteriorly rotated.

AP/PA Rib Projection Analysis Practice

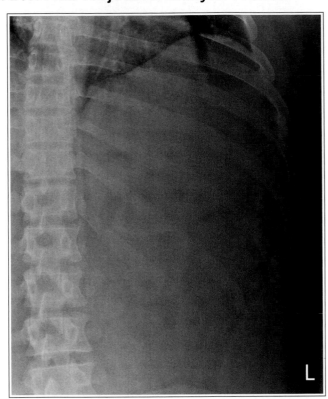

IMAGE 10-1 AP above-diaphragm.

Analysis. The distance from the spinous processes to the left lumbar pedicles is larger than the same distance from the right pedicles to the spinous processes. The patient was rotated toward the left side.

Correction. Rotate the patient toward the right side until the midcoronal plane is parallel with the IR.

RIBS: AP OBLIQUE PROJECTION (RIGHT AND LEFT POSTERIOR OBLIQUE POSITIONS)

See Table 10-5, (Figures 10-23, 10-24, 10-25 and 10-26).

Controlling Magnification. Oblique ribs may be performed using AP and PA oblique projections but, to provide maximum axillary rib detail, the AP oblique projection (right posterior oblique [RPO] and left posterior oblique [LPO] positions) should be routinely performed. In the AP oblique projection (see Figure 10-24), the axillary ribs are placed closer to the IR than in the PA oblique projection (Figure 10-27), resulting in less rib magnification and greater recorded detail.

Patient Obliquity. To open up the curvature of the axillary ribs, rotate the patient toward the affected side until the midcoronal plane is angled 45 degrees with the IR, placing the axillary ribs parallel with the IR (see Figures 10-25 and 10-26). If the patient is rotated in the opposite

TABLE 10-5	AP Oblique Rib Projection
Image Analysis Guidelines (Figures 10-23 and 10-24)	**Related Positioning Procedures (Figures 10-25 and 10-26)**
• Rib magnification is kept to a minimum. • Inferior sternal body is located halfway between the vertebral column and the lateral rib surface. • Axillary ribs are demonstrated without superimposition and are located in the center of the exposure field. • Anterior ribs are located at the lateral edge.	• Use the AP oblique projection. • Begin with the patient in a supine or upright AP projection. • Rotate the thorax toward the affected side until the midcoronal plane is at a 45-degree angle with the IR.
Above Diaphragm • 8 axillary ribs are demonstrated above the diaphragm. • 7th axillary rib is at the center of the exposure field.	**Above Diaphragm** • Take the exposure after deep suspended inspiration. • Center a perpendicular CR halfway between the midsagittal plane and the affected lateral rib surface at a level halfway between the jugular notch and the xiphoid process.
• 1st through 10th axillary ribs of the affected side and thoracic vertebral column are included within the exposure field.	• Center the IR and grid to the CR. • Open the longitudinal collimation to a 17-inch (43 cm) field size. • Transversely collimate to the thoracic vertebral column and the patient's lateral skin line.
Below Diaphragm • 9th through 12th axillary ribs are demonstrated below the diaphragm. • 10th axillary rib is at the center of the exposure field.	**Below Diaphragm** • Take the exposure after full expiration. • Place the lower edge of the IR at the level of the iliac crest. • Center the IR's long axis halfway between the midsagittal plane and the affected lateral rib surface. • Center a perpendicular CR to the IR and grid.
• Part of the thoracic and lumbar vertebral column and the 8th through 12th axillary ribs of the affected side of the patient are included within the exposure field.	• Open the longitudinal collimation to a 17-inch (43 cm) field size. • Transversely collimate to the vertebral column and within 0.5 inch (1.25 cm) of the lateral skin line.

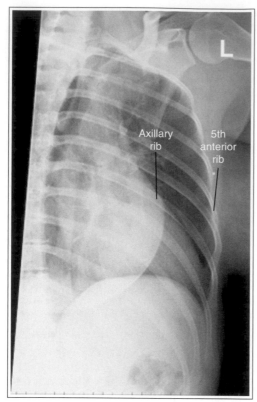

FIGURE 10-23 AP oblique above-diaphragm rib projection (RPO position) with accurate positioning.

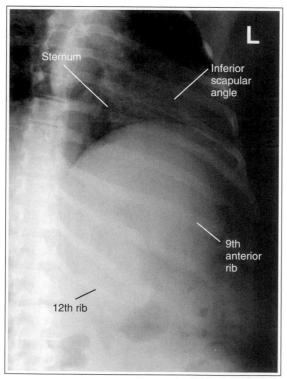

FIGURE 10-24 AP oblique below-diaphragm rib projection (RPO position) with accurate positioning.

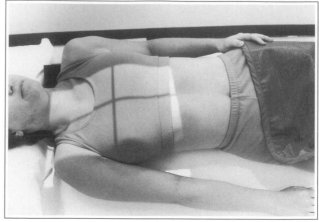

FIGURE 10-25 Proper patient positioning for AP oblique above-diaphragm rib projection (RPO position).

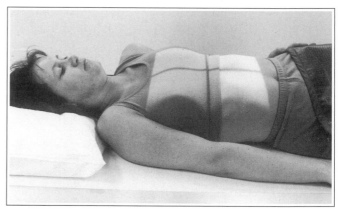

FIGURE 10-26 Proper patient positioning for AP oblique below-diaphragm rib projection (RPO position).

direction, the axillary ribs demonstrate increased foreshortening (see Figure 10-28).

Because the sternum rotates toward the affected axillary ribs on thoracic rotation, the position of the sternum can be used to identify the accuracy of patient rotation. If the inferior sternum is positioned halfway between the vertebral column and the anterior ribs, the patient was rotated 45 degrees and the axillary ribs are "opened." When the desired 45-degree obliquity has not been obtained, view the position of the inferior sternum to determine how to reposition the patient. If the sternal body is demonstrated next to the vertebral column, the patient was insufficiently rotated (Figure 10-29). If the inferior sternal body is demonstrated laterally, the patient was rotated more than 45 degrees.

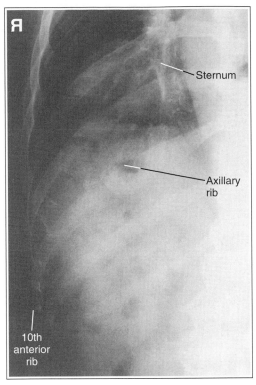

FIGURE 10-27 PA oblique below-diaphragm rib projection demonstrating magnified axillary ribs.

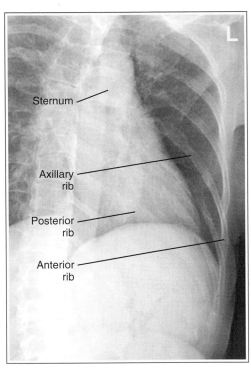

FIGURE 10-29 AP oblique above-diaphragm rib projection demonstrating insufficient obliquity.

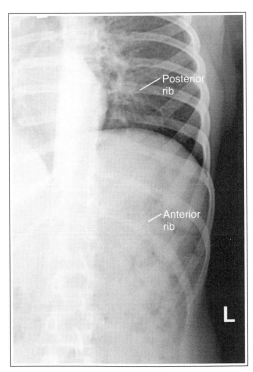

FIGURE 10-28 AP oblique below-diaphragm rib projection with patient rotated in the wrong direction.

Respiration. The number of ribs located above or below the diaphragm is determined by the depth of patient inspiration. In full suspended inspiration, up to 10 axillary ribs may be demonstrated above the diaphragm. In expiration, only seven or eight axillary ribs are clearly visible above the diaphragm, and four or five ribs are demonstrated below the diaphragm. When the above-diaphragm ribs are imaged, take the exposure on full inspiration to maximize the number of ribs located above the diaphragm. Any ribs situated below the diaphragm will not be well demonstrated because the increase in exposure would be needed to demonstrate the abdominal tissue they surround. When below-diaphragm ribs are imaged, it is necessary to use a higher kV and exposure than needed for the above-diaphragm ribs to penetrate the denser abdominal tissue. Any ribs situated above the diaphragm for this projection may have insufficient brightness to evaluate. To maximize the number of ribs located below the diaphragm, take the exposure on full suspended expiration.

AP/PA Oblique Rib Projection Analysis Practice

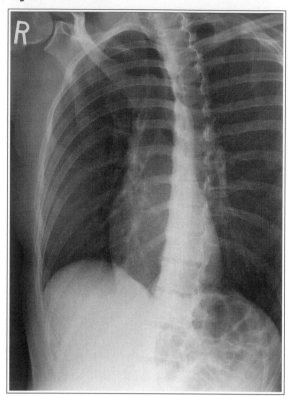

IMAGE 10-2 AP above-diaphragm.

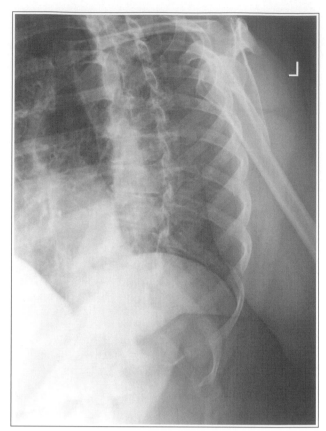

IMAGE 10-3 PA below-diaphragm.

Analysis. The inferior sternal body is demonstrated next to the vertebral column; the patient was insufficiently rotated.

Correction. Increase the degree of rotation until the midcoronal plane is at a 45-degree angle with the IR.

Analysis. The left side axillary ribs demonstrate excessive foreshortening. The patient was rotated the wrong direction.

Correction. Rotate the patient into a RAO 45-degree position.

Cranium, Facial Bones, and Paranasal Sinuses

OUTLINE

Cranium and Mandible: PA or AP
Projection, 462
   PA or AP Analysis Practice, 467
Cranium, Facial Bones, and Sinuses:
PA or AP Axial Projection
(Caldwell Method), 468
   PA/AP Axial Analysis
   Practice, 471
Cranium and Mandible: AP Axial
Projection (Towne Method), 472

AP Axial (Towne) Analysis
Practice, 475
Cranium, Facial Bones, Nasal
Bones, and Sinuses: Lateral
Projection, 476
   Lateral Projection Analysis
   Practice, 478
Cranium, Mandible, and Sinuses:
Submentovertex (SMV) Projection
(Schueller Method), 479

SMV Projection Analysis
Practice, 481
Facial Bones and Sinuses:
Parietoacanthial and
Acanthioparietal Projection
(Waters and Open-Mouth
Methods), 481
   Parietoacanthial and
   Acanthioparietal Projection
   Analysis Practice, 485

OBJECTIVES

After completion of this chapter, you should be able to do the following:

- Identify the required anatomy on cranial, facial bone, nasal bones, mandible, and sinus projections.
- Describe how to position the patient, image receptor (IR), and central ray (CR) properly on cranial, facial bone, nasal bones, mandible, and sinus projections.
- List the analysis guidelines for cranial, facial bone, nasal bones, mandible, and sinus projections with accurate positioning.
- State how to reposition the patient properly when cranial, facial bone, nasal bones, mandible, and sinus projections with poor positioning are produced.
- Discuss how to determine the amount of patient or CR adjustment required to improve cranial, facial bone, nasal bones, mandible, and sinus projections with poor positioning.

- State the kilovoltage routinely used for cranial, facial bone, nasal bones, mandible, and sinus projections, and describe which anatomic structures are visible when the correct technique factors are used.
- State how the CR is adjusted to obtain accurate cranial positioning when the patient has a suspected cervical injury or is unable to adequately align the head with the IR.
- Define and state the common abbreviations used for the cranial positioning lines.
- Discuss why the parietoacanthial (Waters) projection is taken with the mouth open.
- Explain how the patient and CR are positioned to demonstrate accurate air-fluid levels in the sinus cavities.

KEY TERMS

lips-meatal line (LML)   mentomeatal line (MML)   orbitomeatal line (OML)

IMAGE ANALYSIS GUIDELINES

Technical Data. When the technical data in Table 11-1 are followed, or adjusted as needed for additive and destructive patient conditions (see Table 2-6), along with the best practices discussed in Chapters 1 and 2 all upper extremity projections will demonstrate the image analysis guidelines in Box 11-1 unless otherwise indicated.

Cranial Positioning Lines. Lines that connect facial landmarks are used when positioning the patient for cranium, facial bones, and sinus projections. Table 11-2 lists and defines the landmarks used in the information presented.

Trauma Cranial Imaging (Cervical Vertebral Injuries Precaution). For trauma cranial projections, the patient is placed supine on the table. If injury to the cervical

TABLE 11-1 | **Cranium, Facial Bones and Paranasal Sinus Technical Data**

Projection	Structure	kV	Grid	AEC	mAs	SID
AP or PA	Cranium	80-85	Grid	Center		40-48 inches (100-120 cm)
	Mandible	75-85	Grid		10	
PA axial (Caldwell method)	Cranium	80-85	Grid	Center		40-48 inches (100-120 cm)
	Facial bones	75-85	Grid	Center		
	Sinuses	75-85	Grid			
AP axial (Towne method)	Cranium	80-85	Grid	Center		40-48 inches (100-120 cm)
	Mandible	75-85	Grid		12	
Lateral	Cranium	80-85	Grid	Center		40-48 inches (100-120 cm)
	Facial bones	70-80	Grid	Center		
	Sinuses	75-85	Grid		6	
	Nasal bones	60-70			1	
Submentovertex (Schueller method)	Cranium	80-90	Grid	Center		40-48 inches (100-120 cm)
	Mandible	75-90	Grid	Center		
	Sinuses	75-85	Grid	Center		
Parietoacanthial (Waters method)	Facial bones	75-85	Grid	Center		40-48 inches (100-120 cm)
	Sinuses	75-85	Grid		25	

TABLE 11-2 | **Cranial Positioning Landmarks**

Acanthion	Point on the midsagittal plane where the nose and upper lip meet.
External auditory meatus (EAM)	External ear canal opening.
Glabella	Point located on the midsagittal plane at the level of the eyebrows.
Nasion	Point located on the midsagittal plane at the level of the eyes; depression at the bridge of the nose.
Outer canthus	Point where the top and bottom eyelids meet laterally; outer corner of eyelid.
Cranial Positioning Lines	
Infraorbitomeatal line (IOML)	Line connecting the inferior orbital margin and EAM.
Interpupillary line (IPL)	Line connecting the outer corners of the eyelids.
Lips-meatal line (LML)	Line connecting the lips (with mouth closed) and EAM.
Mentomeatal line (MML)	Line connecting the chin and EAM.
Orbitomeatal line (OML)	Line connecting the outer canthus and EAM. Line is 7-8 degrees superior to IOML.

BOX 11-1 | **Cranium, Facial Bone, Nasal Bone, and Paranasal Sinus Imaging Analysis Guidelines**

- The facility's identification requirements are visible.
- A right or left marker identifying the correct side of the patient is present on the projection and is not superimposed over the VOI.
- Good radiation protection practices are evident.
- Bony trabecular patterns and cortical outlines of the anatomic structures are sharply defined.
- Contrast resolution is adequate to demonstrate the air-filled cavities, sinuses, and mastoids, and bony structures of the cranium, facial bones, nasal bones, and mandible, when present.
- No quantum mottle or saturation is present.
- Scattered radiation has been kept to a minimum.
- There is no evidence of removable artifacts.

vertebrae is suspected, do not adjust the patient's head to obtain the positioning as described in the projections below; instead, take the projection with the head positioned as is. If a cervical vertebral injury is not in question or if it has been cleared by the radiologist, adjust the head as indicated. Trauma projections should meet all the requirements listed for the corresponding non-trauma projections following, although some features of the cranium will appear different because of the increased magnification of the structures situated farther from the IR. For example, in the AP projection the orbits are positioned farther from the IR than the lateral parietal bones, whereas in the PA projection the lateral parietal bones are farther from the IR. This difference will cause the projection to demonstrate less distance from the oblique orbital line to the lateral cranial cortices on the AP than on the PA projection. (Compare Figures 11-12 and 11-13, and Figures 11-40 and 11-44.)

CRANIUM AND MANDIBLE: PA OR AP PROJECTION

See Table 11-3, (Figures 11-1, 11-2, and 11-3).

TABLE 11-3	PA or AP Cranium and Mandible Projection
Image Analysis Guidelines (Figures 11-1 and 11-2)	**Related Positioning Procedures (Figure 11-3)**
• Distances from the lateral margin of orbits to the lateral cranial cortices, from the crista galli to the lateral cranial cortices, and from the mandibular rami to the lateral cervical vertebrae on both sides are equal.	• *PA:* Position the patient in a prone or upright PA projection. Rest the nose and forehead against the IR. • *AP:* Position the patient in a supine AP projection. *(Cervical vertebrae injuries must be cleared before proceeding. See precaution above.)* • Adjust head rotation to align the midsagittal plane perpendicular to the IR.
• Anterior clinoids and dorsum sellae are seen superior to the ethmoid sinuses. • Petrous ridges are superimposed over the supraorbital margins. • Internal acoustic meatus is visualized horizontally through the center of the orbits.	• Tuck the chin toward the chest until the OML is aligned perpendicular to the IR.
• *Mandible:* The mouth is closed with the teeth together.	• Instruct the patient to close the jaw, with teeth and lips placed together.
• Crista galli and nasal septum are aligned with the long axis of the exposure field. • Supraorbital margins and TMJs are demonstrated on the same horizontal plane.	• Adjust head tilting to align the midsagittal plane with the collimator's longitudinal light line.
• *Cranium:* Dorsum sellae is at the center of the exposure field. • *Mandible:* A point midway between the mandibular rami is at the center of the exposure field.	• *Cranium:* Center a perpendicular CR to exit (PA) or enter (AP) at the glabella. • *Mandible:* Center a perpendicular CR to exit (PA) or enter (AP) at the acanthion.
• *Cranium:* Outer cranial cortex and the maxillary sinuses are included within the exposure field. • *Mandible:* Entire mandible is included within the exposure field.	• Center the IR and grid to the CR. • *Cranium:* Open the longitudinal and transverse collimation fields to within 0.5 inch (1.25 cm) of the head skin line. • *Mandible:* Open the longitudinal collimation fields to include the orbits and chin, and transversely collimate to within 0.5 inch (1.25 cm) of the lateral skin line.

TMJ, Temporomandibular joint.

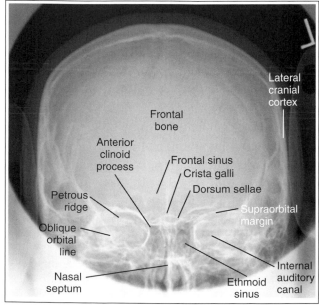

FIGURE 11-1 PA cranial projection with accurate positioning.

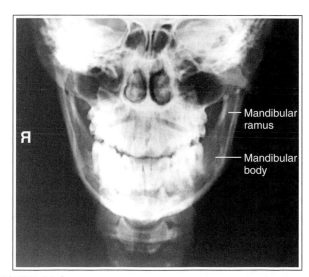

FIGURE 11-2 PA mandible projection with accurate positioning. *(From Ballinger PW, Frank ED:* Merrill's atlas of radiographic positions and radiologic procedures, *vol 2, ed 10, St Louis, 2005, Elsevier, p. 382).*

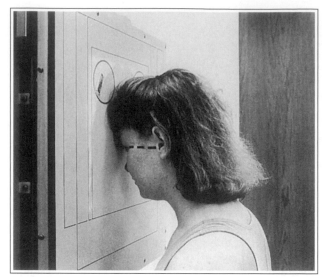

FIGURE 11-3 Proper patient positioning for PA cranial projection.

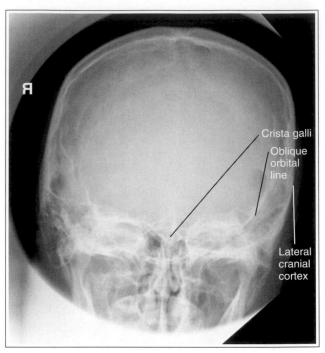

Crista galli

Oblique orbital line

Lateral cranial cortex

FIGURE 11-4 PA cranium projection taken with the patient's face rotated toward the left side.

Head Rotation. Positioning the midsagittal plane perpendicular to the IR prevents cranial rotation. The best method of accomplishing this goal is to place an extended flat palm next to each lateral parietal bone. Then adjust the head rotation until your hands are perpendicular to the IR and parallel with each other. Head rotation is present on a PA/AP projection if the distance from the lateral margins of orbit to the lateral cranial cortices on one side is greater than on the other side, the distance from the crista galli to the lateral cranial margin on one side is greater than on the other side, and the distance from the mandibular rami on one side is greater than on the other side (Figure 11-4). The patient's face was rotated away from the side demonstrating the greater distance.

Orbitomeatal Line and IR Alignment. To position the anterior clinoids and dorsum sellae superior to the ethmoid sinuses, tuck the chin toward the chest until the orbitomeatal line (OML) is perpendicular to the IR. This positioning moves the frontal bone inferiorly, until it is parallel with the IR, and the orbits inferiorly, until the supraorbital margins are situated beneath the petrous ridges, and places the petrous pyramids and internal acoustic meatus within the orbits.

Adjusting CR for Poor OML Alignment. If the patient is unable to tuck the chin adequately to position the OML perpendicular to the IR, the CR angle may be adjusted to compensate. Instruct the patient to tuck the chin to place the OML as close as possible to perpendicular to the IR. Then angle the CR parallel with the OML; this is accomplished by aligning the collimator's transverse light line with the OML.

Detecting Poor OML Alignment. Poor OML alignment can be detected by evaluating the relationship of the petrous ridges and supraorbital margin. If the chin was not adequately tucked to bring the OML perpendicular to the IR, the petrous ridges are demonstrated inferior to the supraorbital margins, the internal acoustic meatus is obscured by the infraorbital margins, and the dorsum sellae and anterior clinoids are demonstrated within the ethmoid sinuses (Figures 11-5 and 11-6). If the chin was tucked more than needed to bring the OML perpendicular to the IR, the petrous ridges are demonstrated superior to the supraorbital margins, the internal acoustic meatus is distorted, and the dorsum sellae and anterior clinoids are clearly visualized superior to the ethmoid sinuses (Figures 11-7 and 11-8). When adjusting for poor OML alignment, because the petrous ridges, dorsum sellae, and anterior clinoids are centrally located in the cranium at the cranial and cervical vertebrae pivot point, the head must be adjusted the full distance demonstrated between the petrous ridges and supraorbital margins to move the patient the needed amount. For example, if the petrous ridges are demonstrated one-half inch inferior to the supraorbital margin on a less than optimal projection the chin would need to be tucked one-half inch to superimpose the petrous ridges and supraorbital margin and obtain an optimal projection. (See the "Steps for Repositioning the Patient for Repeat Projections" section in Chapter 1 for a more complete discussion on this subject.)

Trauma AP Projection. For a trauma AP projection taken on a patient who cannot adjust the head to accurately align the OML, angle the CR until it is aligned with the OML, as shown in Figure 11-9. The angulation required varies according to the chin elevation provided by the cervical collar but is most often between 10 and 15 degrees caudad.

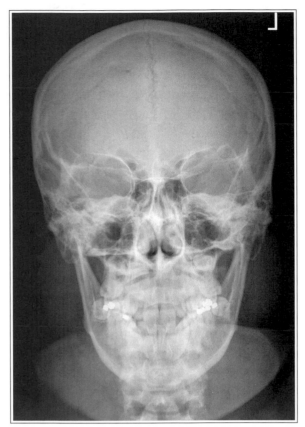

FIGURE 11-5 PA cranial projection taken with the chin insufficiently tucked to bring the OML perpendicular with the IR.

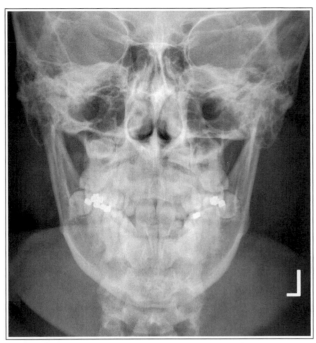

FIGURE 11-6 PA mandible projection taken with the chin insufficiently tucked to bring the OML perpendicular with the IR.

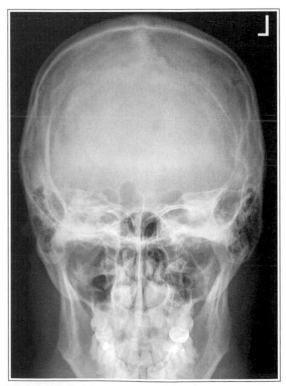

FIGURE 11-7 PA cranial projection taken with the chin tucked more than needed to bring the OML perpendicular with the IR.

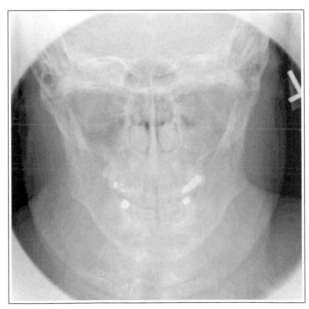

FIGURE 11-8 PA mandible projection taken with the chin tucked more than needed to bring the OML perpendicular with the IR.

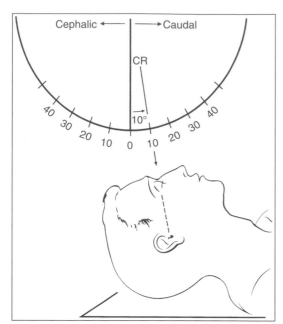

FIGURE 11-9 Proper patient positioning for AP cranial projection. CR, Central ray. *(Reproduced with permission from Martensen K: Trauma Skulls [In-Service Reviews in Radiologic Technology, vol 15, no 5], Birmingham, AL, 1991, Educational Reviews.)*

Correcting the CR Angulation for a Trauma AP Projection. The CR angulation determines the relationship of the petrous ridges and the supraorbital margins on a trauma AP projection. When a trauma AP projection demonstrates poor supraorbital margin and petrous ridge superimposition, adjust the CR angulation in the direction that you need the orbits to move. For example, if the petrous ridges are demonstrated inferior to the supraorbital margins, the CR was angled too cephalically for the projection and should be decreased (adjusted caudally; Figures 11-10 and 11-11) to obtain an optimal projection. If the petrous ridges are demonstrated superior to the supraorbital margins, the CR was not angled cephalically enough and should be increased (see Figure 11-7).

Mandible: Jaw Position. To obtain a PA/AP projection of the mandible, have the patient close the jaw, with teeth and lips placed together. Failing to obtain this jaw position will result in an elongated mandible (see Figure 11-11). If a fracture is suspected or the patient is unable to close the jaw the CR can be angled cephalically until it is aligned with the palpable posterior mandibular rami to obtain a less elongated projection.

Head Tilting and Midsagittal Plane Alignment. Aligning the head's midsagittal plane with the long axis of the IR ensures that the crista galli and nasal septum are aligned with the long axis of the exposure field and the cranium and mandible are demonstrated without tilting. Head tilting does not change any anatomic relationships for this position, although severe tilting prevents tight collimation and makes viewing the projection slightly more awkward.

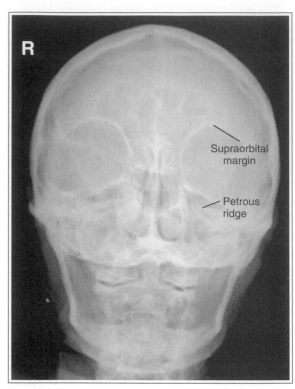

FIGURE 11-10 Trauma AP cranial projection taken with the CR angled too cephalically.

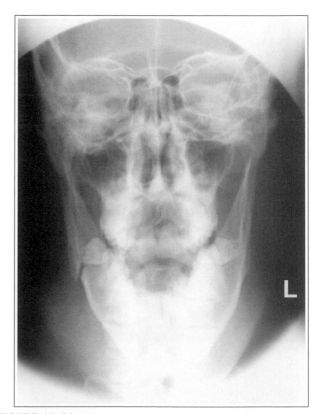

FIGURE 11-11 Trauma AP mandible projection taken with the CR angled too caudally and the mouth open.

PA or AP Analysis Practice

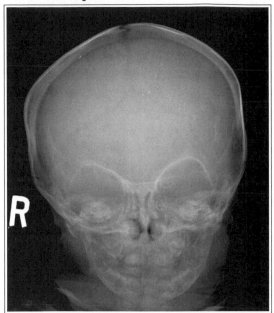

IMAGE 11-1 AP cranium projection.

Analysis. The distances from the lateral orbital margins to the lateral cranial cortices on the right side are greater than the same distances on the left side. The patient's face was rotated toward the left side. The petrous ridges are demonstrated inferior to the supraorbital margins; the patient's chin was not tucked enough to position the OML perpendicular to the IR.

Correction. Rotate the patient's face toward the right side until the midsagittal plane is aligned perpendicular to the IR. Tuck the chin until the OML is aligned perpendicular to the IR or adjust the CR angulation caudally.

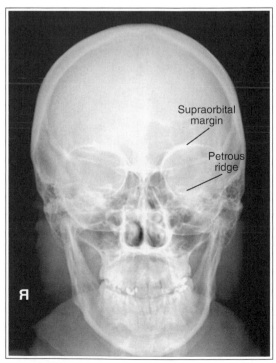

IMAGE 11-2 PA cranium projection.

Analysis. The petrous ridges are demonstrated inferior to the superior orbital margins and the dorsum sellae and anterior clinoids are demonstrated within the ethmoid sinuses. The patient's chin was not tucked enough to position the OML perpendicular to the IR.

Correction. Tuck the chin until the OML is aligned perpendicular to the IR or move it the full distance demonstrated between the petrous ridges and the supraorbital margins.

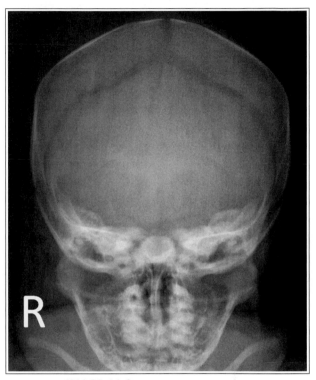

IMAGE 11-3 AP cranium projection.

Analysis. The petrous ridges are demonstrated superior to the supraorbital margins in the internal acoustic meatus are obscured. The patient's chin was tucked more than needed to position the OML perpendicular to the IR.

Correction. Extend the neck, moving the chin away from the thorax until the OML is aligned perpendicular to the IR or move it the full distance demonstrated between the petrous ridges and the supraorbital margins.

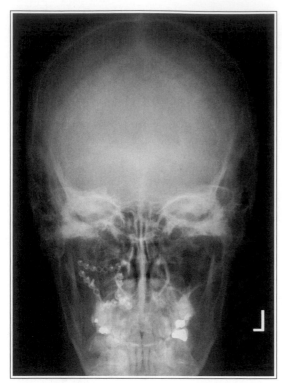

IMAGE 11-4 PA cranium projection.

Analysis. The petrous ridges are demonstrated superior to the supraorbital margins in the internal acoustic meatus are obscured. The patient's chin was tucked more than needed to position the OML perpendicular to the IR.

Correction. Extend the neck, moving the chin away from the thorax until the OML is aligned perpendicular to the IR or move it the full distance demonstrated between the petrous ridges and the supraorbital margins.

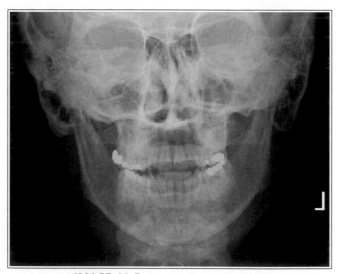

IMAGE 11-5 PA mandible projection.

Analysis. The petrous ridges are demonstrated inferior to the superior orbital margins and the dorsum sellae and anterior clinoids are demonstrated within the ethmoid sinuses. The patient's chin was not tucked enough to position the OML perpendicular to the IR.

Correction. Tuck the chin until the OML is aligned perpendicular to the IR or move it the full distance demonstrated between the petrous ridges and the supraorbital margins.

CRANIUM, FACIAL BONES, AND SINUSES: PA OR AP AXIAL PROJECTION (CALDWELL METHOD)

See Table 11-4, (Figures 11-12, 11-13, and 11-14).

Head Rotation. To prevent rotation on a PA axial projection, the midsagittal plane is positioned perpendicular to the IR. Head rotation is present on an AP axial projection if the distance from the lateral orbital margin to the lateral cranial cortex on one side is greater than that on the other side and if the distance from the crista galli to the lateral cranial cortex is greater on one side than on the other side (Figures 11-15 and 11-16). The patient's face was rotated away from the side demonstrating the greater distance.

OML and IR Alignment. Accurate petrous ridge and pyramid placement within the lowest third of the orbits is accomplished when the chin is tucked toward the chest until the OML is aligned perpendicular to the IR. This alignment positions the cranium as described above in the PA projection. For the PA axial projection, a 15-degree caudal CR angulation is then used to align the CR perpendicular to the frontal and ethmoid sinuses, orbital margins, superior orbital fissures, nasal septum, and anterior nasal spine. This angulation also projects the petrous ridges and pyramids inferiorly onto the lowest third of the orbits.

Adjusting the CR for Poor OML Alignment. For a patient who is unable to tuck the chin adequately to position the OML perpendicular to the IR, the CR angulation may be adjusted to compensate. Instruct the patient to tuck the chin to position the OML as close as possible to perpendicular to the IR. Angle the CR parallel with the OML. Then adjust the CR 15 degrees caudally from the angle that resulted when the CR was parallel with the OML.

Detecting Poor OML and CR Alignment. Poor OML and CR alignment can be detected on the PA axial by evaluating the relationship of the petrous ridges and the orbits. If the chin was not adequately tucked to bring the OML perpendicular to the IR, or if the OML was adequately positioned but the CR was angled more than 15 degrees caudally, the petrous ridges are demonstrated inferior to the infraorbital margins (Figure 11-17). If the chin was tucked more than needed to bring the OML perpendicular to the IR, or if the OML was adequately positioned but the CR was angled less than 15 degrees caudally, the petrous ridges and pyramids are demonstrated in the upper half of the orbits (see Figure 11-16).

CR Angulation for a Trauma AP Axial (Caldwell) Projection. For a trauma AP axial projection taken on a patient who cannot adjust the head to accurately align

TABLE 11-4	PA Axial Cranium, Facial Bone, and Sinus Projection	
Image Analysis Guidelines (Figures 11-12 and 11-13)	**Related Positioning Procedures (Figure 11-14)**	
• Distances from the lateral orbital margins to the lateral cranial cortices on both sides and from the crista galli to the lateral cranial cortices on both sides are equal.	• *PA axial:* Position the patient in a prone or upright PA projection. Rest the nose and forehead against the IR. • *AP axial:* Position the patient in a supine AP projection. *(Cervical vertebrae injuries must be cleared before proceeding. See precaution above.)* • Adjust head rotation to align the midsagittal plane perpendicular to the IR.	
• Petrous ridges are demonstrated horizontally through the lower third of the orbits. • Petrous pyramids are superimposed over the infraorbital margins. • Superior orbital fissures are seen within the orbits.	• Tuck the chin toward the chest until the OML is aligned perpendicular to the IR. • *PA axial:* Place a 15-degree caudal angle on the CR. • *AP axial:* Place a 15-degree cephalic angle on the CR.	
• Crista galli and nasal septum are aligned with the long axis of the exposure field. • Supraorbital margins are demonstrated on the same horizontal plane.	• Adjust head tilting to align the midsagittal plane with the collimator's longitudinal light line.	
• Ethmoid sinuses are at the center of the exposure field.	• Center the CR to exit (PA axial) or enter (AP axial) at the nasion. • Center IR and grid to CR.	
• *Cranium:* Outer cranial cortex and ethmoid sinuses are included within the exposure field. • *Facial bones and sinuses:* Frontal and ethmoid sinuses and lateral cranial cortices are included within the exposure field.	• *Cranium:* Open the longitudinal and transverse collimation fields to within 0.5 inch (1.25 cm) of the head skin line. • *Facial bones and sinuses:* Open the longitudinal and transverse collimation fields to within 1 inch (2.5 cm) of the sinus cavities.	

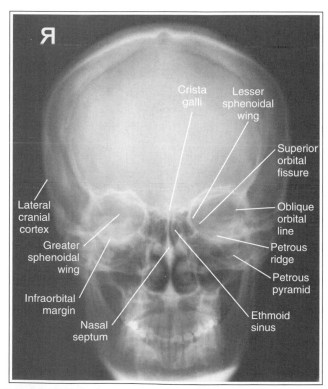

FIGURE 11-12 PA axial (Caldwell) cranial projection with accurate positioning.

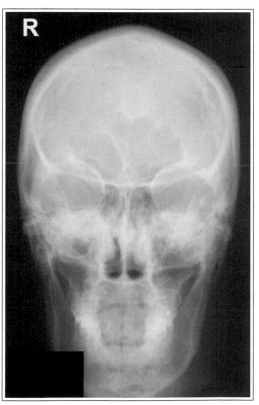

FIGURE 11-13 AP axial (Caldwell) cranial projection with accurate positioning.

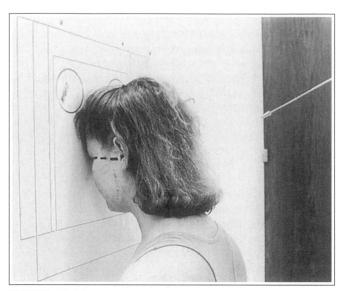

FIGURE 11-14 Proper patient positioning for PA axial (Caldwell) cranial projection.

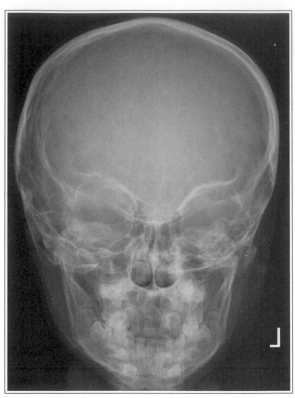

FIGURE 11-15 PA axial cranial projection taken with the face rotated toward the left side.

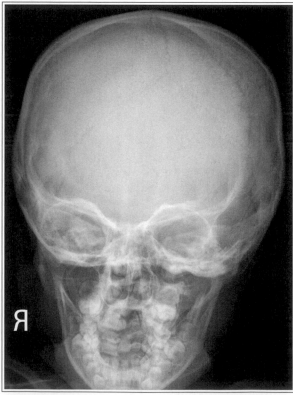

FIGURE 11-16 PA axial cranial projection taken with the face rotated toward the right side and the patient's chin tucked more than needed to bring the OML perpendicular to the IR or with the CR angled too cephalically.

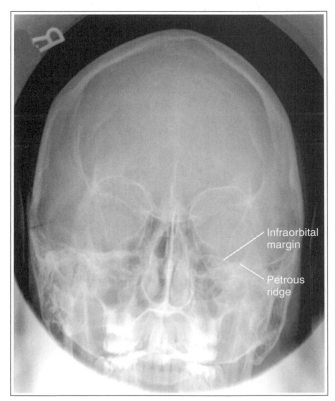

FIGURE 11-17 PA axial cranial projection taken with the chin tucked less than needed to align the OML perpendicular to the IR or with the CR angled too caudally.

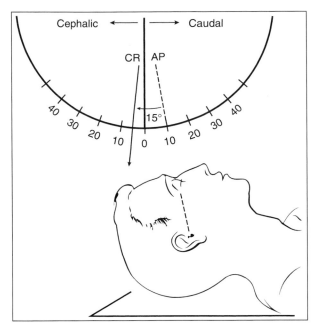

FIGURE 11-18 Determining central ray (CR) angulation for trauma AP axial (Caldwell) cranial projection. *(Reproduced with permission from Martensen K: Trauma Skulls [In-Service Reviews in Radiologic Technology, vol 15, no 5], Birmingham, AL, 1991, Educational Reviews.)*

PA/AP Axial Analysis Practice

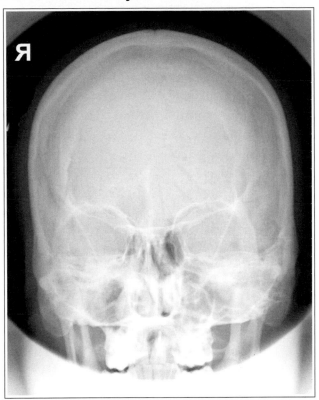

IMAGE 11-6 PA axial cranium projection.

the OML, begin by angling the CR parallel with the OML, as shown in Figure 11-18. The angulation required to do this varies according to the chin elevation provided by the cervical collar, but is most often between 10 and 15 degrees caudad. From this angulation, adjust the CR 15 degrees cephalad (a cephalic angulation is used instead of a caudal angle because the patient is now in an AP projection) to align the angle 15 degrees from the OML, as shown in Figure 11-18. For example, if a 10-degree caudal angle were needed to position the CR parallel with the OML, a 5-degree cephalic angulation would be required for the AP axial projection, 15 degrees cephalad from the OML.

Correcting the CR Angulation for a Trauma AP Axial (Caldwell) Projection. For the trauma AP axial projection, the CR angulation determines the relationship of the petrous ridges and the orbits. For an AP axial projection that demonstrates a poor petrous ridge and orbital relationship, adjust the CR angulation in the direction in which you want the orbits to move. If the petrous ridges are demonstrated inferior to the infraorbital margins, the CR was angled too cephalically and should be decreased. (The petrous ridge and orbital relationship obtained would be similar to that shown in Figure 11-17.) If the petrous ridges are demonstrated in the superior half of the orbits, the CR was not angled cephalically enough and should be increased. (The petrous ridge and orbital relationship obtained would be similar to that shown in Figure 11-16.)

Analysis. The distances from the lateral orbital margins to the lateral cranial cortices and from the crista galli to the lateral cranial cortex are greater on the left side than on the right side. The patient's face was rotated toward the right side. The petrous ridges are demonstrated inferior to the infraorbital margins. The patient's chin was not tight enough to position the OML perpendicular to the IR.

Correction. Rotate the patient's face toward the left side and tuck the chin to bring the OML perpendicular to the IR.

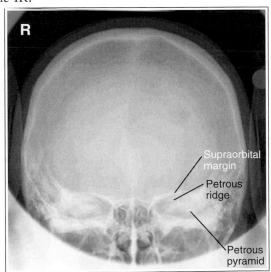

Supraorbital margin

Petrous ridge

Petrous pyramid

IMAGE 11-7 AP axial cranium projection.

Analysis. The petrous ridges and pyramids are demonstrated in the superior half of the orbits. The patient's chin was tucked more than needed to position the OML perpendicular to the IR or the CR was angled too caudally.

Correction. Elevate the chin until the OML is perpendicular to the IR or adjust the CR angulation cephalically.

CRANIUM AND MANDIBLE: AP AXIAL PROJECTION (TOWNE METHOD)

See Table 11-5, (Figures 11-19, 11-20, and 11-21).

Head Rotation. Head rotation is demonstrated on an AP axial projection if the distance from the posterior clinoid process and dorsum sellae to the lateral border of the foramen magnum is greater on one side and the distance from the mandibular neck to the cervical vertebrae is greater on one side than on the other side. The patient's face was rotated toward the side demonstrating the least distance from the posterior clinoid process and dorsum sellae to the lateral foramen magnum (Figure 11-22) and from the mandibular neck to the cervical vertebrae.

OML and Midsagittal Plane Alignment

Cranium and Petromastoid Portion. A combination of patient positioning and CR angulation accurately demonstrates the dorsum sellae and posterior clinoids within the foramen magnum. To accomplish proper patient positioning, tuck the chin until the OML is aligned perpendicular to the IR. This positioning aligns an imaginary line connecting the dorsum sellae and foramen magnum at a 30-degree angle with the IR and the OML.

Mandible. To position the dorsum sellae at the level of the superior foramen magnum and align the CR with the TMJs for an AP axial mandible, the OML is aligned perpendicular to the IR and a 35- to 40-degree caudal angulation.

Poor OML Alignment. If a patient tucked the chin less than needed to position the OML perpendicular to the IR, the dorsum sellae will be demonstrated superior to the foramen magnum (Figures 11-23 and 11-24). If the patient tucked the chin more than needed to align the OML perpendicular to the IR, the dorsum sellae will

TABLE 11-5	AP Axial Cranium and Mandible Projection	
Image Analysis Guidelines (Figures 11-19 and 11-20)		**Related Positioning Procedures (Figure 11-21)**
• Distances from the posterior clinoid process to the lateral borders of the foramen magnum on both sides and the mandibular necks to the lateral cervical vertebrae on both sides are equal. • Petrous ridges are symmetrical. • Dorsum sellae is centered within the foramen magnum.		• *Nontrauma:* Position the patient in an upright or supine AP projection. Rest posterior head against the IR. • *Trauma:* Position the patient in a supine AP projection. *(Cervical vertebrae injuries must be cleared before proceeding. See precaution above.)* • Adjust head rotation to align the midsagittal plane perpendicular to the IR.

• *Cranium and petrosmastoid portion:* Dorsum sellae and posterior clinoids are seen within the foramen magnum without foreshortening and without superimposition of the atlas's posterior arch.
• *Mandible:*
  • The dorsum sellae and posterior clinoids are at the level of the superior foramen magnum.
  • Mandibular condyles and fossae are clearly demonstrated, with minimal mastoid superimposition.
		• Tuck the chin until the OML is aligned perpendicular to the IR.
		• *Cranium:* Place a 30-degree caudal angle on the CR.
		• *Mandible:* Place a 35- to 40-degree caudal angle on the CR.

• Sagittal suture and nasal septum are aligned with the long axis of the exposure field. • Distances from the posterior clinoid process to the lateral borders of the foramen magnum on both sides are equal. • Petrous ridges are at the same transverse level.		• Adjust head tilting to align the midsagittal plane with the collimator's longitudinal light line.
• *Cranium:* The inferior occipital bone is at the center of the exposure field. • *Mandible:* A point midway between the mandibular rami is at the center of the exposure field.		• *Cranium:* Center the CR to the midsagittal plane at a level 2.5 inches (6 cm) above the glabella. • *Mandible:* Center the CR to the midsagittal plane at the level of the glabella.
• *Cranium:* Outer cranial cortex, petrous ridges, dorsum sellae, and foramen magnum are included within the exposure field. • *Mandible:* Mandible and temporomandibular fossae are included within the exposure field.		• Center the IR and grid to the CR. • *Cranium:* Open the longitudinal and transverse collimation fields to within 0.5 inch (1.25 cm) of the head skin line. • *Mandible:* Open the longitudinal collimation to include the EAM and transversely collimate to include the chin.

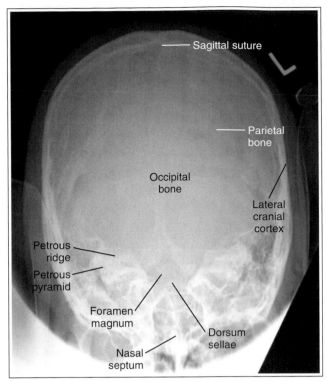

FIGURE 11-19 AP axial (Towne) cranial and mastoid projection with accurate positioning.

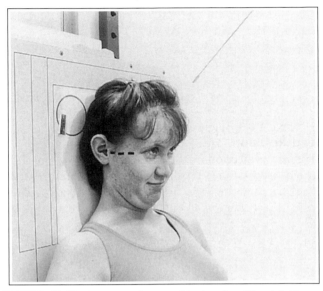

FIGURE 11-21 Proper patient positioning for AP axial (Towne) cranial projection.

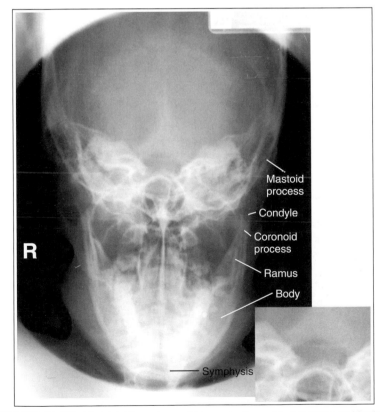

FIGURE 11-20 AP axial (Towne) mandible projection with accurate positioning.

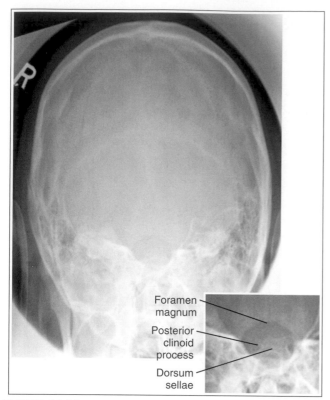

Foramen magnum

Posterior clinoid process

Dorsum sellae

FIGURE 11-22 AP axial cranial projection taken with the patient's face rotated toward the left side.

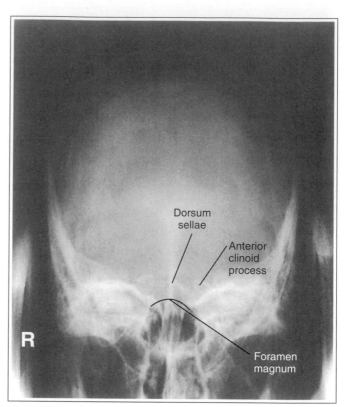

Dorsum sellae

Anterior clinoid process

Foramen magnum

FIGURE 11-23 AP axial cranial projection taken with the patient's chin tucked less than needed to position the OML perpendicular to the IR or with the CR angled too cephalically.

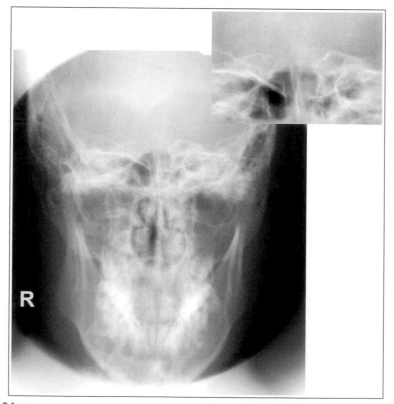

FIGURE 11-24 AP axial mandible projection taken with the patient's chin tucked less than needed to position the OML perpendicular to the IR or with the CR angled too cephalically.

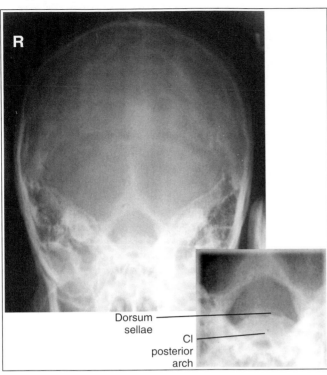

FIGURE 11-25 AP axial cranial projection taken with the patient's chin tucked more than needed to position the OML perpendicular to the IR or with the CR angled too caudally.

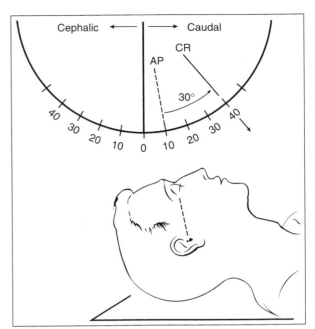

FIGURE 11-26 Determine central ray (CR) angulation for AP axial cranial projection in a trauma patient. *(Reproduced with permission from Martensen K: Trauma Skulls. [In-Service Reviews in Radiologic Technology, vol 15, no 5.] Birmingham, AL: Educational Reviews, 1991.)*

be foreshortened and will be superimposed over the atlas's posterior arch (Figures 11-25).

Adjusting for Poor OML Alignment and Determining CR Angulation for Trauma Patients. In a patient who is unable to adequately tuck the chin to position the OML perpendicular to the IR because of cervical trauma or stiffness, the CR angulation may be adjusted to compensate. Instruct the patient to tuck the chin to position the OML as close as possible to perpendicular to the IR. Angle the CR parallel with the OML and then adjust the CR 30 degrees caudally from the angle obtained when the CR was parallel with the OML to obtain an AP axial cranium and petromastoid projection (Figure 11-26) and 35 to 40 degrees caudally from the angle obtained to obtain an AP axial mandible projection. The angle used for this projection should not exceed 45 degrees or excessive distortion will result.

Head Tilting and Rotation. Head tilting, as with head rotation, is demonstrated on an AP axial projection when the distance from the posterior clinoid process and dorsum sellae to the lateral border of the foramen magnum is greater on one side than on the other. Head tilting though will also demonstrate the petrous ridges at different transverse levels, while head rotation will not. The head is tilted toward the side demonstrating the inferior petrous ridge and the side demonstrating the greatest distance from the posterior clinoid to the foramen magnum. Head rotation and tilting are often demonstrated together on the same projection (see Figure 11-22).

AP Axial (Towne) Analysis Practice

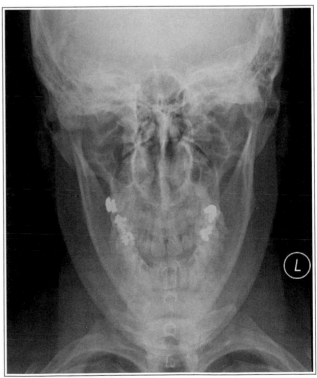

IMAGE 11-8 AP axial mandible projection.

Analysis. The dorsum sellae and anterior clinoids are demonstrated superior to the foramen magnum. Either the patient's chin was not tucked enough or the CR was not angled caudally enough to form a 30-degree angle with the OML.

Correction. Tuck the chin until the OML is perpendicular to the IR. If the patient is unable to tuck the chin any further, leave the chin positioned as is and adjust the CR angulation caudally the needed amount.

CRANIUM, FACIAL BONES, NASAL BONES, AND SINUSES: LATERAL PROJECTION

See Table 11-6, (Figures 11-27, 11-28, 11-29, 11-30, and 11-31).

Air-Fluid Levels in Sinus Cavities. To demonstrate air-fluid levels within the sinus cavities, the lateral projection should be taken in an upright position with a horizontal CR. In this position the thick, gelatin-like sinus fluid settles to the lowest position, creating an air-fluid line that shows the reviewer the amount of fluid present.

Head Rotation. The lateral projection is obtained without head rotation when the head's midsagittal plane is positioned parallel with the IR (see Figure 11-31). It may be necessary to position a sponge beneath the patient's chin or head to help maintain precise positioning.

Positioning for Trauma. A trauma lateral projection is accomplished by placing the IR and grid against the lateral cranium and directing a horizontal CR to a point 2 inches (5 cm) superior to the EAM. For a patient whose head position can be manipulated, elevate the occiput on a radiolucent sponge and adjust the head as indicated for the nontrauma lateral projection. If a cervical vertebral injury is suspected, do not adjust the patient's head until it has been cleared by the radiologist or take the projection with the head positioned as is and the IR positioned 1 inch (2.5 cm) below the occipital bone.

Detecting Head Rotation. Accurate positioning of the head's midsagittal plane is essential to prevent rotation of the cranium, facial bones, sinuses, and nasal bones. If the patient's head was not adequately turned to position the midsagittal plane parallel with the IR, rotation results. Rotation causes distortion of the sella turcica and situates one of the mandibular rami, greater wings of the sphenoid, external acoustic canals, zygomatic bones, and anterior cranial cortices anterior to the other on a lateral projection (Figure 11-32). Because the two sides of the cranium are mirror images, it is very difficult to determine which way the face was rotated when studying lateral projections with poor positioning. Paying close attention to initial positioning may give you an idea as to which way the patient has a tendency to lean. Routinely, patients tend to rotate their faces and lean the tops of their heads toward the IR.

Head Tilting. The lateral projection is obtained without head tilting when the IPL is aligned perpendicular with the IR. If the patient's head was tilted toward or away from the IR, preventing the midsagittal plane from aligning parallel with the IR or the IPL from aligning perpendicular to the IR, tilting of the cranium, facial

TABLE 11-6	Lateral Cranium, Facial Bones, Nasal Bones, and Sinuses Projection
Image Analysis Guidelines (Figures 11-27, 11-28, 11-29, and 11-30)	**Related Positioning Procedures (Figure 11-31)**
• When visualized, the sella turcica is seen in profile. • Orbital roofs, mandibular rami, greater wings of the sphenoid, external acoustic canals, zygomatic bones, and cranial cortices are superimposed.	• Place patient in a prone or upright position, with the affected side of the head against the IR. • Rotate the head and body as needed to place the head's midsagittal plane parallel with the IR. • Adjust head tilting to align the IPL perpendicular to the IR.
• *Cranium:* The posteroinferior occipital bones and posterior arch of the atlas are free of superimposition. • *Cranium:* An area 2 inches (5 cm) superior to the external auditory meatus is at the center of the exposure field. • *Facial bones and sinuses:* Zygoma and greater wings of the sphenoid are at the center of the exposure field. • *Nasal bones:* Nasal bones are at the center of the exposure field.	• Adjust the chin as needed to bring the IOML perpendicular to the front edge of the IR. • *Cranium:* Center a perpendicular CR to a point 2 inches (5 cm) superior to the EAM. • *Facial bones and sinuses:* Center a perpendicular CR midway between the outer canthus and EAM. • *Nasal bones:* Center a perpendicular CR 0.5 inch (1.25 cm) inferior to the nasion.
• *Cranium:* Outer cranial cortex is included within the exposure field. • *Facial bones and sinuses:* Frontal, ethmoid, sphenoid, and maxillary sinuses, greater wings of the sphenoid, orbital roofs, sella turcica, zygoma, and mandible are included within the exposure field. • *Nasal bones:* Nasal bones, with surrounding soft tissue, anterior nasal spine of maxilla, and the most anterior aspects of the cranial cortices, orbital roofs, and zygomatic bones, are included within the exposure field.	• Center the IR and grid to the CR. • *Cranium:* Open the longitudinal and transverse collimation fields to within 0.5 inch (1.25 cm) of the patient's head skin line. • *Facial bones and sinuses:* Open the longitudinal collimation field to include the mandible and frontal sinuses and transversely collimate to within 0.5 inch (1.25 cm) of the anterior skin line. • *Nasal bones:* Open the longitudinal field to include the frontal sinuses, and transversely collimate to within 0.5 inch (1.25 cm) of the nose skin line.

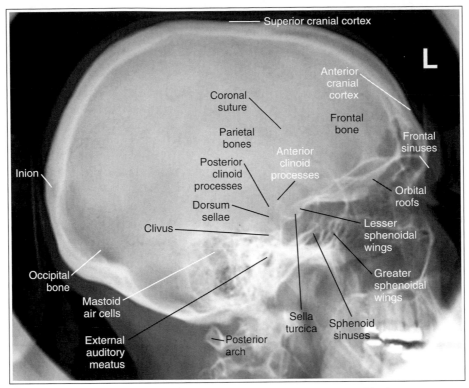

FIGURE 11-27 Lateral cranial projection with accurate positioning.

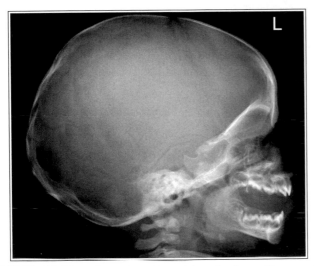

FIGURE 11-28 Pediatric lateral cranial projection with accurate positioning.

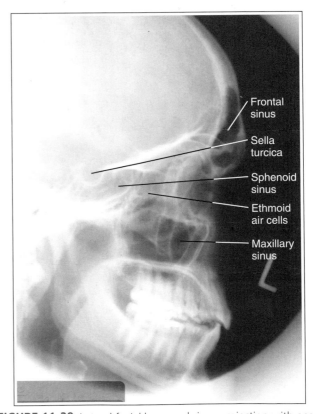

FIGURE 11-29 Lateral facial bone and sinus projection with accurate positioning.

bones, sinuses, and nasal bones results. Tilting can be distinguished from rotation on lateral projections by studying the superimposition of the orbital roofs, the greater wings of the sphenoid, the external acoustic canals, the zygomatic bones, and the inferior cranial cortices. If the patient's head was tilted, one of each corresponding structure is demonstrated superior to the other. The direction of the head tilt, toward or away from the IR, can be determined by evaluating the degree of atlas (C1) vertebral foramen visualization. If the top of the head is tilted toward the IR, the foramen will not be visualized, and if the tip of the head is tilted away from the IR, the foramen will be seen (Figure 11-33).

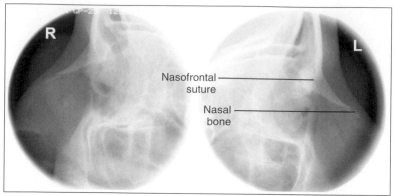

FIGURE 11-30 Lateral nasal bone projection with accurate positioning.

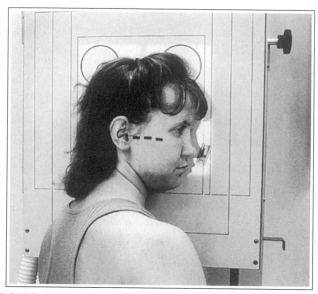

FIGURE 11-31 Proper patient positioning for lateral cranial projection.

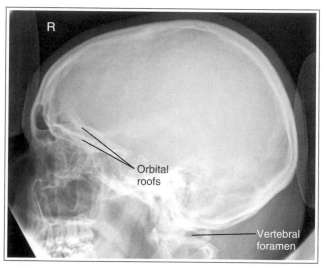

FIGURE 11-33 Lateral cranial projection taken with top of the patient's head tilted away from the IR.

Lateral Projection Analysis Practice

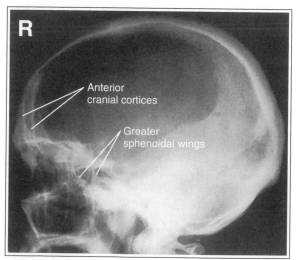

FIGURE 11-32 Lateral cranial projection taken with the patient's head rotated.

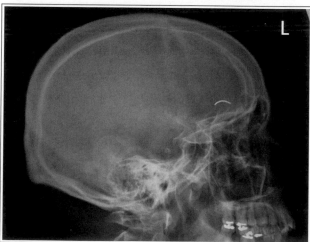

IMAGE 11-9 Lateral cranium projection.

Analysis. The greater wings of the sphenoid and the anterior cranial cortices are demonstrated without superimposition. One of each corresponding structure is demonstrated anterior to the other. The patient's head was rotated. The orbital roofs, EAMs, and inferior cranial cortices are demonstrated without superimposition. One of each corresponding structure is demonstrated superior to the other and the atlas vertebral foramen is visualized. The patient's head was tilted away from the IR.

Correction. Position the cranium's midsagittal plane parallel with the IR and the IPL perpendicular to the IR.

CRANIUM, MANDIBLE, AND SINUSES: SUBMENTOVERTEX PROJECTION (SCHUELLER METHOD)

See Table 11-7, (Figures 11-34, 11-35, and 11-36).

IOML and IR Alignment. The submentovertex (SMV) projection (Schueller method) is accomplished by placing the patient in an upright AP projection, with the cranial vertex resting against the IR and the chin elevated and neck hyperextended until the IOML is parallel to the IR (see Figure 11-36). For a patient with a retracted jaw, it may be necessary to raise the chin and extend the patient's neck beyond the IOML to position the mandibular mentum anterior to the frontal bone. If the patient is unable to align the IOML parallel with the IR, extend the patient's neck as far as possible and angle the CR cephalad until it is aligned perpendicular to the IOML.

Effect of Mispositioning IOML. Mispositioning of the mandibular mentum and ethmoid sinuses on an SMV projection obscures the nasal fossae, ethmoid sinuses, and foramen ovale and spinosum. If the patient's neck was overextended, the mandibular mentum is demonstrated too far anterior to the ethmoid sinuses (Figure 11-37). If the patient's neck was underextended, the mandibular mentum is demonstrated posterior to the ethmoid sinuses (Figures 11-38 and 39).

Head Tilting. The cranium's midsagittal plane is aligned perpendicular to the IR to prevent cranial tilting on an

SMV projection. Cranial tilting can be identified on an SMV projection of the head by comparing the distances from the mandibular ramus and body with the distance to the corresponding lateral cranial cortex on either side. If the head was not tilted, the distances are equal. If the

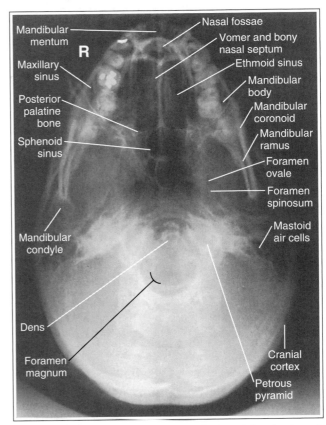

FIGURE 11-34 Submentovertex (Schueller) cranial projection with accurate positioning.

TABLE 11-7	Submentovertex (SMV) Cranium, Mandible, and Sinus Projection	
Image Analysis Guidelines (Figures 11-34 and 11-35)	**Related Positioning Procedures (Figure 11-36)**	
• Mandibular mentum and nasal fossae are demonstrated just anterior to the ethmoid sinuses.	• Position the patient in an upright AP projection, with the cranial vertex resting against the IR. • Elevate the chin and hyperextend the neck until the IOML is aligned parallel to the IR.	
• Distances from the mandibular ramus and body to the lateral cranial cortex on both sides are equal. • Vomer, bony nasal septum, and dens are aligned with the long axis of the exposure field. • *Cranium:* Dens is at the center of the exposure field. • *Sinuses and mandible:* Sphenoid sinuses are at the center of the exposure field.	• Adjust head tilting to align the midsagittal plane perpendicular to the IR. • Adjust head rotation to align the midsagittal plane with the collimator's longitudinal light line. • *Cranium:* Center a perpendicular CR to the midsagittal plane at a level 0.75 inch (2 cm) anterior to the level of the EAM. • *Sinuses and mandible:* Center a perpendicular CR to the midsagittal plane at a level 1.5 to 2 inches (4 to 5 cm) inferior to the mandibular symphysis.	
• *Cranium:* Mandible and the outer cranial cortices are included within the exposure field. • *Sinuses and mandible:* Mandible, lateral cranial cortices, and mastoid air cells are included within the exposure field.	• Center the IR and grid to the CR. • Open the longitudinal and transverse collimation fields to within 0.5 inch (1.25 cm) of the skin lines.	

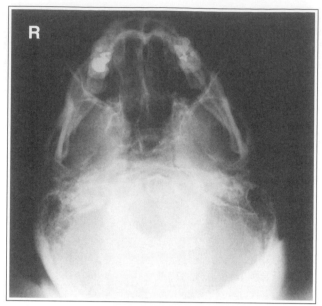

FIGURE 11-35 Submentovertex (Schueller) sinus and mandible projection with accurate positioning.

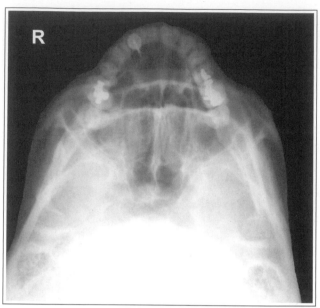

FIGURE 11-37 Submentovertex cranial projection taken with the patient's neck overextended, positioning the chin at a higher level within the forehead.

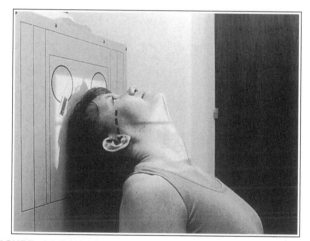

FIGURE 11-36 Proper patient positioning for submentovertex (Schueller) cranial projection.

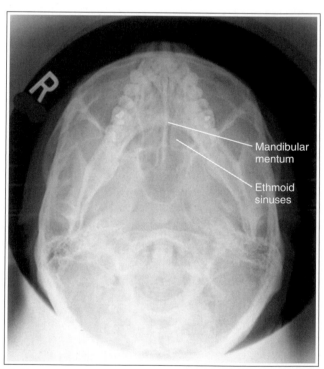

FIGURE 11-38 Submentovertex cranial projection taken with the patient's neck underextended, positioning the chin at a lower level than the forehead.

head was tilted, the distance is greater on the side toward which the cranial vertex was tilted (see Figure 11-39). **Head Rotation.** Aligning the midsagittal plane and the collimator's longitudinal light line ensures that the head is not rotated and that the vomer, bony nasal septum, and dens are aligned with the long axis of the exposure field. Rotation does not change any anatomic relationships for this position, although it does prevent tight collimation and makes viewing of the projection slightly more awkward.

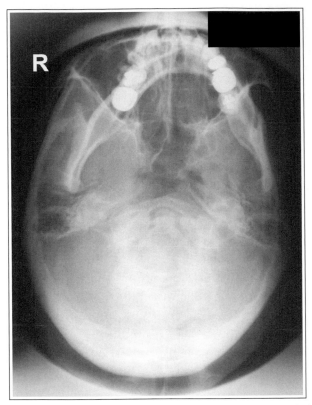

FIGURE 11-39 Submentovertex cranial projection taken with the patient's neck underextended, positioning the chin at a lower level than the forehead, and with the head tilted, positioning the top of the head toward the right side.

SMV Projection Analysis Practice

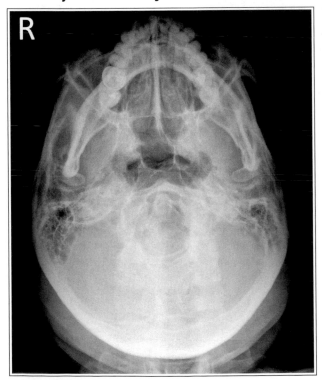

IMAGE 11-10 SMV cranium projection.

Analysis. The distance from the right mandibular ramus and body to its corresponding lateral cranial cortex is greater than the distance from the left mandibular ramus and body to its corresponding lateral cranial cortex. The patient's cranial vertex was tilted toward the right side. The mandibular mentum is demonstrated posterior to the ethmoid sinuses. The patient's neck was underextended, preventing the IOML from being positioned parallel with the IR.

Correction. Tilt the patient's cranial cortex toward the left side until the cranium's midsagittal plane is perpendicular to the IR and elevate the patient's chin until the IOML is aligned parallel with the IR.

FACIAL BONES AND SINUSES: PARIETOACANTHIAL AND ACANTHIOPARIETAL PROJECTION (WATERS METHOD)

See Table 11-8, (Figures 11-40, 11-41, and 11-42).

Demonstrating Air-Fluid Levels. To demonstrate air-fluid levels within the maxillary sinus cavities, this projection must be taken with the patient in an upright position and using a horizontal CR.

Head Rotation. Head rotation is present on a parieto-acanthial and acanthioparietal projections if the distance from the lateral orbital margin to the lateral cranial cortex on one side is greater than on the other side and if the distance from the bony nasal septum to the lateral cranial cortex on one side is greater than on the other side (Figure 11-43). The patient's face was rotated away from the side demonstrating the greater distance.

MML and IR Alignment. To accurately position the petrous ridges inferior to the maxillary sinuses, elevate the patient's chin until the OML is at a 37-degree angle with IR. Chin elevation moves the maxillary sinuses superior to the petrous ridges. This is best accomplished by positioning the MML perpendicular to the IR. If an open-mouth Waters method is required to visualize the sphenoid sinuses through the open mouth, do not have patient drop the jaw until after the MML has been positioned perpendicular to the IR (see Figure 11-42).

Detecting Poor MML Positioning. Poor MML positioning can be detected by evaluating the positions of the petrous ridges and posterior maxillary alveolar process. If the patient's chin was not adequately elevated to bring the MML perpendicular to the IR, the petrous ridges are demonstrated superior to the posterior maxillary alveolar process superimposing the maxillary sinuses (Figures 11-43 and 11-44). If the patient's chin was elevated more than needed to position the MML perpendicular to the IR, the petrous ridges are demonstrated inferior to the maxillary sinuses and posterior maxillary alveolar process, and the maxillary sinuses are superimposed over the posterior molars and alveolar process (Figure 11-45).

TABLE 11-8	Parietoacanthial and Acanthioparietal Facial Bone and Sinus Projection	
Image Analysis Guidelines (Figure 11-40)	**Related Positioning Procedures (Figures 11-41 and 11-42)**	
• Distances from the lateral orbital margin to the lateral cranial cortex and from the bony nasal septum to the lateral cranial cortex on both sides are equal.	• *Parietoacanthial:* Position the patient in a prone or upright PA projection. • *Acanthioparietal:* Position the patient in a supine AP projection. *(Cervical vertebrae injuries must be cleared before proceeding. See precautions below.)* • Adjust head rotation, aligning the midsagittal plane perpendicular to the IR.	
• Petrous ridges are demonstrated inferior to the maxillary sinuses and extend laterally from the posterior maxillary alveolar process.	• Adjust chin elevation until the MML is perpendicular to the IR (OML is at a 37-degree angle with the IR).	
• Bony nasal septum is aligned with the long axis of the exposure field. • Infraorbital margins are demonstrated on the same horizontal plane.	• Adjust head tilting to align the midsagittal plane with the collimator's longitudinal light line.	
• Anterior nasal spine is at the center of the exposure field.	• Using the transverse collimation light line, center a perpendicular CR so it exits at the acanthion. • Center IR and grid to CR.	
• Frontal and maxillary sinuses and lateral cranial cortices are included within the exposure field.	• Open the longitudinal and transverse collimation fields to within 1 inch (2.5 cm) of palpable orbits and zygomatic arches.	

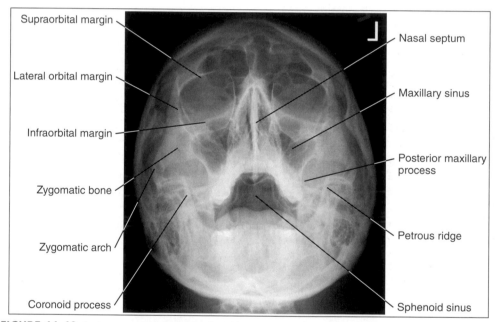

FIGURE 11-40 Parietoacanthial (Waters) facial bone and sinus projection with accurate positioning.

Adjusting the CR for Poor MML Alignment. For a patient who is unable to elevate the chin adequately to position the MML perpendicular to the IR, the CR may be adjusted to compensate. Instruct the patient to elevate the chin to position the MML as close as possible to perpendicular to the IR. Then angle the CR until it is parallel with the OML and then adjust the CR 37 degrees from the OML in the direction that will angle it with the MML (Figure 11-46) (cephalically for the acanthioparietal and caudally for the parietoacanthial projection).

Correcting the CR Angulation for Poor MML Alignment. When an acanthioparietal projection demonstrates poor MML alignment, the CR should be adjusted in the direction that the maxillary sinuses and posterior maxillary alveolar process need to move in relationship to the petrous ridge to obtain an optimal projection. When a parietoacanthial projection demonstrates poor MML alignment, the CR should be adjusted in the direction that the petrous ridges need to move in relationship to the maxillary sinuses and posterior

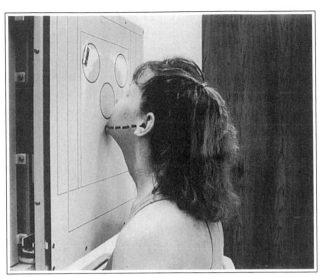

FIGURE 11-41 Proper patient positioning for parietoacanthial (Waters) facial bone and sinus projection.

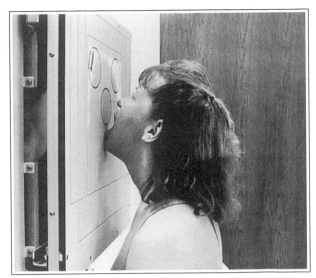

FIGURE 11-42 Proper patient positioning for open-mouth parietoacanthial (Waters) sinus projection.

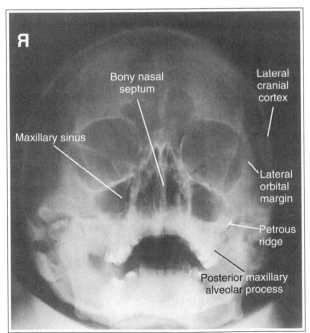

FIGURE 11-43 Parietoacanthial sinus projection taken with the patient's face rotated toward the left side and the chin insufficiently elevated to bring the MML perpendicular to the IR.

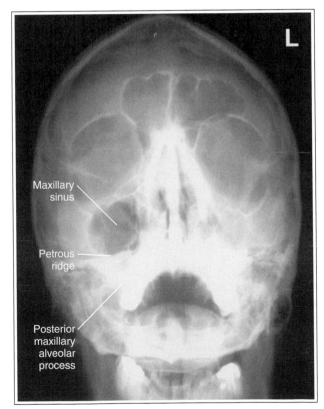

FIGURE 11-44 Acanthioparietal facial bone projection taken with the chin insufficiently elevated to bring the MML perpendicular to the IR.

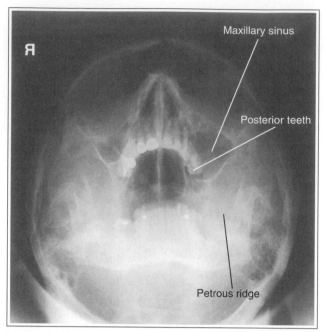

FIGURE 11-45 Parietoacanthial sinus projection taken with the chin elevated more than needed to bring the MML perpendicular to the IR.

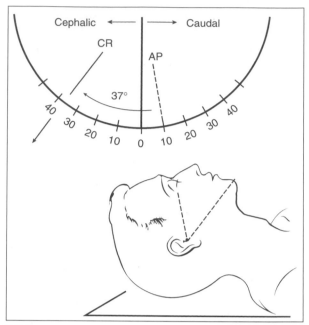

FIGURE 11-46 Determining central ray (CR) angle for acanthioparietal (Waters) facial bone and sinus projection in a trauma patient.

maxillary alveolar process to obtain an optimal projection. If the petrous ridges are demonstrated within the maxillary sinuses and superior to the posterior maxillary alveolar process, the CR was angled too caudally for the acanthioparietal projection and too cephalically for the parietoacanthial projection (see Figures 11-43 and 11-44). If the petrous ridges are demonstrated inferior to the maxillary sinuses and posterior to the maxillary alveolar process, the CR was angled too cephalically for the acanthioparietal projection and too caudally for the parietoacanthial projection (see Figure 11-45).

Modified Waters Method. A modified Waters method is used to position the orbital floors perpendicular to the IR and parallel to the CR for increased demonstration of the orbital floors. This examination is commonly done to rule out fractures of the orbits and demonstrate foreign bodies in the eyes. The modified Waters method is accomplished by positioning the patient as described for the parietoacanthial and acanthioparietal projections, with one exception—the patient's chin is elevated only until the OML is at a 55-degree angle with the IR (LML is perpendicular to IR). In this position the petrous ridges will be demonstrated within the maxillary sinuses rather than inferior to them (Figure 11-47).

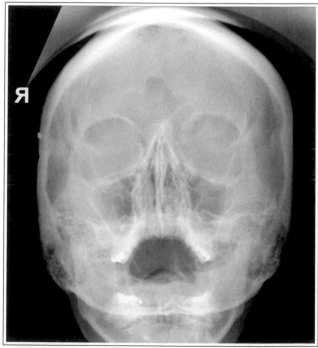

FIGURE 11-47 Modified Waters facial bone and sinus projection with accurate positioning.

Parietoacanthial and Acanthioparietal Projection Analysis Practice

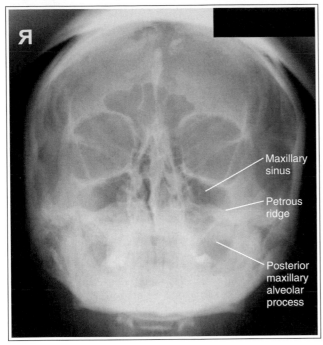

Maxillary sinus

Petrous ridge

Posterior maxillary alveolar process

IMAGE 11-11 Parietoacanthial.

Analysis. The petrous ridges are demonstrated within the maxillary sinuses and superior to the posterior maxillary alveolar process. The patient's chin was not elevated enough to position the MML perpendicular to the IR or the CR was angled too cephalically.

Correction. Elevate the patient's chin until the MML is perpendicular to the IR. If the patient is unable to elevate the chin further, leave the chin positioned as it is and angle the CR caudally until it is aligned with the MML when the patient's mouth is closed.

Digestive System

OUTLINE

Esophagram: Upper GI System, 489
Esophagram: PA Oblique
    Projection (RAO Position), 489
Esophagram: Lateral
    Projection, 490
Esophagram: PA Projection, 492
Stomach and Duodenum: PA
    Oblique Projection (RAO
    Position), 494
Stomach and Duodenum: PA
    Projection, 494

Stomach and Duodenum: Lateral
    Projection (Right Lateral
    Position), 497
Stomach and Duodenum: AP
    Oblique Projection (LAO
    Position), 499
Stomach and Duodenum: AP
    Projection, 501
Small Intestine: PA Projection, 503
Large Intestine: PA or AP
    Projection, 507

Large Intestine (Rectum): Lateral
    Projection, 509
Large Intestine: AP or PA Projection
    (Lateral Decubitus Position), 510
Large Intestine: PA Oblique
    Projection (RAO Position), 512
Large Intestine: PA Oblique
    Projection (LAO Position), 513
Large Intestine: PA Axial Projection
    and PA Axial Oblique Projection
    (RAO Position), 514

OBJECTIVES

After completion of this chapter, you should be able to do the following:

- Identify the required anatomy on upper and lower gastrointestinal projections.
- Describe how to properly position the patient, image receptor (IR), and central ray (CR) for upper and lower gastrointestinal projections.
- Explain the patient preparation procedure used before upper and lower gastrointestinal examinations to prevent residual debris and fluid from obscuring areas of interest.
- List the image analysis guidelines for upper and lower gastrointestinal projections with accurate positioning and state how to reposition the patient when less than optimal projections are produced.

- Describe the differences in size, shape, and position of the stomach and abdominal cavity placement of the small and large intestinal structures among the different types of habitus.
- Define the differences in the barium suspensions that are ingested for upper and lower gastrointestinal projections.
- Describe the differences in the appearance of the stomach on projections of patients with different types of body habitus.
- State where the barium and air will be situated for the different upper and lower gastrointestinal double-contrast projections.
- Explain why the small intestine is imaged at set time intervals for a small intestine study.

KEY TERMS

negative   NPO   positive

IMAGE ANALYSIS GUIDELINES

Technical Data. When the technical data in Table 12-1 are followed, or adjusted as needed for additive and destructive patient conditions (see Table 2-6), along with the best practices discussed in Chapters 1 and 2, all digestive system projections will demonstrate the image analysis guidelines in Box 12-1 unless otherwise indicated.

Using the AEC for Double-Contrast Examinations. For double-contrast examinations, using the AEC may be contraindicated because choosing the cell beneath the barium pool may result in overexposure of the area containing the air contrast.

Pendulous Breasts. Pendulous breasts may overlap and prevent clear visualization of the intestinal structures unless they are shifted superiorly and laterally. Such movement also prevents excessive radiation exposure to the breasts.

Peristaltic Activity and Exposure Times. Short exposure times are needed when imaging the digestive system to control the blur that may result from peristaltic activity within the system. Peristalsis is the contraction

TABLE 12-1	Digestive System Technical Data				
Projection	**kV**	**Grid**	**AEC**	**mAs**	**SID**
Upper Gastrointestinal System					
PA oblique (RAO) position, esophagus	SC = 100-125	Grid	Center		40-48 inches (100-120 cm)
Lateral, esophagus	SC = 100-125	Grid	Center		40-48 inches (100-120 cm)
AP or PA, esophagus	SC = 100-125	Grid	Center		40-48 inches (100-120 cm)
PA oblique (RAO position) stomach	SC = 100-125 DC = 90-100	Grid	Center		40-48 inches (100-120 cm)
PA, stomach	SC = 100-125 DC = 90-100	Grid	Center		40-48 inches (100-120 cm)
Right lateral, stomach	SC = 100-125 DC = 90-100	Grid	Center		40-48 inches (100-120 cm)
AP oblique (LPO position), stomach	SC = 100-125 DC = 90-100	Grid	Center		40-48 inches (100-120 cm)
AP, stomach	SC = 100-125 DC = 90-100	Grid	Center		40-48 inches (100-120 cm)
Small Intestine					
PA or AP	SC = 100-125	Grid	All three		40-48 inches (100-120 cm)
Large Intestine					
AP or PA	SC = 100-125 DC = 80-90	Grid	All three		40-48 inches (100-120 cm)
Lateral, rectum	100-125	Grid	Center		40-48 inches (100-120 cm)
AP or PA (lateral decubitus)	SC = 100-125 DC = 90-100	Grid		6	40-48 inches (100-120 cm)
PA oblique (RAO position)	SC = 100-125 DC = 90-100	Grid	All three		40-48 inches (100-120 cm)
PA oblique (LAO position)	SC = 100-125 DC = 90-100	Grid	All three		40-48 inches (100-120 cm)
PA axial or PA axial oblique (RAO position)	SC = 100-125 DC = 80-90	Grid	All three		40-48 inches (100-120 cm)

DC, Double contrast; SC, single contrast.

BOX 12-1	Digestive System Imaging Analysis Guidelines

- The facility's identification requirements are visible.
- A right or left marker identifying the correct side of the patient is present on the projection and is not superimposed over the VOI.
- Good radiation protection practices are evident.
- The GI structures and cortical outlines of the bony structures are sharply defined.
- Contrast resolution is adequate to demonstrate the barium-coated mucosal surface patterns and intestinal contours.
- No quantum mottle or saturation is present.
- Scatter radiation has been kept to a minimum.
- There is no evidence of removal artifacts.

and relaxation movement of the smooth muscles in the walls of the digestive system that mixes food and secretions and moves the materials through the system. Peristaltic activity of the stomach and large or small intestine can be identified on a projection by sharp bony cortices and blurry gastric and intestinal gases or barium (Figure 12-1).

Body Habitus Positioning Variations. The body habitus determines the size, shape, and position of the stomach and the abdominal cavity placement of the large intestine. Being familiar with these differences will help the technologist adjust the CR centering for optimal demonstration of the required digestive structures.

Hypersthenic. The hypersthenic patient's abdomen is broad and deep from anterior to posterior. The stomach is positioned high in the abdomen and lies transversely at the level of the T9 to T12, with the duodenal bulb at the level of T11 to T12. The colic flexures and transverse colon tend to be positioned high in the abdomen (Figure 12-2). Using the sthenic patient as the reference point, this habitus will require a more superior and medial CR centering and IR placement for AP and PA projections and a more superior and anterior CR centering and IR placement for the lateral projection of the stomach.

Asthenic. The asthenic patient's abdomen is narrow; the stomach is positioned low in the abdomen and runs vertically along the left side of the vertebral column, typically extending from T11 to L5, with the duodenal bulb at the level of L3 to L4. The small and large intestinal structures tend to be positioned low in the abdomen (Figure 12-3). Using the sthenic patient as the reference

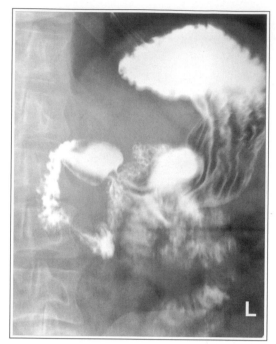

FIGURE 12-1 AP oblique stomach and duodenum projection demonstrating motion caused by peristaltic activity.

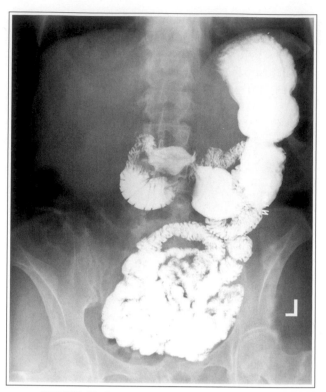

FIGURE 12-3 PA projection of asthenic patient.

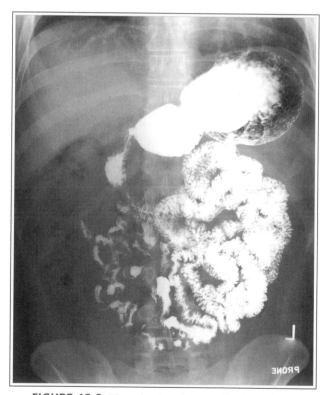

FIGURE 12-2 PA projection of hypersthenic patient.

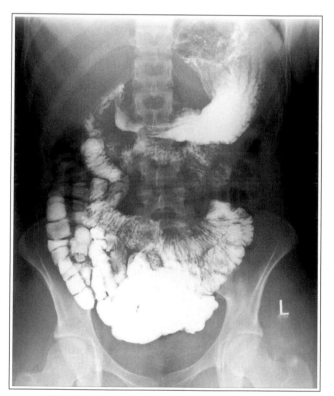

FIGURE 12-4 PA projection of sthenic patient.

point, this habitus will require lower and more lateral centering of the CR for stomach projections.

Sthenic. The sthenic habitus is the most common. The abdomen is less broad than the hypersthenic habitus, yet not as narrow as the asthenic. The stomach also rests at a position between the hypersthenic and asthenic habitus and typically extends from T10 to L2, with the

duodenal bulb at the level of L1-L2. The small and large intestinal structures tend to be centered in the abdomen (Figure 12-4).

Respiration. From full inspiration to expiration the diaphragm position moves from an inferior to a superior

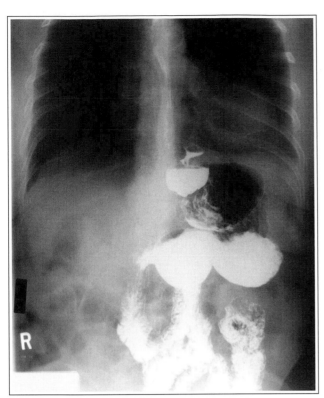

FIGURE 12-5 PA stomach and duodenum projection taken after full inspiration.

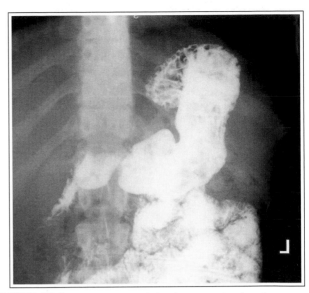

FIGURE 12-6 PA stomach and duodenum projection demonstrating residual food particles in the stomach.

position. This movement also changes the pressure placed on the abdominal structures. On full expiration the right side of the diaphragm dome is at the same transverse level as the eighth thoracic vertebrae, whereas on inspiration it may be found at the same transverse level as the ninth or tenth posterior rib. Exposing upper GI and small and large intestine projections on full expiration allows increased abdominal space for the structures to be demonstrated without segment overlapping and foreshortening (compare Figures 12-4 and 12-5).

ESOPHAGRAM: UPPER GI SYSTEM

Upper GI Preparation Procedure

Esophagram Preparation. No preparation procedures are required when the esophagus is imaged, but if an esophagus and stomach examination is being performed, the stomach and duodenum preparation is to be followed.

Stomach and Duodenum Preparation. Adequate preparation of the upper gastrointestinal (GI) system eliminates residual stomach debris, which may obscure abnormalities, and prevents excessive fluid from accumulating in the stomach, which could dilute the barium suspension enough to interfere with optimal mucosal coating (Figure 12-6). The preparation procedure for the upper GI system includes NPO (nothing orally) after midnight or at least 8 hours before the examination, and avoidance of gum and tobacco products before the procedure.

Contrast Medium. The goal of the esophagram is to demonstrate the workings and appearance of the pharynx and esophagus. This is accomplished through the fluoroscopic procedure and overhead projections that are obtained in an esophagram. Barium is used to demonstrate the pharynx and esophagus during this examination. A 30% to 50% weight or volume barium suspension is ingested continuously during the exposure, or two to three spoonfuls with toothpaste consistency; thick barium is ingested before exposing the esophagus, filling it with barium. The patient may also be asked to swallow cotton balls soaked in thin barium, barium-filled gelatin capsules, barium tablets, or marshmallows when a radiolucent foreign body or stricture is suspected. Adequate filling of the esophagus has occurred when the entire column is filled with barium. Only aspects of the esophagus that are filled with barium will be adequately demonstrated. Figures 12-7 and 12-8 demonstrate a PA oblique and lateral esophagram projections demonstrating the superior and inferior ends of the esophagus that are not filled with barium and cannot be adequately evaluated. For the overhead projections, place a cup full of barium in the patient's hand and place the straw in the patient's mouth so that the patient can ingest barium during the exposure, or ask the patient to swallow two spoonfuls of thick barium and then give a third spoonful that is swallowed immediately before the exposure.

ESOPHAGRAM: PA OBLIQUE PROJECTION (RAO POSITION)

See Table 12-2, (Figures 12-9 and 12-10).

Body Obliquity. Accurate torso obliquity is obtained when the midcoronal plane is at a 35- to 40-degree angle with the IR. This positioning rotates the esophagus from beneath the thoracic vertebrae, positioning it between the vertebrae and heart shadow.

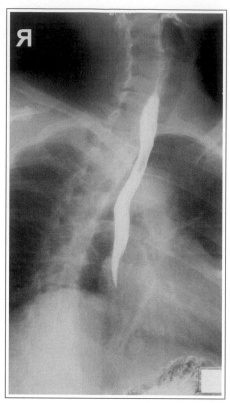

FIGURE 12-7 PA oblique esophagram demonstrating poor barium fill of the superior and inferior ends of the esophagus.

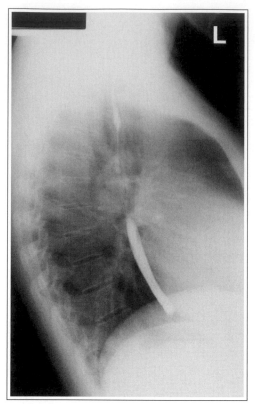

FIGURE 12-8 Lateral esophagram demonstrating poor barium fill of the superior and middle ends of the esophagus.

TABLE 12-2	PA Oblique Esophagram Projection (RAO Position)
Image Analysis Guidelines (Figure 12-9)	**Related Positioning Procedures (Figure 12-10)**
• Esophagus is filled with barium.	• Feed patient appropriately weighted barium suspension before and during exposure.
• Barium-filled esophagus is demonstrated between the vertebrae and heart shadow. • About 0.5 inch (1.25 cm) of the right sternal clavicular end is demonstrated to the left of the vertebrae.	• Place patient in a prone, PA projection. • Rotate the torso toward the right side until the midcoronal plane is at a 35- to 40-degree angle with the IR. • Flex the left elbow and knee as needed to maintain obliquity.
• Midesophagus, at the level of T5 to T6, is at the center of the exposure field.	• Center a perpendicular CR 3 inches (7.5 cm) to the left of the spinous processes and 2-3 inches (5-7.5 cm) inferior to the jugular notch.
• Entire esophagus is included within the exposure field.	• Center the IR and grid to the CR. • Longitudinally collimate to a 17-inch (43 cm) field size. • Transversely collimate to a 6-inch (15 cm) field size.

Inaccurate Patient Rotation. If less than the desired 35 to 40 degrees of obliquity is obtained on a PA oblique esophagram projection, the vertebrae will be superimposed over the esophagus and the right sternal clavicular end (Figure 12-11). If the patient is rotated more than 40 degrees, more than 0.5 inch (1.25 cm) of the right sternal clavicular end will be demonstrated to the left of the vertebrae.

ESOPHAGRAM: LATERAL PROJECTION

See Table 12-3, (Figures 12-12, 12-13, and 12-14).
Rotation. To obtain a lateral esophagram projection, place the patient on the table in a lateral recumbent position. Whether the patient is lying on the right or left side is not significant (see Figure 12-13). Flex the knees and hips for support, and position a pillow or sponge between the knees. The pillow or sponge should be thick enough to prevent the side of the pelvis situated farther from the IR from rotating anteriorly but not so thick as to cause posterior rotation. To avoid vertebral rotation, align the shoulders, posterior ribs, and posterior pelvis perpendicular to the table and IR by resting an extended flat palm against each, respectively, and then adjusting patient rotation until the hand is positioned perpendicular to the IR. The upper and lower thoracic vertebrae can demonstrate rotation independently or simultaneously, depending on which section of the torso was

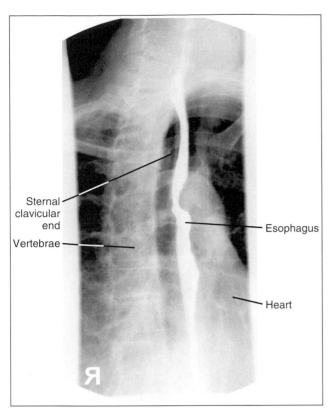

FIGURE 12-9 PA oblique esophagram projection (RAO position) with accurate positioning.

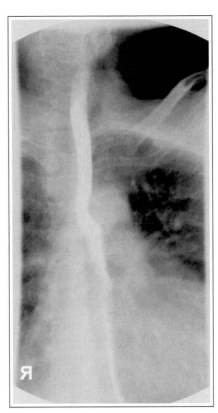

FIGURE 12-11 PA oblique esophagram taken with insufficient patient obliquity.

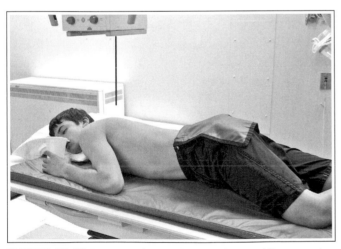

FIGURE 12-10 Proper patient positioning for PA oblique esophagram projection.

rotated if the shoulders were not placed on top of each other, but the ASISs were aligned, the upper thoracic vertebrae demonstrate rotation, and the lower thoracic vertebrae demonstrate a lateral projection. If the ASISs were rotated but the shoulders are placed on top of each other, the lower thoracic vertebrae demonstrate rotation and the upper vertebrae demonstrate a lateral projection.

Detecting Thorax Rotation. Rotation can be detected on a lateral esophagram projection by evaluat-

ing superimposition of the right and left posterior surfaces of the vertebral bodies and superimposition of the posterior ribs. On a nonrotated lateral projection, the posterior surfaces are superimposed and the posterior ribs are almost superimposed. Because the posterior ribs positioned further from the IR were placed at a greater OID than the other side, they demonstrate more magnification. This magnification prevents the posterior ribs from being directly superimposed but positions them approximately 1 inch (2.5 cm) apart. This distance is based on a 40-inch (102-cm) SID. If a longer SID is used, the distance between the posterior ribs is decreased, and if a shorter SID is used, the distance is increased. On rotation, the right and left posterior surfaces of the vertebral bodies are demonstrated one anterior to the other on a lateral projection. Because the two sides of the thorax and vertebrae are mirror images, it is very difficult to determine from a rotated lateral esophagram projection which side of the patient was rotated anteriorly and which posteriorly. If the patient was only slightly rotated, one way of determining which way the patient was rotated is to evaluate the amount of posterior rib superimposition. If the patient's elevated side was rotated posteriorly, the posterior ribs demonstrate more than 0.5 inch (1.25 cm) of space between them (see Figures 8-69 and 8-70). If the elevated side was rotated anteriorly, the posterior ribs are superimposed on slight rotation (Figure 8-71) and demonstrate greater

TABLE 12-3	Lateral Esophagram Projection
Image Analysis Guidelines (Figure 12-12)	**Related Positioning Procedures (Figures 12-13 and 12-14)**
• Esophagus is filled with barium.	• Feed patient appropriately weighted barium suspension before and during exposure.
• Esophagus is positioned anterior to the thoracic vertebrae. • Posterior surfaces of the vertebral bodies are superimposed. • There is no more than 1 inch (2.5 cm) of space demonstrated between the posterior ribs.	• Place patient in a recumbent lateral position. • Flex the knees and hips, and position a pillow or sponge between the knees to prevent anterior rotation. • Position the shoulders, posterior ribs, and ASISs on top of each other, aligning the midcoronal plane perpendicular to the IR.
• Shoulders and humeri do not superimpose the esophagus.	• Position the humeri at a 90-degree angle with the torso or separate the shoulders by positioning the arm and shoulder closer to the table slightly anteriorly and the arm and shoulder farther away from the table posteriorly.
• Midesophagus, at the level of T5-T6, is at the center of the exposure field. • Entire esophagus is included within the exposure field.	• Center a perpendicular CR to the midcoronal plane at a level 2-3 inches (5-7.5 m) inferior to the jugular notch. • Center the IR and grid to the CR. • Longitudinally collimate to a 17-inch (43-cm) field size. • Transversely collimate to a 6-inch (15-cm) field size.

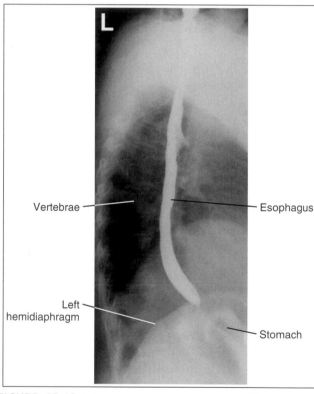

FIGURE 12-12 Lateral esophagram projection with patient on left side.

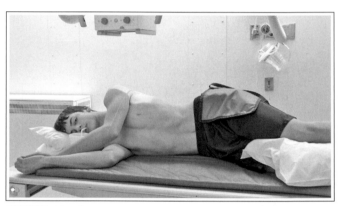

FIGURE 12-13 Proper patient positioning for lateral esophagram projection with arms at 90 degrees.

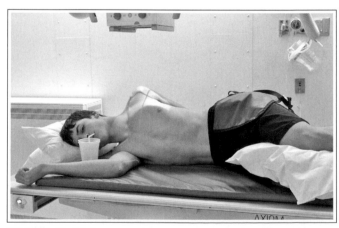

FIGURE 12-14 Proper patient positioning for lateral esophagram projection with shoulders rotated.

separation as rotation of the patient increases in this direction.

ESOPHAGRAM: PA PROJECTION

See Table 12-4, (Figures 12-15 and 12-16).

Rotation. To prevent rotation on a PA esophagus projection, position the shoulders and ASISs at equal distances from the IR. The upper and lower thoracic vertebrae can demonstrate rotation independently or simultaneously, depending on which section of the body is rotated.

Detecting Rotation. Rotation is readily detected on a PA esophagus projection by comparing the distances between the pedicles and spinous processes on the same vertebra and the distances between the vertebral column

TABLE 12-4	PA Esophagram Projection
Image Analysis Guidelines (Figure 12-15)	**Related Positioning Procedures (Figure 12-16)**
• Esophagus is filled with barium.	• Feed patient appropriately weighted barium suspension before and during exposure.
• Distances from the vertebral column to the sternal clavicular ends and from the pedicles to the spinous processes are equal on the two sides.	• Position the patient in a prone, PA projection.
	• Place the shoulders and ASISs at equal distances from the IR, aligning the midcoronal plane parallel with the IR.
• Midesophagus, at the level of T5-T6, is at the center of the exposure field.	• Center a perpendicular CR to the midsagittal plane at a level 2-3 inches (5-7.5 cm) superior to the inferior scapular angle.
• Entire esophagus is included within the exposure field.	• Center the IR and grid to the CR.
	• Longitudinally collimate to a 17-inch (43-cm) field size.
	• Transversely collimate to a 6-inch (15-cm) field size.

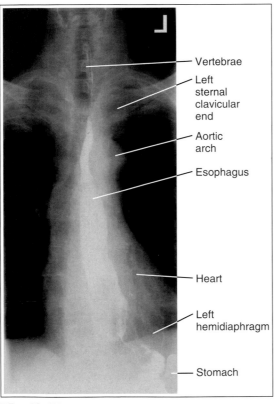

FIGURE 12-15 PA esophagram projection with accurate positioning.

- Vertebrae
- Left sternal clavicular end
- Aortic arch
- Esophagus
- Heart
- Left hemidiaphragm
- Stomach

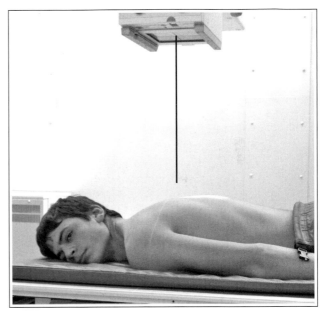

FIGURE 12-16 Proper patient positioning for PA esophagram projection.

and the medial ends of the clavicles. When no rotation is present, the comparable distances are equal. If one side demonstrates a larger distance, vertebral rotation is present. The side demonstrating a larger distance is the side of the patient positioned further from the table and the IR (Figure 12-17).

STOMACH AND DUODENUM

Contrast Medium. Appropriate contrast filling and distribution has been obtained for all of the stomach and duodenum projections presented when the stomach and duodenum demonstrate the following.

Single Contrast. The stomach and duodenum are barium-filled, demonstrating the contour of the stomach and lumen.

The single-contrast PA stomach and duodenum projection demonstrates barium-filled organs with normally present gas. The primary goal of a single-contrast stomach and duodenum study is to demonstrate abnormalities of the stomach and lumen contour. A 30% to 50% weight or volume barium suspension is typically used for this study.

Double Contrast. The stomach and duodenum demonstrate adequate distention and mucosal covering. The rugae (longitudinal gastric folds) are smoothed out, the gastric surface pattern is demonstrated, and a thin, uniform barium line is visible along the contour of the stomach.

The goal of a double-contrast study is to visualize abnormalities in the mucosal details and contour and lumen of the stomach and duodenum. Negative (radiolucent) contrast is most commonly obtained by having the patient swallow effervescent granules, powder, or

TABLE 12-5	Double-Contrast Filling of Upper Gastrointestinal System	
Stomach Projection	**Barium-Filled Structures**	**Air-Filled Structures**
PA oblique (RAO position)	Pylorus, duodenum	Fundus
PA	Pylorus, duodenum	Fundus
Right lateral	Pylorus, duodenum, body	Fundus
AP oblique (LPO position)	Fundus	Pylorus, duodenum
AP	Fundus	Pylorus, duodenum, body

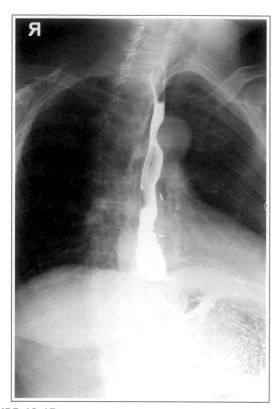

FIGURE 12-17 PA esophagram taken with the right side of the patient positioned closer to the IR than the left side.

tablets that rapidly release 300 to 400 mL of carbon dioxide on contact with the fluid in the stomach. The carbon dioxide causes gastric distention and smoothing of the rugae. Positive (radiopaque) contrast is obtained by having the patient drink a high-density (up to 250% weight or volume) barium suspension. The barium provides the thin coating that covers the mucosal surface. To obtain adequate mucosal coating of the area, the barium is washed over the gastric surface by having the patient turn 360 degrees and then positioning the patient so that the barium pool will be placed away from the area of interest. Because the barium will slowly flow toward the lowest level after coating, the patient should be rotated between projections or the sequence of projections should be taken to optimize coating of the area of interest to maintain an optimal mucosal covering. Table 12-5 indicates where the barium will pool and which aspect of the upper GI tract is best demonstrated in the most commonly obtained stomach and duodenum projections. Failure to obtain good mucosal coating may result in missed or simulated lesions. The quality of the mucosal coating depends on the properties of the barium suspension, the volume of barium and gas, the frequency of washing, and the amount of fluid or secretions and viscosity of mucus in the stomach. Although proper double-contrast filling is primarily the fluoroscopist's responsibility, the technologist's scope of practice does play a part in some of the causes of poor coating, such as using the wrong type of barium, improperly preparing the barium suspension, or performing poor lower intestine preparation. A thorough mixing of the barium suspension is required before the patient ingests the material.

STOMACH AND DUODENUM: PA OBLIQUE PROJECTION (RAO POSITION)

See Table 12-6, (Figures 12-18, 12-19, 12-20, and 12-21). **Patient Obliquity.** To demonstrate the pylorus, duodenal bulb, descending duodenum, and the fundus and stomach body without superimposition the patient is rotated toward the right side until the midcoronal plane is at a 40- to 70-degree angle with the IR. The degree of obliquity needed to accomplish this goal is dependent on the body habitus, as it determines the location and superimposition of these structures. In general, hypersthenic habitus patients require approximately 70 degrees of obliquity, and the asthenic habitus approximately 40 degrees. In the PA oblique the barium pools in the pylorus and duodenal bulb, demonstrating their contour, and air fills the fundus, so the rugae can be evaluated.

If the PA oblique projection does not demonstrate the duodenal bulb and descending duodenum without pyloric superimposition or the fundus without body superimposition, or if the barium is not adequately pooling in the pylorus and duodenum, the degree of obliquity was insufficient. To determine if patient obliquity needs to be increased or decreased, evaluate the location of the zygapophyseal joints within the vertebral bodies. Their appropriate location will vary per the different body types, as indicated in Table 12-6.

STOMACH AND DUODENUM: PA PROJECTION

See Table 12-7, (Figures 12-22, 12-23, 12-24, and 12-25).

TABLE 12-6   PA Oblique Stomach and Duodenum Projection (RAO Position)

Image Analysis Guidelines (Figures 12-18, 12-19, and 12-20)	Related Positioning Procedures (Figure 12-21)
• Air contrast is demonstrated in the fundus and barium is visible in the pylorus, duodenal bulb, and descending duodenum. • Pylorus, duodenal bulb, and descending duodenum are seen without superimposition. • Fundus is seen without body superimposition. • HH: • Left lumbar zygapophyseal joints are in the posterior third of the vertebral bodies. • Long axis of the stomach demonstrates foreshortening, with a closed lesser curvature. • SH: • Left lumbar zygapophyseal joints are at the midline of the vertebral bodies. • Long axis of the stomach is partially foreshortened, with a partially closed lesser curvature. • AH: • Left lumbar zygapophyseal joints are in the anterior third of the vertebral bodies. • Long axis of the stomach is seen without foreshortening. • Lesser curvature is open.	• Place the patient in a prone, PA projection. • Rotate the torso toward the right side until the midcoronal plane is at a 40- to 70-degree angle with the IR. • HH: 70 degrees of obliquity. • SH: 45 degrees of obliquity. • AH: 40 degrees of obliquity. • Flex the left elbow and knee to support and maintain obliquity.
• Pylorus is at the center of the exposure field.	• Center a perpendicular CR halfway between the vertebrae and lateral rib border of the elevated side at the appropriate body type level. • HH: 3-4 inches (7.5-10 cm) superior to the inferior rib margin. • SH: 1-2 inches (2.5-5 cm) superior to the inferior rib margin. • AH: At the inferior rib margin to 1 inch (2.5 cm) inferior to it.
• Stomach and duodenal loop are included within the exposure field.	• Center the IR and grid to the CR. • Longitudinally collimate to a 14-inch (35-cm) field size. • Transversely collimate to the vertebrae and lateral rib border (11-inch [28-cm] field size).

AH, Asthenic habitus; HH, hypersthenic habitus; SH, sthenic habitus.

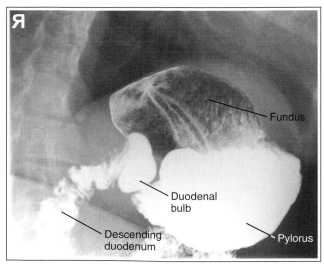

FIGURE 12-18 Hypersthenic PA oblique spot stomach and duodenal projection (RAO position) with accurate positioning.

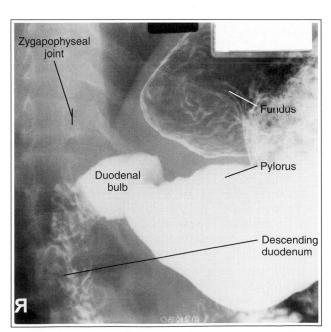

FIGURE 12-19 Sthenic PA oblique spot stomach and duodenal projection (RAO position) with accurate positioning.

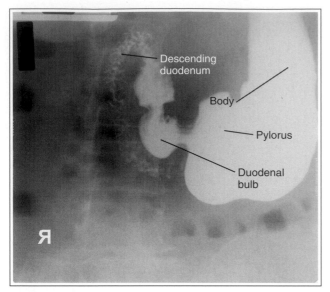

FIGURE 12-20 Asthenic PA oblique spot stomach and duodenal projection (RAO position) with accurate positioning.

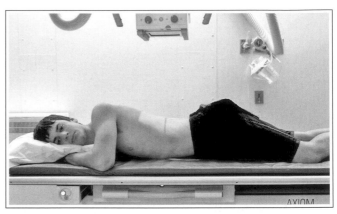

FIGURE 12-21 Proper patient positioning for PA oblique stomach and duodenal projection (RAO position).

TABLE 12-7	PA Stomach and Duodenum Projection

Image Analysis Guidelines (Figures 12-22, 12-23, and 12-24)	Related Positioning Procedures (Figure 12-25)
• Air contrast is demonstrated in the fundus and barium is visible in the body and pylorus. • The spinous processes are aligned with the midline of the vertebral bodies, and the distances from the pedicles to the spinous processes are the same on both sides. • HH: • Stomach is aligned almost horizontally, with the duodenal bulb at the level of T11-T12. • Lesser curvature (posteriorly located) superimposes the greater curvature (anteriorly located), placing the lateral stomach contours in profile. • Stomach body partially superimposes the fundus. • Esophagogastric junction is nearly on end. • SH: • Stomach is aligned almost vertically, with the duodenal bulb at the level of L1-L2. • Stomach is somewhat J-shaped and its long axis is partially foreshortened. • Lesser and greater curvatures, esophagogastric junction, pylorus, and duodenal bulb are in partial profile. • AH: • Stomach is aligned vertically, with the duodenal bulb at the level of L3-L4. • Stomach is J-shaped and its long axis is demonstrated without foreshortening. • Lesser and greater curvatures, esophagogastric junction, pylorus, and duodenal bulb are in partial profile.	• Position the patient in a prone, PA projection. • Place the shoulders and ASISs at equal distances from the table. • Turn the face toward the side that is most comfortable and will avoid rotation of the upper thorax. • Draw arms laterally, away from the thorax.
• Pylorus is at the center of the exposure field.	• Center a perpendicular CR halfway between the vertebrae and left lateral rib border at the appropriate body type level. • HH: 3-4 inches (7.5-10 cm) superior to the inferior rib margin. • SH: 1-2 inches (2.5-5 cm) superior to the inferior rib margin. • AH: at the inferior rib margin to 1 inch (2.5 cm) inferior to it.
• Stomach and descending duodenum are included within the exposure field.	• Center the IR and grid to the CR. • Longitudinally collimate to the full 14-inch (35-cm) field size. • Transversely collimate to the vertebrae and lateral rib border.

AH, Asthenic habitus; HH, hypersthenic habitus; SH, sthenic habitus.

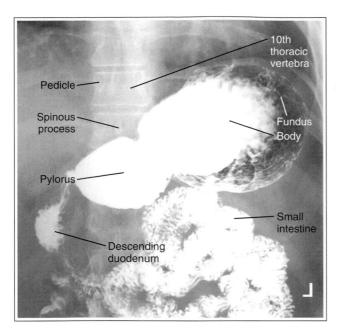

FIGURE 12-22 Hypersthenic PA stomach and duodenum projection with accurate positioning.

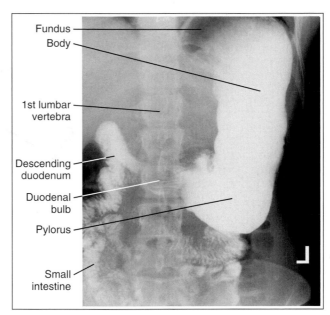

FIGURE 12-24 Asthenic PA stomach and duodenum projection with accurate positioning.

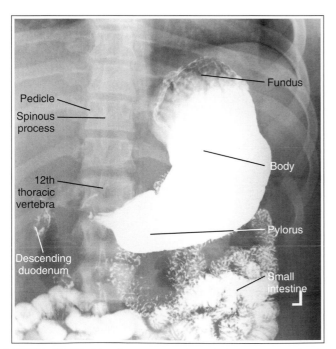

FIGURE 12-23 Sthenic PA stomach and duodenum projection with accurate positioning.

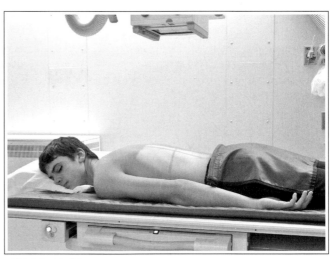

FIGURE 12-25 Proper patient positioning for PA stomach and duodenal projection.

Detecting Rotation. The side demonstrating the greater distance from the pedicles to the spinous processes is the side positioned farther from the IR. The vertebrae demonstrated on the projection should all be evaluated for rotation, since the upper and lower vertebral areas can demonstrate rotation independently or simultaneously.

STOMACH AND DUODENUM: LATERAL PROJECTION (RIGHT LATERAL POSITION)

See Table 12-8, (Figures 12-26, 12-27, 12-28, and 12-29).
Rotation. To obtain a nonrotated lateral stomach projection, position the shoulders, posterior ribs, and ASISs

Patient Obliquity. The PA projection fills the body and pylorus of the stomach with barium, allowing their contours to be evaluated. A nonrotated PA projection is obtained by positioning the shoulders and ASISs at equal distances to the IR. Rotation is effectively detected on a PA stomach by comparing the distance from the pedicles to the spinous processes on both sides.

TABLE 12-8	Lateral Stomach and Duodenum Projection	

Image Analysis Guidelines (Figures 12-26, 12-27, and 12-28)	Related Positioning Procedures (Figure 12-29)
• Air contrast is demonstrated in the fundus, and barium is visible in the pylorus, duodenum bulb, and descending duodenum. • Posterior surfaces of the vertebral bodies are superimposed. • Stomach, duodenal bulb, and descending duodenum are anterior to the vertebrae, demonstrating the retrogastric space. • Pylorus, duodenal bulb, and descending duodenum are in profile. • HH: Long axis of the stomach demonstrates foreshortening, with a closed lesser curvature. • SH: Long axis of the stomach is partially foreshortened, with a partially closed lesser curvature. • AH: Long axis of the stomach is demonstrated without foreshortening, and the lesser curvature is open.	• Position the patient in a recumbent right lateral position. • Flex the knees and hips, and position a pillow or sponge between the knees. • Position the shoulders, the posterior ribs, and the ASISs on top of each other, aligning the midcoronal plane perpendicular to the IR.
• Pylorus is at the center of the exposure field.	• Center a perpendicular CR halfway between the midcoronal plane and anterior abdomen at the appropriate body type level. • HH: 3-4 inches (7.5-10 cm) superior to the inferior rib margin. • SH: 1-2 inches (2.5-5 cm) superior to the inferior rib margin. • AH: At the inferior rib margin to 1 inch (2.5 cm) inferior to it.
• Stomach and duodenal loop are included within the exposure field.	• Center the IR and grid to the CR. • Longitudinally collimate to a 14-inch (35-cm) field size. • Transversely collimate to the vertebrae and lateral rib border.

AH, Asthenic habitus; HH, hypersthenic habitus; SH, sthenic habitus.

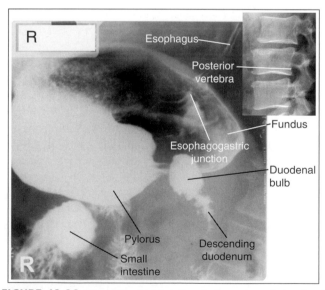

FIGURE 12-26 Hypersthenic lateral spot stomach and duodenal projection (right lateral position) with accurate positioning.

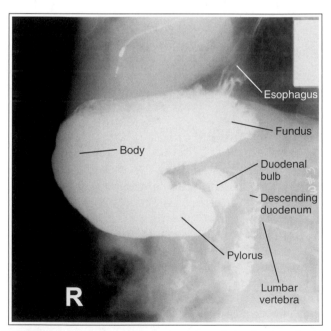

FIGURE 12-27 Sthenic lateral stomach and duodenal projection (right lateral position) with accurate positioning.

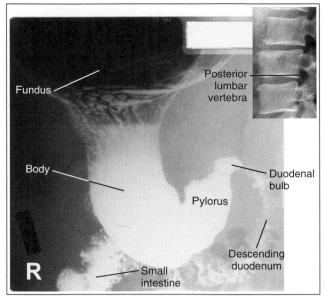

FIGURE 12-28 Asthenic lateral spot stomach and duodenal projection (right lateral position) with accurate positioning.

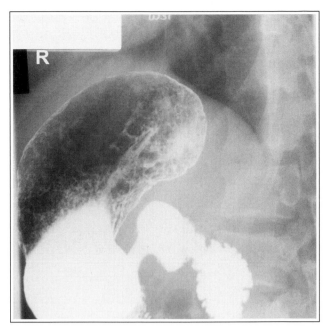

FIGURE 12-30 Lateral stomach and duodenal projection taken with the patient rotated.

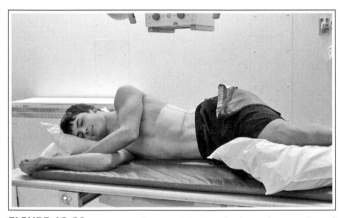

FIGURE 12-29 Proper patient positioning for lateral stomach and duodenal projection (right lateral position).

on top of each other, aligning the midcoronal plane perpendicular to the IR. This is accomplished by resting your extended flat palm against each structure, individually, and then adjusting the patient's rotation until your hand is positioned perpendicular to the table.

Detecting Rotation. On a nonrotated lateral stomach and duodenal projection the vertebral bodies are seen without stomach, duodenum bulb, and descending duodenum superimposition, and the posterior vertebral body surfaces are superimposed, appearing as one. Rotation can be detected on a lateral stomach and duodenal projection when the stomach, duodenum bulb, or descending duodenum superimpose some portion of the vertebral bodies and when the right and left posterior surfaces of the vertebral bodies are demonstrated without superimposition (Figure 12-30).

STOMACH AND DUODENUM: AP OBLIQUE PROJECTION (LAO POSITION)

See Table 12-9, (Figures 12-31, 12-32, 12-33, and 12-34).
Patient Obliquity. The AP oblique (LAO) projection demonstrates the same structures as that demonstrated in the PA oblique (RAO) projection, but because the patient is AP instead of PA the air and barium locations switch. Instead of the air being in the fundus and the barium being in the pylorus and duodenum as it is for the PA oblique, for the AP oblique the barium is in the fundus and air in the pylorus and duodenum. This allows evaluation of the fundus contour and of the rugae of the pylorus and duodenum. To demonstrate the pylorus, duodenal bulb, and descending duodenum and the fundus and stomach body without superimposition the patient is rotated toward the left side until the midcoronal plane is at a 30- to 60-degree angle with the IR. The degree of obliquity needed to accomplish this goal is dependent on the body habitus, as it determines the location and superimposition of these structures. In general, hypersthenic habitus patients require approximately 60 degrees of obliquity, and the asthenic habitus approximately 30 degrees.

If the AP oblique projection does not demonstrate the pylorus without duodenal bulb and descending duodenum superimposition or the body without fundus superimposition, or if the barium is not adequately pooling in the fundus, the degree of obliquity was insufficient. To determine if patient obliquity needs to be increased or decreased, evaluate the location of the zygapophyseal joints within the vertebral bodies. Their appropriate location will vary per the different body types as indicated in Table 12-9.

TABLE 12-9	AP Oblique Stomach and Duodenum Projection (LPO Position)
Image Analysis Guidelines (Figures 12-31, 12-32, and 12-33)	**Related Positioning Procedures (Figure 12-34)**
• Air contrast is demonstrated in the pylorus, duodenal bulb, and descending duodenum, and barium is visible in the fundus. • Pylorus, duodenal bulb, and descending duodenum are seen without superimposition. • Fundus is seen without body superimposition. • HH: • Left lumbar zygapophyseal joints are seen in the posterior third of the vertebral bodies. • Pylorus is superimposed over the vertebrae. • SH: • Left lumbar zygapophyseal joints are seen at the midline of the vertebral bodies. • Vertebrae are demonstrated with little if any pyloric superimposition. • AH: • Left lumbar zygapophyseal joints are seen in the anterior third of the vertebral bodies. • Vertebrae are demonstrated with little if any pyloric superimposition.	• Place the patient in a supine position. • Rotate the patient toward the left side until the midcoronal plane is at a 30- to 60-degree angle with the IR. • HH: 60 degrees of obliquity. • SH: 45 degrees of obliquity. • AH: 30 degrees of obliquity. • Draw the right arm across the chest and have the patient grasp the table edge. • Flex the right knee for support.
• Pylorus is at the center of the exposure field.	• Center a perpendicular CR halfway between the vertebrae and left abdominal margin at the appropriate body type level. • HH: 2 inches (5 cm) superior to the point midway between the xiphoid process and inferior rib margin. • SH: Midway between the xiphoid process and inferior rib margin. • AH: 2 inches (5 cm) inferior to the point midway between the xiphoid process and inferior rib margin.
• Stomach and duodenal loop are included within the exposure field.	• Center the IR and grid to the CR. • Longitudinally collimate to 14-inch (35-cm) field size. • Transversely collimate to the vertebrae and lateral rib border.

AH, Asthenic habitus; HH, hypersthenic habitus; SH, sthenic habitus.

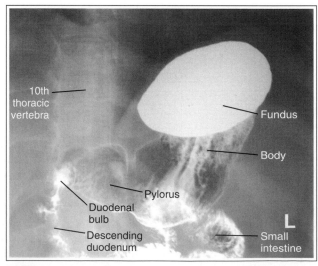

FIGURE 12-31 Hypersthenic AP oblique spot stomach and duodenal projection (LPO position) with accurate positioning.

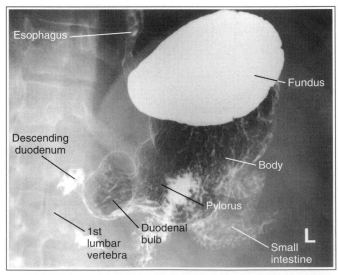

FIGURE 12-32 Sthenic AP oblique spot stomach and duodenal projection (LPO position) with accurate positioning.

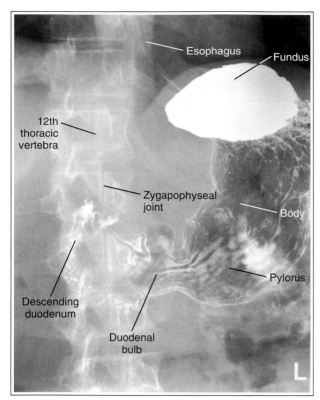

FIGURE 12-33 Asthenic AP oblique spot stomach and duodenal projection (LPO position) with accurate positioning.

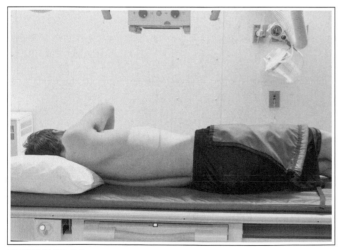

FIGURE 12-34 Proper patient positioning for AP oblique stomach and duodenal projection (LPO position).

STOMACH AND DUODENUM: AP PROJECTION

See Table 12-10, (Figures 12-35, 12-36, 12-37, and 12-38).

Patient Obliquity. The AP projection demonstrates the same structures as those demonstrated in the PA projection, but because the patient is AP instead of PA the air and barium locations switch. Instead of the air being in the fundus and the barium being in the pylorus and duodenum as it is for the PA, for the AP the barium is in the fundus and air in the pylorus and duodenum. This allows evaluation of the fundus contour and of the rugae of the pylorus and duodenum.

Detecting Rotation. A nonrotated AP projection demonstrates the equal distance from the spinous processes to the pedicles on each side and is accomplished when the midcoronal plane is aligned parallel with the IR by positioning the shoulders and ASISs at equal distances from the IR. Rotation is effectively detected on an AP stomach and duodenal projection by comparing the distance from the pedicles to the spinous processes on each side. The side demonstrating the greater distance from the pedicle to the spinous processes is the side positioned closer to the IR.

SMALL INTESTINE

Preparation Procedure

Small Intestine Preparation. Optimal preparation of the small intestine for a small bowel study is obtained through a patient preparation procedure that includes a low-residue diet for 1 to 2 days before the examination, NPO after midnight and until the examination, and avoidance of gum and tobacco products before the examination (these are thought to increase salivation and gastric secretions).

Contrast Medium. For studies of the small intestine, the patient drinks a large amount of barium, then the technologist obtains overhead projections of the stomach and small intestine at timed intervals as peristalsis moves the contrast from the stomach through the small intestine to the cecum. The timing begins when the patient ingests the contrast or as determined by the radiologist. Typically, the first overhead PA projection is obtained at 15 minutes, then at 30 minutes, and then hourly until the barium is demonstrated in the cecum. The barium normally takes 2 to 3 hours to reach the cecum but may vary greatly from patient to patient. Each projection in the timed series must contain a time marker to indicate the amount of time that has passed since the contrast was ingested.

Variations in Positioning Procedure Because of Body Habitus. Because the abdominal cavity varies in size and length because of differences in body habitus and because the abdomen carries much of the fat tissue on the obese patient, there is not a standard protocol that can be followed for all patients for the number of IRs that are needed, the IR size and direction to use, or where the CR is centered. These are chosen so that when all the projections obtained for the exam are combined they together include all of the required image analysis guidelines. Failing to choose correctly will result in clipped structures and an incomplete picture of the small and large intestines (Figure 12-39). The PA and AP projection procedural guidelines for the small and large intestines

TABLE 12-10	AP Stomach and Duodenum Projection	
Image Analysis Guideline (Figures 12-35, 12-36, and 12-37)	**Related Positioning Procedures (Figure 12-38)**
• Air contrast is demonstrated in the pylorus, duodenal bulb, and descending duodenum, and barium is visible in the fundus. • Spinous processes are aligned with the midline of the vertebral bodies and the distances from the pedicles to the spinous processes are the same on both sides. • HH: • Stomach is aligned almost horizontally, with the duodenal bulb at the level of T11-T12. • Lesser curvature (posteriorly located) superimposes the greater curvature (anteriorly located), placing the lateral stomach contours in profile. • Stomach body partially superimposes the fundus. • Esophagogastric junction is almost on end. • SH: • Stomach is aligned almost vertically, with the duodenal bulb at the level of L1-L2. • Stomach is somewhat J-shaped and its long axis is partially foreshortened. • Lesser and greater curvatures, esophagogastric junction, pylorus, and duodenal bulb are in partial profile. • AH: • Stomach is aligned vertically, with the duodenal bulb at the level of L3-L4. • Stomach is J-shaped and its long axis is demonstrated without foreshortening. • Lesser and greater curvatures, esophagogastric junction, pylorus, and duodenal bulb are demonstrated in profile.	• Position the patient in a supine, AP projection. • Place the shoulders and the ASISs at equal distances from the table, aligning the midcoronal plane parallel with the IR.
• Pylorus is at the center of the exposure field.	• Center a perpendicular CR halfway between the vertebrae and left abdominal margin at the appropriate body type level. • HH: 2 inches (5 cm) superior to the point midway between the xiphoid process and inferior rib margin. • SH: midway between the xiphoid process and inferior rib margin. • AH: 2 inches (5 cm) inferior to the point midway between the xiphoid process and inferior rib margin.
• Stomach and duodenal loop are included within the exposure field.	• Center the IR and grid to the CR. • Longitudinally collimate to a 14-inch (35-cm) field size. • Transversely collimate to the lateral rib border.

AH, Asthenic habitus; HH, hypersthenic habitus; SH, sthenic habitus.

(Tables 12-11, 12-13, and 12-15) are for the routine sthenic, hyposthenic, and asthenic, nonobese patient.

Supine Hypersthenic Patient. If using the computed radiography system, two 14 × 17 inch (35 × 43 cm) crosswise IRs are needed to include the required anatomic structures as long as the transverse abdominal measurement is less than 17 inches (43 cm). Take the first projection with the CR centered to the midsagittal plane at a level halfway between the symphysis pubis and ASIS. Position the bottom of the second IR so that it includes 2 to 3 inches (5-7.5 cm) of the same transverse section of the peritoneal cavity imaged on the first projection to ensure that no middle peritoneal information has been excluded. The top of the IR should extend to the patient's xiphoid, to make sure that the twelfth thoracic vertebra is included (Figure 12-40).

If using the DR system, open the longitudinal collimation to a 17-inch (43-cm) field size and transversely collimate to within 0.5 inches (2.5 cm) of the lateral skin line as needed to a 17-inch (43-cm) field size. If more than 17 inches (43 cm) of transverse width is needed for either of these systems, follow the procedure for the obese patient below.

Supine Obese Patient. It may be necessary to obtain three or four projections to demonstrate all of the abdominal structures for the obese patient. Figure 3-125 demonstrates a supine AP abdomen procedure on an obese patient that required three projections to include all of the required abdominal tissue. If using the computed radiography system, take the first projection with the IR crosswise and the CR centered to the midsagittal plane at a level halfway between the symphysis pubis

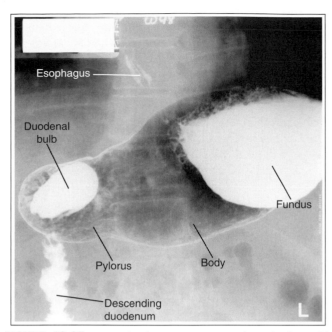

FIGURE 12-35 Hypersthenic AP spot stomach projection with accurate positioning.

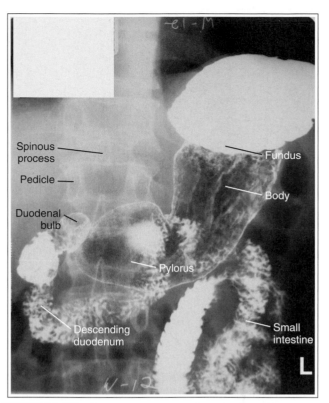

FIGURE 12-36 Sthenic AP spot stomach projection with accurate positioning.

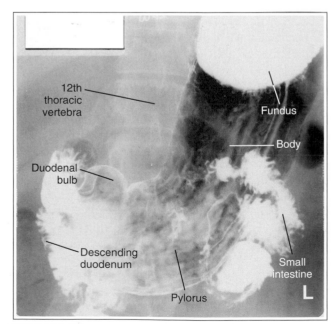

FIGURE 12-37 Asthenic AP spot stomach projection with accurate positioning.

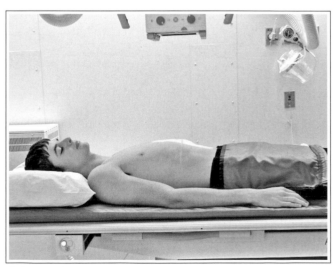

FIGURE 12-38 Proper patient positioning for AP stomach and duodenal projection.

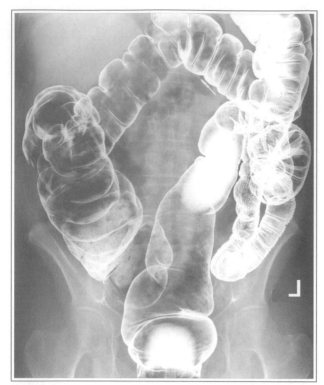

FIGURE 12-39 PA large intestine taken without including the left colic (splenic) flexure and part of the transverse colon.

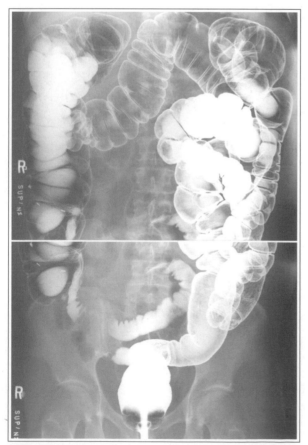

FIGURE 12-40 AP large intestine projections of hypersthenic patient with accurate positioning.

and ASIS. To obtain the second projection, place the IR lengthwise and positioned so the bottom of the IR includes 2 to 3 inches (5-7.5 cm) of the same transverse section of peritoneal cavity imaged on the first projection, center the CR to the IR, and then move the patient (and tabletop) laterally until the CR is centered on the right side halfway between the midsagittal plane and lateral soft tissue. For the third projection, repeat the procedure for the left side of the patient. The second and third projections should include 2 to 3 inches (5-7.5 cm) of overlapping peritoneal tissue at the midsagittal plane.

If using the DR system, follow that used for the computed radiography system with the exception that collimation will need to be less than the full 17-inch (43-cm) field size available or more than 2 to 3 inches (5-7.5 cm) of overlap will result.

SMALL INTESTINE: PA PROJECTION

See Table 12-11, (Figures 12-41, 12-42, 12-43, and 12-44).

CR Centering for Early Versus Later Series Projections. The CR is centered 2 inches higher for the projections obtained early in the series to demonstrate the barium-filled stomach, descending duodenum, and superior small intestines, which are located more superiorly in the abdomen. As the contrast medium works its way through the small intestines to reach the cecum the CR centering is adjusted inferiorly. Failure to adjust the CR centering as the contrast medium progresses may result in clipping of pertinent structures (Figure 12-45).

Rotation. To obtain a nonrotated PA small intestine projection, position the shoulders and ASISs at equal distances from the table. The prone position is chosen to demonstrate the small intestine because it will cause compression of the abdominal structures, increasing image quality.

Detecting Abdominal Rotation. Evaluate all the vertebrae on the projection for rotation, since the upper and lower lumbar vertebrae can demonstrate rotation independently or simultaneously, depending on which section of the body is rotated. Rotation is effectively detected on a PA small intestine projection by comparing the distances from the pedicles to the spinous processes on both sides and the symmetry of the iliac wings. The side demonstrating the greater distance from the pedicles to the spinous processes and the wider iliac wing is the side positioned farther from the IR.

LARGE INTESTINE

Preparation Procedure

Large Intestine Preparation. Adequate cleansing of the large intestine for a barium enema is obtained through a patient preparation procedure including a low-residue diet for 2 to 3 days before the examination, followed by a clear liquid diet 1 day before the

TABLE 12-11	PA Small Intestinal Projection (for Sthenic, Hyposthenic, and Asthenic Nonobese Patients)

Image Analysis Guidelines (Figures 12-41, 12-42, and 12-43)	Related Positioning Procedures (Figure 12-44)
• Marker indicates the amount of time that has elapsed since the patient ingested the contrast medium.	• Place marker on IR that indicates the time since the patient ingested the contrast.
• Spinous processes are aligned with the midline of the vertebral bodies. The distances from the pedicles to the spinous processes are the same on both sides.	• Position the patient in a prone, PA projection.
• Iliac wings are symmetric.	• Place the shoulders and ASISs at equal distances from the table, aligning the midcoronal plane parallel with IR.
• Small intestine is at the center of the exposure field.	• Draw the arms laterally.
	• Earlier in series: Center a perpendicular CR to the midsagittal plane at a level 2 inches (5 cm) superior to the iliac crest.
	• Later in series: Center a perpendicular CR to the midsagittal plane at the level of the iliac crest.
• Early in series: Stomach and proximal aspects of the small intestine are included within the exposure field on projection.	• Center the IR and grid to the CR.
• Later in series: Small intestine and cecum are included within the exposure field on projection.	• Longitudinally collimate to a 17-inch (43-cm) field size.
	• Transversely collimate to within 0.5 inch (1.25 cm) of the patient's lateral skin line.

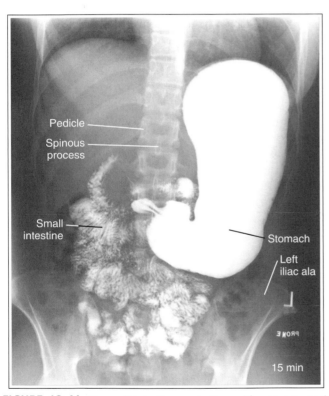

FIGURE 12-41 PA small intestine projection with accurate positioning 15 minutes after ingestion.

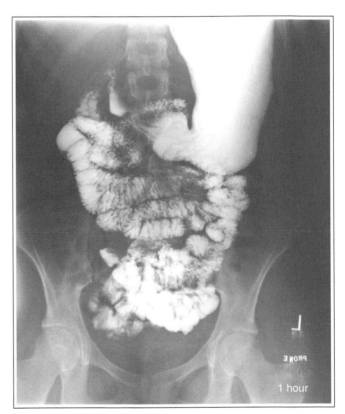

FIGURE 12-42 PA small intestine projection with accurate positioning 1 hour after ingestion.

examination, laxatives the afternoon before the examination, and a suppository or cleansing enema the morning of the examination. Remaining fecal material may obscure the mucosal surfaces and, when barium-coated, may mimic polyps and small tumors. Remaining residual fluid causes dilution of the barium suspension, resulting in poor mucosal coating and coating artifacts (Figure 12-46). On arrival in the fluoroscopic department, the patient should be queried to determine whether proper preparation instructions were given and followed. Adequate preparation can be assumed if the patient's last bowel movement lacked solid fecal material.

Good Double-Contrast Lower Intestinal Filling. Good gaseous distention is demonstrated when:
• Bowel lumina are distended, eliminating the mucosal folds and allowing all parts of the barium-coated mucosal lining of the colon and any small intraluminal lesions to be visualized.

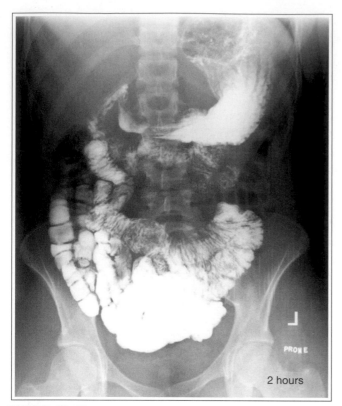

FIGURE 12-43 PA small intestine projection with accurate positioning 2 hours after ingestion.

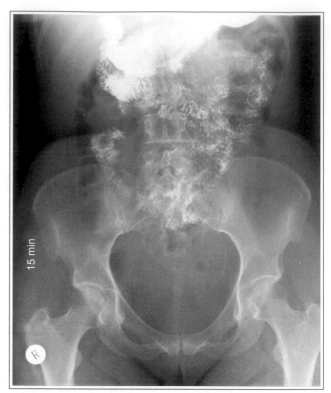

FIGURE 12-45 PA small intestine projection taken early in the series and not including the stomach.

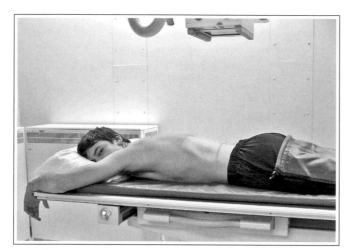

FIGURE 12-44 Proper patient positioning for PA small intestine projection.

Good lower intestinal barium coating is demonstrated when:
- Surface positioned farther from the IR on recumbent projections or superiorly on erect projections, also called the nondependent surface, demonstrates a thin layer of barium coating on the mucosal surface.
- Surface positioned closer to the IR on recumbent projections or inferiorly on erect projections, also called the dependent (decubitus) surface, demonstrates a thin layer of barium coating of the highest structures, with barium pooled in the lower crevices.

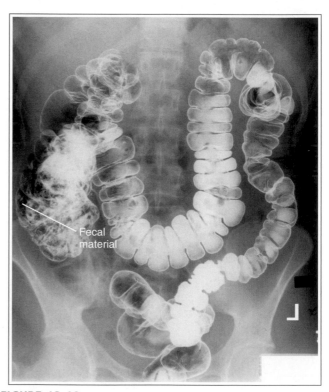

FIGURE 12-46 PA large intestine projection demonstrating fecal matter in the cecum.

Barium Pools. The barium pools are used to wash away residual fecal material from the dependent surface, coat the mucosal surface, and fill any depressed lesions as the patient is rotated. Ideally, barium should fill one third of the large intestine diameter. Overfilling or underfilling may result in obscured lesions or inadequate intestinal washing, respectively. See Table 12-12 to determine where barium pooling will occur on a lower intestine projection. Pooling will occur in the anterior surface on prone projections, posterior surface on supine projections, and inferiorly, between the mucosal folds, on erect projections.

Poor Double Contrast. Poor gaseous distention results in pockets of large barium pools and compacted intestinal segments with tight mucosal folds. Poor mucosal coating is demonstrated by thin, irregular, or interrupted barium coating or excessive barium pooling. Poor coating may cause lesions to be easily missed. Although proper double-contrast filling is primarily the fluoroscopist's responsibility, the technologist's scope of practice may play a part in some of the causes for poor coating, such as using the wrong type of barium, improperly preparing the barium suspension, or performing poor lower intestinal preparation.

LARGE INTESTINE: PA OR AP PROJECTION

See Table 12-13, (Figures 12-47, 12-48, and 12-49).

Detecting Abdominal Rotation. Rotation is effectively detected on a PA or AP lower intestine projection by comparing the distances from the pedicles to the spinous processes on both sides, the symmetry of the iliac wing, and the superimposition of the colic flexures. The x-ray beam divergence causes very different-appearing iliac wings on AP and PA projections as demonstrated by the pelves projections in Figure 12-50. Note that the iliac wings in the AP projection (supine) are wider than those in the PA projection (prone). This information can be used to distinguish whether a projection was taken with the patient in an AP or PA projection. The narrow iliac wings of a PA projection should not be mistaken for narrowness caused by rotation.

PA Projection. For a PA projection the side demonstrating the greater distance from the pedicles to the spinous processes, wider iliac wing, and colic flexure with greater ascending and descending limb superimposition is the side positioned farther from the IR (Figure 12-51).

AP Projection. For an AP projection the side demonstrating the greater distance from the pedicle to the spinous processes, wider iliac wing, and colic flexure with the greater ascending and descending limb superimposition is the side positioned closer to the IR.

TABLE 12-12	Double-Contrast Filling of Large Intestinal Structures	
Large Intestine	**AP Projection (Supine)**	**PA Projection (Prone)**
Cecum	Air	Barium
Ascending colon	Barium	Air
Ascending limb right colic (hepatic) flexure	Barium	Air
Descending limb right colic (hepatic) flexure	Barium	Air
Transverse colon	Air	Barium
Ascending limb left colic (splenic) flexure	Air	Barium
Descending limb left colic (splenic) flexure	Barium	Air
Descending colon	Barium	Air
Sigmoid colon	Air	Barium
Rectum	Barium	Air

TABLE 12-13	PA-AP Large Intestinal Projection (for Sthenic, Hyposthenic, and Asthenic, Nonobese Patients)
Image Analysis Guidelines (Figures 12-47 and 12-48)	**Related Positioning Procedures (Figure 12-49)**
• Spinous processes are aligned with the midline of the vertebral bodies, with the distances from the pedicles to spinous processes the same on both sides. • The iliac wings are symmetric. • Ascending and descending limbs of the colic flexure demonstrate some degree of superimposition. • 4th lumbar vertebra is at the center of the exposure field.	• Position the patient prone, in a PA projection, or in a supine, AP projection. • Place the shoulders and the ASISs at equal distances from the table, aligning the midcoronal plane parallel with the IR. • Center a perpendicular CR to the midsagittal plane at the level of the iliac crest.
• Entire large intestine, including the left colic flexure and rectum, is included within the exposure field.	• Center the IR and grid to the CR. • Longitudinally collimate to a 17-inch (43-cm) field size. • Transversely collimate to within 0.5 inch (1.25 cm) of the lateral skin line.

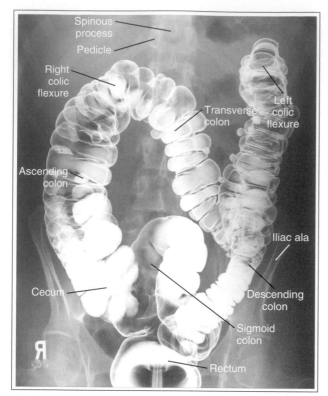

FIGURE 12-47 PA large intestine projection with accurate positioning.

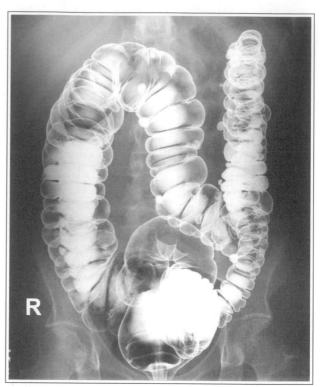

FIGURE 12-48 AP large intestine projection with accurate positioning.

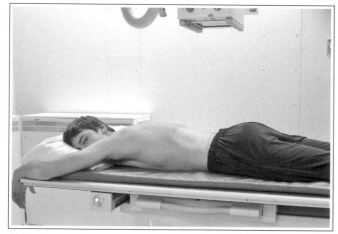

FIGURE 12-49 Proper patient positioning for PA large intestine projection.

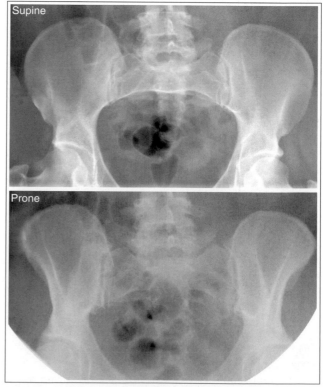

FIGURE 12-50 Iliac alae images of supine and prone patient.

TABLE 12-14 | Lateral Large Intestinal (Rectum) Projection

Image Analysis Guidelines (Figure 12-52)	Related Positioning Procedures (Figure 12-53)
• Scatter radiation is controlled. • Rectum is in profile. • Sacrum demonstrates a lateral projection. • Median sacral crest is in profile and the femoral heads are superimposed.	• Place a lead sheet on the table at the edge of the posteriorly collimated field. • Position the patient in a recumbent lateral position (typically left). • Place the shoulders, the posterior ribs, and ASISs on top of the other, aligning the midcoronal plane perpendicular to the IR. • Flex the knees and hips for support, and position a pillow or sponge that is thick enough to prevent anterior pelvis rotation between the knees.
• Rectosigmoid region is at the center of the exposure field. • Rectum, distal sigmoid, sacrum, and femoral heads are included within the exposure field.	• Center a perpendicular CR to the midcoronal plane at the level of the ASIS. • Center the IR and grid to the CR. • Longitudinally collimate to a 12-inch (30-cm) field size. • Transversely collimate to a 10-inch (24-cm) field size.

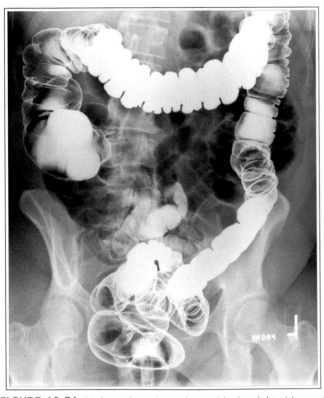

FIGURE 12-51 PA large intestine taken with the right side positioned closer to the IR than the left side.

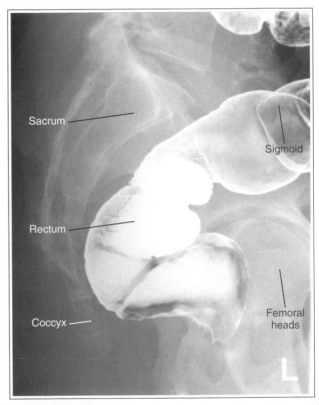

FIGURE 12-52 Lateral large intestine (rectum) projection with accurate positioning.

LARGE INTESTINE (RECTUM): LATERAL PROJECTION

See Table 12-14, (Figures 12-52 and 12-53).

Rotation. To obtain a lateral sacral projection without rotation align the midcoronal plane perpendicular to the IR. Flex the knees and hips for support, and position a pillow or sponge between the knees. The pillow or sponge should be thick enough to prevent the side of the pelvis situated farther from the IR from rotating anteriorly, without being so thick as to cause this side to rotate

posteriorly (Figure 12-53). Rotation can be detected on a lateral rectum projection by evaluating the degree of femoral head superimposition. On a nonrotated lateral rectal projection, the femoral heads are directly superimposed. On rotation, the femoral heads will move away from each other. When rotation has occurred, evaluate the placement of the femoral heads to determine the way in which the patient was rotated. The femoral head that demonstrates the greater magnification is the one situated farther from the IR (Figures 12-54 and 12-55).

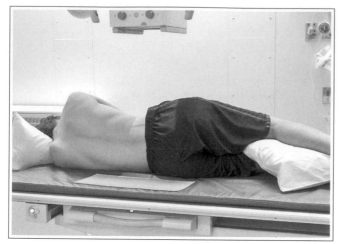

FIGURE 12-53 Proper patient positioning for lateral large intestine projection.

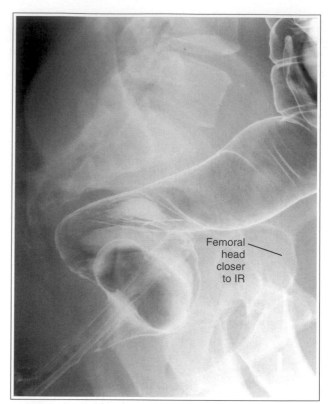

FIGURE 12-55 Lateral large intestine (rectum) taken with the right side of the patient rotated posteriorly to the left.

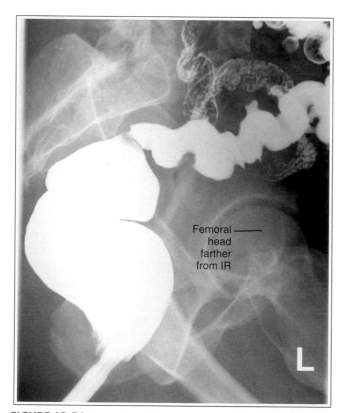

Femoral head farther from IR

L

FIGURE 12-54 Lateral large intestine (rectum) taken with the right side of the patient rotated anterior to the left side.

LARGE INTESTINE: AP OR PA PROJECTION (LATERAL DECUBITUS POSITION)

See Table 12-15, (Figures 12-56, 12-57, and 12-58).
IR Size and Direction for Hypersthenic and Obese Patients. Take two projections using 14- × 17-inch (35- × 43-cm) crosswise field sizes (IR cassettes for computed radiography) on hypersthenic patients and obese patients

who have a transverse abdominal measurement of 14 inches (35 cm) or more to include all the necessary lower intestinal structures. Take the first projection with the CR centered to the midsagittal plane at a level halfway between the symphysis pubis and ASIS. Position the bottom of the second projection so that it includes 2 to 3 inches (5-7.5 cm) of the same transverse section of the peritoneal cavity imaged on the first projection to ensure that no middle peritoneal information has been excluded. The top of the IR should extend to the patient's xiphoid (which is at the level of the tenth thoracic vertebra) to make sure that the left colic (splenic) flexure is included.
Rotation. Rotation is effectively detected on a PA or AP lower intestine projection (lateral decubitus position) by comparing the distance from the pedicles to the spinous processes on each side, the symmetry of the iliac wings, and the superimposition of the colic flexures.

PA Decubitus Projection. The side demonstrating the greater distance from the pedicles to the spinous processes, wider iliac ala, and colic flexure with greater ascending and descending limb superimposition is the side positioned farther from the IR (Figure 12-59).

AP Decubitus Projection. The side demonstrating the greater distance from the pedicle to the spinous processes, wider iliac ala, and colic flexure with greater ascending and descending limb superimposition is the side positioned closer to the IR (Figure 12-60).

TABLE 12-15	AP-PA Large Intestinal Projection (Lateral Decubitus Position) (for Sthenic, Hyposthenic, and Asthenic, Nonobese Patients)
Image Analysis Guideline (Figures 12-56 and 12-57)	**Related Positioning Procedures (Figure 12-58)**
• An arrow or word marker indicating the side of patient that was positioned up and away from the table is present.	• Add an arrow or "word" marker that indicates the side that is up and away from the table superiorly, away from the anatomic structures of interest, and within the collimated field.
• Spinous processes are aligned with the midline to the vertebral bodies, with equal distances from the pedicles to the spinous processes on both sides. • Iliac wings are symmetric. • Ascending and descending limbs of the colic flexures demonstrate some degree of superimposition.	• Position the patient in a left (right) recumbent lateral projection on the imaging table or cart with the back (AP) or abdomen (PA) resting against a grid cassette or the upright IR holder. • Align the shoulders, the posterior ribs, and the pelvic wings so they are at equal distances with the IR.
• Abdominal field positioned against the table is seen in its entirety and without artifact lines.	• Flex knees and place a pillow between them to prevent rotation. • Elevate the patient on a radiolucent sponge or hard surface such as a cardiac board to position the abdomen above the IR's border.
• 4th lumbar vertebra is at the center of the exposure field.	• Center a perpendicular CR to the midsagittal plane at the level of the iliac crest.
• Entire large intestine, including the left colic flexure and rectum, is included within the exposure field.	• Center the IR and grid to the CR. • Longitudinally collimate to a 17-inch (43-cm) field size. • Transversely collimate to within 0.5 inches (1.25 cm) of the lateral skin line.

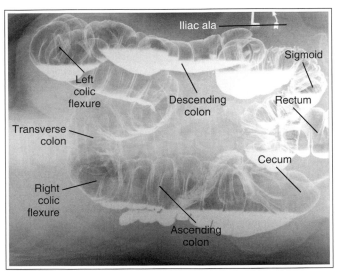

FIGURE 12-56 AP large intestine projection (right lateral decubitus position) with accurate positioning.

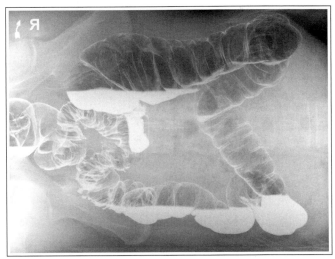

FIGURE 12-57 PA large intestine projection (left lateral decubitus position) with accurate positioning.

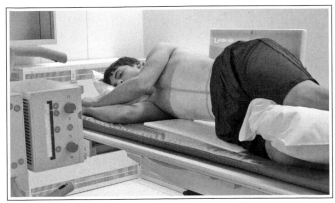

FIGURE 12-58 Proper patient positioning for AP large intestine projection (right lateral decubitus position).

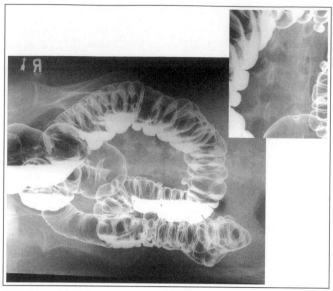

FIGURE 12-59 PA large intestine (lateral decubitus) taken with the right side of the patient positioned closer to the IR than the left side.

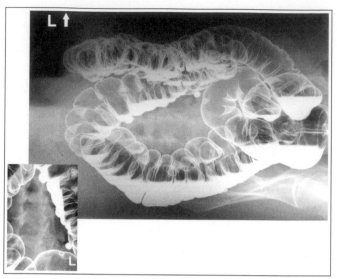

FIGURE 12-60 AP large intestine (lateral decubitus) taken with the left side of the patient positioned closer to the IR than the right side.

TABLE 12-16	PA Oblique Large Intestinal Projection (RAO Position)
Image Analysis Guidelines (Figure 12-61)	**Related Positioning Procedures (Figure 12-62)**
• Ascending and descending limbs of the right colic flexure are seen with decreased superimposition when compared with the PA projection, whereas the limbs of the left colic flexure demonstrate increased superimposition and the rectosigmoid segments are seen without transverse superimposition. • Right iliac ala is narrower than the left, and the distances from the right pedicles to the spinous processes are narrower than the distances from the left pedicles to the spinous processes.	• Position the patient prone on the table. • Rotate the torso toward the right side until the midcoronal plane is at a 35- to 45-degree angle with the table. • Flex the left elbow and knee as needed to support the patient and maintain accurate obliquity.
• Midabdomen is at the center of the exposure field.	• Center a perpendicular CR 1-2 inches (2.5-5 cm) to the left of the midsagittal plane at the level of the iliac crest.
• Entire large intestine is included within the exposure field.	• Center the IR and grid to the CR. • Longitudinally collimate to a 17-inch (43-cm) field size. • Transversely collimate to within 0.5 inch (1.25 cm) of the lateral skin line.

LARGE INTESTINE: PA OBLIQUE PROJECTION (RAO POSITION)

See Table 12-16, (Figures 12-61 and 12-62).

Patient Obliquity. A PA oblique large intestine projection (RAO position) is obtained by positioning the patient prone on the table and then rotating the torso toward the right side until the midcoronal plane is at a 35- to 45-degree angle with the imaging table. In the PA projection, the descending limb of the right colic (hepatic) flexure is superimposed over the ascending limb and the rectum is superimposed over the distal sigmoid. Rotating the patient toward the right side moves the ascending right colic limb from beneath the descending limb and the distal sigmoid from beneath the rectum (transversely), allowing better visualization of these structures. The left elbow and knee are partially flexed and are used to support the patient and maintain accurate obliquity (Figure 12-62).

Detecting Inadequate Obliquity. Insufficient obliquity of the large intestine is demonstrated on the PA oblique projection when the ascending and descending limbs of the right colic flexure are superimposed and the rectum is superimposed over the distal sigmoid (Figure 12-63).

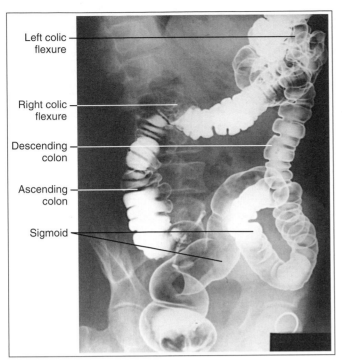

FIGURE 12-61 PA oblique large intestine projection (RAO position) with accurate positioning. *(From Frank ED, Long BW, Smith BJ. Merrill's atlas of radiographic positions and radiologic procedures, vol 2, ed 10, St. Louis, 2007, Mosby, p. 179.)*

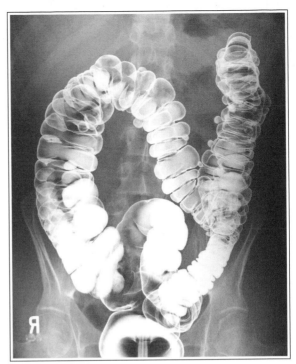

FIGURE 12-63 PA oblique large intestine taken with the patient insufficiently rotated.

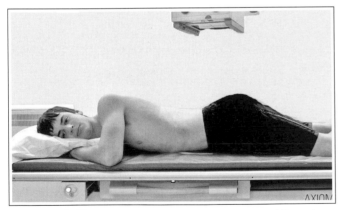

FIGURE 12-62 Proper patient positioning for PA oblique large intestine projection (RAO position).

LARGE INTESTINE: PA OBLIQUE PROJECTION (LAO POSITION)

See Table 12-17, (Figures 12-64 and 12-65).

Patient Obliquity. A PA oblique large intestine projection (LAO) is obtained by positioning the patient prone on the table and then rotating the torso toward the left side until the midcoronal plane is at a 35- to 45-degree angle with the table. In the PA projection, the descending limb of the left colic (splenic) flexure is superimposed over the ascending limb, and the rectum is superimposed over the distal sigmoid. Rotating the patient toward the left side moves the descending left colic limb from beneath the ascending limb, allowing better visualization of these structures. The right elbow and knee are partially flexed and are used to support the patient and maintain accurate obliquity (Figure 12-65).

Detecting Inadequate Obliquity. Insufficient obliquity of the colon is demonstrated on the PA oblique projection when the ascending and descending limbs of the left colic flexure are superimposed.

TABLE 12-17	**PA Oblique Large Intestinal Projection (LAO Position)**
Image Analysis Guidelines (Figure 12-64)	**Related Positioning Procedures (Figure 12-65)**
• Ascending and descending limbs of the left colic flexure are seen with decreased superimposition when compared with a PA projection, whereas the limbs of the right colic flexure demonstrate increased superimposition. • Left iliac ala is narrower than the right and the distances from the left pedicles to the spinous processes are narrower than the distances from the right pedicles to the spinous processes.	• Position the patient prone on the table. • Rotate the torso toward the left side until the midcoronal plane is at a 35- to 45-degree angle with the table. • Flex the left elbow and knee as needed to support the patient and maintain accurate obliquity.
• Midabdomen is at the center of the exposure field.	• Center a perpendicular CR 1-2 inches (2.5-5 cm) to the right of the midsagittal plane at the level 1-2 inches (2.5-5 cm) superior to the iliac crest.
• Entire large intestine is included within the exposure field.	• Center the IR and grid to the CR. • Longitudinally collimate to a 17-inch (43-cm) field size. • Transversely collimate to within 0.5 inch (1.25 cm) of the lateral skin line.

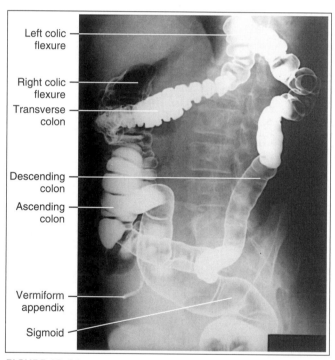

FIGURE 12-64 PA oblique large intestine projection (LAO position) with accurate positioning. *(From Frank ED, Long BW, Smith BJ. Merrill's atlas of radiographic positions and radiologic procedures, vol 2, ed 10, St. Louis, 2007, Mosby, p. 179.)*

Left colic flexure

Right colic flexure

Transverse colon

Descending colon

Ascending colon

Vermiform appendix

Sigmoid

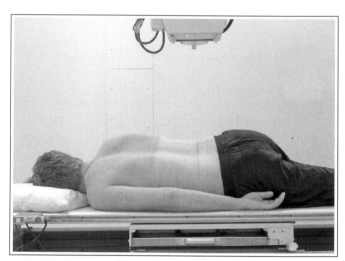

FIGURE 12-65 Proper patient positioning for PA oblique large intestine projection (LAO position).

LARGE INTESTINE: PA AXIAL PROJECTION AND PA AXIAL OBLIQUE PROJECTION (RAO POSITION)

See Table 12-18, (Figures 12-66, 12-67, and 12-68).

PA Axial: Rotation. A PA axial large intestine projection is demonstrated without rotation when the midcoronal plane is aligned perpendicular to the IR (Figure 12-67). Rotation is effectively detected on a PA axial large intestine projection by evaluating the symmetry of the iliac wings and obturator foramen. If the patient was

rotated away from the prone position, the iliac wing positioned farther from the IR will increase in width, the iliac wing positioned closer to the IR will narrow, the obturator foramina positioned farther from the IR will narrow, and the obturator foramina positioned closer to the IR will widen.

PA Axial Oblique Projection (RAO Position): Patient Obliquity. A PA axial oblique large intestine projection (RAO position) is obtained by positioning the patient prone on the table and then rotating the torso toward the right side until the midcoronal plane is at a 35- to 45-degree angle with the table. In the PA projection, the rectum is superimposed over the distal sigmoid, obscuring the rectosigmoid junction. Rotating the patient toward the right side moves the sigmoid from beneath the rectum (transversely), allowing better demonstration of this area (Figure 12-68).

Detecting Inadequate Obliquity. Insufficient patient rotation of the rectosigmoid and pelvic area is

TABLE 12-18	PA Axial and PA Axial Oblique (RAO Position) Large Intestinal Projection
Image Analysis Guidelines (Figure 12-66)	**Related Positioning Procedures (Figures 12-67 and 12-68)**
• PA axial: Iliac wings and obturator foramen are symmetric. • PA axial oblique: • Rectosigmoid segments are seen without transverse superimposition. • Right sacroiliac (SI) joint is shown just medial to the ASIS. • Left obturator foramen is open. • Rectosigmoid segment is demonstrated without inferosuperior superimposition, the pelvis is elongated, and the left inferior acetabulum is at the level of the distal rectum.	• Position the patient prone on the table. • PA axial: Place the shoulders and ASISs at equal distances from the table, aligning the midcoronal plane parallel with the IR. • PA axial oblique: • Rotate the torso toward the right side until the midcoronal plane is at a 35- to 45-degree angle with the IR. • Flex the left elbow and knee as needed to support the patient and maintain obliquity. • Angle the CR 30 to 40 degrees caudally.
• Rectosigmoid area is at the center of the exposure field.	• PA axial: Center the CR to exit at the level of the ASIS and to the midsagittal plane. • PA axial oblique: Center the CR to exit at the level of the ASIS and 2 inches (5 cm) to the left of the spinous processes.
• Rectum, sigmoid, and pelvic structures are included within the exposure field.	• Center the IR and grid to the CR. • Longitudinally collimate to a 14-inch (35-cm) or 17-inch (43-cm) field size. • Transversely collimate to an 11-inch (28-cm) or 14-inch (35-cm) field size.

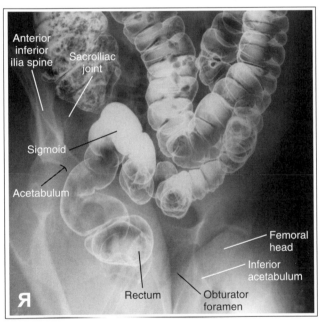

FIGURE 12-66 PA axial oblique large intestine projection (RAO position) with accurate positioning.

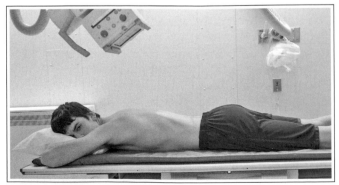

FIGURE 12-67 Proper patient positioning for PA axial oblique large intestine projection (RAO position).

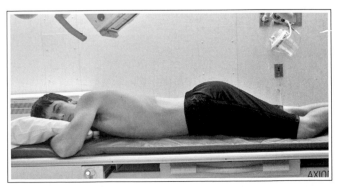

FIGURE 12-68 Proper patient positioning for PA axial large intestine projection.

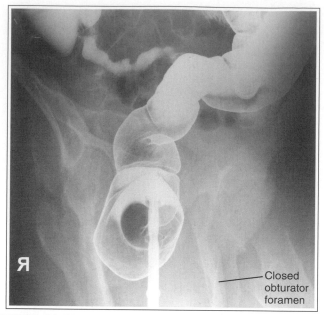

FIGURE 12-69 PA axial oblique large intestine taken with the pelvis rotated more than 45 degrees and with insufficient cephalic CR angulation.

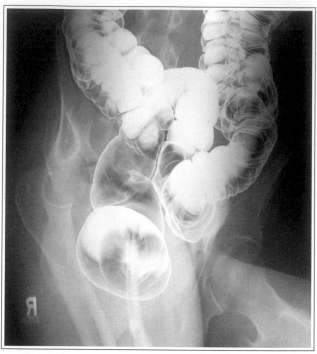

FIGURE 12-70 PA axial oblique large intestine taken with the pelvis rotated more than 45 degrees and with excessive cephalic CR angulation.

demonstrated on the PA axial oblique projection when the rectum is superimposed over the sigmoid colon, the right SI joint is too medial to the ASIS, and the left obturator foramen is narrowed. Too much pelvic rotation is demonstrated when the right SI joint is obscured and the left obturator foramen is closed (Figures 12-69 and 12-70).

CR Angulation. The PA axial oblique (RAO position) and PA axial projections of the large intestine are obtained to demonstrate the rectosigmoid area with less superimposition. To move the posteriorly situated rectum inferiorly and off the distal sigmoid, a 30- to 40-degree caudal angulation is used, decreasing rectosigmoid superimposition and better demonstrating the area. This angulation also elongates the pelvic structures.

Detecting Inadequate CR Angulation. When the rectosigmoid segment demonstrates inferosuperior overlap, the CR angulation used was inadequate. If the inferior aspect of the left acetabulum is demonstrated superior to the distal rectum, the CR was insufficient (see Figure 12-69). If the inferior aspect of the left acetabulum is demonstrated inferior to the distal rectum, the CR angulation was too great (see Figure 12-70).

Adler A, Carlton R: In *Introduction to radiologic sciences and patient care*, ed 5, St Louis, 2011, Elsevier.

Bontrager K, Lampignano J: In *Textbook of radiographic positioning and related anatomy*, ed 8, St Louis, 2013, Elsevier.

Bushberg JT, Seibert JA, Leidholdt EM, et al: In *The essential physics of medical imaging*, ed 3, Philadelphia, 2011, Lippincott Williams & Wilkins.

Bushong SC: In *Radiologic science for technologists*, ed 10, St Louis, 2012, Elsevier.

Carroll QB: In *Radiography science for technologists*, ed 10, Springfield, IL, 2012, Charles C Thomas.

Carter CE, Veale BL: In *Digital Radiography and PACS*, ed 2, St Louis, 2013, Elsevier.

Ehrlich RA, McCloskey ED, Daly JA: In *Patient care in radiography*, ed 8, St Louis, 2012, Mosby.

Eisenberg RL: In *Gastrointestinal radiology: A pattern approach*, ed 4, Philadelphia, 2002, Lippincott Williams & Wilkins.

Fauber TL: In *Radiographic imaging and exposure*, ed 4, St Louis, 2012, Elsevier.

Frank ED, Long BW, Smith BJ: In *Merrill's atlas of radiographic positioning and radiologic procedures*, ed 12, St Louis, 2011, Elsevier.

Frank ED, et al: Mayo Clinic: Radiography of the ankle mortise. *Radiol Technol* 62:354–359, 1991.

Fraser RG, Colman N, Muller N, et al: In *Synopsis of diseases of the chest*, ed 3, Philadelphia, 2005, Saunders.

Hobbs DL: Chest radiography for radiologic technologists, *Radiol Technol* 78:494–516, 2007.

Jeffrey RB, Ralls PW, Leung AN, et al: In *Emergency imaging*, Philadelphia, 1999, Lippincott Williams & Wilkins.

Levine MS, Rubesin SE, Laufer I: In *Double contrast gastro-intestinal radiology*, ed 3, Philadelphia, 2000, Saunders.

Moore QT, Steven D, Goske MJ, et al: *Image gently: Using exposure indicators to improve pediatric digital radiography.* Radiol Technol 2012 84(1):93–99, 2012.

Rogers LF: In *Radiology of skeletal trauma*, ed 3, New York, 2002, Churchill Livingstone.

Shephard CT: In *Radiographic image production and manipulation*, New York, 2003, McGraw-Hill.

Standring S: In *Gray's anatomy: The anatomical basis of clinical practice*, ed 39, St Louis, 2004, Churchill Livingstone.

Statkiewicz MA, Visconti PJ, Ritenour ER, et al: In *Radiation protection in medical radiography*, ed 7, St Louis, 2013, Elsevier.

Thornton A, Gyll C: In *Children's fracture: A radiological guide to safe practice*, London, 2000, Baillière Tindall.

Tortora GJ, Derrickson BH: In *Principles of anatomy and physiology*, ed 13, New York, 2011, John Wiley & Sons.

Ward R, Blickman H: In *Pediatric imaging*, St Louis, 2005, Mosby.

Williamson SL: In *Primary pediatric radiology*, Philadelphia, 2002, Saunders.

abduct To move an extremity outward, away from the torso. The humerus is abducted when it is elevated laterally.

abductor tubercle Round bony structure located posteriorly on the medial aspect of the femur, just superior to the medial condyle.

acanthiomeatal line Imaginary line connecting the point where the upper lip and nose meet with the external ear opening.

additive condition Condition that results in change to the normal bony structures, soft tissues, or air or fluid content of the patient; may require technical changes to compensate for them prior to exposing the patient. Additive diseases cause the tissues to increase atomic density or thickness, resulting in them being more radiopaque.

adduct To move an extremity toward the torso. The humerus is adducted when it is positioned closer to the torso after being abducted.

ALARA Acronym for keeping radiation exposure "*as low as reasonably achievable.*"

algorithm Set of rules or directions used by the computer for getting a specific outcome from a specific input.

annotation Adding markers (e.g., R or L side, text words) to the radiograph after the exposure has been made from the computer display monitor.

anode heel effect Absorption of radiation in the heel of the anode that results in less x-ray intensity at the anode side of a long IR when compared with the cathode side.

anterior (antero-) Refers to the front surface of the patient, used to express something situated at or directed toward the front; includes the palms and tops of the feet as in anatomic position. *The sternum is anterior to the vertebral column.*

anterior shoulder dislocation Condition in which the humeral head is demonstrated anteriorly beneath the coracoid.

artifact Undesirable structure or substance recorded on the image. It may or may not be covering the VOI.

atomic density The concentration of atoms within a given tissue space.

automatic exposure control (AEC) System used in radiography that automatically stops the exposure time when adequate IR exposure has been reached.

automatic implantable cardioverter defibrillator (ICD) Used to detect heart arrhythmias and then deliver an electrical shock to the heart to convert it to a normal rhythm.

automatic rescaling Final phase of image processing in digital radiography during which the computer compares the image histogram with the selected lookup table (LUT) and applies algorithms to the raw data to align the image histogram with the LUT.

axilla Armpit.

backup timer Maximum time that the AEC x-ray exposure will be allowed to continue before automatically shutting off.

bilateral Both sides.

bit depth Determines the maximum range of pixel values the computer can store. The values signify the gray scale that is available to create the digital image.

body habitus Body physique or type. Hypersthenic, sthenic, asthenic, and hyposthenic habitus are discerned in radiography to determine the size of IR to use and locations of the thoracic and peritoneal structures.

bony trabeculae Supporting material in cancellous bone. It is demonstrated on images as thin white lines throughout a bony structure and is evaluated for changes.

breathing technique Technique in which a long exposure time (3-4 seconds) is used with costal breathing to blur the lung details surrounding the bony structures of interest.

brightness Describes the degree of luminance seen on the display monitor and refers to the degree of lightness (white) or lack of lightness (black) of the pixels in the image.

carpal canal Wrist passageway formed anteriorly by the flexor retinaculum, posteriorly by the capitate, laterally by the scaphoid and trapezium, and medially by the pisiform and hamate.

caudal Foot end of the patient. *A caudally angled central ray is directed toward the patient's feet.*

central ray (CR) Center of the x-ray beam. It is used to center the anatomic structure and IR.

central venous catheter (CVC) Catheter used to allow infusion of substances that are too toxic for peripheral infusion, such as for chemotherapy, total parenteral nutrition, dialysis, or blood transfusions.

cephalic Head end of the patient. A cephalically angled CR is directed toward the patient's head.

concave Curved or rounded inward. *The anterior surface of the metacarpals is concave.*

contrast Difference in brightness levels between tissues that represents the differential absorption.

contrast mask A postprocessing manipulation that adds a black background over the areas outside the VOI to eliminate them and provide a perceived enhancement of image contrast.

contrast resolution The degree of difference in brightness levels between adjacent tissues on the displayed image. The higher the contrast resolution, the greater are the gray shade differences, and the lower the contrast resolution, the lower are the gray shade differences.

convex Curved or rounded outward. *The posterior surface of the metacarpals is convex.*

cortical outline Outer layer of a bone demonstrated on an image as the white outline of an anatomic structure.

costal breathing Slow, shallow breathing; used with a long exposure time to blur chest details.

decubitus Refers to the patient lying down on a table or cart while a horizontally directed CR is used; also used with the term *decubitus* is the surface (lateral, dorsal, or ventral) placed adjacent to the table or cart. *The patient is in a left lateral decubitus position.*

density Degree of darkness in an image.

depress To lower or sink down, positioning at a lower level.

destructive condition Condition that results in change to the normal bony structures, soft tissues, or air or fluid content of the patient; may require technical changes to compensate for them prior to exposing the patient. Destructive diseases cause the tissues to decrease tissue density or thickness, resulting in them being more radiolucent.

detector element (DEL) Element in the DR image receptor that contains the electronic components that store the detected energy.

deviate To move away from the normal or routine.

differential absorption Radiographic contrast caused by the atomic density, atomic number, and thickness composition differences of the patient's body parts and how differently each tissue composition will absorb x-ray photons.

distal (disto-) Refers to a structure that is situated away from the source or beginning. *The foot is distal to the ankle.* Or, *The splenic flexure is distal to the hepatic flexure.*

distortion The misrepresentation of the size or shape of the structure being examined.

dorsal (dorso-) See *posterior.*

dorsiflexion Backward bending, as of the hand or foot; brings toes and forefoot upward.

dorsoplantar projection X-ray beam that enters the top of the patient's foot and exits through the bottom of the foot.

dose creep When technique values (mAs, kV) are elevated more than necessary because of fear of producing images with quantum noise.

dose equivalent limits Maximum permissible radiation dose limits; used for radiation protection purposes.

dynamic range Range of gray shades that the imaging system can display; measured by the bit depth for each pixel.

external auditory meatus (EAM) External ear opening.

elevate To lift up or raise, positioning at a higher level.

elongation To make one axis of an anatomic structure appear disproportionately longer on the image than the opposite axis. Angling the CR while the part and IR remain parallel with each other will elongate the axis toward which the CR is angled.

endotracheal tube (ETT) Stiff thick-walled tube used to inflate the lungs.

entrance skin exposure (ESE) Absorbed dose to the most superficial layers of skin.

eversion Act of turning the plantar foot surface as far laterally as the ankle will allow.

exposure field recognition Computed radiography process in which the computer distinguishes the raw data representative of information within the exposure field from that which comes from outside the exposure field so that proper automatic rescaling can occur.

exposure indicator (EI) Readings obtained in digital radiography that express the amount of IR exposure given off by the imaging plate; indicates the amount of radiation exposure to the patient and imaging plate.

exposure maintenance formula Formula used to adjust the mAs the needed amount to maintain the required IR exposure and prevent quantum noise: (new mAs) / (old mAs) = (new distance squared) / (old distances squared).

extension Movement that results in straightening of a joint. With extension of the elbow, the arm is straightened. Extension of the cervical vertebrae shifts the patient's head posteriorly in an attempt to separate the vertebral bodies.

external (lateral) rotation Act of turning the anterior surface of an extremity outward or away from the patient's torso midline.

fat pads Accumulation of adipose or fatty tissue that by its displacement can indicate joint effusion on radiographic images.

field of view (FOV) Area of the image receptor from where the image data are collected. For computed radiography, the area is the entire imaging plate, and for direct or indirect capture radiography it is the detectors that are included in the exposure field, as determined by collimation.

flexion Movement that bends a joint. With flexion of the elbow, the arm is bent. Flexion of the cervical vertebrae shifts the patient's head forward in an attempt to bring the vertebral bodies closer.

foreshorten To make one axis of an anatomic structure appear disproportionately shorter on the image than the See opposite axis. Positioning the long axis of the lower leg at a 45-degree angle with the IR while the CR is perpendicular to the IR foreshortens the image of the lower leg on the image.

frog-leg position Position where the affected leg(s) is flexed and abducted to demonstrate a lateral projection of the hip and proximal femur.

glabelloalveolar line Imaginary line connecting the glabella and alveolar ridge.

gluteal fat plane Fat plane that is superior to the femoral neck.

gray scale Number of gray shades used between white and black to display the radiographic image. A long gray scale indicates that there are many shades and a short gray scale indicates that there are few shades.

grid Device consisting of lead strips that is placed between the patient and IR to reduce the amount of scatter radiation reaching the receptor.

grid cutoff Reduction in the amount of primary radiation reaching the IR because of grid misalignment.

Hill-Sachs defect Posterolateral humeral head notch defect created by impingement of the articular surface of the humeral head against the anteroinferior rim of the glenoid cavity.

histogram Graph that is generated from the raw data that has the pixel brightness value on the x-axis and the number of pixels with that brightness value on the y-axis.

histogram analysis error Image histogram that includes raw data values in the VOI that should not be included; this results in a misshapen histogram that will not match the lookup table closely enough for the computer to rescale the data accurately.

homogeneous Refers to uniformity between structures.

iliopsoas fat plane Fat plane that lies within the pelvis medial to the lesser trochanters.

image acquisition Process of collecting x-ray transmission measurements from the patient.

image receptor (IR) Device that receives the radiation leaving the patient. Computed radiography uses an imaging plate and the DR system uses detector elements.

imaging plate (IP) 1. Plate used in computed radiography that is coated with a photostimulable phosphor material that absorbs the photons exiting the patient, resulting in the formation of a latent image that is released and digitized before being sent to a computer. 2. Thin flexible sheet of plastic with a photostimulable phosphor layer that is placed inside the computed radiography cassette to record the radiographic image; computed radiography's image receptor.

inferior (infero-) Refers to a structure within the patient's torso that is situated closer to the feet; used when comparing the locations of two structures. *The symphysis pubis is inferior to the iliac crest.*

infraorbital Below the orbits.

infraorbitomeatal line (IOML) Imaginary line connecting the inferior orbital margin and external auditory meatus (EAM).

interiliac line Imaginary line connecting the iliac crests.

intermalleolar line Imaginary line drawn between the medial and lateral malleoli.

internal (medial) rotation Act of turning the anterior surface of an extremity inward or toward the patient's torso midline.

interpupillary line Imaginary line connecting the outer corners of the eyelids.

intraperitoneal air Presence of free air in the abdominal cavity.

inverse square law Law that states that radiation intensity is inversely proportional to the square of its distance from the x-ray source.

inversion Act of turning the plantar foot surface as far medially as the ankle will allow.

involuntary motion Movement that the patient cannot control.

ionization chamber Chamber in the AEC system that collects radiation. For adequate IR exposure to result, the appropriate chamber must be selected for the part being imaged.

joint effusion Escape of fluid into the joint.

kyphosis Excessive posterior convexity of the thoracic vertebrae.

lateral (latero-) Refers to the patient's sides; used to express something that is directed or situated away from the patient's median plane or to express the outer side of an extremity. *The kidneys are lateral to the vertebral column.* Or, *Place the IR against the lateral surface of the knee.*

lateral mortise Talofibular joint.

lateral position Refers to positioning of the patient so that the side of the torso or extremity being imaged is placed adjacent to the IR. When a lateral position of the torso, vertebrae, or cranium is defined, the term *right* or *left* is also included to state which side of the patient is placed closer to the IR. *The patient was in a left lateral position when the chest projection was taken.*

law of isometry Used to minimize shape distortion when imaging long bones when the bone and IR cannot be positioned parallel. The law of isometry indicates that the CR should be set at half the angle formed between the bone and IR.

lips-meatal line Imaginary line connecting the lips (with mouth closed) with the external auditory meatus (EAM).

longitudinal foreshortening Long axis of the structure appears disproportionately shorter on the image than the short axis.

lookup table (LUT) Histogram of the brightness and contrast values of the ideal image. It is used as a reference to evaluate the raw data of similar images and automatically rescales their values when needed to match those in the LUT.

magnification Proportionately increasing or enlarging both axes of a structure. The gonadal contact shield is magnified on the image if it is placed on top of the patient.

mammary line Imaginary line connecting the nipples.

manual exposure When the technical factors (mAs, kV) are set based on the patient thickness measurement.

matrix Columns and rows of pixels (array) that divide a digital pixel.

medial (medio-) Refers to the patient's median plane; used to express something that is directed or situated toward the patient's median plane or to express the inner side of an extremity. *The sacroiliac joints are medial to the anterior superior iliac spines (ASISs).* Or, *Place the IR against the medial surface of the knee.*

mentomeatal line Imaginary line connecting the chin with the external auditory meatus (EAM).

midcoronal plane Imaginary plane that passes through the body from side to side and divides it into equal anterior and posterior sections or halves.

midsagittal or median plane Imaginary plane that passes through the body anteroposteriorly or posteroanteriorly and divides it into equal right and left sections or halves.

minimum response time Shortest exposure time to which the AEC can respond and still produce an acceptable image.

moiré grid artifact Wavy line artifact that occurs when a stationary grid is used in computed radiography and the imaging plate is placed in the plate reader so that the grid's lead strips align parallel with the scanning direction.

nonstochastic effect Biologic response of radiation exposure that can be directly related to the dose received.

object–image receptor distance (OID) Distance from the object being imaged to the IR.

oblique Refers to rotation of a structure away from an AP or PA projection. When obliquity of the torso, vertebrae, or cranium is defined, the terms *right* or *left* and *anterior* or *posterior* are used with the term *oblique* to indicate which side of the patient is placed closer to the IR. In a right anterior oblique (RAO) position the patient is rotated so that the right anterior surface is placed closer to the IR. When obliquity of an extremity is defined, the term *medial* (internal) or *lateral* (external) is used with the term *oblique* to indicate which way the extremity is rotated from anatomic position and which side of the extremity is positioned closer to the IR. For a medial oblique position of the wrist, the medial side of the arm is placed closer to the IR.

obturator internus fat plane Fat plane that lies within the pelvic inlet next to the medial brim.

occlusal plane Chewing surface of maxillary teeth.

orbitomeatal line Imaginary line connecting the outer eye canthus and external auditory meatus (EAM).

pacemaker Used to regulate the heart rate by supplying electrical stimulation to the heart. This electrical signal will stimulate the heart the amount needed to maintain an effective rate and rhythm.

palmar Anterior surface of the hand.

pericapsular fat plane Fat plane.

phantom image Artifact that occurs in computed radiography when the imaging plate is not erased adequately before the next image is exposed on it and two images are recorded onto the plate phosphor.

picture archival and communication system (PACS) A system where the digitized images from all the different modalities in a facility (RT, CT, MRI, etc.) are stored and can be retrieved, displayed, and transmitted to computers on the local area network (LAN).

pixel Single cell within a matrix.

plantar Pertaining to the sole of the foot.

plantar flexion Act of moving the toes and forefoot downward.

pleural drainage tube Thick-walled tube used to remove fluid or air from the pleural space that could result in collapse of the lung.

pleural effusion Fluid in the pleural cavity.

pneumectomy Removal of a lung.

pneumothorax Presence of air in the pleural cavity.

postprocessing Adjustments made to the image at the console by the technologist, including windowing for brightness and contrast, edge enhancement, adding annotations, image reorientation (turning or flipping), and zooming.

posterior (postero-) Refers to the back of the patient; used to express something that is situated at or directed toward the back and includes the backs of the hands and bottoms of the feet, as in anatomic position. *The knee joint is posterior to the patella.*

posterior shoulder dislocation Shoulder condition in which the humeral head is demonstrated posteriorly, beneath the acromion process.

prevertebral fat stripe Fat stripe located anterior to the cervical vertebrae.

procedural algorithm Computer software that indicates the dynamic range and average brightness levels for the computer to use when displaying a projection. These are embedded in the LUTs that are used when the histogram is automatically rescaled to optimize the anatomic structures for that projection.

profile Outline of an anatomic structure. *The glenoid fossa is demonstrated in profile on a Grashey method image.*

project The act of throwing the image of an anatomic structure forward. *An angled CR projects the anatomic part situated farther away from the IR farther than the anatomic part situated closer to the IR.*

projection Term used to describe the entrance and exit points of the x-ray beam as it passes through the body when an image is taken. In a projection, the path from the first location to the second must be a straight line. These include anteroposterior, inferosuperior, lateromedial, mediolateral, posteroanterior, and superoinferior projections.

pronate To rotate or turn the upper extremity medially until the hand's palmar surface is facing downward or posteriorly.

pronator fat stripe Soft tissue structure demonstrated on lateral wrist images located parallel to the anterior surface of the distal radius.

protract To move a structure forward or anteriorly. *The shoulder is protracted when it is drawn forward.*

proximal (proximo-) Refers to a structure that is closest to the source or beginning. *The shoulder joint is proximal to the elbow joint.* Or, *The hepatic flexure is proximal to the splenic flexure.*

pulmonary arterial catheter Catheter used to measure atrial pressures, pulmonary artery pressure, and cardiac output.

quantum noise (mottle) Graininess or random pattern that is superimposed on the image, obscuring information. It is present when photon flux is insufficient.

radial deviation While maintaining PA projection, the distal hand is moved toward the radial side as much as the wrist will allow.

radiolucent Allowing the passage of x-radiation. A radiolucent object appears dark on an image.

radiopaque Preventing the passage of x-radiation. A radiopaque object appears white on an image.

raw data Brightness values that have come from the digital IR before rescaling occurs.

recorded detail Sharpness of structures that have been included on the image.

recumbent Lying down.

resolution Differentiation of individual structures or details from one another on an image.

retract To move a structure backward or posteriorly. *The shoulder is retracted when it is drawn backward.*

saturation Demonstrated on an image as a loss of contrast resolution, with some or all of the structures demonstrating a black shade. The postprocessing technique of windowing cannot restore the saturated area.

scaphoid fat stripe Soft tissue structure demonstrated on wrist images located just lateral to the scaphoid.

scatter radiation Radiation that has changed in direction from the primary beam because of an interaction with the patient or other structure. Because it is emitted in a random direction, it carries no useful signal or subject contrast.

scoliosis Spine condition that results in the vertebral column's curving laterally instead of running straight.

source–image receptor distance (SID) Distance from the anode's focal spot to the IR.

source–object distance (SOD) Distance from the anode's focal spot to the patient.

source–skin distance (SSD) Distance from the source of radiation (anode) to the patient's skin. Good radiation practices dictate that this distance must be at least 12 inches (30 cm) to prevent unacceptable entrance skin exposure.

spatial frequency Used to define spatial resolution; refers to how often the number of details change in a set amount of space. It is expressed as line pairs per millimeter (lp/mm).

spatial resolution Ability of an imaging system to distinguish small adjacent details from each other in the image.

stochastic effect Biologic response to radiation in which the chance of occurrence of the effect, rather than the severity of the effect, is proportional to the dose of radiation received.

subject contrast Contrast caused by the x-ray attenuating characteristics (atomic density and number, and thickness) of the subject being imaged.

subluxation Partial dislocation.

superimpose To lie over or above an anatomic structure or object.

superior (supero-) Refers to a structure within the patient's torso that is situated closer to the head; used when comparing the locations of two torso structures. *The thoracic cavity is superior to the peritoneal cavity.*

supination Rotating or turning the upper extremity laterally until the hand's palmar surface is facing upwardly or anteriorly.

supraorbital Above the orbit.

supraspinatus outlet Opening formed between the lateral clavicle, acromion process, and superior scapula when the patient is positioned for a tangential outlet projection of the shoulder.

symmetrical Refers to structures on opposite sides demonstrating the same size, shape, and position.

talar dome Dome shape formed by the most medial and lateral aspects of the talus's trochlear surface when it is in a lateral position.

tarsi sinus Opening between the calcaneus and talus.

thin-film transistor (TFT) Component in direct/indirect capture radiography that collects the electric chargers produced in the detector elements when the remnant radiation strikes it.

trabecular pattern Supporting material within cancellous bone. It is demonstrated on an image as thin white lines throughout a bony structure.

transverse foreshortening Short axis of a structure appears disproportionately shorter on the image than the long axis.

ulnar deviation While maintaining a PA projection, the distal hand is turned toward the ulnar side as much as the wrist will allow.

umbilical artery catheter (UAC) Found only in neonates because the cord has dried up and fallen off in older infants. It is used to measure oxygen saturation.

umbilical vein catheter (UVC) Catheter used to deliver fluids and medications.

unilateral One side.

valgus deformity Knee deformity in which the lateral side of the knee joint is narrower than the medial side.

varus deformity Knee deformity in which the medial side of the knee joint is narrower than the lateral side.

vascular lung markings White markings in the lung fields that indicate blood vessels on a chest x-ray.

ventral (ventro-) See *anterior*.

volume of interest (VOI) Brightness values (raw data) that represent only the anatomic structures of interest in digital radiography.

voluntary motion Motion that the patient is able to control.

weight-bearing Putting weight on the structure, as with a standing lateral foot or AP knee projection.

windowing Postprocessing manipulation of the image's brightness and contrast to better demonstrate the VOI.

Page numbers followed by "f" indicate figures, "t" indicate tables, and "b" indicate boxes.

A

Abdomen, 129-141
  abdominal body habitus, 132
  abdominal lines/devices/tubes/
    catheters, 130-131
  abdominal rotation
    detection, 140
    scoliosis, differences, 136-137
  abdominal tissue (exclusion),
    supine AP abdomen (impact),
    132f
  AEC chamber/respiration, 137
  anteroposterior (AP) neonate/infant
    abdomen projection, patient
    positioning, 142f
  AP abdomen analysis, 138-139
    correction, 138-139
    practice, 138-139
  AP (lateral decubitus) abdomen
    projection, 139t
  AP (right lateral decubitus) chest
    projection, patient positioning,
    129f
  AP left lateral decubitus abdomen
    free intraperitoneal air
      demonstration, 140f
    left side rotation, 140f
    positioning accuracy, 139f
    projection, patient positioning,
    140f
  AP left lateral decubitus abdomen
    analysis, 141
    correction, 141
    practice, 141
  AP projection (left lateral decubitus
    position), 139-141
    intraperitoneal air, demonstration,
    140
    IR size/direction, 139-140
    midcoronal plane positioning/
      rotation, 140
  AP projection (supine/upright),
    132-139
  ascites, 130
  asthenic abdomen, 132
  body habitus, IR size/placement
    variations, 132-135
  bowel gas, impact, 130
  bowel obstruction, 130
  child AP (left lateral decubitus)
    abdomen projection, 146t
  child supine AP abdomen
    projection, positioning,
    144f

Abdomen (Continued)
  child upright AP abdomen
    projection, positioning,
    144f-145f
  free intraperitoneal air, 131
  hypersthenic abdomen, 132
  hypersthenic patient
    left lateral decubitus position,
    139-140
    supine AP abdomen, crosswise IR
      cassettes (usage), 135f
  IR size/direction, 139-140
  kidneys, location, 129-130
  midcoronal plane positioning/
    rotation, 135-137, 140
  nasogastric (NG) tubes, subject
    contrast, 130-131
  obese patient, left lateral decubitus
    position, 139-140
  obesity, consideration, 130, 132
  patient, wide hips, 140
  pediatric abdomen, 141-148
  pendulous breasts
    lateral movement (brightness
      comparison), AP abdomens
      (usage), 130f
  pendulous breasts, interference,
    130
  positioning procedure (variations),
    body habitus (impact), 131
  psoas major muscles, location,
    129-130
  respiration, impact, 137
  scoliosis, supine AP abdomen,
    137f
  soft tissue masses, 130
  spinal stimulator implant, 131
    AP abdomen/lateral vertebrae
      demonstration, 131f
  sthenic abdomen, 132
  subject contrast/brightness, 129
  supine AP abdomen
    bowel gas excess demonstration,
    130f
    nasogastric tube placement,
      accuracy, 131f
    projection, 133t
    projection, patient positioning,
    133f
    right side, rotation, 137f
    scoliosis, presence, 137f
  supine hypersthenic patient,
    134-135
  supine obese patient, 135

Abdomen (Continued)
  technical data, 129-130, 129t
    adjustment, 130
    imaging analysis guidelines, 129b
  uniform density, wedge-
    compensating filter (usage),
    140-141
  upright AP abdomen
    full expiration, 139f
    full respiration, 138f
    left side rotation, 136f
  upright AP abdomen projection,
    134t
    patient positioning, 135f
    positioning accuracy, 134f
  upright hypersthenic patient, 135
  upright obese patient, 135
Acanthioparietal facial bones, chin
  elevation (insufficiency), 483f
Acanthioparietal (Waters) facial bone/
  sinus projection, central ray (CR)
  angle (determination), 484f
Acetabulum, inclusion, 384-385
Acromioclavicular (AC) joint: AP
  projection, 267-270
  AP axial projection (Alexander
    method), 270
  bilateral AC joint projection, 270
  clavicle rotation, 267
  CR centering, 269-270
  exam indication, 267
  exam variations, 270
  kyphotic patient, 269
  midcoronal plane positioning, 267
  midcoronal plane tilting, 269
  trauma, positioning, 272-273
Additive patient conditions, 53
Adjacent finger overlap, 158-159
Aeration, appearance, 115-116
Air levels (demonstration), positioning
  (usage), 104-105
Aliasing artifact, 62-64
Alternate mediolateral wrist
  projection, 191
Alternate transthoracic lateral humerus
  projection, 232-233
Analog-to-digital converter (ADC), 38
Anatomical distortion, causes, 23f
Anatomic alignment, CR placement
  (impact), 20f
Anatomic artifacts, 36, 59-60
  AP abdomen projection, hand
    superimposition, 60f
  radiation protection, problem, 35f

Anatomic relationships, 17-25
  positioning procedures, correlation,
    18-19
Anatomic structure
  computed radiography, usage, 14
  digital radiography, 14
  identification, 19-20
  requirements/placement, 14
Angled central ray, 21-22
Ankle
  anatomic position, AP projections
    (differences), 322-323
  external rotation, 312f
  flexion, 291
  internal rotation, 312f
Ankle: AP oblique projection (medial
    rotation), 314-318
  anteroposterior (AP) 45-degree
    oblique ankle projection
    distal lower leg, elevation,
      317f
    foot, dorsiflexion, 318f
    obliquity, insufficiency, 317f
    positioning accuracy, 316f
  anteroposterior (AP) oblique
    (mortise) ankle projection, foot
    inversion, 316f
  anteroposterior (AP) oblique
    (mortise) ankle projection,
    obliquity
    excess, 316f
    insufficiency, 315f
  anteroposterior oblique ankle
    projection, patient positioning,
    315f
  anteroposterior (45-degree) oblique
    ankle projection, positioning
    accuracy, 315f
  anteroposterior (mortise) oblique
    ankle projection, positioning
    accuracy, 314f
  calcaneus, 317
  15- to 20-degree AP oblique
    (mortise), 314-315
  foot inversion, ankle rotation
    (differences), 315
  45-degree AP oblique, 315-316
  intermalleolar line, IR alignment,
    315f
  internal foot rotation, 316f
  rotation, inadequacy (repositioning),
    314-315
  tibiotalar joint
    openness, evaluation, 316-317
    space, 316-317
Ankle: AP projection, 311-314
  ankle
    external rotation, 312f
    internal rotation, 312f
  medial mortise, 311-312
  rotation, 312
  ruptured ligament variation, 312

Ankle: AP projection (Continued)
  tibiotalar joint
    openness, evaluation, 313
    space, 312-313
    visualization, foot positioning
      (effect), 313
Ankle: lateral projection
    (mediolateral), 318-322
  anterior pretalar/posterior
    pericapsular fat pads,
    demonstration, 318
  calcaneus, depression, 321f
  fifth metatarsal base, 321
  foot dorsiflexion, 318-320
  medial/lateral talar domes, 320-321
    anterior/posterior alignment,
      320-321
    proximal alignment, 320
Anode heel effect, 52-53
  positioning guidelines, 53t
  thoracic vertebrae: AP projection,
    414-415
  usage, 53f
Anterior abdominal tissue, impact, 93f
Anterior ankle, anatomy, 312f
Anterior distal radial margins,
    identification, 178-179
Anterior lung visualization, 96-97
Anterior pretalar/posterior
    pericapsular fat pads,
    demonstration, 313
Anterior superior iliac spine (ASIS),
    index finger (placement), 34
Anteroinferior lung/heart visualization,
    91
Anteroinferior lungs (compression),
    anterior abdominal tissue
    (impact), 93f
Anteroposterior (AP) abdomen
    analysis, 138-139, 318
  correction, 138-139, 283
  practice, 138-139
Anteroposterior (AP) abdomen oblique
    projection (Grashey Method),
    248t
Anteroposterior (AP) abdomen
    projections
  contrast masking, 7f
  exposure, 55f
  external artifact, 61f
  hands, superimposition, 60f
  involuntary patient motion, 30f
  position, CR placement effect, 21f
Anteroposterior (AP) above-
    diaphragm, 457f
Anteroposterior (AP) above-diaphragm
    rib projection
  patient rotation, 455f
  positioning accuracy, 454f
  spinal scoliosis, 456f
Anteroposterior (AP) above/diaphragm
    rib projection, 456f

Anteroposterior (AP)
  acromioclavicular joint
    positioning, 268f
Anteroposterior (AP)
  acromioclavicular joint projection,
    268t
  upper midcoronal plane
    anterior tilt, 269f
    posterior tilt, 269f
    weights, 269f
      absence, 269f
      usage, 269f
Anteroposterior (AP)
  acromioclavicular joint projection,
    positioning (accuracy), 268f
Anteroposterior (AP) analysis,
    467-468
Anteroposterior (AP) ankle analysis,
    313-314
  correction, 309-310, 313
  practice, 313-314
Anteroposterior (AP) ankle projection,
    311t
  ankle, external rotation, 312f
  distal lower leg, elevation, 313f
  obtaining, 29f
  patient positioning, 311f
  positioning accuracy, 311f
  proximal lower leg, elevation,
    313f
  rupture ligament, 312f
Anteroposterior (AP) atlas/axis
    (open-mouthed) projection
  caudal CR angulation
    excess, 399f
    insufficiency, 399f
  CR cephalic angle, 398f
  face, rotation, 397f
  head, tilt, 398f
  patient positioning, 397f
    trauma evaluation, 399f
  positioning accuracy, 397f
  upper incisors/mastoid tip,
    alignment, 398f
Anteroposterior (AP) atlas/axis
    (open-mouthed) projection
    exposure, 56f
Anteroposterior (AP) axial (Towne)
    analysis, 475-476
Anteroposterior (AP) axial cervical
    projection
  cephalic CR angulation, excess, 395f
  cervical column, lateral flexion,
    395f
  chin tuck, 395f
  head, tilt, 395f
  kyphotic patient, 394f
  patient positioning, 393f
  positioning accuracy, 392f
  thorax, rotation, 393f
Anteroposterior (AP) axial cervical
    vertebrae projection, 392t

Anteroposterior (AP) axial (lordotic) chest projection, 108t
  computed radiography angle, patient positioning, 109f
  computed radiography angulation, 45-degree midcoronal plane, 109f
  45-degree midcoronal plane, 109f
  patient positioning, 108f
  positioning accuracy, 108f
Anteroposterior (AP) axial clavicle projection, 266t
Anteroposterior (AP) axial clavicular positioning, 267f
Anteroposterior (AP) axial clavicular projection
  fractured clavicle, demonstration, 267f
  positioning, 267f
Anteroposterior (AP) axial coccygeal projection, 443t
  bladder, contents (presence), 443f
  patient positioning, 443f
  positioning accuracy, 443f
Anteroposterior (AP) axial coccyx projection
  caudal CR angulation, insufficiency, 444f
  fecal matter, superimposition, 444f
Anteroposterior (AP) axial (Towne) cranial/mastoid projection, positioning accuracy, 473f
Anteroposterior (AP) axial cranial projection
  central ray (CR) angulation, determination, 475f
  chin tuck, 474f
  face rotation, 474f
Anteroposterior (AP) axial cranial projection, chin tuck, 475f
Anteroposterior (AP) axial (Towne) cranial projection, cranial projection, 473f
Anteroposterior (AP) axial (Caldwell method) cranial projection, positioning problems, 27f
Anteroposterior (AP) axial cranium/mandible projection, 472t
Anteroposterior (AP) axial cranium projection, 471f
Anteroposterior (AP) axial foot analysis, 294
  correction, 294
  practice, 294
Anteroposterior (AP) axial foot projection, 290t
  patient positioning, 291f
  positioning accuracy, 291f
Anteroposterior (AP) axial intercondylar fossa (Béclère method), 349t

Anteroposterior (AP) axial knee projection
  distal lower leg
    depression, 350f
    elevation, 350f
  knee
    external rotation, 351f
    internal rotation, 351f
  knee flexion
    excess, 350f
    insufficiency, 350f
  patient positioning, 349f
  positioning accuracy, 349f
Anteroposterior (AP) axial mandible projection, chin tuck, 474f
Anteroposterior (AP) axial (Towne) mandible projection, positioning accuracy, 473f
Anteroposterior (AP) axial oblique cervical vertebrae projection, 407t
  patient positioning, 408f
    trauma, evaluation, 411f
  trauma, evaluation, 411f
Anteroposterior (AP) axial sacral projection, 438t
  fecal material, superimposition, 439f
  left side, rotation, 439f
  patient positioning, 439f
  positioning accuracy, 438f
  right side, rotation, 439f
Anteroposterior (AP) axial sacroiliac joints analysis, 387
  correction, 387
  practice, 387
Anteroposterior (AP) axial sacroiliac joints projection, 386t
  cephalic angulation
    excess, 387f
    insufficiency, 387f
  patient positioning, 387f
  positioning accuracy, 386f
Anteroposterior (AP) axial (Stryker Notch) shoulder analysis, 261
  correction, 261
  practice, 260-261
Anteroposterior (AP) axial shoulder projection (Stryker "Notch" method), 258t
Anteroposterior (AP) axial (Stryker) shoulder projection
  cephalic CR angulation, 259f
  distal humerus, medial tilt, 260f
  humerus, abduction, 259f-260f
  positioning, 259f
    accuracy, 258f
Anteroposterior (AP) axial toe(s) analysis, 283
  correction, 283-284
  practice, 283-284

Anteroposterior (AP) axial toe(s) projection, 280t
  CR alignment, absence, 283f
  lateral rotation, 282f
  medial rotation, 282f
  patient positioning, 281f
Anteroposterior (AP) below-diaphragm rib projection, patient positioning, 455f
Anteroposterior (AP) cervical atlas/axis analysis, 400
  correction, 400
  practice, 400
Anteroposterior (AP) cervical atlas/axis projection, 396t
Anteroposterior (AP) cervical vertebrae analysis, 396
  correction, 396
  practice, 396
Anteroposterior (AP) cervical vertebral mobility, evaluation, 403
Anteroposterior (AP) chest (portable) analysis, 103-104
  correction, 103
  practice, 103-104
Anteroposterior (AP) chest
  demonstration, 80f
  central venous catheter (CVC) placement, 81f-82f
  CR angle, 100f-101f
  endotracheal tube placement, 81f
  external monitoring lines, 84f
  implanted cardioverter defibrillator (ICD) placement, 84f
  left side, positioning, 100f
  pacemaker placement, 83f
  pulmonary arterial catheter placement, 83f
  right side, positioning, 100f
Anteroposterior (AP) chest projection, 49f
  equipment-related artifact, display, 62f-63f
  external artifacts, display, 60f
  patient arms, 60f
  patient positioning, 99f
  pleural drainage tubes, placement, 82f
  positioning accuracy, 99f
  right lateral decubitus, 5f
    patient positioning, 105f
  supine/portable, 99t
Anteroposterior (AP) clavicle analysis, 266
  correction, 266
  practice, 266
Anteroposterior (AP) clavicle projection, 264t
Anteroposterior (AP) clavicular positioning, 265f

Anteroposterior (AP) clavicular projection
  fracture clavicle, demonstration, 267f
  patient rotation, 265f
  positioning accuracy, 264f
  upper midcoronal plane
    anterior tilt, 265f
    posterior tilt, 265f
Anteroposterior (AP) coccyx analysis, 444
  correction, 444
  practice, 444
Anteroposterior (AP) cranial projection, patient positioning, 466f
Anteroposterior (AP) cranium/mandible projection, 463t
Anteroposterior (AP) distal femur projection, 355t
  external rotation, 356f
  internal rotation, 356f
  patient positioning, 356f
  positioning accuracy, 356f
Anteroposterior (AP) elbow analysis, 212
  correction, 212
  practice, 212
Anteroposterior (AP) elbow projections, 208t
  CR centering, 211f
    effects, 27f
  external rotation, 209f
  hand/wrist pronation, 210f
  humerus, parallel position, 210f
  internal rotation, 209f
  patient positioning, 209f
  positioning accuracy, 208f
  proximal humerus, elevation, 211f
Anteroposterior (AP) external oblique knee projection, external obliquity
  excess, 337f
  insufficiency, 336f
Anteroposterior (AP) female pelvis projection, positioning accuracy, 368f
Anteroposterior (AP) femur analysis, 359
  correction, 360
  practice, 359-360
Anteroposterior (AP) femur projection, overexposure, 50f
Anteroposterior (AP) finger projection
  closed joints, presence, 27f
  open joints, presence, 26f
Anteroposterior (AP) flexed finger projection. See Finger (AP projection)
Anteroposterior (AP) foot projection, upside down display, 7f

Anteroposterior (AP) forearm analysis, 203
  correction, 203
  practice, 203
Anteroposterior (AP) forearm positioning, 201f
Anteroposterior (AP) forearm projection, 200t
  PA projection, wrist (presence), 201f
  patient positioning, 202f
  positioning accuracy, 200f
  skin line collimation, 16f
  wrist, internal rotation, 201f
Anteroposterior (AP) frog-leg hip analysis, 382
  correction, 382
  practice, 382
Anteroposterior (AP) frog-leg hip projection
  knee/hip flexion, 380f
  leg abduction, 381f
    femur, angle, 381f
  patient positioning, 379f
  patient rotation, 379f
  positioning accuracy, 379f
Anteroposterior (AP) frog-leg (mediolateral) hip projection, 378t
Anteroposterior (AP) frog-leg pelvis analysis, 374
  practice, 374
Anteroposterior (AP) frog-leg pelvis projection, 371t
  femoral shafts, abduction, 373f
  patient positioning, 371f
  pelvis, left side (rotation), 372f
  positioning accuracy, 371f
Anteroposterior (AP) hip analysis, 377-378
  correction, 377-378
  practice, 377-378
Anteroposterior (AP) hip, metal apparatus (presence), 377f
Anteroposterior (AP) hip projection, 374t
  backboard, usage, 68f
  femoral neck fracture, 376f
  foot, vertical placement, 376f
  internal artifact, prosthesis (impact), 61f
  leg, external rotation, 376f
  patient positioning, 375f
  patient rotation, 375f
  positioning accuracy, 375f
  radiopaque prosthesis exposure, 56f
Anteroposterior (AP) hip projection, marker placement, 13f
Anteroposterior (AP) humerus projection, 226t
  arm
    external rotation, 227f
    internal rotation, 228f

Anteroposterior (AP) humerus projection (Continued)
  fractured humerus, demonstration, 228f
  patient positioning
    collimator head rotation, 227f
    fracture, 228f
    positioning accuracy, 227f
Anteroposterior (AP) infant chest projection (patient positioning), immobilization equipment (usage), 114f
Anteroposterior (AP) knee analysis, 333
  correction, 333
  practice, 333
Anteroposterior (AP) knee projections, 328t
  bright spots, 66f
  cephalic CR angulation
    excess, 332f
    inadequacy, 333f
  external rotation, 329f
  internal rotation, excess, 330f
  knee flexion, 331f
  low subject contrast, demonstration, 59f
  patellar subluxation, 330f
  positioning accuracy, 329f
  valgus deformity, 332f
  varus deformity, 332f
Anteroposterior (AP) knee projections, fluid demonstration, 58f
Anteroposterior (AP) large intestinal projection, patient types, 511t
Anteroposterior (AP) large intestine projections, 504f
  patient positioning, 511f
  patients, types, 507t
  position accuracy, 508f, 511f
Anteroposterior (AP) lateral decubitus abdomen projection, 139t
Anteroposterior (AP) lateral decubitus projections, marker placement guidelines, 10
Anteroposterior (AP) left lateral decubitus neonate abdomen, intraperitoneal air demonstration, 146f
Anteroposterior (AP) like toe projections, soft tissue/phalanx concavity comparison, 282f
Anteroposterior (AP) lordotic chest analysis, 109-110
  correction, 110
  practice, 109-110
Anteroposterior (AP) lower leg analysis, 324
  correction, 324
  practice, 324

Anteroposterior (AP) lower leg
projection, 53f, 322t
ankle, AP projection, 323f
distal lower leg fracture, 324f
knee, internal rotation, 323f
leg/sternal rotation, 324f
patient positioning, 323f
positioning accuracy, 323f
x-ray divergence, impact, 325f
Anteroposterior (AP) lumbar analysis,
428
correction, 428
practice, 428
Anteroposterior (AP) lumbar
projection
intervertebral disk space alignment,
427f
knees/hips, flexion (absence), 428f
scoliosis, 426f
Anteroposterior (AP) lumbar vertebrae
projection, 5f, 424t
exposure, 55f
patient positioning, 425f
positioning accuracy, 425f
right side, closeness, 425f
scoliosis, 433f
Anteroposterior (AP) male pelvis
projection, positioning accuracy,
368f
Anteroposterior (AP) medial oblique
knee projection
cephalic CR angulation
excess, 336f
inadequacy, 336f
internal obliquity, excess, 336f
Anteroposterior (AP) neonate/infant
abdomen projection, patient
positioning, 142f
Anteroposterior (AP) oblique above-
diaphragm rib projection (RPO
position)
obliquity, insufficiency, 459f
patient positioning, 458f
positioning accuracy, 458f
Anteroposterior (AP) oblique ankle
analysis, 317-318
practice, 317-318
Anteroposterior (AP) oblique ankle
projection, 314t
patient positioning, 315f
Anteroposterior (AP) oblique (mortise)
ankle projection
intermalleolar line, IR alignment,
315f
obliquity
excess, 316f
insufficiency, 315f
Anteroposterior (AP) oblique below-
diaphragm rib projection (RPO
position)
patient positioning, 458f
positioning accuracy, 458f

Anteroposterior (AP) oblique chest
projections, 111-112
Anteroposterior (AP) oblique elbow
analysis, 216
correction, 216
practice, 216
Anteroposterior (AP) oblique elbow
projection, 213t
Anteroposterior (AP) oblique foot
analysis, 297-298
correction, 297-298
practice, 297-298
Anteroposterior (AP) oblique foot
projection, 294t
high contrast, 57f
low contrast, 57f
obliquity
excess, 297f
insufficiency, 297f
patient positioning, 296f
positioning accuracy, 295f
medial foot arch, types (impact),
296f
Anteroposterior (AP) oblique knee
analysis, 337
correction, 337
practice, 337
Anteroposterior (AP) oblique knee
projection, 334t
impact, 30f
Anteroposterior (AP) (external)
oblique knee projection
patient positioning, 335f
positioning accuracy, 335f
Anteroposterior (AP) (internal) oblique
knee projection
patient positioning, 335f
positioning accuracy, 334f
Anteroposterior (AP) oblique lumbar
analysis, 430
correction, 430
practice, 430
Anteroposterior (AP) oblique lumbar
projection, patient rotation
excess, 430f
insufficiency, 430f
Anteroposterior (AP) oblique
lumbar vertebrae projection,
428t
marker placement, 12f
positioning accuracy, 429f
Anteroposterior (AP) (posterior)
oblique lumbar vertebral
projection, patient positioning,
429f
Anteroposterior (AP) oblique
projection, 255
marker placement guidelines,
10
Anteroposterior (AP) oblique ribs
projection, 457t
analysis, 460

Anteroposterior (AP) oblique sacroiliac
joint analysis, 389
correction, 389
practice, 389
Anteroposterior (AP) oblique sacroiliac
joint projection
patient positioning, 388f
pelvic obliquity
excess, 389f
insufficiency, 389f
positioning accuracy, 388f
Anteroposterior (AP) oblique sacroiliac
joints guidelines, 388t
Anteroposterior (AP) oblique shoulder
analysis, 252
correction, 252
practice, 252
Anteroposterior (AP) oblique shoulder/
hip projections, marker placement
guidelines, 10
Anteroposterior (AP) oblique
(Grashey) shoulder projection
coracoid/acromion processes,
alignment, 249f
IR, patient leaning, 251f
obliquity
excess, 250f
insufficiency, 250f
positioning, 249f
upper midcoronal plane
anterior tilt, 250f
posterior tilt, 250f
Anteroposterior (AP) oblique (scapular
Y) shoulder projection, 232f
Anteroposterior oblique (Grashey
method) shoulder projection,
41f
Anteroposterior (AP) oblique (Grashey
method) shoulder projection
exposure, 56f
Anteroposterior (AP) oblique (Grashey
method) shoulder projection,
inverted grid artifact
demonstration, 63f
Anteroposterior (AP) oblique (scapular
Y) shoulder projection,
positioning, 257f
Anteroposterior (AP) oblique stomach/
duodenal projection (LPO
position), 501f
Anteroposterior (AP) oblique stomach/
duodenum projection
LPO position, 500t
motion demonstration, 488f
Anteroposterior (AP) oblique toe
analysis, 286
correction, 286
practice, 286
Anteroposterior (AP) oblique toe(s)
projection, 284t
CR alignment, absence, 286f
obliquity, excess, 285f

Anteroposterior (AP) oblique toe(s)
projection *(Continued)*
patient positioning, 285f
positioning accuracy, 284f
separation, 286f
Anteroposterior (AP) pelvis analysis,
370
correction, 370
practice, 370
Anteroposterior (AP) pelvis projection,
367t
equipment-related artifact, presence,
64f
exposure/overexposure, 50f
feet, vertical placement, 369f
femoral epicondyles, placement,
369f
high subject contrast, 57f
impact, 22f
internal artifact, 62f
leg, external rotation, 369f
obese patient, low subject contrast,
58f
patient positioning, 368f
pelvis rotation, 368f
penetrated/underpenetrated
accuracy, 48f
right femoral neck fracture,
370f
soft tissue overlap, 74f
Anteroposterior (AP) projection, 2, 4
differences, cervical vertebrae
(usage), 105-106
elongation, presence/absence, 23f
gonadal shielding, 33-34
marker placement guidelines, 10
posteroanterior projection,
difference, 98
Anteroposterior (AP) proximal femur
projection, 357t
foot, vertical position, 359f
fracture, demonstration, 359f
leg, external rotation, 358f
patient positioning, 357f
pelvis, rotation, 358f
positioning accuracy, 357f
Anteroposterior (AP) ribs projection,
453t-454t
Anteroposterior (AP) ribs projection
analysis, 457
Anteroposterior (AP) sacral projection,
collimation, 17f
Anteroposterior (AP) sacrum analysis,
440
correction, 440
practice, 440
Anteroposterior (AP) scapula
projection, 270t
Anteroposterior (AP) scapular analysis,
273
correction, 273
practice, 273

Anteroposterior (AP) scapular
positioning, 271f
Anteroposterior (AP) scapular
projection
abduction, absence, 271f
positioning, 271f
scapular fracture, demonstration,
272f
shoulder retraction, inadequacy,
272f
Anteroposterior (AP) shoulder
analysis, 241
correction, 241
practice, 241
Anteroposterior (AP) shoulder
projection, 235t
anterior dislocation, 241f
anterior shoulder dislocation,
240f
equipment-related artifact, display,
63f
humeral epicondyles
IR parallel position, 239f
positioning, 236f
marker placement, 13f
midcoronal plane
anterior tilt, 238f
posterior tilt, 238f
mobility, 240
patient rotation, 237f
phantom image artifact, CR
demonstration, 64f
proximal humeral head fracture,
240f
Anteroposterior (AP) skull projection,
quantum noise (demonstration),
49f
Anteroposterior (AP) stomach/
duodenum projection, 502t
patient positioning, 503f
Anteroposterior (AP) thoracic
projection
full inspiration, 416f
leg extension, 417f
patient positioning, compensating
filter (absence), 415f
positioning accuracy, 415f
spinal scoliosis, demonstration,
417f
upper thorax, left side position,
416f
Anteroposterior (AP) thoracic
vertebrae analysis, 418
correction, 418
practice, 418
Anteroposterior (AP) thoracic
vertebrae projection,
415t
Anteroposterior (AP) thumb analysis,
162
correction, 162
practice, 162

Anteroposterior (AP) thumb
projection, 159t
hand, internal rotation, 160f
MC, absence, 161f
MP joint elevation, 161f
patient positioning, 160f
positioning accuracy, 159f
Arms
elevation, 275f
positioning, 96-97
Artifacts, 59-66
aliasing artifact, 62-64
anatomic artifacts, 36, 59-60
cart pad artifact, 105
external artifact, 60-61
internal artifact, 61-62
lines, prevention, 124
Moiré artifact, 62-64
pad artifact, demonstration, 126f
Ascites, 130
As low as reasonably achievable
(ALARA) philosophy, 32
Asthenic abdomen, 132
Asthenic anteroposterior oblique spot
stomach/duodenal projection
(LPO position), 501f
Asthenic anteroposterior spot stomach
projection, 503f
Asthenic lateral spot stomach/
duodenal projection, positioning
accuracy, 499f
Asthenic PA oblique spot stomach/
duodenal projection (RAO
position), 496f
Asthenic PA stomach/duodenum
projection, positioning accuracy,
497f
Asthenic patient
PA chest, 86f
PA projection, 488f
Augmentation mammoplasty, 84-85
PA/lateral chest, 85f
Automatic exposure control (AEC)
backup timer, 35
center AEC chamber, usage, 56f
chamber
AP abdomen projection exposure,
55f
AP lumbar vertebrae projection
exposure, 55f
respiration, relationship, 137
exposure-related factor, 53-56
images, correction, 56
ionization chamber, 41-42
obese patients, 75
peripheral positioning, 56f
right AEC chamber activation, 79f
setting, 67
use, best practice guidelines, 54b
Automatic implantable cardioverter
defibrillator (automatic ICD),
83-84

Automatic rescaling, 39-40
Axial calcaneal analysis, 307
    correction, 307
    practice, 307
Axial calcaneal projection
    CR/talocalcaneal joint alignment,
        problem, 307f
    external ankle rotation, 308f
    positioning, 306f
Axial calcaneus projection, 305t
Axiolateral analysis, 386
    correction, 386
    practice, 386
Axiolateral elbow (Coyle Method)
        analysis, 226
    correction, 226
    practice, 226
Axiolateral elbow projection, 223t
    distal forearm
        depression, 225f
        positioning, 225f
    elbow flexion, 225f
    proximal humerus, elevation, 224f
    wrist, PA projection, 225f
Axiolateral (Coyle method) elbow
        projection
    positioning accuracy, 224f
Axiolateral elbow projection, proximal
        humerus (depression), 224f
Axiolateral hip projection, 383t
    femoral neck, fracture
        (demonstration), 385f
    femur-to-CR angulation, 384f
    leg, external rotation, 385f
    patient positioning, 384f
    positioning accuracy, 383f
    unaffected leg, flexion/abduction
        insufficiency, 384f

B

Background radiation
    fogging, 44, 64f
    values, excess, 43f
Backup time, setting, 54
Beam divergence, off-centering, 20
Béclère method, 348-351, 349t
Bilateral AP acromioclavicular joint
        projection, 270f
    rotation, 269f
Bilateral PA hand projections, marker
        placement, 12f
Body habitus
    abdominal body habitus, 132
    IR placement, 85, 98
    IR size/placement variations,
        132-135
Bone age (assessment), pediatric PA
        hand projections (usage), 169f
Bowel gas
    excess, supine AP abdomen
        demonstration, 130f
    impact, 130

Bowel obstruction, 130
Breasts
    positioning situations, 84-85
Brightness, abdomen, 129

C

Calcaneal fracture, demonstration,
        309f
Calcaneal tuberosity, 305-307
    dorsiflexion, compensation, 305
    foot positioning, 305
    plantar flexion, compensation,
        305-307
Calcaneus, 317
    depression, 321f
Calcaneus: axial projection
        (plantodorsal), 305-307
    axial/lateral calcaneal projections,
        308f
    calcaneal tuberosity, 305-307
    CR angle, 306f-307f
    plantar flexion, compensation,
        305-307
    rotation/tilting, 307
    talocalcaneal joint space, 305-307
Calcaneus: lateral projection
        (mediolateral), 301
    foot dorsiflexion, 308
    foot positioning, 310
    lower leg positioning, 309
        problems, repositioning, 309-310
    repositioning, tibia/fibular
        relationship (usage), 310
    talar dome, alignment, 309-310
Caldwell method, 27f, 468-472
CareStream DRX-Revolution portable
        AP chest projection, 65f
Carpal canal visualization, 198-199
Carpometacarpal (CMC) joint
        visualization (differences), PA
        wrist projections (usage), 3f
Cart pad artifact, 105
Centering
    offcentering, 20-21
    side-to-side centering, 34
Central ray
    centering, 42
    repositioning steps, 28-36
    structure location, CR adjustment
        guidelines, 28b
Central venous catheter (CVC), 81-82
    placement, 81f
    AP chest demonstration, 82f
Cephalic angulation
    excess, 387f
    insufficiency, 387f
Cephalic-caudal CR alignment,
        100-101
Cephalic CR angulation
    absence, 340f
    excess, 332f, 341f
    inadequacy, 333f

Cervical atlas/axis: AP projection
        (open-mouth position), 396-400
    CR positioning, 397-399
    occipital base positioning, 397-399
    rotation, 396-397
        direction, detection, 397
    trauma, positioning, 398-399
    upper incisor positioning, 397-399
Cervical vertebrae
    AP projection, 106f
    image analysis guidelines, 391-422,
        391b
    PA projection, 106f
    technical data, 391, 391t
    usage, 105-106
Cervical vertebrae: AP axial
        projection, 391-396
    cervical column/exposure field
        alignment, 395
    CR/intervertebral disk alignment,
        391-394
    CR misalignment, effect, 394
    kyphotic patient, 393-394
    mandibular mentum positioning,
        394
    occipital base positioning, 394
    occiput-mentum mispositioning,
        effect, 394
    rotation, 391
    trauma, 395
    upright position, supine position
        (differences), 392-393
Cervical vertebrae: lateral projection,
        400-406
    C1/C2 visualization, elevation
        (effect), 400-402
    C7/T1 vertebrae, demonstration,
        404-405
    cervical column/exposure field
        alignment, 403
    clivus, inclusion (importance), 404
    head positioning, 400-403
    lateral cervicothoracic projection
        (twinning method), 405
    lateral flexion/extension projections,
        403
    lateral head detection, 402-403
    mandibular rotation, effect,
        400-402
    prevertebral fat stripe visualization,
        400
    rotation, 400
    shoulder tilting, detection,
        402-403
    trauma/recumbency, 404-405
Cervical vertebrae: PA/AP axial
        oblique projection (anterior/
        posterior oblique positions),
        406-412
    CR/intervertebral disk space
        alignment, 406-409
    head positioning, 410

Cervical vertebrae: PA/AP axial oblique projection (anterior/posterior oblique positions) *(Continued)*
  interpupillary line positioning, 409-410
  problem, detection, 410
  kyphosis, positioning, 408-409
  midcoronal plane rotation, 406
  rotation, problem (effect), 406
  trauma, 410-411
  vertebral column alignment, inaccuracy, 406-408
Cervicothoracic vertebrae: lateral projection (Twining method; Swimmer's technique), 412-414
  C7 identification, 412
  exam indication, 412
  IPL/midsagittal plane positioning, 412
  rotation, 412
  trauma, 412
Chest
  anteroposterior axial projection (lordotic position), 107-110
  anteroposterior chest projection, right lateral decubitus, 105f
  anteroposterior projection, 98-107, 104t
  central venous catheter (CVC), 81-82
  devices, 78-84, 80t
  endotracheal tube (ETT), 79-81
  free intraperitoneal air, 78
  image analysis guidelines, 77-84
  lateral decubitus, 104t
  lateral projection (left lateral position), 91-98
  left side, rotation (PA chest), 87f
  pleural drainage tube, 81
  pleural effusion, 77-78
  pneumothorax/pneumectomy, 77
  posteroanterior oblique projection, right/left anterior oblique positions, 110-113
  posteroanterior projection, 84-91, 104-107, 104t
  projection, histogram, 39f
  pulmonary arterial catheter, 82
  right/left lateral decubitus projection, 104-107
  source-to-IR distance (SID), 77
  technical data, 77, 78t
    imaging analysis guidelines, 78b
  tracheostomy, 79
  tubes/lines/catheters, 78-84, 80t
  umbilical artery catheter, 82-83
  vascular lung markings, 77
    visualization, 77-78
  ventilated patient, 77
Child abdomen, AP projection (left lateral decubitus position), 145-148

Child abdomen, AP projection (supine/upright), 143
Child AP (left lateral decubitus) abdomen
  analysis, 148
    practice, 148
  correction, 148
  projection, 146t
    positioning, 147f
Child AP abdomen projection, 144t
Child AP abdominal analysis, 143
  correction, 143
  practice, 143
Child AP chest projection, positioning, 118f
Child AP/PA (lateral decubitus) chest
  analysis, 128
  correction, 129
  practice, 128-129
Child AP/PA (lateral decubitus) chest projection, 128t
Child chest
  AP/PA projection (right/left lateral decubitus position), 127-129
  lateral projection, left lateral position, 122-124
  PA/AP (portable) chest analysis, 117, 119
    correction, 117, 119
    practice, 117-119
  PA/AP (portable) projections, 117-119
Child lateral chest analysis, 122-124
  correction, 122-124
  practice, 122-124
Child lateral chest projection, positioning, 123f
  accuracy, 123f
Child PA/AP (portable) chest projection, 118t
Child PA (right lateral decubitus) chest projection, positioning (accuracy), 128f
Child supine AP abdomen projection, positioning, 144f
Child upright AP abdomen projection, positioning, 144f-145f
Clavicle: AP axial projection (lordotic position), 266-267
  CR angulation, 266-267
  midcoronal plane positioning, 266
  rotation, 266
Clavicle: AP projection, 264-266
  midcoronal plane positioning, 264-265
  rotation, 264-265
Clavicles, 87, 101
  midcoronal plane, 108-109
Clivus, inclusion (importance), 404
Closed joints, presence, 27f

Clothing artifacts
  demonstration, lateral femur projection (impact), 61f
  lateral knee projection, usage, 73f
  pediatric imaging, 72-73
CM joint spaces, wrist (PA projection), 179
Coccygeal vertebrae
  image analysis guidelines, 424-438, 424b
  technical data, 424, 424t
Coccyx: AP axial projection, 443-444
  CR/coccyx alignment, 444
  emptying bladder/rectum, 443
  rotation, 443-444
Coccyx: lateral projection, 444-446
  collimation, 446
  CR/vertebral column, 444-445
  lateral lumbar flexion, detection, 444
  rotation, 444
  vertebral column, sagging (adjustment), 445
Collimated borders, usage, 15f
Collimation, 14-17, 35, 52
  anteroposterior (AP) sacral projection, 17f
  determination, hand's shadow (viewing), 18f
  guidelines, 16b
  histogram analysis errors, 42
  humerus: AP projection, 228
  overcollimation, 16-17
  problem, 43f, 195f
  tightness, obtaining, 17f
Collimator guide
  example, 13f
  usage, 12
Collimator head, rotation, 16, 227f
Collimator light field, IR coverage (differences), 16f
Compartments, 332
Compensating filter, absence, 415f
Computed radiography (CR)
  alignment, 427f
    accuracy, 26f, 152f
    problem, 27f, 152f
    problem, identification, 100
  anatomic structure, 14
  angulation
    degree, determination, 109
    inadequacy, identification, 109
    placement, 28
  anteroposterior chest projection, 65f
  anteroposterior oblique (Grashey method) shoulder projection, 41f
  axiolateral hip projection, 44f
  background radiation fogging, 44
  cassette, barcode label, 8

Computed radiography (CR) (Continued)
  centering, 180-181
    effects, comparison, 27f
    impact, 21f
  effect (demonstration), AP pelvis projections (impact), 22f
  exposure, cassette location, 65
  histogram, 43f
    scatter radiation values, presence, 44f
  image/data acquisition, 38
  image receptor
    multiple projections, 43-44
    patient orientation, 4
  lumbar vertebral column, alignment, 433f
  marker placement, collimator guide (usage), 12
  phosphor plate, equipment-handling artifact, 65f
  placement, 14-15
    impact, 20f-21f
    location, collimated borders (usage), 15f
  posteroanterior chest projection histogram, 41f
    30% coverage, 43
    usage, 32f
  volume of interest, defining, 42-43
Contact shield, usage (avoidance), 51f
Contrast differences, 57b
Contrast making, 59
Contrast mask, 6
Contrast resolution, 56-58
  alignment, 70
    guidelines, 69-72
  inadequacy, kV (adjustment), 48-49
  scatter radiation fogging, impact, 50f
Coracoid process, location, 249f
Cranium
  image analysis guidelines, 461-462, 462b
  positioning landmarks, 462t
  positioning lines, 461
  technical data, 461, 462t
  trauma cranial imaging (cervical vertebral injuries), 461-462
Cranium/facial bones/nasal bones/ sinuses: lateral projection, 476-479
  head rotation, 476
    detection, 476
  head tilting, 476-477
  sinus cavities, air-fluid levels, 476
  trauma, positioning, 476
Cranium/facial bones/sinuses: PA/AP axial projection (Caldwell method), 468-472
  analysis, 471
  correction, 471

Cranium/facial bones/sinuses: PA/AP axial projection (Caldwell method) (Continued)
  CR alignment, detection, 468
  head rotation, 468
  OML alignment, detection (CR adjustment), 468
  OML alignment, problem (CR adjustment), 468
  OML/IR alignment, 468-471
  trauma AP axial (Caldwell) projection, CR angulation, 468-471
  correction, 471
Cranium/mandible: AP axial projection (Towne method), 472-476
  analysis, 475
  cranium portion, 472
  head rotation, 472
  head tilting, 475
  mandible, 472
  OML alignment, problem, 472-475
    adjustment, 475
  OML/midsagittal plane alignment, 472-475
  petromastoid portion, 472
  trauma patients, CR angulation (determination), 475
Cranium/mandible: PA/AP projection, 462-468
  CR adjustment, OML alignment problem, 464
  head rotation, 464
  head tilt, 466
  mandible, jaw position, 466
  midsagittal plane alignment, 466
  OML alignment problems, detection, 464
  orbitomeatal line/IR alignment, 464-466
  trauma AP projection, 464
    CR angulation correction, 466
Cranium/mandible/sinuses: submentovertex projection (Schueller method), 479-481
  head rotation, 480
  head tilt, 479-480
  IOML/IR alignment, 479
  IOML mispositioning, effect, 479
Crosstable lateral distal femur projection, patient positioning, 361f
Cross-table lateral infant chest projection (patient positioning), immobilization equipment (usage), 121f
Cross-table lateral knee projection, fractured patella (presence), 339f
Cross-table lateral projection, left lateral position, 120-122

Cross-table lateral projection, overhead lateral projection (differences), 120
Cross-table lateral projections, marker placement guidelines, 10
Crosstable lateral proximal femur projection
  patient positioning, 364f
  positioning accuracy, 364f
Crosstable lateromedial knee projection
  leg abduction, 344f
  leg adduction, 343f
Crosswise (CW) direction, 85
Crosswise IR cassettes, usage, 135f
Curved vertebral column, sagging (adjustment), 437f

D
Danelius-Miller method, 382-386
Data acquisition, 38
Decubitus chest analysis, 107
  correction, 107
  practice, 107
Demographic requirements, 8-10
Destructive patient conditions, 53-56
Detector elements (DELs), 32
Digestive system
  AEC, usage, 486
  asthenic patient, 487-488
  body habitus positioning variables, 487-488
  hypersthenic patient, 487
  image analysis guidelines, 486-493, 487b
  pendulous breasts, relationship, 486
  peristaltic activity/exposure times, 486-487
  respiration, 488-489
  sthenic patient, 488
  technical data, 486-487, 487t
Digital anteroposterior femur projection, 52f
Digital posteroanterior hand projection, 43f
Digital radiography, 38-75
  anatomic structure, 12f
  post-processing, 58-59
Digital system artifact, 65-66
Direct-indirect capture digital radiography (DR), 5
  patient examination, 8-10
Direct-indirect radiography, image/ data acquisition, 38
Distal femurs, 355-356
  artifacts, lateral knee projection, 73f
  depression, 354f
  elevation, 363f

Distal forearm
　depression, 220f-221f
　fracture alignment (demonstration),
　　lateral/PA wrist projection
　　(usage), 19f
　positioning, 199-200
Distal humeral fracture, 231
Distal humeral tilting, 260
Distal humerus
　alignment, problem, 230f
　AP/lateral projections, 219f
Distal lower leg
　depression, 347f, 350f
　elevation, 302f, 310f, 313f, 317f,
　　320f
　fracture, 324f
　　lateral lower leg projection, 327f
Distal radius joint
　wrist: PA oblique projection (lateral
　　rotation), 183-184
　wrist: PA projection, 178-179
Distal scaphoid
　anterior alignment, 187-188
　distal alignment, 188-189
　fracture, wrist: ulnar deviation, PA
　　axial projection (scaphoid),
　　196f
Diverged x-ray beam, usage, 15f
Dorsiflexion, compensation, 305
Dose creep, avoidance, 35-36
Double-contrast examination, AEC
　usage, 486
Double-exposed AP abdomen
　projections, barium (presence),
　31f
Double-exposed AP vertebral
　projections, 31f
Double-exposed lateral vertebral
　projections, 31f
Double exposure, 30
Duodenum, 493-501
　contrast medium, 493-494
　double contrast, 493-494
　single contrast, 493
Duodenum: AP oblique projection
　(LAO position), 499
Duodenum: AP projection, 501
Duodenum: lateral projection (right
　lateral position), 497-499
Duodenum: PA oblique projection
　(RAO position), 494
Duodenum: PA projection, 494-497

E

Elbow
　external rotation, 209f
　flexed elbow, positioning, 211
　flexion, 208-211
　　forearm: AP projection, 202
　internal rotation, 209f
　joint spaces, 216
　　CR centering, 216

Elbow (Continued)
　positioning, 186-187, 201-202
　soft tissue structures, 217
Elbow: AP oblique projections
　　(medial/lateral rotation), 212-216
　AP oblique elbow projection, flexed
　　elbow (patient positioning),
　　215f
　elbow flexion, 213-215
　elbow joint spaces, 216
　external AP oblique elbow
　　projection
　　distal forearm, elevation, 229f
　　elbow obliquity, 215f
　　patient positioning, 214f
　externally rotated AP oblique elbow
　　projection, positioning
　　(accuracy), 213f
　flexed elbow, positioning, 215
　humeral epicondyles, 212-213
　internal AP oblique elbow
　　projection
　　elbow obliquity, 214f
　internal AP oblique elbow
　　projection, patient positioning,
　　214f
　internally rotated AP oblique elbow
　　projection, positioning
　　(accuracy), 213f
　lateral oblique (external rotation),
　　212-213
　medial oblique (internal rotation),
　　212
Elbow: AP projection, 207-212
　humeral epicondyles, 207
　radial head/ulna relationship,
　　207
　radial tuberosity, 207-208
Elbow: axiolateral elbow projection
　　(Coyle method), 223-226
　CR alignment, 224
　CR angulation, 223-224
　elbow flexion, 224
　forearm, 224-225
　humerus, 223-224
　patient positioning, 224f
　wrist/hand, 225
Elbow joint space
　CR centering/openness, 205-206
　openness, 205-206
Elbow: lateral projection
　　(lateromedial), 217-223
　distal forearm
　　depression, 221f
　　mispositioning, 218-220
　　positioning, IR/wrist
　　　(relationship), 221f
　elbow flexion, 217-218
　elbow soft tissue structures, 217
　fat pad visualization, 217-218
　humeral epicondyles, 218-220
　patient positioning, 218f

Elbow: lateral projection
　　(lateromedial) (Continued)
　proximal humerus, elevation, 219f
　radial head fractures, positioning,
　　220-222
　radial tuberosity, 220
Electric charge, collection, 38
Eleventh thoracic vertebra,
　identification, 97
Endotracheal tube (ETT), 79-81
　placement, 81f
Equipment-handling artifact, 65f
Equipment-related artifact
　AP chest projection, usage, 62f-63f
　AP pelvis projection, 64f
　AP shoulder projection, usage, 63f
Equipment-related artifact-Moiré grid
　artifact, 64f
Esophagram: lateral projection,
　490-492
　rotation, 490-492
　thorax rotation, detection, 491-492
Esophagram: PA oblique projection
　　(RAO position), 489-490
　body obliquity, 489-490
　patient rotation, inaccuracy, 490
Esophagram: PA projection, 492-493
　rotation, 492-493
　　detection, 492-493
Esophagram: UGI system, 489
　contrast medium, 489
　esophagram preparation, 489
　stomach/duodenum preparation,
　　489
　Ugi preparation procedure, 489
Expiration chest, 90-91
Exposed AP pelvis projections, 50f
Exposure indicators (EIs), 40-41
　parameters, 40t
Exposure-related factors, 50-56
External artifact, 60-61
　display, pillow (involvement), 61f
　lateral knee projection, 61f
Externally rotated AP shoulder
　projection, positioning, 239f
External monitoring lines, 84f
External monitoring tubes/lines, 84
Extremity flexion, degree
　determination, 25
　estimation, 26f
Extremity projections, marker
　placement guidelines, 10

F

Facial bones
　imaging analysis guidelines, 462b
　projection, 476t
Facial bones/sinuses: parietoacanthial/
　acanthioparietal projection
　(Waters method), 481-485
　air-fluid levels, demonstration, 481
　head rotation, 481

Facial bones/sinuses: parietoacanthial/
acanthioparietal projection
(Waters method) *(Continued)*
MML alignment problem, CR
adjustment, 482
MML alignment problem, CR
angulation correction, 482-484
MML/IR alignment, 481-484
MML positioning problem,
detection, 481
modified Waters method, 484
Facial bones, technical data, 462t
Family members, radiation exposure,
36
Fat pads
anterior pretalar/posterior
pericapsular fat pads, 298-299
anterior pretalar/posterior
pericapsular fat pads,
demonstration, 318
location, 299f, 319f
lateral elbow projection, 218f
suprapatellar fat pads, location,
338f
visualization, elbow: lateral
projection (lateromedial),
217-218
Fat planes, location, 368f
Female patients, gonadal shielding, 34f
AP projection, 33-34
lateral projection, 34, 35f
Female pelves, male pelves
(differences), 367, 368t
Femoral abudction, 373f
Femoral condyles
antcrior/postcrior alignment,
340-344
distal alignment, 343-344
superior position, 351-353
Femoral head, inclusion, 384-385
Femoral inclination
reduction, supine position, 340f
upright position, 339f
Femoral neck
fracture, 384
demonstration, 385f
localization, 377f
location, 384f
misalignment, 383
visualization, 380-383
Femoral shafts, abduction, 373f
Femur abduction, 372f, 381f
effect, 362-363
maximum, 381f
Femur: AP projection, 355-360
distal femur, 355-356
epicondyles, 355-356
femoral condyle shape, 355-356
femoral neck, 357-359
femoral shaft overlap, 356
fracture, positioning, 356, 359
pelvis rotation, 357

Femur: AP projection *(Continued)*
proximal femur, 357-359
soft tissue, 359
trochanters, 357-359
Femur: lateral projection
(mediolateral), 360-365
anterior/posterior femoral condyle
alignment, 360
femoral condyles, 360-362
femur abduction, effect, 362-363
fracture, positioning, 361-365
greater/lesser trochanter, 362
midfemur/grid midline alignment,
363
proximal femur, 362-365
Femur positioning, problem, 353f
Fibula, presence, 24f
Fibular head, tibial superimposition
(absence), 343f
Field of view (FOV), 31
Fifth toe, lateral projection (patient
positioning), 288f
Finger
adjacent overlap, 158-159
extension, PA oblique hand
projection (patient positioning),
172f
flexion
PA hand projection, 169f
PA oblique hand projection, 173f
fractures, 158-159
lateral projection, 157-159
phalangeal midshaft concavity,
157
Finger (AP projection), flexed fingers,
153f
patient positioning, 153f
Finger (PA oblique projection),
154-157
alternate second finger positioning,
155
joint space, 155
phalangeal soft tissue width/
midshaft concavity, 154-155
phalanges, 155
soft tissue overlap, 155
Finger (PA projection), 150-154,
151t
CR, parallel alignment (absence),
153f
flexed fingers, 153f
joint spaces/phalanges, 151
medial rotation, 152f
phalangeal soft tissue width/
midshaft concavity, 150-151
positioning, 151f
unextendable finger, positioning,
151
First AP axial toe projection,
positionng (accuracy), 281f
First lateral toe projection, posititing
(accuracy), 287f

First toe, lateral projection (patient
positioning), 288f
Flexed elbow, positioning, 211
Flexed fingers
AP projection, 153f
PA projection, 153f
Fluid levels (demonstration),
positioning (usage), 104-105
Focal spot
size, 29
usage, 29
Focal spot size, 75
Foot: AP axial projection
(dorsoplantar), 290-294
ankle flexion, 291
CR angulation, determination, 291
medial arch/rotation, 290
metatarsal/cuneiform/talar/calcaneal
spacing, 290
projections, changes, 292f
tarsometatarsal/navicular-cuneiform
joint spaces, 291
third metatarsal, base (location),
291
weight-bearing AP, 290-291
Foot: AP oblique projection (medial
rotation), 294-298
ankle flexion, 295
cuboid-cuneiform/intermetatarsal
joints, 294-295
obliquity
degree, determination, 294-295
inadequacy, 295
Foot dorsiflexion, 308, 318-320, 318f
absence, 319f
Foot inversion, ankle rotation
(differences), 315
Foot: lateral projection (mediolateral/
lateromedial), 298-305
anterior pretalar/posterior
pericapsular fat pads,
298-299
fat pads, location, 299f
foot dorsiflexion, 299-300
foot positioning, 301-302
lower leg, positioning, 300,
300f
repositioning, 300-301
repositioning, tibia/fibula (usage),
303
talar domes, 300
anterior/posterior alignment,
294-295
proximal alignment, 300-301
weight-bearing lateromedial foot,
301
weight-bearing lateromedial
projection, 304
weight-bearing mediolateral foot,
301
Foot positioning, 385f
problems, 321f, 369f

Foot rotation
examples, 351-354, 358f
problems, 376f
Forearm
metacarpals, alignment, 189
positioning, 179
thumb, alignment, 189
Forearm: AP projection, 199-203
CR centering, 202
distal forearm, 202
proximal forearm, 202
elbow flexion, 202
elbow joint spaces, 202
fracture, positioning, 202-203
distal forearm, 202
proximal forearm, 203
humerus/elbow positioning, 201-202
radial tuberosity, 200
ulnar styloid, 201-202
wrist/distal forearm positioning, 199-200
wrist, openness, 202
Forearm: lateral projection (lateromedial), 203-207
CR centering, 205-206, 211
elbow joint space, openness, 205-206
elbow positioning, 205
elbow soft tissue, placement, 205f
fracture, positioning, 206
humerus, positioning, 205
radius/ulna alignment, 204
soft tissue structures, 203-204
wrist/distal forearm positioning, 204-205
wrist, placement, 205f
Foreshortening, 23
absence/presence, 24f
45-degree PA oblique (LAO) chest projection, 111f
rotation (45 degrees), 112f
45-degree PA oblique (RAO) chest projection, 111f
superior midcoronal plane, posterior tilt, 112f
Fourth metacarpal, posterior displacement, 67f
Fractured distal humerus, lateral distal humerus projection demonstration, 232f
Fractured humerus, demonstration, 228f
Fractured patella, presence, 339f
Fractured proximal humerus, demonstration, 232f
Fracture lines, demonstration, 25
Free intraperitoneal air, 78
abdomen, 131
AP left lateral decubitus abdomen demonstration, 140f
PA chest demonstration, 80f

Full lung aeration (absence), PA chest (usage), 90f

G

Glenoid cavity: AP oblique projection (Grashey Method), 248-252
kyphotic patient, 250-251
midcoronal plane
positioning, 248-250
tilting, 250-251
recumbent position, 251
shoulder protraction, 251
shoulder rotation, 248-250
Glenoid cavity, placement, 244f
arm, abduction, 244f
Gonadal shielding, 33, 435
female patients, anteroposterior projection, 33-34
lateral projection, 35f
lateral vertebral/sacral/coccygeal projections, 435f
Greater trochanter, 362, 379-380, 383-384
alignment, 382-383
visualization, 368-371, 380-381
Grid cutoff
artifact, 62
causes, 62b, 62f
off-centered grid cutoff, 64f
Grids, 51
conversion factor, 51t
line artifacts, digital AP femur projection (impact), 52f

H

Hand
external rotation, 175f
flexion
adequacy, 163f
PA hand projection, 169f
obliquity, inadequacy, 172f
overflexion, 164f
shadow, viewing, 18f
Hand: fan lateral projection (lateromedial), 173-176
fanned fingers, 174-175
lateral hand, extension, 174-175
metacarpal superimposition, 173-174
Hand: PA oblique projection (lateral rotation), 170-173
joint spaces, 171
metacarpal spacing, 170-171
phalanges, 171
soft tissue overlap, 171
thumb positioning, 171
Hand: PA projection, 167-170
conditions, 169
joint spaces, 167
metacarpals, 167
pediatric bone age assessment, 169

Hand: PA projection (Continued)
phalangeal/metacarpal midshaft concavity, 167
phalanges, 167
soft tissue width, 167
thumb/hand closeness, 167-169
Heart
anteroinferior lung/heart visualization, 91
magnification, SID (relationship), 98
penetration, optimum, 83f
visualization, obliquity (impact), 110
Hemidiaphragm visualization, 94-96
Hickey method, 378
usage, 379f
Hill-Sachs defect, 245f
Hip
dislocation, positioning, 369
image analysis guidelines, 366-389, 367b
joint, localization, 377f
technical data, 366, 367t
Hip: AP frog-leg (mediolateral) projection (modified Cleaves method), 378-382
femoral neck visualization, 380-381
greater trochanter visualization, 380-381
hip flexion problem, 380
knee flexion problem, 380
Lauenstein/Hickey methods, 378
leg abduction problem, 381
lesser/greater trochanter, 379-380
pelvis rotation, 378
Hip: AP projection, 374-378
compact ray (CR) centering, 376-377
dislocated hip positioning, 375-376
femoral head/neck, localization, 376-377
femoral neck, 374-376
fractured femoral neck/proximal femur, 375-376
leg rotation problem, identification, 374-375
marker placement, 13f
orthopedic apparatuses, inclusion, 377
pelvis rotation, 374
rotation, identification, 374
Hip: axiolateral (inferosuperior) projection (Danelius-Miller method), 382-386
acetabulum, inclusion, 384-385
CR centering, 385
CR/femoral neck misalignment, effect, 383
femoral head, inclusion, 384-385
femoral neck, fracture, 384
femoral neck visualization, 382-383

Hip: axiolateral (inferosuperior) projection (Danelius-Miller method) *(Continued)*
  greater/lesser trochanter alignment, 382-383
  hip dislocation, 384
  IR placement, 385f
  lateral hip, metal apparatus (usage), 385f
  leg rotation problem, identification, 384
  lesser/greater trochanter, 383-384
  obese patients, 385
  orthopedic apparatuses, inclusion, 385
  proximal femur, fracture, 384
  unaffected leg position, 382
Hip flexion, 380f
  problem, 380
Histogram, 38f
  analysis error (demonstration), digital PA hand projection (impact), 43f
  chest projection, 39f
  formation, 38-39
  image histograms, production (guidelines), 39b
  part selection, workstation menu (usage), 42
Histogram analysis errors, 41-44
  collimation, 42
  demonstration, computed radiography anteroposterior oblique shoulder projection, 41f
  demonstration, computed radiography axiolateral hip projection, 44f
  demonstration, digital posteroanterior hand projection (usage), 43f
Holmblad method, 345-348, 346t
Honeycomb pattern, computed radiography AP chest projection demonstration, 65f
Humeral abduction, absence, 188f
Humeral epicondyles
  elbow: AP projection, 207-212
  humerus: AP projection, 226-228
  IR parallel alignment, 187f
Humeral fracture
  positioning, 228, 231-233
  shoulder: AP projection, 240
Humeral head fracture, demonstration, 245f
Humerus (humeri)
  nonelevation, 96f
  positioning, 186-187, 201-202, 239-241
  rotation, 245-246

Humerus: AP projection, 226-228
  collimation, 228
  humeral epicondyles, 226-228
  IR length, 228
Humerus bones (AP projection)
  elongation, absence/presence, 23f
  foreshortening, absence/presence, 24f
Humerus: lateral projection (lateromedial/medioateral), 229-233
  distal humeral fracture, 231
  distal humerus fracture, patient positioning, 231f
  mediolateral projections, lateromedial projections (differences), 229-231
  proximal humeral fracture, 231-232
Hypersthenic abdomen, 132
Hypersthenic anteroposterior oblique spot stomach/duodenal projection (LPO position), 500f
Hypersthenic anteroposterior spot stomach projection, 503f
Hypersthenic lateral spot stomach/duodoneal projection, positioning accuracy, 498f
Hypersthenic PA oblique spot stomach/duodenal projection (RAO position), 495f
Hypersthenic PA stomach/duodenum projection, positioning accuracy, 497f
Hypersthenic patient
  anteroposterior large intestine projections, 504f
  PA chest, 86f
  PA projection, 488f
  supine AP abdomen, crosswise IR cassettes (usage), 135f
Hyposthenic patient, PA chest, 87f
Hysterosalpingogram, 33f

I

Iliac alae images (supine/prone patients), 508f
Image acceptaibility, defining, 66
Image acquisition, 38
Image analysis
  form, 8-25, 8b-9b
  guidelines
    chest/abdomen, 77-113
    shoulder, 235-277
    upper extremity, 150-233, 150b
  optimal image, characteristics, 3-8
  reason, 2-3
  terminology, 3
Image display, 4-6
  adjustment, 6
  guidelines, 4b
Image histograms, production (guidelines), 39b

Image matrix, 31f
Image modification, procedural algorithms (selection), 59
Image receptor (IR)
  adjustments, causes, 46t-47t
  alignment, 70, 95f
    guidelines, 69-72
  anteroposterior (right lateral decubitus) chest, 106f
  computed radiography image receptor, patient orientation, 4
  conditions, contrast differences, 57b
  coverage, collimator light field (differences), 16f
  CW-LW position, 73
  exposure, 45-50
    maintenance, 73-74
  long bones, diagonal positioning, 15f
  magnification, 22f
  multiple projections, 43-44
  overexposed projection, evaluation, 47t
  overexposure
    causes, 47t
    identification, 49-50
  placement, body habitus, 85, 98
  post-processing, 58-59
  projection, angulation, 21f
  right side, anteroposterior (left lateral decubitus) chest, 106f
  size, 31f, 139-140
    comparison, 32f
  subject contrast, 48
  underexposure
    causes, 46t
    identification, 45-47
    technical adjustment, determination, 48
  usage, 2-3
Imaging
  mobile imaging, 66-69
  situations, 66-69
  trauma imaging, 66-69
Imaging plate (IP), trapped electron storage, 38
Immobilization devices, 32
Immobilization equipment, usage, 114f, 121f
Implanted cardioverter defibrillator (ICD), placement, 84f
Infant abdomen, AP projection (left lateral decubitus position), 143-145
  intraperitoneal air demonstration, 143-144
  midcoronal plane positioning/rotation, 144
Infant abdomen, AP projection (supine), 141-143
  lumbar vertebrae alignment, IR (usage), 141

Infant abdomen, AP projection
    (supine) (Continued)
  midcoronal plane/rotation, 141
  respiration, 141-142
  ventilated patient, 142
Infant abdomen projection, AP (left
    lateral decubitus) neonate
    positioning, 146f
Infant AP abdomen projection, 141t
Infant AP (left lateral decubitus)
    abdominal analysis, 145
  correction, 145
  practice, 145
Infant AP chest
  analysis, 116-117
    correction, 116-117
    practice, 116-117
  full lung aeration, absence, 116f
  pleural drainage tube placement, 82f
  projection, 113t
  right side, rotation, 115f
Infant AP (lateral decubitus) chest
    projection, 124t-125t
Infant AP decubitus chest analysis,
    127
  correction, 127
  practice, 127
Infant chest
  AP projection, 113-117
    right/left lateral decubitus
        position, 124-127
  AP (left lateral decubitus)
      projection, patient positioning,
      126f
  arm positioning, 124-125
  chin position, 115, 124-125
  CR/IR alignment, 125-126
    alternates, 115
    perpendicular/cephalic angle, 115
  cross-table lateral projection
      arms/chin, 121
    left lateral position, 120-122
    respiration, 121-122
  IR alignment, 125-126
    alternate, 125-126
  lung field, artifact lines (prevention),
      124
  lungs/aeration, appearance, 115-116
  midcoronal plane positioning/
      rotation, 124
  midsagittal plane tilting, 124
  patient alignment, 125-126
  patient positioning, 113
  right/left lungs, identification, 121
  rotation, 113-115
    identification, IR/side-to-side CR
        alignment (problem),
        114-115
    identification, patient positioning
        (problem), 114
    prevention, side-to-side CR
        alignment, 114

Infant lateral chest
  exposure field, chin (presence), 121f
  projection, 120t
  right lung, posterior rotation, 121f
Inferior midsaggital plane, IR tilt, 95f
Inferosuperior axial shoulder analysis,
    247-248
  correction, 247-248
  practice, 247-248
Inferosuperior axial shoulder
    positioning, 243f
  shoulder, nonelevation, 247f
Inferosuperior axial shoulder
    projection, 242t
  anterior dislocation, 245f
  arm
    abduction, 246f
    external rotation, 246f
  CR size, problem, 245f
  Hill-Sachs defect, 245f
  humeral epicondyles, positioning,
      243f
  humeral head fracture
      demonstration, 245f
  IR position, 247f
  lateral neck flexion, inadequacy,
      247f
  positioning accuracy, 242f
  upper thoracic vertebrae, upward
      arch, 247f
Inferosuperior (axial) shoulder
    projection, 6f
Injury, physical signs (site assessment),
    67
Intercondylar fossa: AP axial
    projection (Béclère method),
    348-351
  knee joint/tibial plateau, 350
  knee magnification, 351
  medial/lateral intercondylar fossa
      surface, 351
  proximal intercondylar fossa
      surface, 348-350
Intercondylar fossa: PA axial
    projection (Holmblad method),
    345-348
  femur positioning problem,
      repositioning, 345
  foot positioning problem,
      repositioning, 346
  foot rotation, 348
  knee joint/tibial plateau, 345-346
  medial/lateral surfaces, 347-348
    femoral inclination, 347-348
  proximal intercondylar fossa
      surface/patella, 345
Intercondylar fossa visualization, knee
    flexion (inclusion), 330
Intercondylar sulci, superior position,
    351-353
Intermalleolar line, IR alignment,
    315f

Internal AP oblique elbow projection,
    trauma positioning, 70f
Internal artifacts, 61-62
  AP pelvis projection, 62f
  display, lateral knee projection,
      61f
  prosthesis, impact, 61f
Internal foot positioning, 369f
Internal foot rotation, 376f
Internal leg rotation, absence, 353f
Internally rotated AP shoulder
    projection, positioning, 239f
Interpupillary line positioning,
    409-410
Intervertebral disk spaces, CR
    alignment, 426, 431-432
Intraperitoneal air, demonstration, 140
  AP (left lateral decubitus) neonate
      abdomen demonstration, 146f
  neonate/infant abdomen, AP
      projection (left lateral decubitus
      position), 143-144
Inverted grid artifact (demonstration),
    AP oblique (Grashey method)
    should projection (usage), 63f
Involuntary patient motion, 30f

J

Joint effusion, visualization, 338-339
Joint flexion, degree (estimation), 26f
Joint mobility, demonstration, 180
Joint spaces, 151
  alignment, 26f, 152f
    problems, 27f, 152f
  anterior thigh soft tissue, projection,
      353
  demonstration, 25
  finger (PA oblique projection), 155
  hand: PA oblique projection (lateral
      rotation), 171
  thumb
    AP projection, 160-161
    lateral projection, 162-163
Joint visualization, CR centering
    (effects), 27f
Jones fracture, demonstration, 321f

K

Kidneys, location, 129-130
Kilovoltage (kV)
  setting, 67
Kilovoltage (kV), adjustment, 48-49
Knee: AP oblique projection (medial/
    lateral rotation), 333-337
  CR angulation problems,
      adjustment, 334
  knee joint, 333-334
  lateral (external) oblique position,
      334
  medial (internal) oblique position,
      334
  rotation, 334

Knee: AP projection, 328-333
  condylar margins, 331-332
  CR angulation problems,
      adjustment, 332
  femoral epicondyle, tibia/fibular
      head relationship, 328-329
  rotation, 328-329
  joint space, 331-332
    narrowing, 332
  patella/intercondylar fossa
      demonstration, 329-331
    intercondylar fossa visualization,
        knee flexion (inclusion), 330
    knee flexion, impact, 329-330
    nonextendable knee, 330-331
    patellar subluxation, 330
  tibial plateau, CR alignment (supine
      position), 331-332
Knee flexion, 354f, 380f
  anteroposterior (AP) knee
      projection, 331f
  impact, 329-330
  lateral knee projection, 343f
  patella, movement, 330f
  problem, 380
Knee: lateral projection (mediolateral),
    337-345
  alternate positioning method,
      340-341
  compact ray (CR) angulation
    degree, determination, 340
    problems, adjustment, 340
  femoral condyles
    anterior/posterior alignment,
        340-344
    distal alignment, 343-344
  fracture, positioning, 339
  joint effusion visualization,
      338-339
  knee flexion, 338-339, 343
  knee joint space, 339-340
  knee rotation, 341-342
  lateral/medialcondyles, distinction,
      340
  patella position, 338-339
  patellofemoral joint, 338-339
  supine (cross-table) lateromedial
      knee projection, 343-344
Knees
  anatomic position, AP projections
      (differences), 322-323
  cathode end position, 53f
  external rotation, 351f
  internal rotation, 351f
  joints, detector alements (impact),
      66f
  magnification, 351
  overflexion, 347f
  positioning problems, patella
      (locations), 342f
  silhouettes, CR centering, 355f
  underflexion, 347f

Kodak CR system, usage, 42f
Kyphotic anteroposterior shoulder
    projections, 238f

L
L5-S1 lateral lumbosacral junction
    projection, 437f
  right side, 437f
L5-S1 lumbar region, supplementary
    projection, 434-435
L5-S1 lumbosacral junction: lateral
    projection, 436-438
  central ray/L5-S1 disk space
      alignment, 436-437
  lateral lumbar flexion, detection,
      437
  rotation, 436
Large intestine, 504-516
  barium pools, 507
  double-contrast lower intestinal
      filling, 505-507
  double contrast problems, 507
  preparation, 504-505
    procedure, 504-505
  structures, double-contrast filling,
      507t
Large intestine: AP/PA projection
    (lateral decubitus position)
  AP decubitus projection, 510
  hypersthenic/obese patients, IR size/
      direction, 510
  PA decubitus projection, 510
  rotation, 510
Large intestine (rectum): lateral
    projection, 509
  rotation, 509
Large intestine: PA/AP projection,
    507
  abdominal rotation, detection, 507
  AP projection, 507
  PA projection, 507
Large intestine: PA axial projection/PA
    axial oblique projection (RAO
    position), 514-516
  CR angulation, 516
    inadequacy, detection, 516
  inadequate obliquity, detection,
      514-516
  PA axial oblique projection (RAO
      position): patient obliquity,
      514-516
  PA axial rotation, 514
Large intestine: PA oblique projection
    (LAO position), 513
  obliquity, inadequacy (detection),
      513
  patient obliquity, 513
Large intestine: PA oblique projection
    (RAO position), 512
  obliquity, inadequacy (detection),
      512
  patient obliquity, 512

Lateral ankle analysis, 322
  correction, 322
  practice, 322
Lateral ankle projection, 319t
  central ray centering/collimation,
      319f
  distal lower leg, elevation, 320f
  foot dorsiflexion, absence,
      319f-320f
  Jones fracture, demonstration, 321f
  knee positioning, 320f
  lateral foot surface positioning, 321f
  leg
    external rotation, 321f
    internal rotation, 321f
  lower leg positioning, 320f
  low subject contrast, 58f
  positioning accuracy, 319f
  proximal lower leg, elevation, 320f
Lateral anteroposterior lumbar
    projections, intervertebral disk
    apace alignment, 427f
Lateral calcaneal analysis, 311
  correction, 311
  practice, 311
Lateral calcaneal projection
  calcaneal fracture, demonstration,
      309f
  CR centering/collimation, 309f
  distal lower leg, elevation, 310f
  leg
    external rotation, 310f
    internal rotation, 311f
  positioning accuracy, 309f
  proximal lower leg, elevation, 309f
Lateral calcaneus projection, 308t
Lateral cervical projection
  causes, 402-403
  head/upper cervical vertebral
      column, tilt, 403f
  hyperextension, patient positioning,
      404f
  hyperflexion, 404f
    patient positioning, 404f
  IOML/dens/atlantoaxial joint
      alignment visualization, 399f
  shoulder depression, 405f
  supine patient, 393f
  trauma, evaluation (patient
      positioning), 405f
  upper incisor/dens/atlantoaxial joint
      space/posterior occiput
      relationship, 397f
  upright patient, 393f
Lateral cervical vertebrae analysis,
    405-406
  correction, 405-406
  practice, 405-406
Lateral cervicothoracic projection
    (twinning method), 405
  head/upper cervical vertebrae, tilt,
      414f

Lateral cervicothoracic projection
(twinning method) *(Continued)*
left shoulder
anterior position, 413f
posterior position, 414f
patient positioning, 414f
positioning accuracy, 413f
Lateral cervicothoracic vertebrae
analysis, 414
correction, 414
practice, 414
Lateral cervicothoracic vertebrae
projection, 412t
Lateral chest
anteroinferior lungs (compression),
anterior abdominal tissue
(impact), 93f
full lung aeration, absence, 97f
humeri, nonelevation, 96f
inferior midsaggital plane, IR tilt,
95f
positioning, midsagittal plane/IR
alignment, 95f
right thorax, anterior rotation,
93f
scoliosis, presence, 95f
Lateral chest analysis, 97-98
correction, 98
practice, 97-98
Lateral chest demonstration
pacemaker placement, 84f
tracheostomy placement, 81f
Lateral chest projection, 92t
patient positioning, 93f
positioning accuracy, 92f
skin line collimation, 16f
tilted lateral chest projection,
nonrotated/rotated collimator
head, 17f
Lateral coccygeal projection, 445t
patient positioning, 445f
positioning, accuracy, 445f
Lateral coccyx projection
collimation, excess, 446f
rotation, 445f
Lateral cranial projection
head rotation, 478f
head tilt, 478f
patient positioning, 478f
positioning accuracy, 477f
Lateral cranium projection, 476t
Lateral distal femur projection
crosstable lateral distal femur
projection, patient positioning,
361f
leg
external rotation, 361f
internal rotation, 361f
patient positioning, 361f
positioning accuracy, 360f
Lateral distal humerus projection,
demonstration, 232f

Lateral elbow analysis, 222-223
correction, 222-223
practice, 222-223
Lateral elbow projection, 217t
distal forearm
depression, 220f-221f
elevation, 221f
position, IR/wrist (relationship),
221f
elbow extension, 218f
fat pads, locations, 218f
patient positioning, 218f
positioning accuracy, 217f
proximal humerus
depression, 220f
elevation, 219f
proximal humerus, elevation, 219f
wrist
external rotation, 222f
internal rotation, 222f
Lateral esophagram
barium fill demonstration, 490f
projection, 492t
left side, 492f
patient positioning, 492f
shoulder rotation, 492f
Lateral facial bone/sinus projection,
positioning accuracy, 477f
Lateral femur image analysis
practice, 365
Lateral femur projection, clothing
artifact demonstration, 61f
Lateral finger analysis, 159
correction, 159
practice, 159
Lateral finger projection, 157t
flexion, impact, 158f
obliquity, insufficiency, 158f
patient positioning, 158f
positioning accuracy, 157f
proximal phalanx fracture,
demonstration, 158f
Lateral flexion/extension projections,
usage, 403
Lateral foot, 293f
positioning, calcaneus
depression, 303f, 310f
elevation, 303f, 310f
surface, positioning
accuracy, 302f
usage, 310f
Lateral foot analysis, 304-305
correction, 305
practice, 304-305
Lateral (lateromedial) foot positioning,
problem, 304f
Lateral foot projections, 292f,
298t
CR alignment, problem, 293f
CR centering/collimation, 299f
distal lower leg, elevation, 302f
dorsiflexion/plantar flexion, 299f

Lateral foot projections *(Continued)*
leg
external rotation, 303f
internal rotation, 303f
lower leg, positioning accuracy,
300f
medial foot arch, types, 301f
plantar flexion, 300f
proximal lower leg, elevation,
302f
weight-bearing positions, non-
weight-bearing positions
(differences), 293f
Lateral (lateromedial) foot projection,
standing positioning, 69f
Lateral (mediolateral) foot projection,
tabletop positioning, 69f
Lateral (mediolateral) foot projection,
wheelchair positiioning, 70f
Lateral forearm analysis, 207
correction, 207
practice, 207
Lateral forearm projection, 204t
muscular/proximal forearm,
207f
patient positioning, 204f
positioning accuracy, 204f
proximal humerus, elevation,
206f
wrist, internal rotation, 205f
Lateral hand analysis, 176
correction, 176
practice, 176
Lateral hand flexion, 175
Lateral hand projections, 174t
anatomical alignment, CR centering
(impact), 21f
display, 6f
foreign body location, 18f
fourth metacarpal, posterior
displacement, 67f
hand
external rotation, 175f
internal rotation, 175f
hand/fingers
flexion, 176f
full extension, 176f
patient positioning, 175f
positioning accuracy, 174f
Lateral hip
metal apparatus, usage, 385f
projection, Lauenstein/Hickey
methods (usage), 379f
Lateral humeral analysis, 233
correction, 233
practice, 233
Lateral humerus projection, 229t
fractured humerus, demonstration,
231f
Lateral knee analysis, 344-345
correction, 344-345
practice, 344-345

Lateral knee projection, 337t
  alternate CR alignment, 341f
  cephalic CR angulation
    absence, 340f
    excess, 341f
  compact ray (CR) alignment, 341f
  external/internal artifacts, display,
    61f
  femur, CR alignment, 341f
  knee flexion (30 degrees), 339f
  knee flexion (90 degrees), 343f
  leg
    external rotation, 342f
    internal rotation, 342f
  medial condyle, posterior
    demonstration, 343f
  patient positioning, 329f
    medial femoral epicondyle,
      location, 338f
Lateral (mediolateral) knee projection,
    positioning accuracy, 338f
Lateral knee projections, fluid
    demonstration, 58f
Lateral knee projection, usage, 73f
Lateral L5:S1 analysis, 438
  correction, 438
  practice, 438
Lateral L5-S1 lumbosacral junction
  positioning, 436f
  projection, 436t
    positioning accuracy, 436f
Lateral large intestinal (rectum)
    projection, 509t
Lateral large intestine (rectum)
  patient rotation, 510f
  projection, 509f
  right side, 510f
Lateral large intestine projection,
    patient positioning, 510f
Lateral lower leg analysis, 328
  correction, 328
  practice, 328
Lateral lower leg projection, 325t
  distal lower leg fracture, 327f
  external rotation
    excess, 327f
    insufficiency, 327f
  fiberglass cast, usage, 68f
  patient positioning, 326f
  positioning accuracy, 326f
Lateral lumbar flexion, detection, 437,
    441
Lateral lumbar projection
  extension, 434f
  flexion, 434f
Lateral lumbar vertebrae analysis, 435
  correction, 435
  practice, 435
Lateral lumbar vertebrae projection,
    431t
  marker placement, 11f
  overcollimation, 18f

Lateral lumbar vertebrae projection
    (Continued)
  patient positioning, 431f
  positioning accuracy, 431f
  right side, posterior rotation, 432f
  scoliosis, 433f
Lateral (extension) lumbar vertebral
    projection, patient positioning,
    434f
Lateral (flexion) lumbar vertebral
    projection, patient positioning,
    434f
Lateral nasal bone projection,
    positioning accuracy, 478f
Lateral projections, 69-70
  analysis, 478-479
  left lateral position, 91-98
  marker placement guidelines, 10
Lateral proximal femur projection
  distal femur, elevation, 363f
  leg/pelvis, rotation
    excess, 363f
    insufficiency, 363f
  patient positioning, 363f
  positioning accuracy, 362f
Lateral sacral projection, 441t
  patient positioning, 441f
  positioning accuracy, 441f
  right side, posterior rotation,
    442f
Lateral sacrum analysis, 442
  correction, 442
  practice, 442
Lateral scapula positioning, arm
    abduction, 274f
Lateral scapula projection, 273t
Lateral scapular analysis, 277
  correction, 277
  practice, 277
Lateral scapular positioning,
    274f
Lateral scapular projection
  arm abduction, 274f
  arm elevation, 276f
  arm resting, 275f
  obliquity
    excess, 276f
    insufficiency, 276f
Lateral sternal projection, left thorax
    (anterior rotation), 452f
Lateral sternal rotation, right thorax
    (anterior rotation), 453f
Lateral sternum projection, 450t
  patient positioning, 451f
  positioning, accuracy, 451f
  superior sternum, positioning
    accuracy, 451f
Lateral stomach/duodenum projection,
    498t
  patient positioning, 499f
  patient rotation, 499f
Lateral talar dome, presence, 24f

Lateral thoracic projection
  deep breathing, 419f
  lower thoracic vertebrae positioning,
    419f, 422f
  patient positioning, 419f
  positioning accuracy, 419f
  respiration, suspension, 420f
  right side
    anterior rotation, 421f
    posterior rotation, 420f
  spinal scoliosis, 421f
Lateral thoracic vertebrae analysis,
    422
  correction, 422
  practice, 422
Lateral thoracic vertebrae projection,
    418t
Lateral thumb analysis, 164
  correction, 164
  practice, 164
Lateral thumb projection, 162t,
    163f
  abduction, absence, 164f
  hand, overflexion, 164f
  patient positioning, 163f
  positioning accuracy, 163f
Lateral toe analysis, 289-290
  correction, 289-290
  practice, 289-290
Lateral toe projection, 287t
  obliquity, excess, 289f
  toe obliquity, inadequacy, 288f
  unaffected toes, affected toe
    (relationship), 289f
Lateral vertebral/sacral/coccygeal
    projections, gonadal shielding,
    435f
Lateral wrist
  analysis, 191-192
    correction, 191-192
    practice, 191-192
  flexion, 180f
  radial deviation/ulnar deviation,
    189f
Lateral wrist projection, 186t
  alternate mediolateral wrist
    projection, 191
  CR centering, 190
  CR positioning, 190f
  distal scaphoid
    anterior alignment, 187-188
    distal alignment, 188-189
  elbow/humerus positioning,
    186-187
  humeral abduction, absence, 188f
  humeral epicondyles, IR parallel
    alignment, 187f, 189f
  patient positioning, 187f
  pisiform
    anterior alignment, 187-188
    distal alignment, 188-189
  positioning accuracy, 187f

Lateral wrist projection *(Continued)*
 proximal forearm, patient
   positioning, 189f
 radial deviation, 189f
 thumb, IR paralelism, 190f
 usage, 3f, 19f
 wrist
   extension, 190f
   external rotation, 205f
   flexion, 190f
   ulnar deviation, 189f
Lateromedial foot projection
 leg, internal rotation, 304f
Lateromedial foot projection,
   positioning accuracy, 304f
Lateromedial humerus projection
 internal rotation, insufficiency, 231f
 patient positioning, 230f
   distal humerus alignment,
     problem, 230f
 positioning accuracy, 215f
Lauenstein method, 378
 usage, 379f
Law of isometry, usage, 71f
Left anterior oblique positions,
   110-113
Left lateral chest projection, 23f
 right lateral chest projection,
   differences, 95-96
Left lateral knee projection,
   positioning, 24f
Left lateral lumbar vertebrae
   projection
 display, 5f
 marker superimposing VOI, 11f
Left lateral position, 91-98
Left lungs
 anterior rotation, 452f
 anterior, rotation, 94f
 right lungs, differences, 93-94
Left side pleural effusion,
   demonstration, 126f
Legs
 abduction, 380f
   problem, 381
 extension, 417f
 external rotation, 303f, 310f, 321f,
   342f
 internal rotation, 303f-304f, 311f,
   321f, 342f
 rotation problem, identification,
   384
Lengthwise (LW) direction, 85
Lesser trochanter, 362, 379-380,
   383-384
 alignment, 382-383
 visualization, 368-370
Lesser tubercle, 245
Long bones
 diagonal position, 15f
 imaging, 70-72
   isometry law, usage, 71f

Long bones *(Continued)*
 positioning, diverged x-ray beam
   (usage), 15f
 projections, optimum (creation),
   71f
Long bones, anatomic structure, 14
Lookup table (LUT), 39-40
 application, 38
 usage, 59
Lordotic curvature, effect, 426
Lordotic position, 107-110
Lower extremity
 image analysis guidelines, 279-365
 technical data, 279, 280t
   imaging analysis guidelines,
     280b
Lower left jaw, orthopantomogram
   image, 65f
Lower leg: AP projection, 322-324
 ankle/knee, anatomic position/AP
   projections (differences),
   322-323
 fracture, positioning, 323
 leg, IR placement, 324
 rotation, 323
Lower leg: lateral projection
   (mediolateral), 325-328
 fracture, positioning, 325-327
 leg, IR placement, 327
 rotation, 327
 true lateral knee/ankle projections,
   variation, 325-327
Lower leg positioning problem,
   repositioning, 309-310
Lumbar vertebrae
 alignment, 427f
 image analysis guidelines, 424-438,
   424b
 technical data, 424, 424t
Lumbar vertebrae, AP mobility
   (evaluation), 432-434
Lumbar vertebrae: AP oblique
   projection (right/left posterior
   oblique positions), 428-430
 AP/PA projection, 428
 obliquity problems, identification,
   429
 rotation, 428-429
 Scottie dogs
   identification, lumbar anatomy,
     429f
   lumbar obliquity accuracy,
     428-429
Lumbar vertebrae: AP projection,
   424-428
 intervertebral disk spaces, CR
   alignment, 426
 lordotic curvature, effect, 426
 psoas muscle demonstration,
   424-425
 rotation, 425-426
   scoliosis, distinction, 426

Lumbar vertebrae: lateral projection,
   430-435
 CR centering/long axis placement,
   435f
 gonadal shielding, 435, 435f
 intervertebral disk spaces, CR
   alignment, 431-432
 IR center alignment, 434
 L5-S1 lumbar region, supplementary
   projection, 434-435
 rotation
   detection, 430-431
   effect, 430
 scoliotic patient, 432
Lung aeration, 90-91, 102, 107
 maximum, 97
 problem, identification, 90, 116
Lung field
 artifact lines, prevention, 124
 scapulae, demonstration, 109f
Lungs
 appearance, 115-116
 conditions, impact, 77-78
 development, 113

M

Magnification (size distortion), 22
 image receptor, 22f
Male patients, gonadal shielding, 34f
 AP projection, 34-36
 lateral projection, 34, 35f
Male pelves, female pelves
   (differences), 367, 368t
Mandible, jaw position, 466
Mandibular mentum positioning,
   394
Manubrium, location, 91
Marker annotation, 14f
Marker magnification/distortion,
   11f
Marker placement
 collimated image, tightness, 13f
 collimator guide, usage, 12
 digital radiography, usage, 12-13
 guidelines, 10b
Medial condyle
 lateral knee projection
   demonstration, 343f
 left lateral knee projection, 24f
Medial foot arch, types, 294-295,
   301f
Medial mortise, 311-312
Mediastinal widening, PA chest
   projection (evaluation), 2f
Mediolateral foot projection,
   positioning accuracy, 298f
Mediolateral humerus projection
 patient positioning, 230f
 positioning accuracy, 229f
 torso, rotation, 230f
Mediolateral projections, lateromedial
   projections (differences), 229-231

Mediolateral wrist projection, 191f
  alternate mediolateral wrist
    projection, 191
Metacarpal bases, wrist (PA
    projection), 178
Metacarpal midshaft concavity
  hand: PA projection, 167
  thumb (lateral projection), 162
  thumb (PA oblique projection),
    164
Metacarpals, alignment, 189
Metacarpal spacing, hand: PA oblique
    projection (lateral rotation),
    170-171
Metaphalangeal (MP) joint, elevation,
    161f
Midcoronal plane alignment, problem
    (identification), 100
Midcoronal plane positioning/rotation,
    85-87, 92-94, 105-106
  abdomen, 135-137
  neonate/infant abdomen, AP
    projection (left lateral decubitus
    position), 144
Midcoronal plane/rotation, neonate/
    infant abdomen AP projection
    (supine), 141
Midcoronal plane tilting, 87-90, 107,
    112
  distinction, 89-90
  identification, 88-89
  superior midcoronal plane, anterior
    tilt, 89f
Midfemur, grid midline alignment,
    363
Midforearm alignment, 179-180
  wrist: PA oblique projection (lateral
    rotation), 182
Midsagittal plane
  alignment, 95f
  lateral tilting, demonstration, 126f
  positioning, 94-96
  tilting, 124
Midshaft concavity, 150-151
  finger (PA oblique projection),
    154-157
Milliamperage (mAs), setting, 67
Mobile imaging, 66-69
Modified Waters facial bone/sinus
    projection, positioning accuracy,
    484f
Modified Waters method, 484
Moiré artifact, 62-64
Mortise
  anteroposterior (mortise) oblique
    ankle projection, positioning
    accuracy, 314f
  15- to 20-degree AP oblique
    (mortise), 314-315
  medial mortise, 311-312
Motion, 30
  sharpness, 30

N

Nasal bone projection, 476t
Nasogastric (NG) tubes
  placement, accuracy (supine AP
    abdomen), 131f
  subject contrast, 130-131
Navicular-cuneiform joint spaces, 291
Neonatal AP abdomen, positioning
    accuracy, 142f
Neonatal AP (left lateral decubitus)
    abdomen projection, positioning,
    146f
Neonate abdomen
  AP (left lateral decubitus),
    intraperitoneal air
    demonstration, 146f
  AP (left lateral decubitus), left side
    (rotation), 147f
  AP projection, left lateral decubitus
    position, 143-145
Neonate abdomen, AP projection
    (supine), 141-143
  lumbar vertebrae alignment, IR
    (usage), 141
  midcoronal plane/rotation, 141
  respiration, 141-142
  ventilated patient, 142
Neonate AP abdomen
  analysis, 142-143
    correction, 143
  long axis alignment, absence,
    142f
  projection, 141t
  right side, rotation, 143f
Neonate AP (left lateral decubitus)
  abdominal analysis, 145
  correction, 145
  practice, 145
Neonate AP chest
  analysis, 116-117
    correction, 116-117
    practice, 116-117
  caudal CR angle/low CR centering,
    absence, 115f
  central venous catheter (CVC)
    placement, 82f
  ETT placement, 81f
  5-degree caudal CR angle,
    116f
  left side, rotation, 114f
  projection, 113t
    positioning accuracy, 114f
  right side, rotation, 115f
  umbilical vein catheter (UVC),
    placement, 83f
Neonate AP (left lateral decubitus)
    chest
  demonstration, 126f
  left arm, nonelevation, 127f
  left side rotation, 126f
  lordotic appearance, 127f
  right side rotation, 126f

Neonate AP (right lateral decubitus)
    chest
  projection, positioning (accuracy),
    125f
  upper chest position, 127f
Neonate AP (lateral decubitus) chest
    projection, 124t-125t
Neonate AP decubitus chest analysis,
    127
  correction, 127
  practice, 127
Neonate chest
  AP projection, 113-117
    right/left lateral decubitus
      position, 124-127
  AP (left lateral decubitus)
    projection, patient positioning,
    126f
  arm position, 124-125
  chin position, 115, 124-125
  CR/IR alignment, 125-126
    alternates, 115
    perpendicular/cephalic angle, 115
  cross-table lateral projection
    arms/chin, 121
    left lateral position, 120-122
    respiration, 121-122
  IR alignment, 125-126
    alternate, 125-126
  lung field, artifact lines (prevention),
    124
  lungs/aeration, appearance, 115-116
  midcoronal plane positioning/
    rotation, 124
  midsagittal plane tilting, 124
  patient alignment, 125-126
  patient positioning, 113
  right/left lungs, identification, 121
  rotation, 113-115
    identification, IR/side-to-side CR
      alignment (problem),
      114-115
    identification, patient positioning
      (problem), 114
    prevention, side-to-side CR
      alignment, 114
Neonate cross-table lateral chest
    projection, positioning (accuracy),
    120f
Neonate lateral chest
    projection, 120t
  right lung, posterior rotation, 121f
Nipple shadows, 84
Nonextendable AP elbow positioning,
    211f
Nonextendable AP elbow projection
  anteroposterior (AP) elbow
    projections, 210f
  forearm, patient positionng, 210f
Nonextendable AP elbow projection,
    patient positioning, 210f
Nonextendable knee, 330-331

Nonextendable toes, CR angulation, 280, 285
Nonkyphotic anteroposterior shoulder projections, 238f

O

Obese patients, 73-75
  anteroposterior abdomen/lateral knee projections, 74f
  AP pelvis projection, low subject contrast, 58f
  automatic exposure control, 75
  focal spot size, 75
  left lateral decubitus position, 139-140
  scatter radiation control, 74-75
  supine AP abdomen, lengthwise/crosswise IR cassettes (usage), 136f
  technical considerations, 73-74
Obesity, consideration (abdomen), 130
Object-image receptor distance (OID), 22, 52
  anteroposterior ankle projection, traction device (impact), 29f
  increase, right lung field (magnification increase), 23f
Oblique projections, 70
Obliquity
  accuracy, 110-112
  problem, repositioning, 110-111
  usage, 110
Obscured CM joint spaces, causes (identification), 179
Occipital base positioning, 394
Occiput-mentum mispositioning, effect, 394
Off-centered grid cutoff, 64f
Off-centering, 20-21
Open joints, presence, 26f
Open-mouth parietocanthial (Waters) sinus projection, patient positioning, 483f
Open radioscaphoid joint (demonstration)
  forearm, positioning, 179
  patient positioning, 184
Optimal image, characteristics, 3-8
Orthopantomogram image, 65f
Overcollimation, 16-17
  lateral lumbar vertebral projection, 18f
Overexposed AP pelvis projections, 50f
Overexposed projection, evaluation, 47t
Overexposure
  causes, 47t
  identification, 49-50

P

Pacemakers, 83
  placement, 83f-84f

Pad artifact, demonstration, 126f
Palmar soft tissue, thumb (AP projection), 161
Paranasal sinus
  imaging analysis guidelines, 462b
  technical data, 462t
Parietoacanthial/acanthioparietal facial bones/sinus projection, 482t
Parietoacanthial/acanthioparietal projection analysis, 485
Parietoacanthial (Waters) facial bone/sinus projection
  open-mouth parietoacanthial (Waters) sinus projection, patient positioning, 483f
  patient positioning, 483f
  positioning accuracy, 464f
Parietoacanthial sinus projection
  chin elevation, 484f
  face rotation, 483f
Patella (patellae)
  movement, 330f
  superior position, 351-353
Patella/patellofemoral joint: tangential projection (Merchant method), 351-355
  femoral condyles, superior position, 351-353
  intercondylar sulci, superior position, 351-353
  joint space
    anterior thigh soft tissue, projection, 353
    patellae/tibial tuberosities, 353
    visualization, 353-354
  large calves, positioning, 354
  patellae, superior position, 351-353
  patellar subluxation, 353
  positioning accuracy, light field silhouette (indication), 354
  rotation, 351-353
  scatter radiation control, 351
Patellar subluxation, 330, 330f, 353
  presence, 353f
Patient conditions, technical factors (adjustment), 54t
Patient exposure (minimization), exposure factors (impact), 35
Patient obliquity, degree
  determination, 24-25
  estimation, 25f
Patient obliquity, repositioning, 110-111
Patient positioning
  anode heel effect guidelines, 53t
  45-degree PA oblique (LAO) chest projection, 111f
  posteroanterior oblique (RAO) chest projection, 111f
  60-degree PA oblique (LAO) chest projection, 111f
Patient repositioning, steps, 25-27

Pediatric abdomen, 141-148
Pediatric anteroposterior elbow projection, external rotation/flexion, 209f
Pediatric anteroposterior humerus projection, positioning accuracy, 227f
Pediatric anteroposterior shoulder projection, midcoronal plane (anterior tilt), 238f
Pediatric AP oblique foot projection, positioning accuracy, 295f
Pediatric AP oblique (Grashey) shoulder projection, positioning (accuracy), 249f
Pediatric bone age assessment, 169
Pediatric chest, 113-129
  shape/size, 113
Pediatric imaging, 72-73
  clothing artifacts, 72-73
  technical considerations, 72
Pediatric inferosuperior axial shoulder projection, positioning (accuracy), 243f
Pediatric lateral cranial projection, positioning accuracy, 477f
Pediatric lateral elbow projection, distal forearm (depression), 221f
Pediatric lateral foot projection, positioning accuracy, 298f
Pediatric lateral hand projection, hand (internal rotation), 175f
Pediatric lateral knee projection, positioning accuracy, 338f
Pediatric lateral lower leg projection, positioning accuracy, 326f
Pediatric lateral thumb projection, positioning (accuracy), 163f
Pediatric lateral wrist projection, wrist (internal rotation), 188f
Pediatric patients, technical factors (guidelines), 73b
Pediatric posteroanterior hand projections
  bone age assessment, 169f
  skeletal development, 72f
Pediatric posteroanterior oblique thumb projection, positioning (accuracy), 165f
Pediatric posteroanterior thumb projection, positioning (accuracy), 160f
Pediatric posteroanterior wrist projections (skeletal development), 72f
Pelvis
  image analysis guidelines, 366-389, 367b
  male/female pelves, differences, 367, 368t
  projections, position, 21f

Pelvis (Continued)
rotation, 370
technical data, 366, 367t
Pelvis: AP frog-leg projection
(modified Cleaves method),
370-374
femoral neck visualization, 370-371
femurs, abduction, 372f
greater trochanter visualization,
370-371
knee/hip flexion, 372f
problems, identification, 370
lesser/greater trochanter
visualization, 370
pelvis rotation, 367-368
symmetrical femoral abduction,
importance, 371
Pelvis: AP projection, 366-370
fat planes, 366-367
femoral neck
fracture, positioning, 369
visualization, 368-369
foot positioning problem, 369f
greater/lesser trochanter,
visualization, 368-369
hip dislocation, positioning, 369
hip joint mobility, analysis (CR
centering usage), 369-370
internal foot positioning, 369f
leg positioning problem, detection,
369
male/female pelves, differences, 367
proximal femoral fracture,
positioning, 369
rotation, 367-368
Pendulous breasts, 84
digestive system, relationship, 486
interference (abdomen), 130
lateral movement (brightness
comparison), AP abdomens
(usage), 130f
PA chest, 85f
Penetrated AP pelvis projection,
accuracy, 48f
Personnel, radiation exposure, 36
Phalangeal midshaft concavity
hand: PA projection, 167
lateral finger projection, 157
thumb (AP projection), 159-160
thumb (PA oblique projection), 164
toe: AP axial projection, 279-280
Phalangeal soft tissue width/midshaft
concavity, 150-151
finger (PA oblique projection),
154-155
Phalanges, 151
finger (PA oblique projection), 155
hand: PA oblique projection (lateral
rotation), 171
thumb (AP projection), 160-161
Phalanx, thumb (lateral projection),
162

Phantom image artifact, 64
computed radiograph AP should
projection demonstration, 64f
Phosphor plate-handling artifact, 65
Photomultiplier tube (PMT), 38
Picture archival and communication
system (PACS), 6
projection, impact, 10
Pillow, external artifact, 61f
Pisiform
anterior alignment, 187-188
distal alignment, 188-189
Pixel sizes, 31f
Plantar flexion, compensation,
305-307
Pleural drainage tube, 81
placement, 82f
Pleural effusion, 77-78
Pneumectomy, 77
Pneumothorax, 77
posteroanterior chest demonstration,
78f
Positioning
devices, determination, 67
PA chest projection, 89f
procedures, anatomic relationships
(correlation), 18-19
routines, 17-18
Posterior ankle, anatomy, 312f
Posterior collimated border, contact
shield (absence), 51f
Posterior distal radial margins,
identification, 178-179
Posterior knee
axial viewer positioning, 354f
curve, location, 354f
positioning, 354f
Posterior rib, superimposition,
120-121
Posteroanterior (PA) above-diaphragm
rib projection
patient positioning, 455f
patient rotation, 455f
Posteroanterior (PA) analysis,
467-468
Posteroanterior (PA) axial (scaphoid)
analysis, 197
correction, 197
practice, 197
Posteroanterior (PA) axial cranial
projection
chin tuck, 470f
face rotation, 470f
Posteroanterior (PA) axial (Caldwell)
cranial projection
patient positioning, 470f
positioning accuracy, 469f
Posteroanterior (PA) axial cranium/
facial bones/sinuses projection,
469t
Posteroanterior (PA) axial cranium
projection, 471f

Posteroanterior (PA) axial knee
analysis, 348
correction, 348
practice, 348
Posteroanterior (PA) axial knee
position, 347f
Posteroanterior (PA) axial knee
projection (Holmblad method),
346t
distal lower leg
depression, 347f
elevation, 347f
femur, vertical position, 348f
knee
overflexion, 347f
underflexion, 347f
patient positioning, 347f
positioning accuracy, 346f
proximal femur, medial position,
347f
Posteroanterior (PA) axial large
intestine projection, patient
positioning, 515f
Posteroanterior (PA) axial oblique
cervical vertebrae analysis,
411-412
correction, 411-412
practice, 411-412
Posteroanterior (PA) axial oblique
cervical vertebrae projection,
407t
cervical vertebral column, tilt, 409f
cranium
lateral projection, 407f
PA oblique projection, 407f
head
oblique position, 410f
tilt, 410f
kyphosis, 409f
patient positioning, 408f
patient rotation
excess, 408f
insufficiency, 408f
upper cervical vertebrae, rotation,
409f
Posteroanterior (PA) axial oblique
(RAO position) large intestinal
projections, 515t
Posteroanterior (PA) axial oblique
large intestine
pelvis, rotation, 516f
projection (RAO position), 515f
patient positioning, 515f
Posteroanterior (PA) axial (scaphoid)
wrist projection, 192t
Posteroanterior (PA) axial wrist
projection, ulnar deviation
maximum, 194f
Posteroanterior (PA) below-diaphragm
rib projection
full inspiration, 456f
positioning accuracy, 454f

Posteroanterior (PA) chest analysis, 91
  correction, 91
  practice, 91
Posteroanterior (PA) chest
    demonstration
  free intraperitoneal air, 80f
  tracheostomy placement, 81f
Posteroanterior (PA) chest projection,
    88t
  histogram, 41f
  Kodak CR system, usage, 42f
  patient positioning, 89f
Posteroanterior (PA) cranial projection
  chin insufficiency, 465f
  chin tuck, 465f
  positioning accuracy, 463f
Posteroanterior (PA) cranium/mandible
    projection, 463t
Posteroanterior (PA) cranium
    projection, 5f
Posteroanterior (PA) esophagram,
    patient (right side), 494f
Posteroanterior (PA) esophagram
    projection, 493t
  patient positioning, 489
  positioning, accuracy, 493f
Posteroanterior (PA) finger analysis,
    154
  correction, 154
  practice, 154
Posteroanterior (PA) finger projection,
    151t. *See also* Finger (PA
    projection)
Posteroanterior (PA) hand analysis,
    170
  correction, 170
  practice, 170
Posteroanterior (PA) hand projections,
    167t
  foreign body location, 18f
  fourth metacarpal, posterior
      displacement, 67f
  hand/finger flexion, 169f
  medial rotation, 168f
  patient positioning, 168f
  positioning, 169f
    accuracy, 168f
Posteroanterior (PA) large intestinal
    projection, patient types, 511t
Posteroanterior (PA) large intestine
  lateral decubitus, 512f
  left colic (splenic) flexure, 504f
  right side, 509f
Posteroanterior (PA) large intestine
    projection, 506f
  left lateral decubitus position, 511f
  patient positioning, 508f
  patients, types, 507t
  positioning accuracy, 508f
Posteroanterior (PA) lateral decubitus
    projections, marker placement
    guidelines, 10

Posteroanterior (PA) mandible
    projection
  chin insufficiency, 465f
  chin tuck, 465f
  positioning accuracy, 463f
Posteroanterior (PA) oblique below-
    diaphragm rib projection
  axillary ribs, magnification, 459f
  patient rotation, 459f
Posteroanterior (PA) oblique chest
    analysis, 112-113
  correction, 113
  practice, 112-113
Posteroanterior (PA) oblique chest
    projection, 110t
Posteroanterior (PA) oblique (RAO)
    chest projection, patient
    positioning, 111f
Posteroanterior (PA) oblique
    esophagram
  barium fill demonstration, 490f
  patient obliquity, insufficiency,
      491f
  projection (RAO position), 490t
    positionng accuracy, 491f
  projection, patient positioning,
      491f
Posteroanterior (PA) oblique finger
    analysis, 157
  correction, 157
  obliquity, 156f
  practice, 157
  soft tissue, 156f
Posteroanterior (PA) oblique finger
    projection, 155t
  parallel positioning, absence, 156f
  patient positioning, 155f
Posteroanterior (PA) oblique hand
    analysis, 173
  correction, 173
  practice, 173
Posteroanterior (PA) oblique hand
    projection, 171t
  fingers
    extension, 172f
    parallel positioning, absence, 173f
    spread, absence, 172f
  hand obliquity, inadequacy, 172f
  obliquity, 172f
  patient positioning, finger flexion,
      173f
  positioning accuracy, 171f
Posteroanterior (PA) oblique large
    intestinal projection (LAO
    position), 514t
Posteroanterior (PA) oblique large
    intestinal projection (RAO
    position), 512t
Posteroanterior (PA) oblique large
    intestine projection (LAO
    position), 514f
  patient positioning, 514f

Posteroanterior (PA) oblique large
    intestine projection (RAO
    position), 513f
  patient positioning, 513f
Posteroanterior (PA) oblique (scapular
    Y) positioning, 253f
Posteroanterior (PA) oblique
    projections
  right/left anterior oblique positions,
      110-113
Posteroanterior (PA) oblique
    projections, marker placement
    guidelines, 10
Posteroanterior (PA) oblique rib
    projection analysis, 460
Posteroanterior (PA) oblique (Scapular
    Y) shoulder analysis
  correction, 257-258
  practice, 257-258
Posteroanterior (PA) oblique (scapular
    Y) shoulder analysis, 257-258
  practice, 257-258
Posteroanterior (PA) oblique (scapular
    Y) shoulder projection, 253t
  anterior dislocation, 255f
  obliquity
    excess, 254f
    insufficiency, 254f
  positioning accuracy, 253f
  posterior demonstration, 256f
  proximal humeral fracture,
      demonstration, 256f
    obliquity, insufficiency, 256f
  upper mid-coronal plane
    anterior tilt, 255f
    posterior tilt, 255f
Posteroanterior (PA) oblique sternal
    projection
  breathing technique, 449f
  patient obliquity, insufficiency,
      450f
Posteroanterior (PA) oblique sternal
    projection, LAO position, 449f
Posteroanterior (PA) oblique sternum
    projection, 448t
  deep breathing, 449f
  RAO position, 448f
  patient positioning, 449f
Posteroanterior (PA) oblique stomach/
    duodenum projection (RAO
    position), 495t
  patient positioning, 496f
Posteroanterior (PA) oblique thumb
    analysis, 167
  correction, 167
  practice, 167
Posteroanterior (PA) oblique thumb
    projection, 165t
  palmar surface/thumb position, 166f
  palm, placement, 166f
  patient positioning, 166f
  positioning accuracy, 165f

Posteroanterior (PA) oblique thumb projection (Continued)
thumb, long axis (alignment absence), 166f
Posteroanterior (PA) oblique wrist
analysis, 186
correction, 186
practice, 186
Posteroanterior (PA) oblique wrist projection, 183t
patient positioning, 183f-184f
positioning accuracy, 183f
proximal forearm
elevation, 185f
lower position, 185f
wrist
obliquity, 184f
radial deviation, 185f
Posteroanterior (PA) projection
anteroposterior projection, difference, 98
differences, cervical vertebrae (usage), 105-106
Posteroanterior (PA) projection, marker placement guidelines, 10
Posteroanterior (PA) rib projection analysis practice, 460f
Posteroanterior (PA) ribs projection, 453t-454t
Posteroanterior (PA) small intestinal projection
contrast media demonstration, 49f
patients, types, 505t
Posteroanterior (PA) small intestine projection, 506f
patient positioning, 506f
Posteroanterior (PA) small intestine projection, positioning accuracy, 505f
Posteroanterior (PA) stomach/duodenum projection, 496t
full inspiration, 489f
patient positioning, 497f
residual food particles, 489f
Posteroanterior (PA) thumb projection, positioning accuracy, 162f
Posteroanterior (PA) wrist
radial deviation/ulnar deviation, 181f
Posteroanterior (PA) wrist analysis, 182
correction, 182
practice, 182
Posteroanterior (PA) wrist projections, 177t, 184f
closed second/third/open fourth/fifth CM joint, 181f
hand/fingers
extension, 180f
overflexion, 180f
humerus, vertical position, 178f
patient positioning, 177f

Posteroanterior (PA) wrist projections (Continued)
positioning accuracy, 177f
proximal forearm, positioning, 179f
radial deviation, 181f
ulnar deviation, 182f
usage, 3f, 19f
wrist
external rotation, 178f
internal rotation, 179f
obliquity, 184f
Posterolateral humeral head, profile, 245-246
Post-exam annotation, 13-14
Postprocedure requirements, 66
Pregnancy, radiation, 33
Primary beam, radiosensitive cells (shielding), 35
Projections, marking, 10-14
Pronator fat stripe
location, 187f
wrist: lateral projection (lateromedial), 186
Proximal femur, 357-359
fracture, 384
projection
CR centering, 364f
fracture, presence, 364f
Proximal forearm
elevation, 185f, 195f
distal forearm elevation, comparison, 185f
patient positioning, 179, 184
lateral wrist projection, 189f
wrist: ulnar deviation, PA axial projection (scaphoid), 194
PA wrist projection, 179f
Proximal humeral fracture, 231-232
demonstration, 256f
detection, 254-255
transthoracic lateral positioning, 232f
Proximal humeral head fracture, 240f
Proximal humerus
depression, 220f
elevation, 206f
patient positioning, 219f
mispositioning, 218
transthoracic lateral projection, positioning accuracy, 233f
Proximal humerus: AP axial projection (Stryker "Notch" method), 258-261
CR angulation, 259
distal humeral tilting, 260
humeral abduction, 259-260
humeral head positioning, 258-260
humerus positioning, 258-260
midcoronal plane positioning, 258-259
shoulder rotation, 258

Proximal intercondylar fossa surface, 348-350
Proximal lateral femur projection, 362t
Proximal lower leg, elevation, 302f, 313f, 320f
Proximal phalanx
fracture, demonstration, 158f
superimposition, prevention, 158f
Proximal tibia, slope, 331f
Psoas major muscles, location, 129-130
Psoas muscle demonstration, 424-425
Pulmonary arterial catheter (Swan-Ganz catheter), 82
placement, 83f
Pulmonary arterial line placement, AP chest demonstration, 80f

Q

Quantum noise
adjustment, 49
demonstration, 49f

R

Radial head
elbow: AP projection, 207
fractures, positioning, 220-222
Radial styloid, wrist: PA projection, 178
Radial tuberosity, 200, 204-205
elbow: AP projection, 207-208
elbow: lateral projection (lateromedial), 220
Radiation projection practices, demonstration, 7f
Radiation protection, 32-34
patient communication, 32
practices, usage, 68
problem, 35f
Radiolunate joints
demonstration, forearm positioning, 179
patient positioning, 184
wrist: PA oblique projection (lateral rotation), 183-184
Radiolunate joints, wrist: PA projection, 178-179
Radiopaque materials, atomic number, 55-56
Radioscaphoid joints
space, 194
wrist: PA oblique projection (lateral rotation), 183-184
wrist: PA projection, 178-179
Radiosensitive cells, shielding, 35
Radioulnar articulation, wrist (PA projection), 178
Radius, alignment, 204

Recorded details
  distances, 29-30
  sharpness, 28-32
  sharpness, comparison, 29f
Recumbent lateral cervicothoracic
  projection, patient positioning,
  413f
Repeat projections
  central ray repositioning steps,
    28-36
  patient repositioning, 25-27
Ribs, 453-460
  imaging analysis guidelines, 448b
  midcoronal plane, 108-109
  posterior rib, superimposition,
    120-121
  technical data, 448t
Ribs: AP oblique projection (right/left
    posterior oblique positions),
    457-460
  magnification, control, 457
  patient obliquity, 457-458
  respiration, 459
Ribs: AP/PA projection (above/below
    diaphragm), 453-457
  AP projection/PA projection,
    differences, 453-454
  CR positioning, 456
  inferior scapula, location, 456
  respiration, 455-456
  rotation, 454-455
  scapula, removal, 456
  scoliosis, rotation (differences), 455
  soft tissue structures, 453
Right anterior oblique positions,
    110-113
Right femoral neck fracture, 370f
Right lateral ankle projection, position
    (problems), 24f
Right lateral chest projection
  left lateral chest projection,
    differences, 95-96
  positioning accuracy, 96f
Right lateral decubitus
  AP chest, 112f
    projection, patient positioning,
      105f
Right lateral wrist projection, diagonal
    display, 6f
Right lung
  anterior rotation, 452f
  field, magnification (increase), 23f
  left lung, differences, 93-94
Right lungs
  anterior, rotation, 94f
Right PA hand projections, display, 6f
Right-sided mastectomy, PA chest, 85f
Right-sided pleural effusion, PA/lateral
    chest, 79f
Right-sided pneumectomy
  AP chest, 79f
  PA chest, 79f

Right thorax
  anterior rotation, 93f
  posterior rotation, 93f
Rotated PA chest projection, 2f
Rotation
  identification, 86, 94, 106
  prevention, patient positioning, 113
  scoliosis, differences, 94

S

Sacral vertebrae
  image analysis guidelines, 424-438,
    424b
  technical data, 424
Sacroiliac (SI) joints
  image analysis guidelines, 366-389
  rotation, detection, 386-387
  technical data, 366
Sacroiliac (SI) joints: AP axial
    projection, 386-387
  CR angulation
    adjustment, 387
    problem, identification, 387
  median sacral crest alignment,
    386-387
  sacral alignment/CR centering, 387
  sacroiliac joints
    rotation, detection, 386-387
    visualization, distortion (absence),
      387
  sacrum/pelvic brim alignment,
    386-387
  symphysis pubis alignment, 386-387
Sacroiliac (SI) joints: AP oblique
    projection (left/right posterior
    oblique positions)
  alternate marking, 388
  ilium/sacrum, 388
Sacroiliac (SI) joints; AP oblique
    projection (left/right posterior
    oblique positions), 388-389
Sacrum, 438-446
  imaging analysis guidelines, 424b
  technical data, 424t
Sacrum: AP axial projection, 438-440
  CR effect, 440
  CR/sacral alignment, 439-440
  sacral misalignment, 440
Sacrum: lateral projection, 440-442
  CR/L5-S1 disk space/sacral
    alignment, 441-442
  lateral lumbar flexion, detection,
    441
  rotation, 440-441
  vertebral column, sagging
    (adjustment), 442
Scaphoid fat stripe
  location, 178f
  wrist (PA projection), 177
Scaphoid fracture, sites, 196f
Scaphoid visualization, wrist (PA
    projection), 179

Scaphotrapezial joint spaces, wrist: PA
    oblique projection (lateral
    rotation), 184
Scaphotrapezium/scaphotrapezoidal
    joint spaces, wrist: ulnar
    deviation, PA axial projection
    (scaphoid), 192
Scapula: AP projection, 270-273
  breathing technique, 272
  exam variations, 272-273
  humeral abduction, 270-271
  kyphotic patient, 272
  midcoronal plane tilting, 271-272
  respiration, 272
  shoulder retraction, 271
Scapulae, 87, 107
  demonstration, 109f
  positioning, 101-102
Scapula: lateral projection
    (lateromedial/mediolateral),
    273-277
  humerus positioning, 273-274
  laberal border, 276f
  midcoronal plane positioning,
    274-275
  obliquity, inaccuracy (detection),
    275
  scapular obliquity, 274-275
Scapular body, long axis, 274f
Scapular Y, PA oblique projection,
    252-258
  AP oblique projection, 255
    recumbent patient, 255
  kyphotic patient, 254
  midcoronal plane, 254
    positioning, 252-254
  patient positioning, 232f
  proximal humeral fracture,
    254-255
    detection, 254-255
  shoulder dislocation, 254-255
    detection, 254
  shoulder rotation, 252-254
Scapula, vertebral border, 275f
Scatter radiation
  control, 42, 74-75, 351
  creation, 50-51
  fogging, 64
    impact, 50f
  reduction, 451
  values, inclusion, 44f
Scoliosis
  abdominal rotation, differences,
    136-137
  distinction, rotation (usage),
    86-87
  PA chest, 87f
  presence, 95f
  rotation, differences, 94, 416
  supine AP abdomen, 137f
Scoliotic lumbar vertebral column,
    alignment, 433f

Scottie dogs
  identification, lumbar anatomy, 429f
  lumbar obliquity accuracy, 428-429
Second AP axial toe projection, positioning (accuracy), 281f
Second CM spaces, wrist: PA oblique projection (lateral rotation), 184
Second finger positioning, alternate, 155
Second lateral toe projection, positioning accuracy, 287f
Shoulder
  depression
    lateral cervical projection, 405f
    midcoronal plane tilting, 89-90
  dislocations, 240-241, 244
  elevation
    PA chest, 88f
    supine AP chest, 102f
  image analysis guidelines, 235-277, 236b
  protraction (absence), PA chest (usage), 88f
  rotation, scapular Y (PA oblique projection), 252-254
  tangential (supraspinatus outlet) projection, 19f
  technical data, 235, 235t
Shoulder: AP projection, 235-241
  dislocations, 240-241
  humeral epicondyles, 239-240
  humeral fractures, 240
  humerus positioning, 239-241
  kyphotic patients, 237-239
  marker placement, 13f
  midcoronal plane positioning, 236
  midcoronal plane tilting, 237-239
  movements, 235-236
  rotation, 236
  supine AP shoulder projection, positioning accuracy, 236f
  supine, upright (differences), 235-236
  upright AP shoulder projection, positioning accuracy, 236f
Shoulder: inferosuperior axial projection (Lawrence method), 242-248
  coracoid process/base, 246
  humeral fracture, 244
  humerus foreshortening, 244-245
  humerus rotation, 245-246
  medial coracoid, inclusion, 246
  posterior surface, 246
  shoulder dislocation, 244
Side-to-side centering, 34
Side-to-side CR alignment, 98-100
  identification, IR (usage), 100
Singular mastectomy, 84
Sinuses projection, 476t
60-degree PA oblique (LAO) chest projection, 111f

Size distortion (magnification), 22
Skeletal bones, positioning, 19f
Skeletal development, pediatric PA hand/wrist projections, 72f
Skeletal structure, placement, 74f
Skin line collimation, 16f
Small intestine, 501-504
  contrast medium, 501
  positioning procedure, variations, 501-504
  preparation, 501
    procedure, 501
  supine hypersthenic patient, 502
  supine obese patient, 502-504
Small intestine: PA projection, 504
  abdominal rotation, detection, 504
  CR centering, 504
  rotation, 504
Soft tissue
  anteroposterior pelvis projection, 74f
  femur: AP projection, 359
  masses, impact, 130
  overlap
    finger (PA oblique projection), 155
    hand: PA oblique projection (lateral rotation), 171
    structures, forearm: lateral projection (lateromedial), 203-204
    superimposition, prevention, 158f
Soft tissue width
  hand (PA projection), 167
  thumb (AP projection), 159-160
  thumb (PA oblique projection), 164-167
  toe: AP axial projection, 279-280
Source-image receptor distance (SID), 12
  heart magnification, 98
  increase, 51-52
  length, 29
Source-skin distance, 32-33
Source-to-IR distance (SID), chest, 77
Spatial resolution, 30-32
  comparison, 32f
Spinal kyphosis, 101
  AP/lateral chest, 101f-102f
  midcoronal plane, position, 101f
Spinal scoliosis
  demonstration, 417f
  lateral thoracic projection, 421f
Spinal stimulator implant, 131
Standing lateral scapular positioning, 274f
Sternum, 447-452
  image analysis guidelines, 447, 448b
  technical data, 447, 448t
Sternum: lateral projection, 450-452
  homogeneous brightness, positioning, 450-451

Sternum: lateral projection
  (Continued)
  humerus positioning, 452
  respiration, 452
  rotation, 451-452
  scatter radiation, reduction, 451
  source-image distance (SID), 452
  supine patient, 452
Sternum: PA oblique projection (right anterior oblique position), 447-450
  blurring overlying sternal structures, 447-449
  field size, 450
  obliquity
    accuracy, evaluation, 450
    determination, 450
  patient obliquity, 449-450
  RAO position, reason, 447
Sthenic abdomen, 132
Sthenic anteroposterior oblique spot stomach/duodenal projection (LPO projection), 500f
Sthenic anteroposterior spot stomach/duodenal projection, 503f
Sthenic lateral stomach/duodenal projection, positioning accuracy, 498f
Sthenic PA oblique spot stomach/duodenal projection (RAO position), 495f
Sthenic PA stomach/duodenum projection, positioning accuracy, 497f
Sthenic patient
  PA chest, 86f
  PA projection, 488f
Stomach, 493-501
  contrast media, 493-494
    penetration, PA small intestinal projection (demonstration), 49f
  double contrast, 493-494
  single contrast, 493
Stomach: AP oblique projection (LAO position), 499
Stomach: AP projection, 501
Stomach: lateral projection (right lateral position), 497-499
Stomach: PA oblique projection (RAO position), 494
Stomach: PA projection, 494-497
Structures
  CR adjustment guidelines, 28b
  distinguishing, 23-24
Subject contrast, 48
  abdomen, 129
  demonstration, destructive disease (impact), 58f
  knee joint, impact, 58f

Submentovertex (SMV) (Schueller)
    cranial projection
    neck overextension, 480f
    neck underextension, 480f-481f
    patient positioning, 480f
    positioning accuracy, 479f
Submentovertex (SMV) cranium/
    mandible/sinuses projection,
    479t
Submentovertex (SMV) (Schueller)
    projection analysis, 481
Submentovertex (SMV) (Schueller)
    sinus/mandible projection,
    positioning accuracy, 480f
Superior midcoronal plane
    anterior tilt, 89f
    PA chest, 89f
    IR tilt
        anteroposterior (left lateral
            decubitus) chest, 107f
        anteroposterior (right lateral
            decubitus) chest, 107f
    posterior tilt, 90f
        45-degree PA oblique (RAO)
            chest, 112f
    PA chest, 90f
Supine AP abdomen
    obese patient, lengthwise/
        crosswise IR cassettes
        (usage), 136f
    projection, 133t
Supine AP chest
    projection, 101
        positioning accuracy, 102f
        shoulder, elevation, 102f
Supine AP oblique (Grashey) shoulder
    projection
    glenoid cavity, 251f
    obliquity
        excess, 252f
        insufficiency, 252f
Supine AP shoulder projection,
    positioning accuracy, 236f
Suprapatellar fat pads, location,
    338f
Supraspinatus "outlet": tangential
    projection (Neer method),
    261-264
    arm position, 261-263
    CR alignment, 263
    midcoronal plane, 263
        tilting, 265
    obliquity (determination),
        palpable structures (usage),
        263
    shoulder obliquity, 261-263
    tangential (outlet) shoulder
        projection, positioning
        (accuracy), 261f
Swan-Ganz catheter (pulmonary
    arterial catheter), 82
Swimmer's technique, 412-414

T
Talar domes, 300
    alignment, 309-310
    anterior/posterior alignment,
        301-304
    medial/lateral talar domes,
        320-321
        anterior/posterior alignement,
            320-321
        proximal alignment, 320
    proximal alignment, 300-301
Talocalcaneal joint space, 305-307
Tangential inferosuperior (carpal
    canal) wrist projection, 198t
Tangential (Merchant) patella analysis,
    355
    correction, 355
    practice, 355
Tangential patella/patellofemoral joint
    projection (Merchant method),
    352t
Tangential (Merchant) patella
    projection
    distal femurs, depression, 354f
    internal leg rotation, absence,
        353f
    knees
        extension, 354f
        flexion, 354f
    patellar subluxation, presence, 353f
Tangential (supraspinatus outlet)
    projection, 19f
Tangential (axial) projection knee
    projection
    patient positioning, 352f
    positioning accuracy, 352f
Tangential (outlet) shoulder analysis,
    263-264
    correction, 264
    practice, 263-264
Tangential (outlet) shoulder projection
    arm abduction, 262f
    arm dangling (nonabducted),
        262f
    caudal CR angulation, 263f
    CR cephalic angle, 264f
    obliquity, excess, 262f
    positioning accuracy, 261f
Tangential (supraspinatus outlet)
    shoulder projection, positioning,
    20f
Tangential supraspinatus outlet
    projection (Neer method), 261t
Tarsometatarsal joint spaces, 291
Thigh thickness, central ray (CR)
    angle determination, 331f,
    335f
Thin-film transistor (TFT), electric
    charge collection, 38
Third MC alignment, 179-180
    wrist: PA oblique projection (lateral
        rotation), 182

Thoracic vertebrae
    image analysis guidelines, 391-422,
        391b
    technical data, 391, 391t
Thoracic vertebrae: AP projection,
    414-418
    anode heel effect, 414-415
    brightness uniformity, obtaining,
        414-416
    CR/intervertebral disk space
        alignment, 416-417
    expiration, inspiration (differences),
        415-416
    kyphosis positioning, 417
    rotation, 416
    scoliosis, differences, 416
Thoracic vertebrae: lateral projection,
    418-422
    breathing technique, 418
    CR intervertebral disk space
        alignment, 421
    inclusion, verification, 421-422
    lateral cervicothoracic (Twining
        method) projection, 422
    rotation, 418-421
        scoliosis, differences, 421
    scoliotic patient, 421
    T7 location, 421
Thorax
    arm resting, 275f
    rotation, 393f
        detection, 491-492
Thumb
    abduction, 163
    alignment, 189
    alternate PA thumb projection,
        161
    collimator alignment, 161
    lateral thumb projection, 162t
    positioning
        hand: PA oblique projection
            (lateral rotation), 171
        lateral wrist projection, 189
Thumb: AP projection, 159-162
    joint spaces, 160-161
    palmar soft tissue, 161
    phalangeal/metacarpal midshaft
        concavity/soft tissue width,
        159-160
    phalanges, 160-161
Thumb: lateral projection, 162-164
    abduction, 163
    joint spaces, 162-163
    phalangeal, 162-163
    phalanx/metacarpal midshaft
        concavity, 162
Thumb: PA oblique projection,
    164-167
    joint space (phalangeal/metacarpal),
        165
    longitudinal thumb alignment,
        165

Thumb: PA oblique projection
(Continued)
phalangeal/metacarpal midshaft
concavity, 164
soft tissue width, 164
Tibiotalar joint
openness, evaluation, 316-317
space, 312-313
ankle: AP oblique projection
(medial rotation), 316-317
Tilted lateral chest projection,
nonrotated/rotated collimator
head, 17f
Toe: AP axial projection, 279-284
joint spaces, 280
nonextendable toes, CR angulation,
280
phalangeal midshaft concavity,
279-280
phalanges, 280
soft tissue width, 279-280
Toe: AP oblique projection, 284-286
bony/soft tissue overlap, 286
joint spaces, 284-285
nonextendable toes, CR angulation,
285
phalangeal midshaft concavity,
284
phalanges, 284-285
rotation accuracy, 284
soft tissue width, 284
Toe: lateral projection (mediolateral/
lateromedial), 286-290
bony overlap, 286
condyle superimposition, 286
phalanx concavity, 286
soft tissue overlap, 286
Toes, anteroposterior (AP) axial
projection, 281f
Torso, rotation, 230f
Towne method, 472-476
Tracheostomy, 79
placement, PA/lateral chest
demonstration, 81f
Traction device, impact, 29f
Transthoracic lateral humerus
projection, alternate, 232-233
Trapeziotrapezoidal joint space, wrist:
PA oblique projection (lateral
rotation), 185
Trapezium
visualization, lateral wrist
projections (usage), 3f, 189-190
wrist: PA oblique projection (lateral
rotation), 185
Trapezoid space, wrist: PA oblique
projection (lateral rotation),
185
Trauma anteroposterior axial
(Caldwell) cranial projection,
central ray (CR) angulation
determination, 471f

Trauma anteroposterior cranial
projection, CR cephalic angle,
466f
Trauma anteroposterior lower leg
projection, joint position, 72f
Trauma anteroposterior mandible
projection, CR caudal angle,
466f
Trauma cranial imaging (cervical
vertebral injuries), 461-462
Trauma imaging, 66-69
Trauma lateral ankle projection,
69f
Trauma patients, technical
adjustments, 67t
Trochanters, 357-359
greater/lesser trochanter, 362
alignment, 382-383
visualization, 370-371
Twelfth thoracic vertebra,
identification, 97f
Twining method, 412-414, 422
Twinning method, 405

U

Ulna
alignment, 204
elbow: AP projection, 207
Ulnar-deviated PA axial (scaphoid)
wrist projection
patient positioning, 193f
positioning, 192f
Ulnar deviation, 181f
Ulnar styloid
forearm: AP projection, 201-202
wrist (PA projection), 177
wrist: lateral projection
(lateromedial), 186-187
wrist: PA oblique projection (lateral
rotation), 182
Umbilical artery catheter (UAC),
82-83
Umbilical vein catheter (UVC), 83
placement, 83f
Underexposed projection, evaluation,
46t
Underexposure
causes, 46t
identification, 45-47
technical adjustment, determination,
48
Underpenetrated AP pelvis projection,
accuracy, 48f
Unextendable finger, positioning, 151
Unilateral finger projections, marker
placement, 12f
Upper extremity
image analysis guidelines, 150-233,
150b
technical data, 150t
Upper gastrointestnial system, double-
contrast filling, 494t

Upright AP abdomen
full expiration, 139f
full inspiration, 138f
projection, 134t

V

Valgus deformity, 332f
Varus deformity, 332f
Vascular lung markings, 77
Vertebral column, alignment, 421f,
432f
Volume of interest (VOI), 4
defining, 42-43
excess background radiation values,
43f
identification, 38-39
identification, accuracy, 38
superimposition, 11f
Voluntary patient motion,
anteroposterior oblique knee
projection (impact), 30f

W

Wedge-compensating filter, usage,
140-141
Windowing, 58-59
Wrist
external rotation, 205f, 222f
internal rotation, 205f
joint mobility, lateral projections,
189
obliquity, insufficiency/excess
(identification), 185
positioning, 199-200
radial deviation
PA oblique wrist projection, 185f
PA wrist projection, 181f
ulnar deviation, PA wrist projection,
182f
Wrist: carpal canal (tunnel)
(tangential, inferosuperior
projection), 198-199
carpal canal anatomy, 198f
carpal canal projection, positioning
accuracy, 198f
carpal canal visualization, 198-199
carpal canal wrist
CR/IR acute angle, 199f
CR/palmar surface angle, 199f
positioning, 198f
fifth MC/IR, perpendicular
alignment, 199f
pisiform/hamulus process, 199
wrist extension, CR alignment, 199f
Wrist: lateral projection (lateromedial),
186-192
pronator fat stripe, 186
ulnar styloid, 186-187
Wrist: PA oblique projection (lateral
rotation), 182-186
distal radius joints, 183-184
radiolunate joints, 183-184

Wrist: PA oblique projection (lateral rotation) *(Continued)*
  radioscaphoid joints, 183-184
  second CM/scaphotrapezial joint spaces, 184
  third MC/midforearm, alignment, 182
  trapezoid/trapezium/ trapeziotrapezoidal joint space, 185
  ulnar styloid, 182
Wrist: PA projection, 177-182
  CM joint spaces, 179
  distal radius joints, 178-179
  MC bases, 178
  posterior/anterior distal radial margins, identification, 178-179
  radial styloid, 178
  radiolunate joints, 178-179
  radioscaphoid joints, 178-179
  radioulnar articulation, 178
  scaphoid fat stripe, 177
  scaphoid visualization, 179
  ulnar styloid, 177

Wrist: ulnar deviation, PA axial projection (scaphoid), 192-197
  collimation, 196
  CR alignment, 195f
    problem, 195f
  CR angulation, 195-196
    adjustment, 195-196
  CR/fracture, alignment, 193f
  distal scaphoid fracture, 196f
  lateral wrist, neutral position, 193f
  medial wrist rotation, 194
  PA axial wrist projection
    hand extension, absence, 169f
    scaphoid waist fracture, 194f
  PA axial wrist projection, ulnar deviation maximum (absence), 194f
  posteroanterior axial wrist projection
    collimation, problems, 195f
    15-degree proximal CR angle, 196f
    5-degree proximal CR angle, 196f
    proximal forearm, elevation, 195f

Wrist: ulnar deviation, PA axial projection (scaphoid) *(Continued)*
    30-degree proximal CR angle, 197f
  wrist, external rotation, 194f
  proximal forearm, patient positioning, 194
  scaphoid fracture, sites, 196f
  scaphoid/scaphocapitate/ scapholunate joint spaces, 192-194
  scaphotrapezium/scaphotrapezoidal joint spaces, 192
  ulnar deviation, 193f
    inadequacy, compensation, 193-194

X

X-rays
  divergence, impact, 325f
  emission, 20
  tube
    anode/cathode ends, identification, 53f
    housing, top, 53f